GRAY'S ATLAS
OF ANATOMY

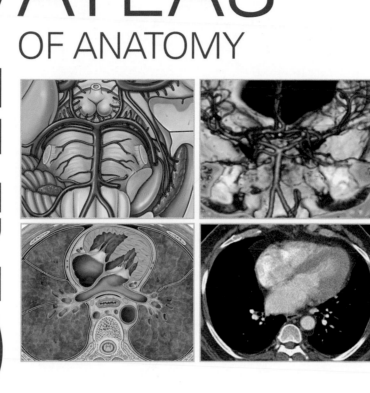

GRAY'S ATLAS
OF ANATOMY

Third Edition

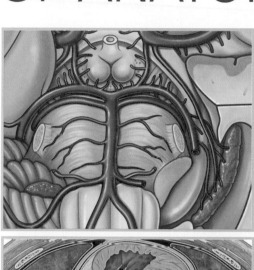
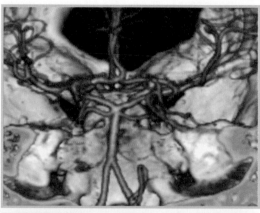
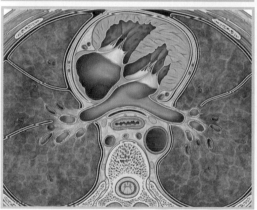
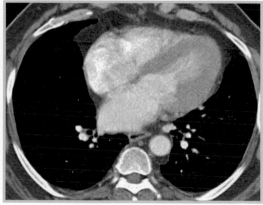

Richard L. Drake
PhD, FAAA

Director of Anatomy
Professor of Surgery
Cleveland Clinic Lerner College
  of Medicine
Case Western Reserve
  University
Cleveland, Ohio, USA

A. Wayne Vogl
PhD, FAAA

Professor of Anatomy
  and Cell Biology
Department of Cellular
  and Physiological Sciences
Faculty of Medicine
University of British Columbia
Vancouver, British Columbia,
  Canada

Adam W.M. Mitchell
MBBS, FRCS, FRCR

Consultant Radiologist and Senior
  Lecturer Imperial College
Chelsea and Westminster Hospital
London, UK

Illustrated by

Richard M. Tibbitts
Saffron Walden, UK

Paul E. Richardson
Cambridge, UK

Photographs by

Ansell Horn

ELSEVIER

Elsevier
1600 John F. Kennedy Blvd.
Ste 1800
Philadelphia, PA 19103-2899

GRAY'S ATLAS OF ANATOMY, THIRD EDITION
INTERNATIONAL EDITION

ISBN: 978-0-323-63639-1
ISBN: 978-0-323-63640-7

Notices

Practitioners and researchers must always rely on their own experience and knowledge in evaluating and using any information, methods, compounds or experiments described herein. Because of rapid advances in the medical sciences, in particular, independent verification of diagnoses and drug dosages should be made. To the fullest extent of the law, no responsibility is assumed by Elsevier, authors, editors or contributors for any injury and/or damage to persons or property as a matter of products liability, negligence or otherwise, or from any use or operation of any methods, products, instructions, or ideas contained in the material herein.

Previous editions copyrighted 2015 and 2008.

Library of Congress Control Number: 2019957237

Content Strategist: Jeremy Bowes
Director, Content Development: Rebecca Gruliow
Publishing Services Manager: Catherine Jackson
Senior Project Manager: Daniel Fitzgerald
Design and Art Direction: Antbits Ltd.
Cover design: Amy Buxton

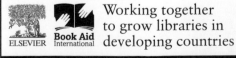

Printed in India

Last digit is the print number: 9   8   7   6   5   4

To my wife who supports me and to my parents who are always with me.
Richard L. Drake

To my family, to my professional colleagues and role models, and to my students.
A. Wayne Vogl

Thanks, to Cathy, Max and Elsa
Adam W.M. Mitchell

To my family – my inspiration, Evi, Zoë, and Nicholas
Richard M. Tibbitts

To my wife Fern, Junior, Ava and Henry, to Lesley and in memory of AMR and JER
Paul E. Richardson

ACKNOWLEDGMENTS

The following reviewers helped enormously with their detailed critiques and suggestions for every chapter. Their assistance was invaluable.

Mark Hankin, PhD, University of Toledo College of Medicine, Toledo, Ohio

Marios Loukas, MD, PhD, St. George's University School of Medicine, Grenada

James J. Rechtien, DO, PhD, Michigan State University School of Medicine, East Lansing, Michigan

William A. Roy, PT, PhD, Touro University, Henderson, Nevada

Susan Standring, MBE, PhD, DSc, FKC, Hon FRCS, Emeritus Professor of Anatomy, King's College London, London

William Swartz, PhD, Louisiana State University Health Sciences Center, Baton Rouge, Louisiana

Mark F. Teaford, PhD, Johns Hopkins University School of Medicine, Baltimore, Maryland

We want to thank Dr. Bruce Crawford for a radiograph of the head and neck and Dr. Murray Morrison for laryngoscopic images of the larynx; Dr. Jerry Healy for three images in the Abdomen section: the celiac artery, the bile duct system, and a three-dimensional view of abdominal vessels; and Siemens Medical Solutions USA and the following individuals with that company: Mollie Beaver, Director, CT Clinical Solutions, and Dr. Louise McKenna, Global Clinical Marketing Manager, CT Oncology, who supplied a *syngo* Multi-modality Workplace, which was used to acquire the majority of the clinical images.

Stuart Morrison, MD, helped with all aspects of coordinating the collection of the radiographic material. Radiological assistance and images were contributed in each of the following areas:

Back
Mark Kayanja, MD, PhD
Jeffrey S. Ross, MD

Thorax
Mario Garcia, MD
A. Michael Lincoff, MD

Abdomen
Namita Gandhi, MD
Michelle Inkster, MD, PhD
Brian R. Lane, MD
Anand Rao, MD
James S. Wu, MD

Pelvis
Matthew Barber, MD, MHS
Tommaso Falcone, MD
J. Stephen Jones, MD
Eunice Moon, MD
James S. Newman, MD, PhD

Extremities
Hakan Ilaslan, MD
Bradford J. Richmond, MD
Joshua Polster, MD

Head and Neck
Todd W. Stultz, DDS, MD
J. Martin Paloma, DDS, MSD
Cindy McConnaughy
Ronald Lemmo, DDS

A working knowledge of anatomy is not an "optional extra" for health care professionals – it is fundamental. Acquiring that knowledge has always challenged even the most motivated students. Over many generations, learning materials that aid the process effectively have been warmly welcomed by students and their teachers (and by patients, who are the ultimate beneficiaries of that knowledge). I remember my own students' response when I first included illustrations from *Gray's Anatomy for Students* in a lecture—afterward, I was asked repeatedly for the source of the marvelous pictures. Looking beyond the "wow" factor that leapt from the pages of the book, it was clear that an enormous amount of thought and skill had gone into producing the artwork.

This atlas contains a series of additional outstanding pieces of anatomical art from the illustrative team of Richard Tibbitts and Paul Richardson that will complement those in *Gray's Anatomy for Students*, combined with relevant clinical pictures, surface anatomy, and images from a range of modern imaging procedures. Of course, anatomy cannot be learned from books and interactive DVDs alone, no matter how excellent they may be. Anatomy is a practical subject, best learned by gaining hands-on experience of the body. Students should spend as much time as they can examining cadaveric dissections (if they do not have the opportunity to dissect themselves) and should always read from screen or page with the appropriate bones in front of them. They need to combine and correlate information from a wide variety of sources in order to gain the working knowledge mentioned earlier.

This atlas will provide a valuable companion to their studies, and I am confident that it will remain in their libraries long after they have completed the early stages of their training.

Susan Standring, MBE, PhD, DSc, FKC, Hon FRCS
Emeritus Professor of Anatomy
King's College, London

FOREWORD

We began working on *Gray's Atlas of Anatomy* in 2005 following the publication of our textbook, *Gray's Anatomy for Students*. We wanted to produce an atlas that would build on themes and concepts established in the textbook and that would couple artistic renderings of "internal" gross anatomy with actual "living" anatomy, as visualized with modern imaging techniques and with surface anatomy. We believe that the final atlas , now in its third edition, presents a fresh and integrated approach to anatomy that is accessible to entry-level students in anatomy, as well as to students at more advanced levels.

Because an atlas is used in a much different way than a textbook, we could not simply repackage figures used in *Gray's Anatomy for Students* and put them in the atlas. Consequently, most of the figures in the atlas are new and were designed to present structures in a more complete context than in the textbook, even though the color palette and overall look of the figures in both the atlas and textbook are similar. Also, figures in the atlas provide additional detail not included in the textbook and directly correlate artistic representations of anatomy with computed tomography (CT) and magnetic resonance imaging (MRI). Where appropriate, we have included endoscopic, laryngoscopic, and laparoscopic views of the anatomy and have included examples of ultrasound images. In a number of regions, we also have reconstructed the internal anatomy of patients by abstracting specific information from multiple MR or CT images, and we present these reconstructions together with artwork of the same anatomy. Although the artwork was done independently of the reconstructed images, the two types of representations are strikingly similar.

Each page of this atlas was planned prior to beginning work on the figures, and all of the artwork was generated digitally. Most of the figures were created from an extensive digital database created for the textbook. In this third edition, we have updated the images and added a few new ones in response to feedback from our readers.

We hope that the textbook and this edition of the atlas used together will provide powerful learning tools for students of human gross anatomy.

The Authors

This 3rd edition of *Gray's Atlas of Anatomy* continues in the tradition of the first two editions, coupling artistic rendering with actual living anatomy as visualized with modern imaging techniques and surface anatomy. The combination of modern illustrations, imaging, and surface anatomy is unique among atlases available today.

At the end of every chapter, tables and schematic drawings allow for quick review of subject matter. These include major nerves plexuses throughout the body, branching patterns of major arteries, summaries of muscles organized into compartments or regions, and other helpful information. This material is designed to provide the reader quick access to information.

It's our hope that the 3rd edition of *Gray's Atlas of Anatomy* will become a valuable learning aid for students encountering anatomy for the first time or for the individual seeking to review information critical to their daily experiences.

The Authors

CONTENTS

CONTENTS

4 ABDOMEN

CONTENTS

CONTENTS

7 UPPER LIMB

CONTENTS

CONTENTS

THE BODY

1

CONTENTS

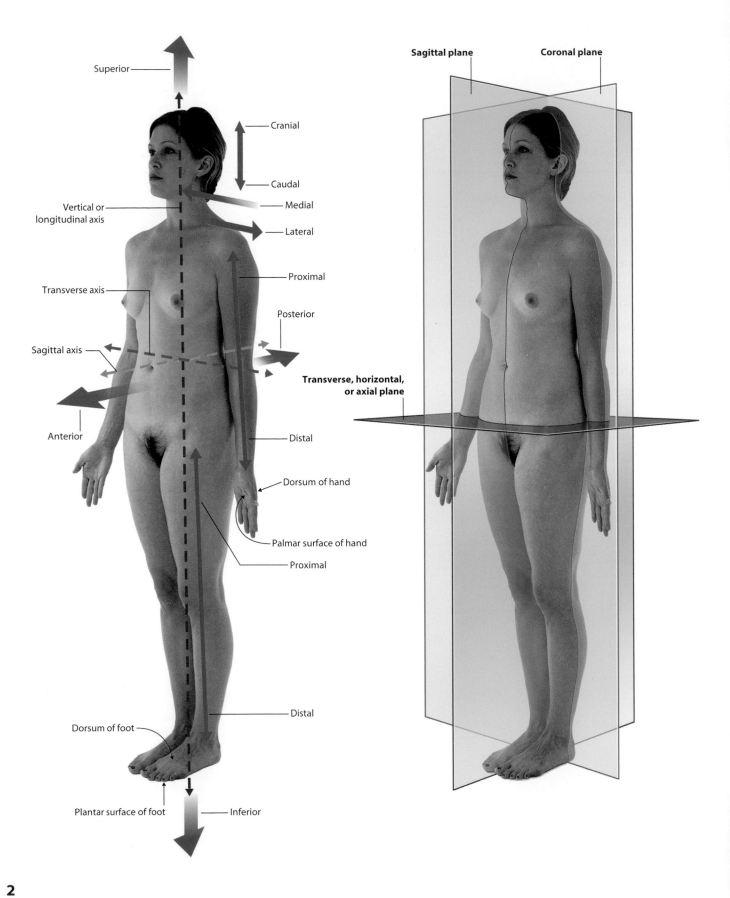

Superior

Cranial

Caudal

Medial

Vertical or
longitudinal axis

Lateral

Proximal

Transverse axis

Posterior

Sagittal axis

Anterior

Distal

Dorsum of hand

Palmar surface of hand

Proximal

Distal

Dorsum of foot

Plantar surface of foot

Inferior

Sagittal plane

Coronal plane

**Transverse, horizontal,
or axial plane**

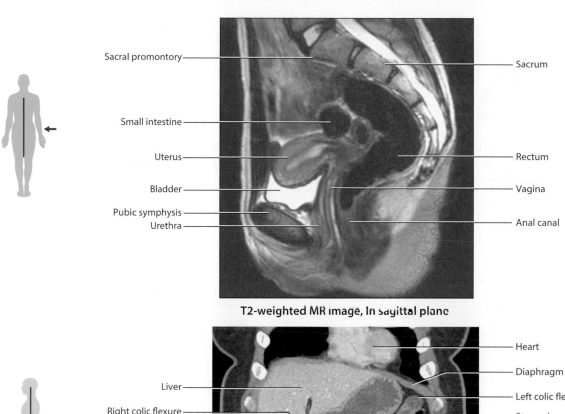

Sacral promontory

Small intestine

Uterus

Bladder

Pubic symphysis

Urethra

Sacrum

Rectum

Vagina

Anal canal

T2-weighted MR image, in sagittal plane

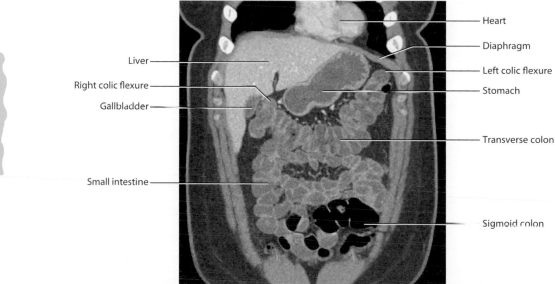

Liver

Right colic flexure

Gallbladder

Small intestine

Heart

Diaphragm

Left colic flexure

Stomach

Transverse colon

Sigmoid colon

CT image, with contrast, in coronal plane

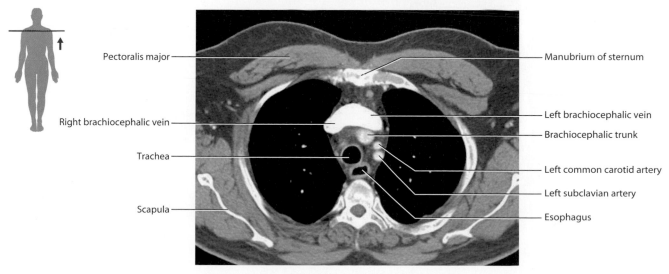

Pectoralis major

Right brachiocephalic vein

Trachea

Scapula

Manubrium of sternum

Left brachiocephalic vein

Brachiocephalic trunk

Left common carotid artery

Left subclavian artery

Esophagus

CT image, with contrast, in axial plane

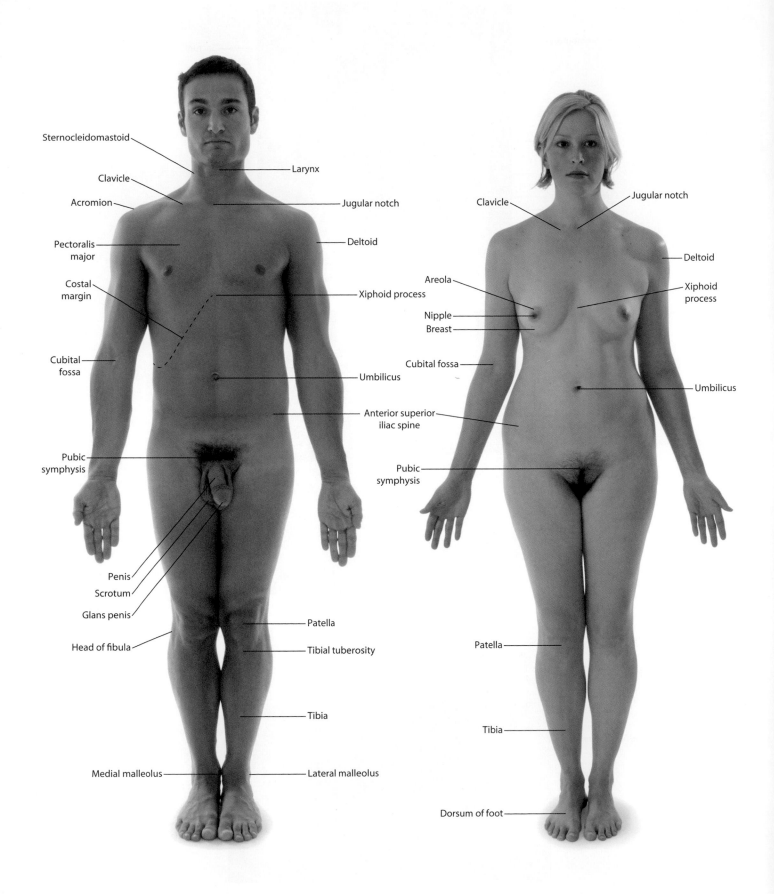

Sternocleidomastoid

Clavicle

Acromion

Pectoralis major

Costal margin

Cubital fossa

Pubic symphysis

Penis

Scrotum

Glans penis

Head of fibula

Medial malleolus

Larynx

Jugular notch

Deltoid

Xiphoid process

Umbilicus

Anterior superior iliac spine

Patella

Tibial tuberosity

Tibia

Lateral malleolus

Clavicle

Jugular notch

Areola

Nipple

Breast

Cubital fossa

Pubic symphysis

Patella

Tibia

Dorsum of foot

Deltoid

Xiphoid process

Umbilicus

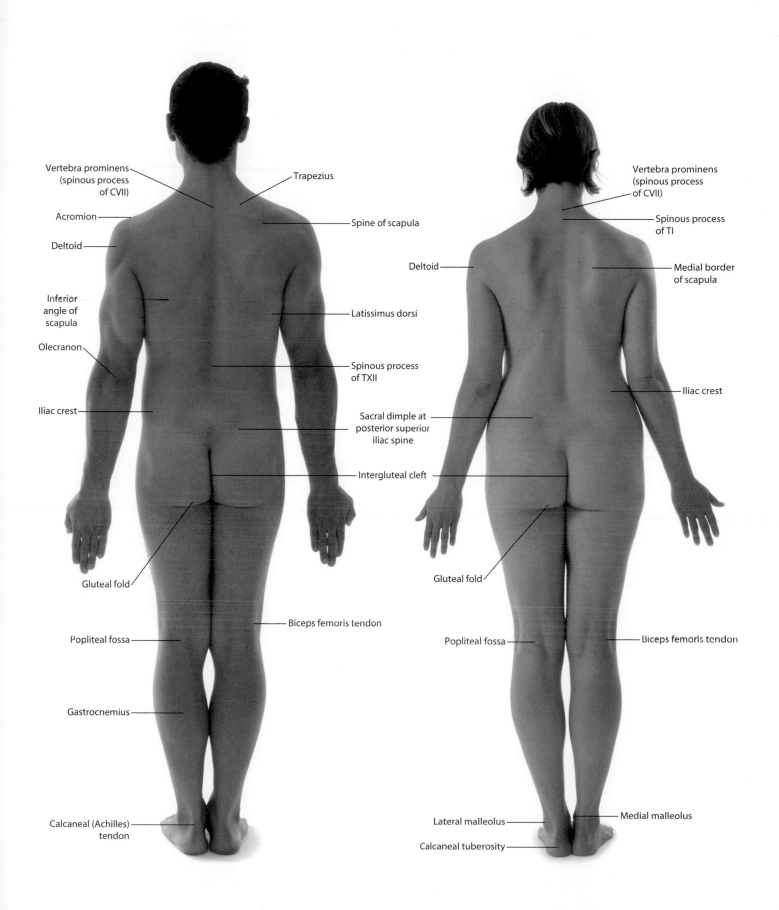

Vertebra prominens (spinous process of CVII)

Acromion

Deltoid

Inferior angle of scapula

Olecranon

Iliac crest

Gluteal fold

Popliteal fossa

Gastrocnemius

Calcaneal (Achilles) tendon

Trapezius

Spine of scapula

Latissimus dorsi

Spinous process of TXII

Sacral dimple at posterior superior iliac spine

Intergluteal cleft

Biceps femoris tendon

Vertebra prominens (spinous process of CVII)

Spinous process of TI

Deltoid

Medial border of scapula

Iliac crest

Gluteal fold

Popliteal fossa

Biceps femoris tendon

Lateral malleolus

Medial malleolus

Calcaneal tuberosity

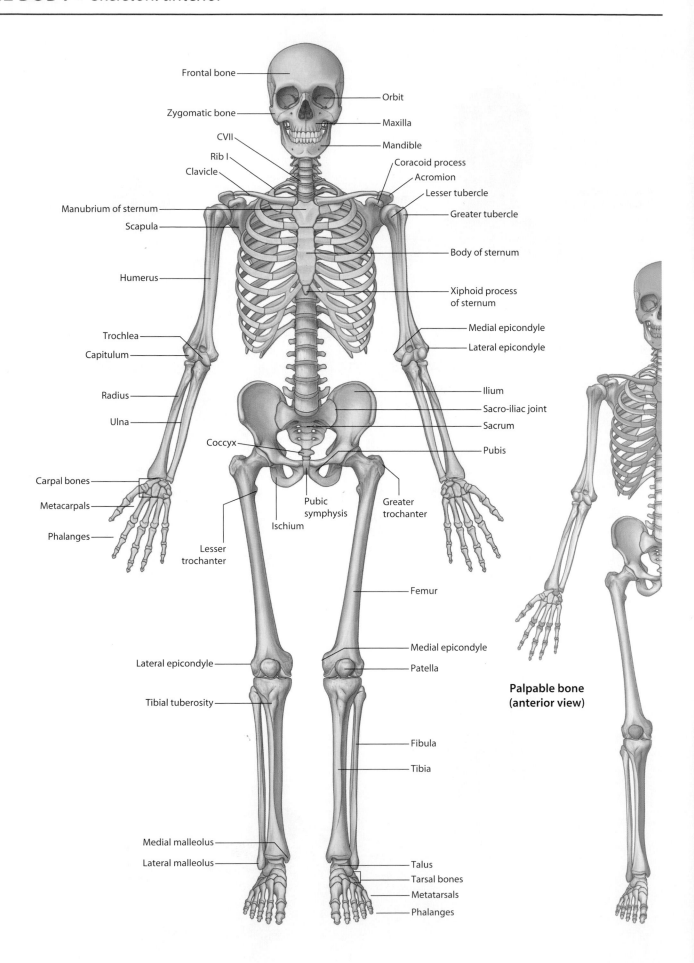

Frontal bone
Orbit
Zygomatic bone
Maxilla
CVII
Mandible
Rib I
Coracoid process
Clavicle
Acromion
Lesser tubercle
Manubrium of sternum
Greater tubercle
Scapula
Body of sternum
Humerus
Xiphoid process of sternum
Medial epicondyle
Trochlea
Lateral epicondyle
Capitulum
Radius
Ilium
Ulna
Sacro-iliac joint
Sacrum
Coccyx
Pubis
Carpal bones
Pubic symphysis
Greater trochanter
Metacarpals
Ischium
Phalanges
Lesser trochanter
Femur
Medial epicondyle
Lateral epicondyle
Patella
Tibial tuberosity
Fibula
Tibia
Medial malleolus
Lateral malleolus
Talus
Tarsal bones
Metatarsals
Phalanges

Palpable bone (anterior view)

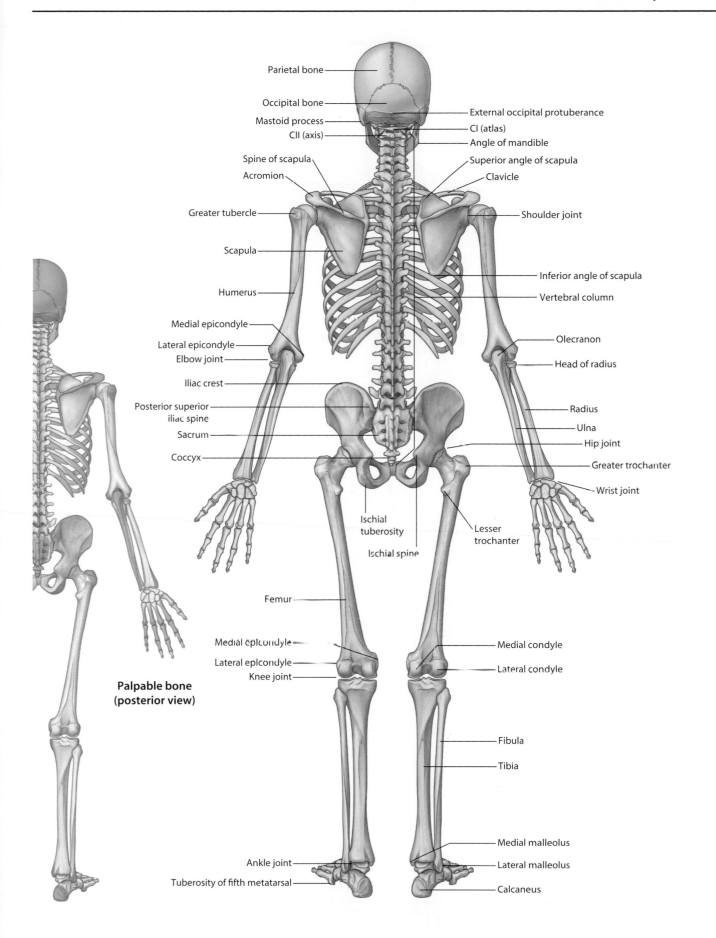

Parietal bone

Occipital bone

Mastoid process

CII (axis)

External occipital protuberance

CI (atlas)

Angle of mandible

Spine of scapula

Acromion

Superior angle of scapula

Clavicle

Greater tubercle

Shoulder joint

Scapula

Inferior angle of scapula

Humerus

Vertebral column

Medial epicondyle

Olecranon

Lateral epicondyle

Head of radius

Elbow joint

Iliac crest

Posterior superior iliac spine

Radius

Ulna

Sacrum

Hip joint

Coccyx

Greater trochanter

Wrist joint

Ischial tuberosity

Lesser trochanter

Ischial spine

Femur

Medial epicondyle

Medial condyle

Lateral epicondyle

Lateral condyle

Knee joint

Palpable bone (posterior view)

Fibula

Tibia

Medial malleolus

Ankle joint

Lateral malleolus

Tuberosity of fifth metatarsal

Calcaneus

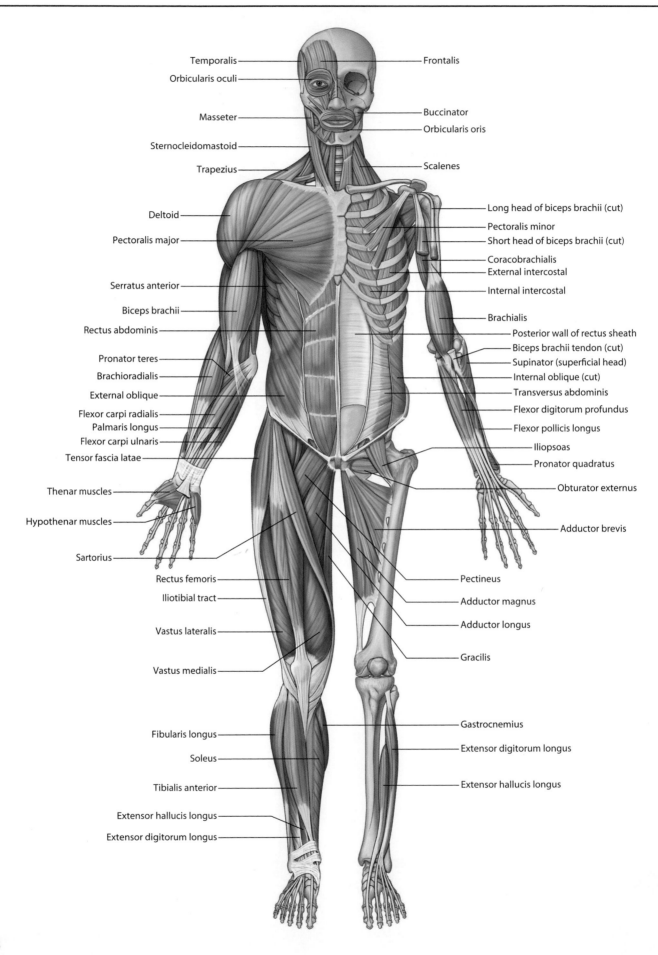

Temporalis — Frontalis

Orbicularis oculi

Masseter — Buccinator
— Orbicularis oris

Sternocleidomastoid

Trapezius — Scalenes

Deltoid — Long head of biceps brachii (cut)
— Pectoralis minor

Pectoralis major — Short head of biceps brachii (cut)
— Coracobrachialis
— External intercostal

Serratus anterior — Internal intercostal

Biceps brachii — Brachialis

Rectus abdominis — Posterior wall of rectus sheath
— Biceps brachii tendon (cut)

Pronator teres — Supinator (superficial head)

Brachioradialis — Internal oblique (cut)

External oblique — Transversus abdominis

Flexor carpi radialis — Flexor digitorum profundus

Palmaris longus — Flexor pollicis longus

Flexor carpi ulnaris — Iliopsoas

Tensor fascia latae — Pronator quadratus

Thenar muscles — Obturator externus

Hypothenar muscles — Adductor brevis

Sartorius

Rectus femoris — Pectineus

Iliotibial tract — Adductor magnus

Vastus lateralis — Adductor longus

Vastus medialis — Gracilis

Fibularis longus — Gastrocnemius

Soleus — Extensor digitorum longus

Tibialis anterior — Extensor hallucis longus

Extensor hallucis longus

Extensor digitorum longus

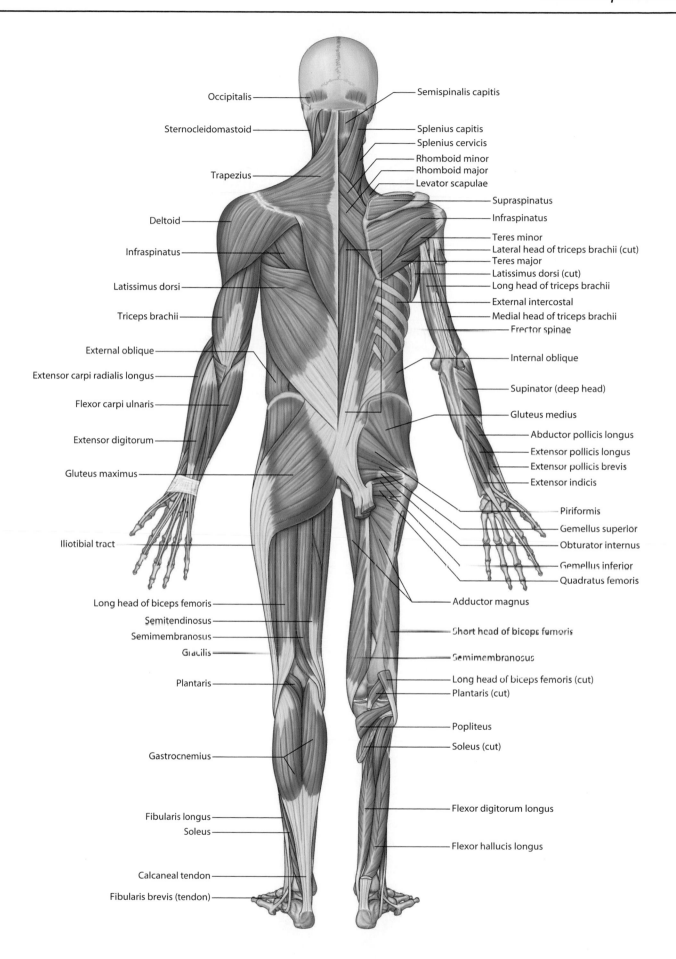

Occipitalis

Sternocleidomastoid

Trapezius

Deltoid

Infraspinatus

Latissimus dorsi

Triceps brachii

External oblique

Extensor carpi radialis longus

Flexor carpi ulnaris

Extensor digitorum

Gluteus maximus

Iliotibial tract

Long head of biceps femoris

Semitendinosus

Semimembranosus

Gracilis

Plantaris

Gastrocnemius

Fibularis longus

Soleus

Calcaneal tendon

Fibularis brevis (tendon)

Semispinalis capitis

Splenius capitis

Splenius cervicis

Rhomboid minor

Rhomboid major

Levator scapulae

Supraspinatus

Infraspinatus

Teres minor

Lateral head of triceps brachii (cut)

Teres major

Latissimus dorsi (cut)

Long head of triceps brachii

External intercostal

Medial head of triceps brachii

Erector spinae

Internal oblique

Supinator (deep head)

Gluteus medius

Abductor pollicis longus

Extensor pollicis longus

Extensor pollicis brevis

Extensor indicis

Piriformis

Gemellus superior

Obturator internus

Gemellus inferior

Quadratus femoris

Adductor magnus

Short head of biceps femoris

Semimembranosus

Long head of biceps femoris (cut)

Plantaris (cut)

Popliteus

Soleus (cut)

Flexor digitorum longus

Flexor hallucis longus

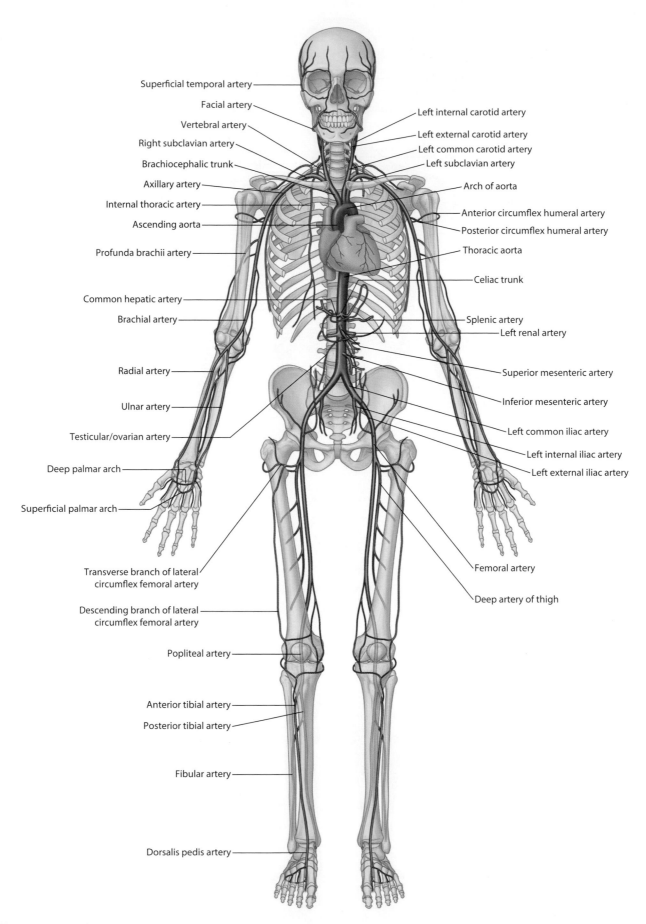

Superficial temporal artery

Facial artery

Vertebral artery

Right subclavian artery

Brachiocephalic trunk

Axillary artery

Internal thoracic artery

Ascending aorta

Profunda brachii artery

Common hepatic artery

Brachial artery

Radial artery

Ulnar artery

Testicular/ovarian artery

Deep palmar arch

Superficial palmar arch

Transverse branch of lateral circumflex femoral artery

Descending branch of lateral circumflex femoral artery

Popliteal artery

Anterior tibial artery

Posterior tibial artery

Fibular artery

Dorsalis pedis artery

Left internal carotid artery

Left external carotid artery

Left common carotid artery

Left subclavian artery

Arch of aorta

Anterior circumflex humeral artery

Posterior circumflex humeral artery

Thoracic aorta

Celiac trunk

Splenic artery

Left renal artery

Superior mesenteric artery

Inferior mesenteric artery

Left common iliac artery

Left internal iliac artery

Left external iliac artery

Femoral artery

Deep artery of thigh

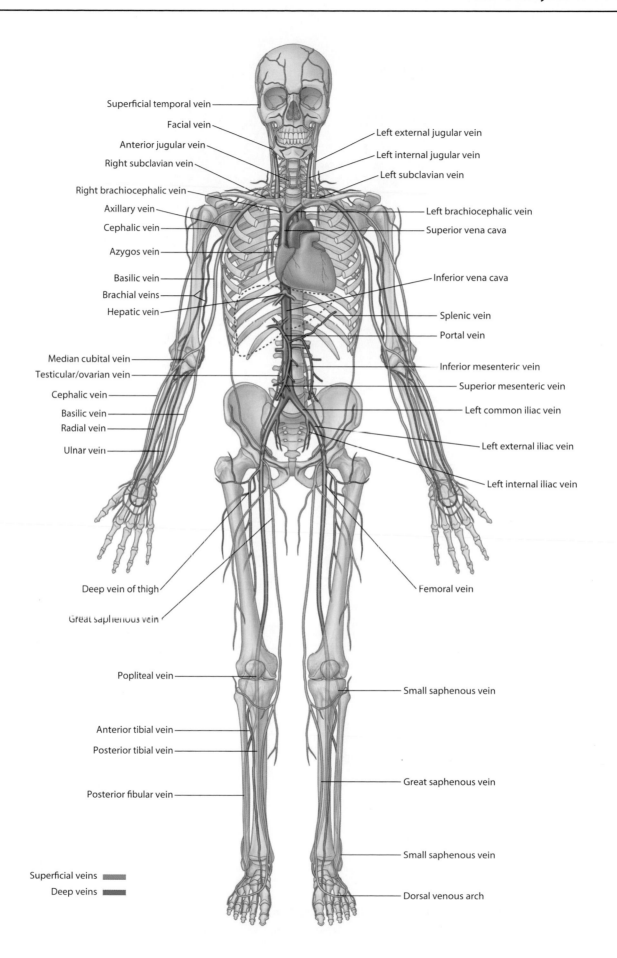

Superficial temporal vein

Facial vein

Anterior jugular vein

Right subclavian vein

Right brachiocephalic vein

Axillary vein

Cephalic vein

Azygos vein

Basilic vein

Brachial veins

Hepatic vein

Median cubital vein

Testicular/ovarian vein

Cephalic vein

Basilic vein

Radial vein

Ulnar vein

Deep vein of thigh

Great saphenous vein

Popliteal vein

Anterior tibial vein

Posterior tibial vein

Posterior fibular vein

Left external jugular vein

Left internal jugular vein

Left subclavian vein

Left brachiocephalic vein

Superior vena cava

Inferior vena cava

Splenic vein

Portal vein

Inferior mesenteric vein

Superior mesenteric vein

Left common iliac vein

Left external iliac vein

Left internal iliac vein

Femoral vein

Small saphenous vein

Great saphenous vein

Small saphenous vein

Dorsal venous arch

Superficial veins

Deep veins

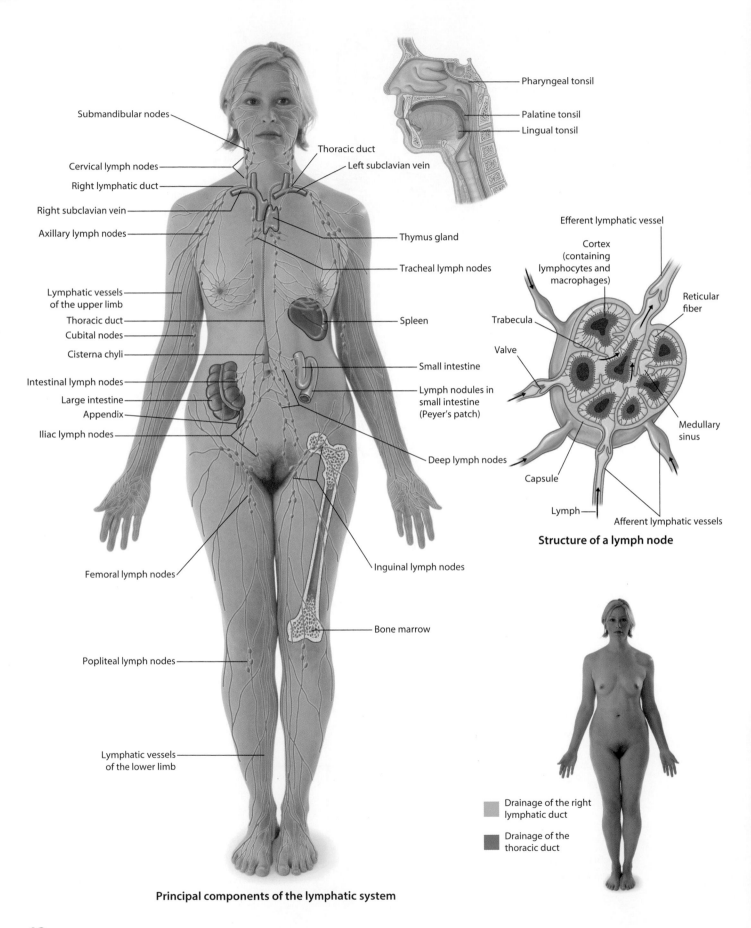

Submandibular nodes

Cervical lymph nodes

Right lymphatic duct

Right subclavian vein

Axillary lymph nodes

Lymphatic vessels of the upper limb

Thoracic duct

Cubital nodes

Cisterna chyli

Intestinal lymph nodes

Large intestine

Appendix

Iliac lymph nodes

Femoral lymph nodes

Popliteal lymph nodes

Lymphatic vessels of the lower limb

Thoracic duct

Left subclavian vein

Thymus gland

Tracheal lymph nodes

Spleen

Small intestine

Lymph nodules in small intestine (Peyer's patch)

Deep lymph nodes

Inguinal lymph nodes

Bone marrow

Pharyngeal tonsil

Palatine tonsil

Lingual tonsil

Efferent lymphatic vessel

Cortex (containing lymphocytes and macrophages)

Trabecula

Valve

Capsule

Lymph

Reticular fiber

Medullary sinus

Afferent lymphatic vessels

Structure of a lymph node

Drainage of the right lymphatic duct

Drainage of the thoracic duct

Principal components of the lymphatic system

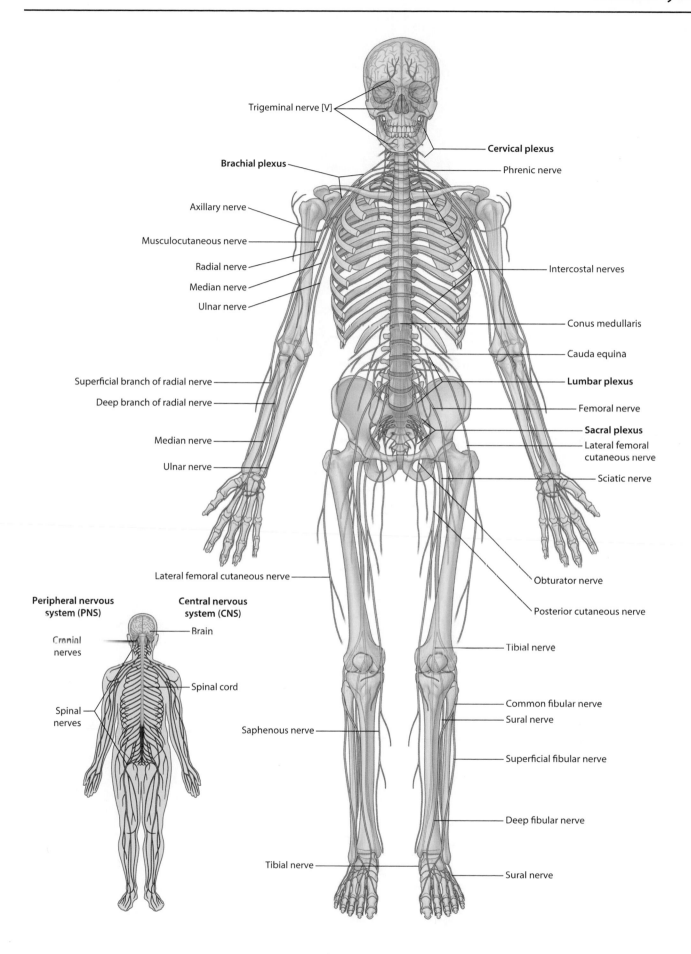

Trigeminal nerve [V]

Cervical plexus

Brachial plexus

Phrenic nerve

Axillary nerve

Musculocutaneous nerve

Radial nerve

Median nerve

Ulnar nerve

Intercostal nerves

Superficial branch of radial nerve

Deep branch of radial nerve

Conus medullaris

Cauda equina

Lumbar plexus

Femoral nerve

Sacral plexus

Median nerve

Ulnar nerve

Lateral femoral cutaneous nerve

Sciatic nerve

Lateral femoral cutaneous nerve

Obturator nerve

Posterior cutaneous nerve

Tibial nerve

Peripheral nervous system (PNS)

Central nervous system (CNS)

Cranial nerves

Brain

Spinal cord

Spinal nerves

Saphenous nerve

Common fibular nerve

Sural nerve

Superficial fibular nerve

Deep fibular nerve

Tibial nerve

Sural nerve

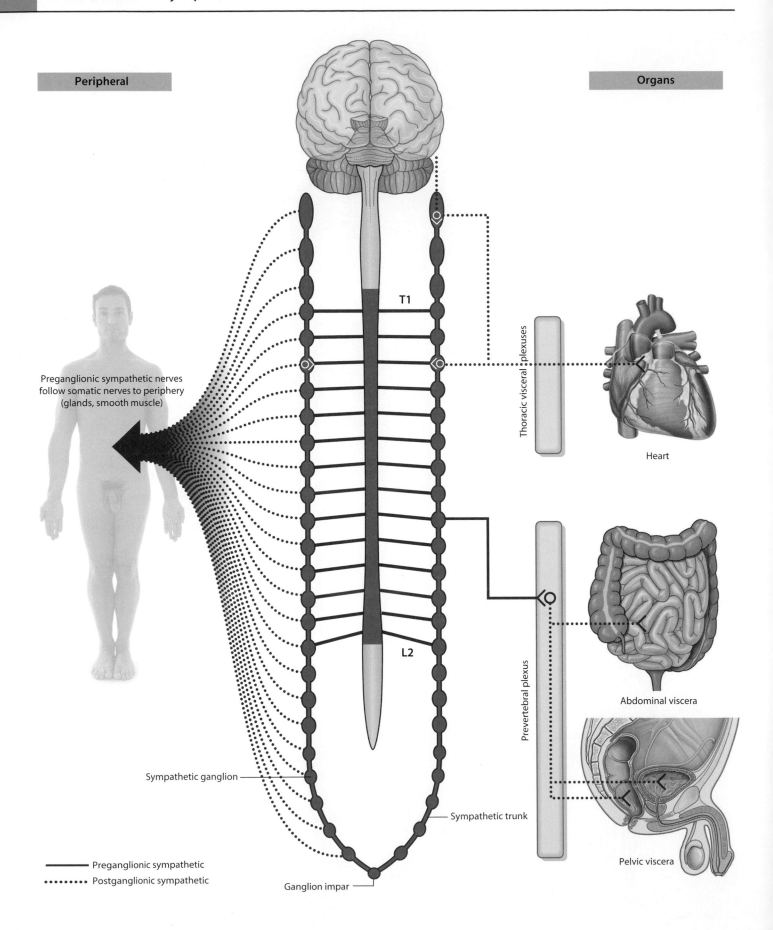

Peripheral

Organs

Preganglionic sympathetic nerves follow somatic nerves to periphery (glands, smooth muscle)

T1

L2

Thoracic visceral plexuses

Heart

Prevertebral plexus

Abdominal viscera

Pelvic viscera

Sympathetic ganglion

Sympathetic trunk

Ganglion impar

———— Preganglionic sympathetic

·········· Postganglionic sympathetic

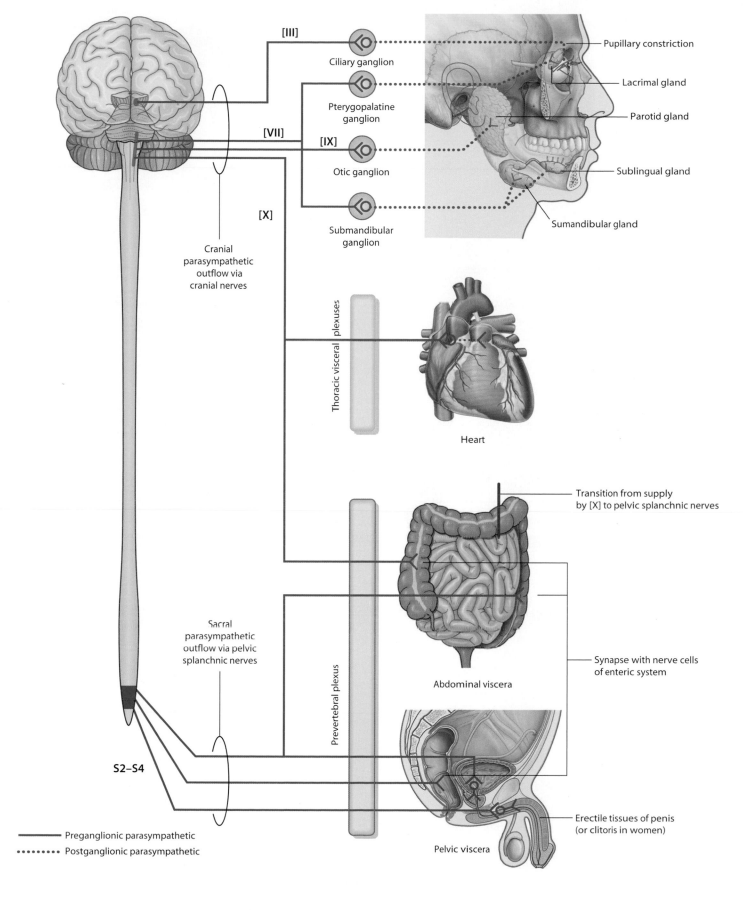

[III]

Ciliary ganglion

Pterygopalatine ganglion

[VII]

[IX]

Otic ganglion

[X]

Submandibular ganglion

Cranial parasympathetic outflow via cranial nerves

Pupillary constriction

Lacrimal gland

Parotid gland

Sublingual gland

Sumandibular gland

Thoracic visceral plexuses

Heart

Transition from supply by [X] to pelvic splanchnic nerves

Sacral parasympathetic outflow via pelvic splanchnic nerves

Prevertebral plexus

Abdominal viscera

Synapse with nerve cells of enteric system

S2–S4

———— Preganglionic parasympathetic

·········· Postganglionic parasympathetic

Erectile tissues of penis (or clitoris in women)

Pelvic viscera

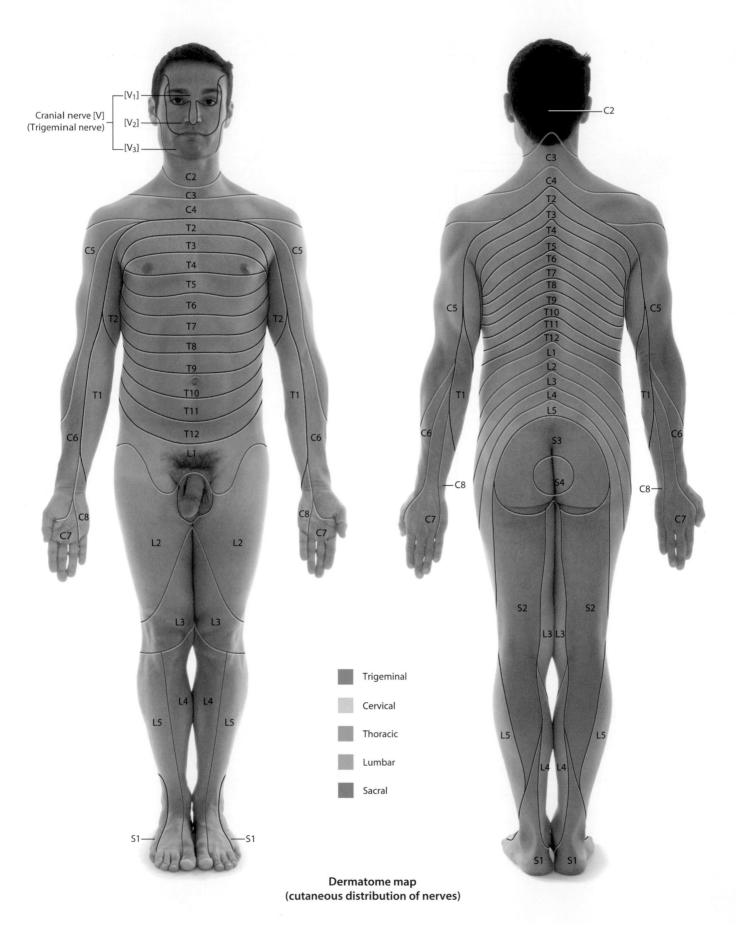

Dermatome map
(cutaneous distribution of nerves)

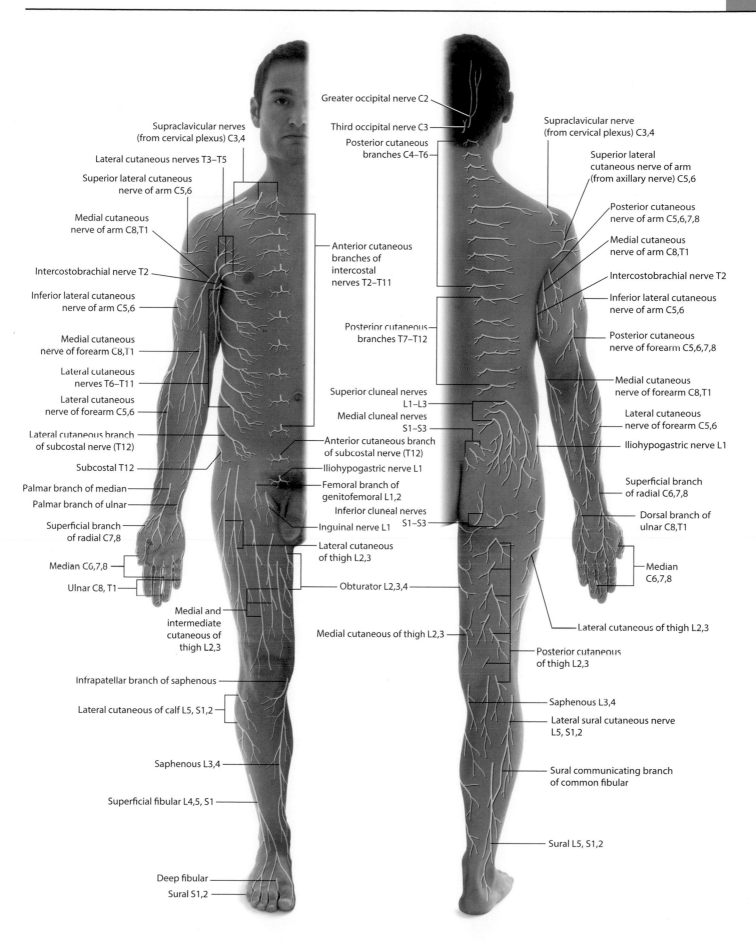

Greater occipital nerve C2

Third occipital nerve C3

Supraclavicular nerves
(from cervical plexus) C3,4

Lateral cutaneous nerves T3–T5

Superior lateral cutaneous
nerve of arm C5,6

Medial cutaneous
nerve of arm C8,T1

Intercostobrachial nerve T2

Inferior lateral cutaneous
nerve of arm C5,6

Medial cutaneous
nerve of forearm C8,T1

Lateral cutaneous
nerves T6–T11

Lateral cutaneous
nerve of forearm C5,6

Lateral cutaneous branch
of subcostal nerve (T12)

Subcostal T12

Palmar branch of median

Palmar branch of ulnar

Superficial branch
of radial C7,8

Median C6,7,8

Ulnar C8, T1

Medial and
intermediate
cutaneous of
thigh L2,3

Infrapatellar branch of saphenous

Lateral cutaneous of calf L5, S1,2

Saphenous L3,4

Superficial fibular L4,5, S1

Deep fibular

Sural S1,2

Posterior cutaneous
branches C4–T6

Anterior cutaneous
branches of
intercostal
nerves T2–T11

Posterior cutaneous
branches T7–T12

Superior cluneal nerves
L1–L3

Medial cluneal nerves
S1–S3

Anterior cutaneous branch
of subcostal nerve (T12)

Iliohypogastric nerve L1

Femoral branch of
genitofemoral L1,2

Inferior cluneal nerves
S1–S3

Inguinal nerve L1

Lateral cutaneous
of thigh L2,3

Obturator L2,3,4

Medial cutaneous of thigh L2,3

Supraclavicular nerve
(from cervical plexus) C3,4

Superior lateral
cutaneous nerve of arm
(from axillary nerve) C5,6

Posterior cutaneous
nerve of arm C5,6,7,8

Medial cutaneous
nerve of arm C8,T1

Intercostobrachial nerve T2

Inferior lateral cutaneous
nerve of arm C5,6

Posterior cutaneous
nerve of forearm C5,6,7,8

Medial cutaneous
nerve of forearm C8,T1

Lateral cutaneous
nerve of forearm C5,6

Iliohypogastric nerve L1

Superficial branch
of radial C6,7,8

Dorsal branch of
ulnar C8,T1

Median
C6,7,8

Lateral cutaneous of thigh L2,3

Posterior cutaneous
of thigh L2,3

Saphenous L3,4

Lateral sural cutaneous nerve
L5, S1,2

Sural communicating branch
of common fibular

Sural L5, S1,2

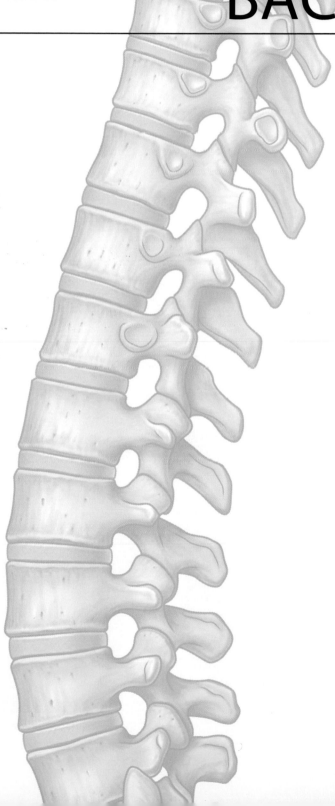

CONTENTS

2
BACK

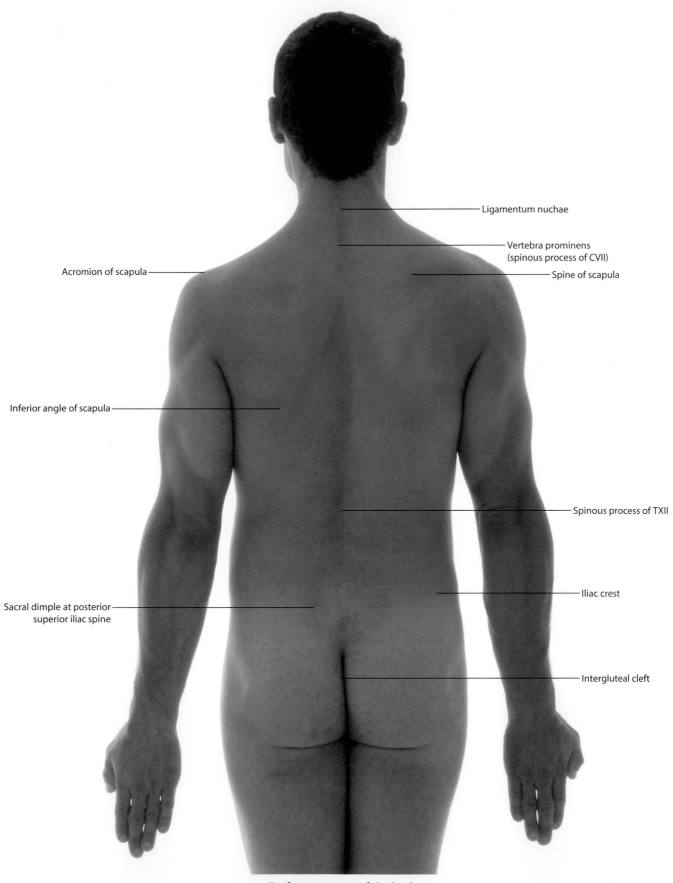

Ligamentum nuchae

Vertebra prominens
(spinous process of CVII)

Acromion of scapula

Spine of scapula

Inferior angle of scapula

Spinous process of TXII

Iliac crest

Sacral dimple at posterior
superior iliac spine

Intergluteal cleft

Surface anatomy of the back

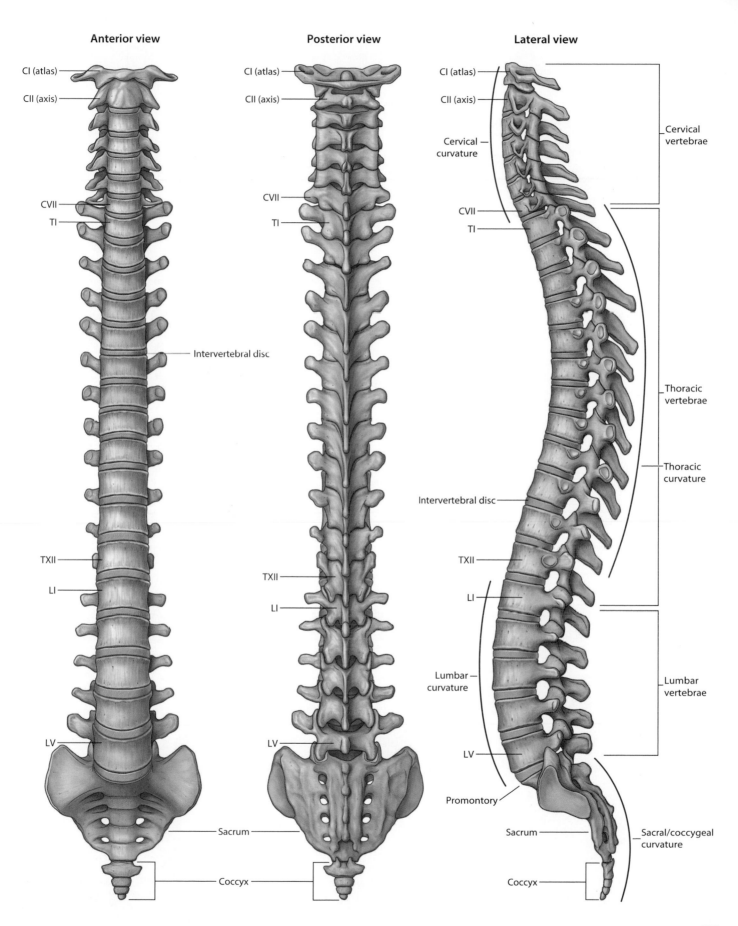

Anterior view

CI (atlas)
CII (axis)
CVII
TI
Intervertebral disc
TXII
LI
LV
Sacrum
Coccyx

Posterior view

CI (atlas)
CII (axis)
CVII
TI
TXII
LI
LV
Sacrum
Coccyx

Lateral view

CI (atlas)
CII (axis)
Cervical curvature
CVII
TI
Cervical vertebrae
Intervertebral disc
Thoracic vertebrae
Thoracic curvature
TXII
LI
Lumbar curvature
Lumbar vertebrae
LV
Promontory
Sacrum
Coccyx
Sacral/coccygeal curvature

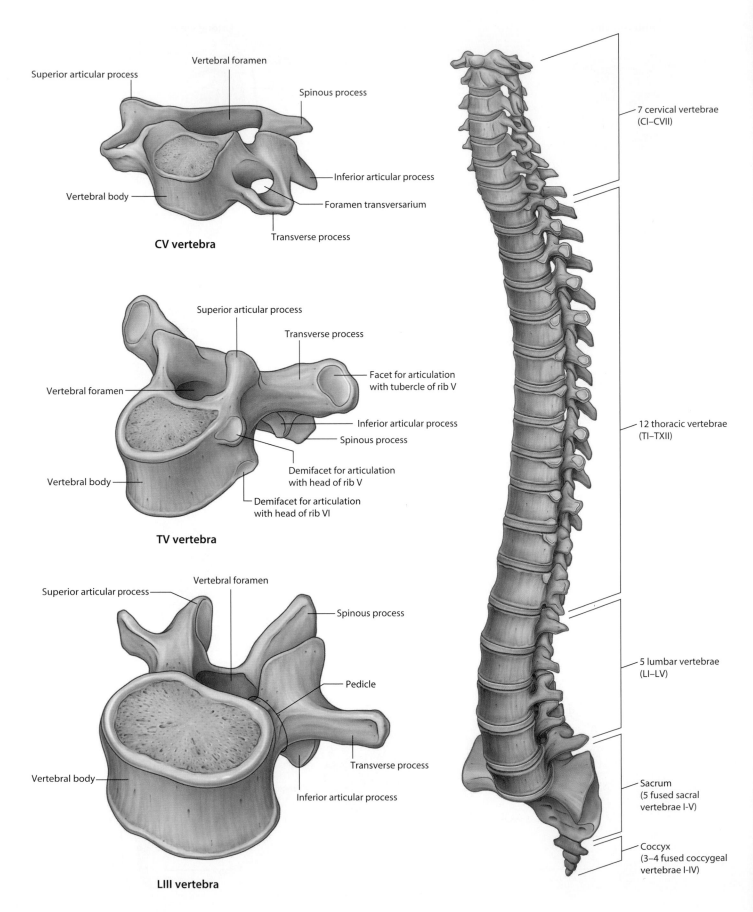

Superior articular process

Vertebral foramen

Spinous process

Inferior articular process

Foramen transversarium

Vertebral body

Transverse process

CV vertebra

Superior articular process

Transverse process

Facet for articulation with tubercle of rib V

Vertebral foramen

Inferior articular process

Spinous process

Demifacet for articulation with head of rib V

Vertebral body

Demifacet for articulation with head of rib VI

TV vertebra

Vertebral foramen

Superior articular process

Spinous process

Pedicle

Transverse process

Vertebral body

Inferior articular process

LIII vertebra

7 cervical vertebrae (CI–CVII)

12 thoracic vertebrae (TI–TXII)

5 lumbar vertebrae (LI–LV)

Sacrum (5 fused sacral vertebrae I-V)

Coccyx (3–4 fused coccygeal vertebrae I-IV)

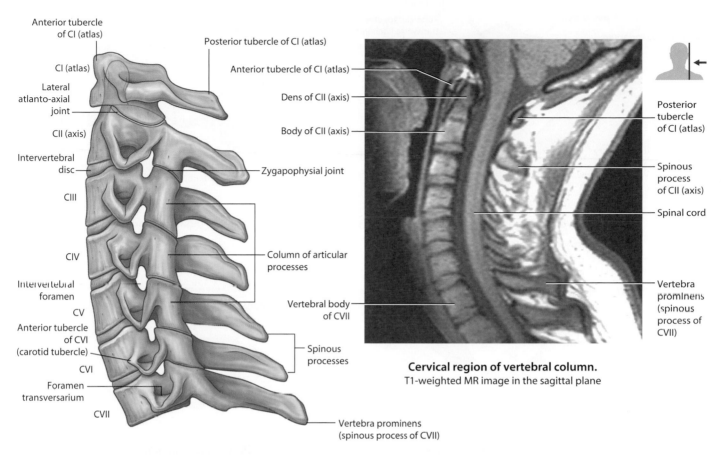

Anterior tubercle of CI (atlas)

CI (atlas)

Lateral atlanto-axial joint

CII (axis)

Intervertebral disc

CIII

CIV

Intervertebral foramen

CV

Anterior tubercle of CVI (carotid tubercle)

CVI

Foramen transversarium

CVII

Posterior tubercle of CI (atlas)

Anterior tubercle of CI (atlas)

Zygapophysial joint

Column of articular processes

Vertebral body of CVII

Spinous processes

Vertebra prominens (spinous process of CVII)

Cervical vertebrae lateral view

Anterior tubercle of CI (atlas)

Dens of CII (axis)

Body of CII (axis)

Posterior tubercle of CI (atlas)

Spinous process of CII (axis)

Spinal cord

Vertebra prominens (spinous process of CVII)

Cervical region of vertebral column.
T1-weighted MR image in the sagittal plane

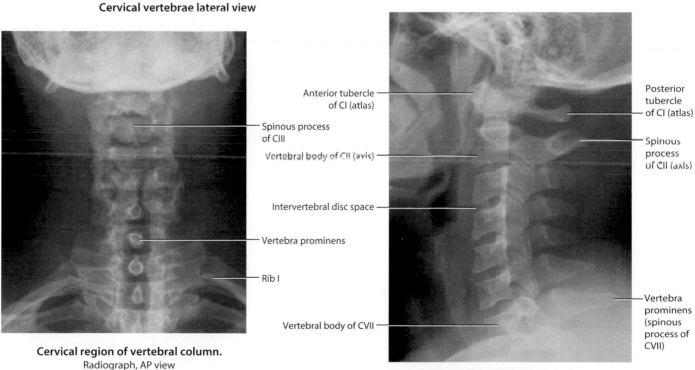

Spinous process of CIII

Vertebral body of CII (axis)

Vertebra prominens

Rib I

Cervical region of vertebral column.
Radiograph, AP view

Anterior tubercle of CI (atlas)

Vertebral body of CII (axis)

Intervertebral disc space

Vertebral body of CVII

Posterior tubercle of CI (atlas)

Spinous process of CII (axis)

Vertebra prominens (spinous process of CVII)

Cervical region of vertebral column.
Radiograph, lateral view

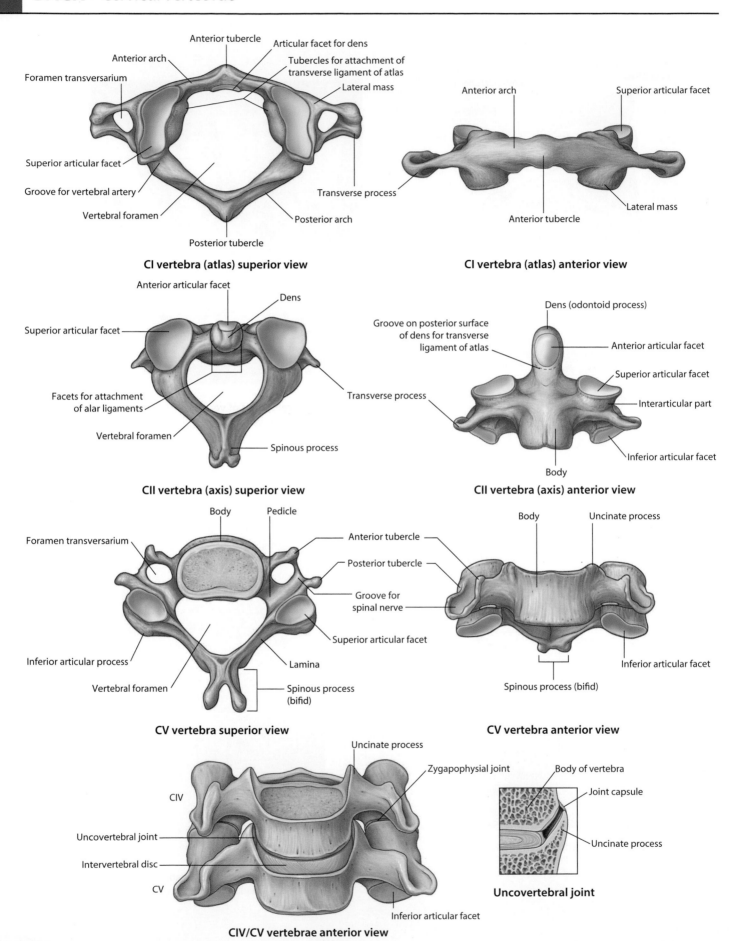

CI vertebra (atlas) superior view

Anterior tubercle
Articular facet for dens
Anterior arch
Tubercles for attachment of transverse ligament of atlas
Foramen transversarium
Lateral mass
Superior articular facet
Groove for vertebral artery
Transverse process
Vertebral foramen
Posterior arch
Posterior tubercle

CI vertebra (atlas) anterior view

Anterior arch
Superior articular facet
Anterior tubercle
Lateral mass

CII vertebra (axis) superior view

Anterior articular facet
Dens
Superior articular facet
Facets for attachment of alar ligaments
Transverse process
Vertebral foramen
Spinous process

CII vertebra (axis) anterior view

Dens (odontoid process)
Groove on posterior surface of dens for transverse ligament of atlas
Anterior articular facet
Superior articular facet
Interarticular part
Transverse process
Inferior articular facet
Body

CV vertebra superior view

Body
Pedicle
Foramen transversarium
Anterior tubercle
Posterior tubercle
Groove for spinal nerve
Superior articular facet
Inferior articular process
Lamina
Vertebral foramen
Spinous process (bifid)

CV vertebra anterior view

Body
Uncinate process
Inferior articular facet
Spinous process (bifid)

CIV/CV vertebrae anterior view

Uncinate process
Zygapophysial joint
Body of vertebra
CIV
Joint capsule
Uncovertebral joint
Intervertebral disc
Uncinate process
CV
Inferior articular facet

Uncovertebral joint

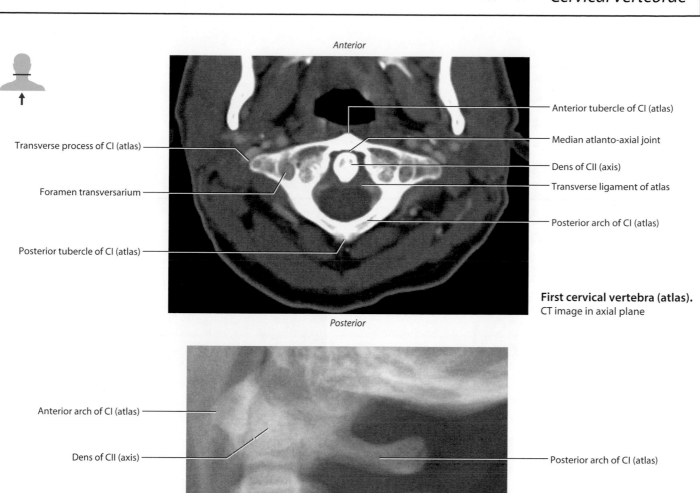

Anterior

Transverse process of CI (atlas)

Foramen transversarium

Posterior tubercle of CI (atlas)

Anterior tubercle of CI (atlas)

Median atlanto-axial joint

Dens of CII (axis)

Transverse ligament of atlas

Posterior arch of CI (atlas)

Posterior

First cervical vertebra (atlas).
CT image in axial plane

Anterior arch of CI (atlas)

Dens of CII (axis)

Vertebral body of CII (axis)

Intervertebral disc space

Posterior arch of CI (atlas)

Spinous process of CII (axis)

Cervical vertebrae CI–CIII.
Radiograph, lateral view

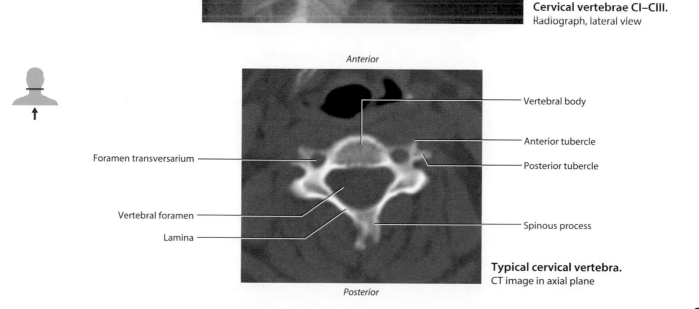

Anterior

Foramen transversarium

Vertebral foramen

Lamina

Vertebral body

Anterior tubercle

Posterior tubercle

Spinous process

Typical cervical vertebra.
CT image in axial plane

Posterior

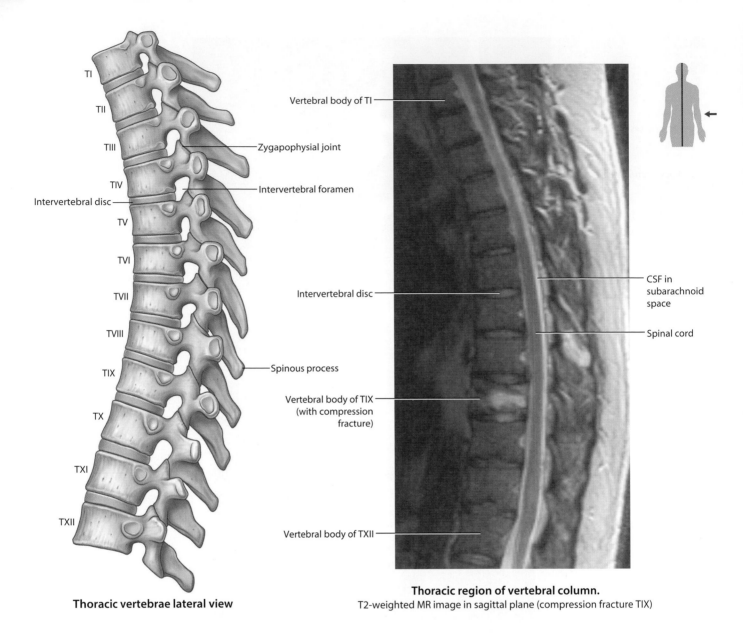

TI

TII

TIII — Zygapophysial joint

TIV — Intervertebral foramen

Intervertebral disc —

TV

TVI

TVII

TVIII

TIX — Spinous process

TX

TXI

TXII

Thoracic vertebrae lateral view

Vertebral body of TI

Intervertebral disc

CSF in subarachnoid space

Spinal cord

Vertebral body of TIX (with compression fracture)

Vertebral body of TXII

Thoracic region of vertebral column.
T2-weighted MR image in sagittal plane (compression fracture TIX)

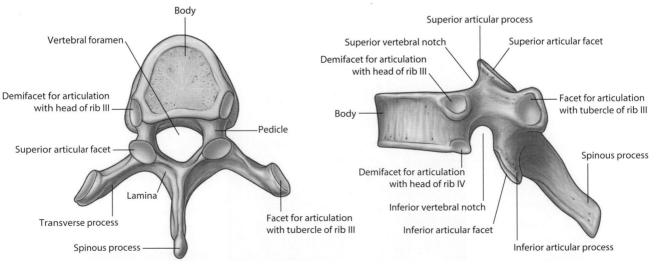

Body

Vertebral foramen

Demifacet for articulation with head of rib III

Superior articular facet

Transverse process

Spinous process

Lamina

Pedicle

Facet for articulation with tubercle of rib III

TIII vertebra superior view

Superior articular process

Superior vertebral notch

Demifacet for articulation with head of rib III

Body

Demifacet for articulation with head of rib IV

Inferior vertebral notch

Inferior articular facet

Inferior articular process

Superior articular facet

Facet for articulation with tubercle of rib III

Spinous process

TIII vertebra lateral view

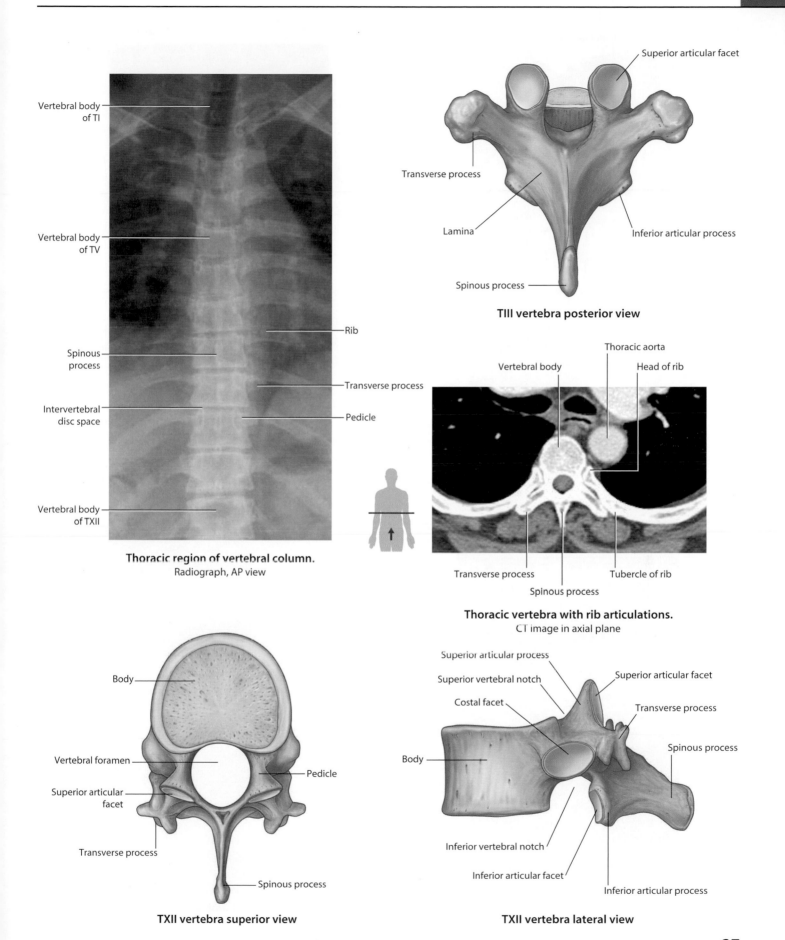

Vertebral body of TI

Vertebral body of TV

Spinous process

Intervertebral disc space

Vertebral body of TXII

Rib

Transverse process

Pedicle

Thoracic region of vertebral column.
Radiograph, AP view

Superior articular facet

Transverse process

Lamina

Inferior articular process

Spinous process

TIII vertebra posterior view

Thoracic aorta

Vertebral body

Head of rib

Transverse process

Spinous process

Tubercle of rib

Thoracic vertebra with rib articulations.
CT image in axial plane

Body

Vertebral foramen

Superior articular facet

Transverse process

Pedicle

Spinous process

TXII vertebra superior view

Superior articular process

Superior vertebral notch

Costal facet

Body

Inferior vertebral notch

Inferior articular facet

Superior articular facet

Transverse process

Spinous process

Inferior articular process

TXII vertebra lateral view

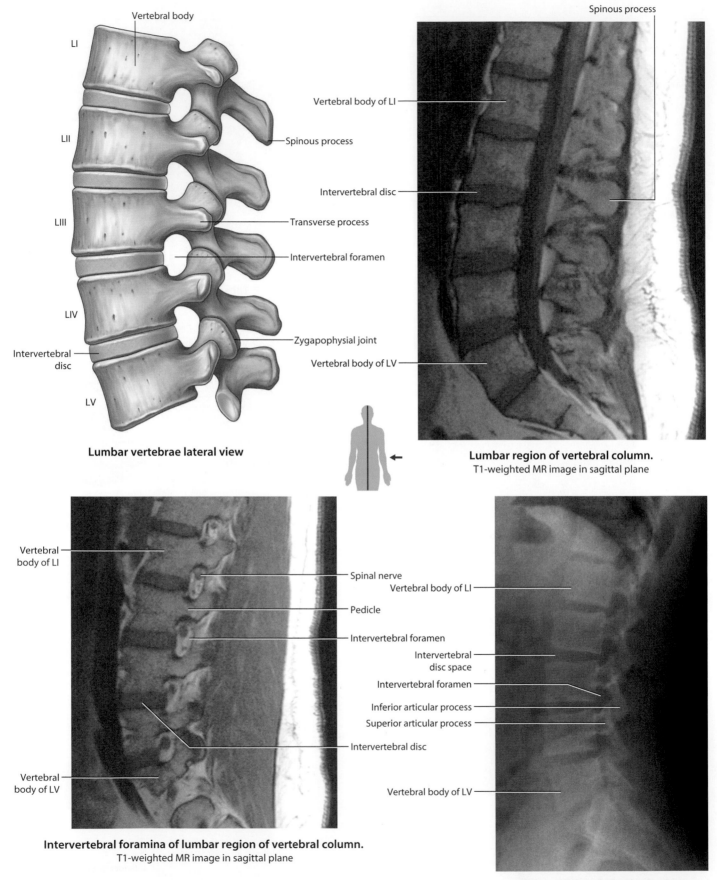

Lumbar vertebrae lateral view

Vertebral body
LI
LII
LIII
LIV
Intervertebral disc
LV

Spinous process
Transverse process
Intervertebral foramen
Zygapophysial joint

Lumbar region of vertebral column.
T1-weighted MR image in sagittal plane

Spinous process
Vertebral body of LI
Intervertebral disc
Vertebral body of LV

Intervertebral foramina of lumbar region of vertebral column.
T1-weighted MR image in sagittal plane

Vertebral body of LI
Vertebral body of LV
Spinal nerve
Pedicle
Intervertebral foramen
Intervertebral disc

Lumbar region of vertebral column.
Radiograph, lateral view

Vertebral body of LI
Intervertebral disc space
Intervertebral foramen
Inferior articular process
Superior articular process
Vertebral body of LV

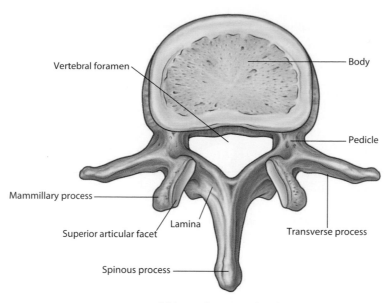

Vertebral foramen

Body

Pedicle

Mammillary process

Lamina

Superior articular facet

Transverse process

Spinous process

LIV vertebra superior view

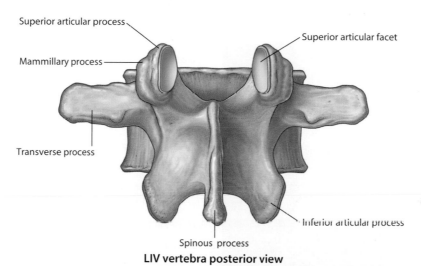

Superior articular process

Superior articular facet

Mammillary process

Transverse process

Inferior articular process

Spinous process

LIV vertebra posterior view

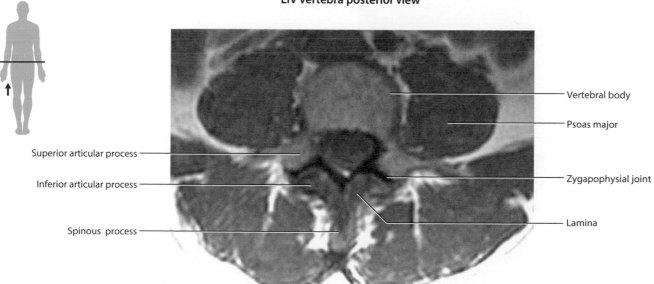

Superior articular process

Inferior articular process

Spinous process

Vertebral body

Psoas major

Zygapophysial joint

Lamina

Articulation of lumbar vertebrae.
T1-weighted MR image in axial plane

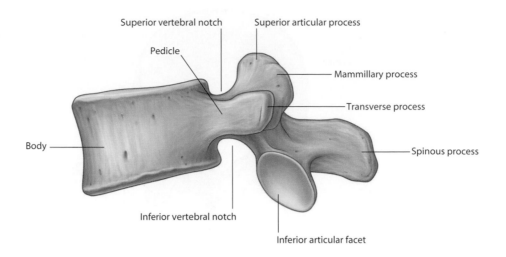

LIV vertebra lateral view

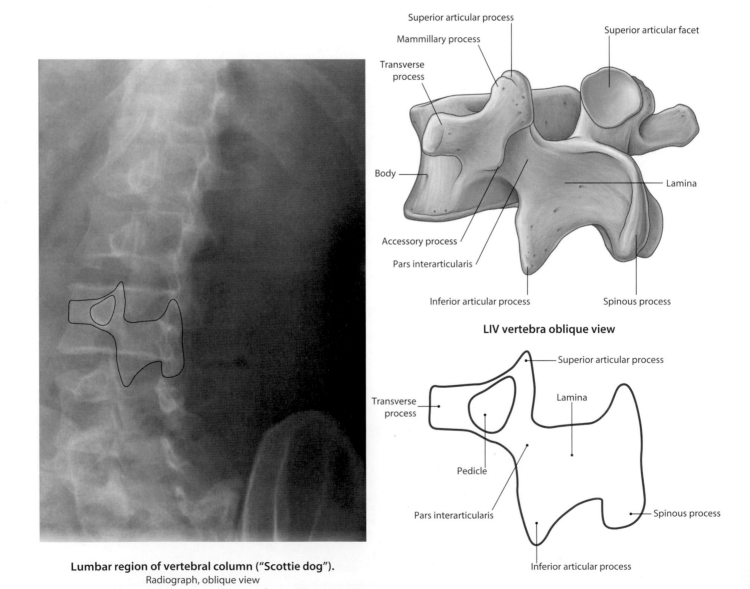

Lumbar region of vertebral column ("Scottie dog").
Radiograph, oblique view

LIV vertebra oblique view

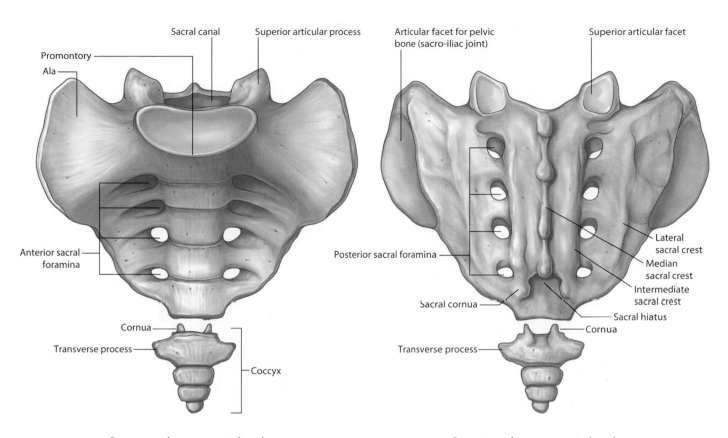

Sacral canal

Superior articular process

Promontory

Ala

Anterior sacral foramina

Cornua

Transverse process

Coccyx

Sacrum and coccyx anterior view

Articular facet for pelvic bone (sacro-iliac joint)

Superior articular facet

Posterior sacral foramina

Lateral sacral crest

Median sacral crest

Intermediate sacral crest

Sacral cornua

Sacral hiatus

Cornua

Transverse process

Sacrum and coccyx posterior view

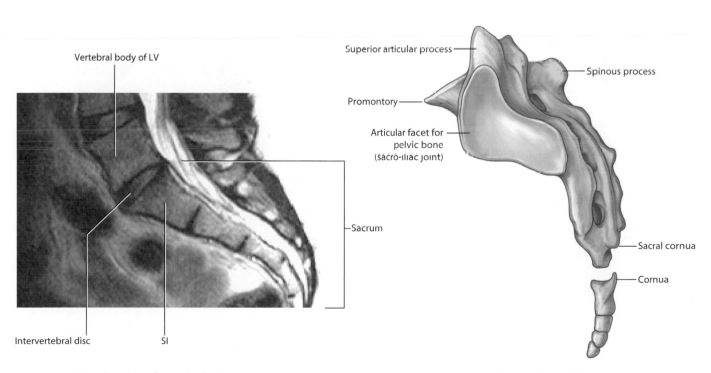

Vertebral body of LV

Intervertebral disc

SI

Sacrum

Sacral region of vertebral column.
T2-weighted MR image in sagittal plane

Superior articular process

Spinous process

Promontory

Articular facet for pelvic bone (sacro-iliac joint)

Sacral cornua

Cornua

Sacrum and coccyx lateral view

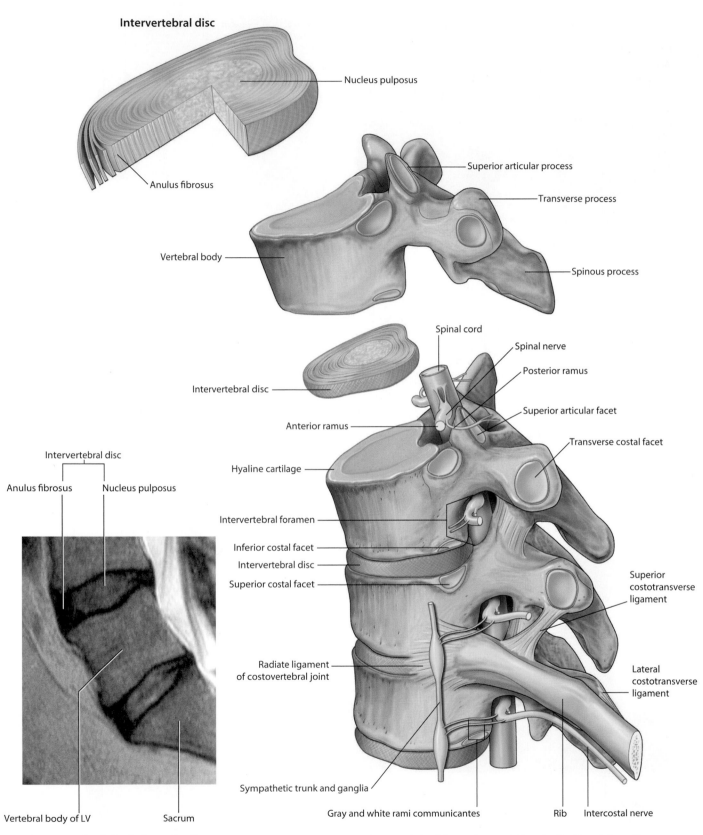

Intervertebral disc

Nucleus pulposus

Anulus fibrosus

Superior articular process

Transverse process

Vertebral body

Spinous process

Spinal cord

Spinal nerve

Posterior ramus

Intervertebral disc

Superior articular facet

Anterior ramus

Transverse costal facet

Hyaline cartilage

Intervertebral foramen

Inferior costal facet

Intervertebral disc

Superior costal facet

Superior costotransverse ligament

Radiate ligament of costovertebral joint

Lateral costotransverse ligament

Sympathetic trunk and ganglia

Gray and white rami communicantes

Rib

Intercostal nerve

Intervertebral disc

Anulus fibrosus   Nucleus pulposus

Vertebral body of LV   Sacrum

Intervertebral disc in lower lumbar region of vertebral column.
T2-weighted MR image in sagittal plane

Intervertebral foramina and discs in the thoracic region

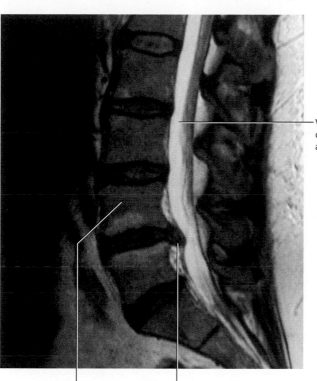

Vertebral canal containing CSF and cauda equina

LIV vertebra

Disc protrusion

Intervertebral disc protrusion in lower lumbar region of vertebral column.
T2-weighted MR image in sagittal plane

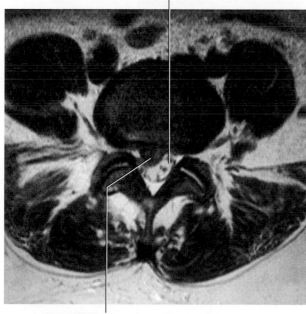

Vertebral canal containing CSF and cauda equina

Disc protrusion

Intervertebral disc protrusion in lower lumbar region of vertebral column.
T2-weighted MR image in axial plane

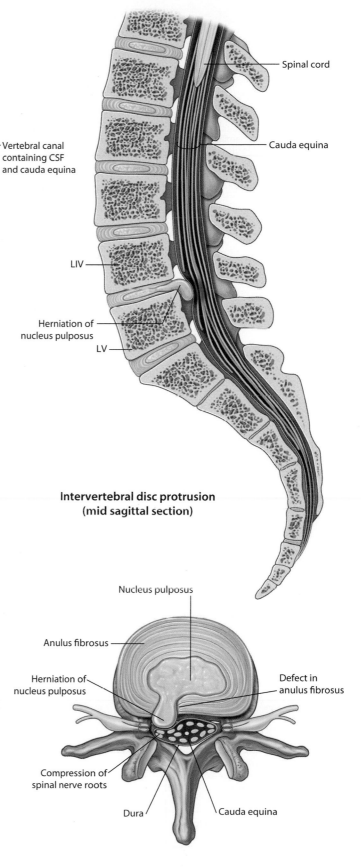

Spinal cord

Cauda equina

LIV

Herniation of nucleus pulposus

LV

Intervertebral disc protrusion (mid sagittal section)

Nucleus pulposus

Anulus fibrosus

Herniation of nucleus pulposus

Defect in anulus fibrosus

Compression of spinal nerve roots

Dura

Cauda equina

Intervertebral disc protrusion (superior view)

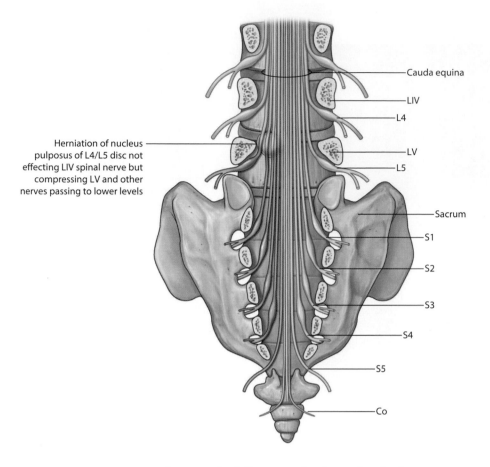

Herniation of nucleus pulposus of L4/L5 disc not effecting LIV spinal nerve but compressing LV and other nerves passing to lower levels

Cauda equina
LIV
L4
LV
L5
Sacrum
S1
S2
S3
S4
S5
Co

Intervertebral disc protrusion (posterior view)

Nerve root	Main weakness	Reflex decreased	Area of sensory decrease	Disc involved
C5	Deltoid (biceps)	(biceps, pectoralis)	Shoulder, upper lateral arm	C4–C5
C6	Wrist extension	(biceps, brachioradialis)	1st and 2nd digits (lateral forearm)	C5–C6
C7	Triceps	Triceps	Third finger	C6–C7
C8	Intrinsic hand muscles		4th and 5th digits (medial forearm)	C7–T1

C5
C5–C6
C7
C6

Clinically important nerve roots in the upper limb

Nerve root	Main weakness	Reflex decreased	Area of sensory decrease	Disc involved
L4	Iliopsoas and quadriceps	Patellar tendon (knee jerk)	Knee, medial lower leg	L3–L4
L5	Dorsiflexion of foot at ankle (big toe extension, foot eversion and inversion		Dorsum of foot, big toe	L4–L5
S1	Plantar flexion of foot at ankle	Achilles tendon (ankle jerk)	Lateral foot, small toe, sole	L5–S1

L4
L5
S1

Clinically important nerve roots in the lower limb

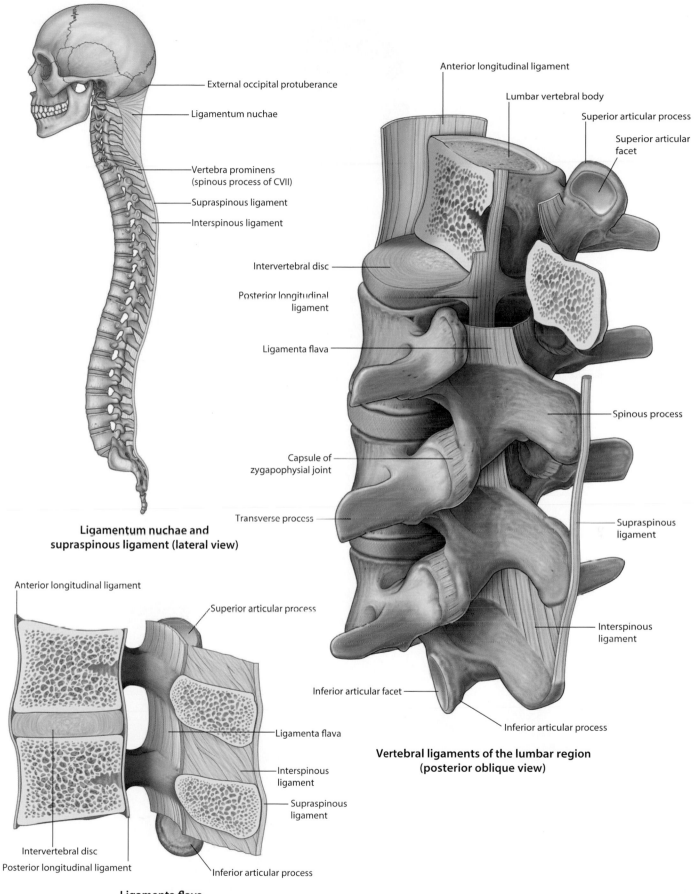

External occipital protuberance

Ligamentum nuchae

Vertebra prominens
(spinous process of CVII)

Supraspinous ligament

Interspinous ligament

**Ligamentum nuchae and
supraspinous ligament (lateral view)**

Anterior longitudinal ligament

Lumbar vertebral body

Superior articular process

Superior articular
facet

Intervertebral disc

Posterior longitudinal
ligament

Ligamenta flava

Spinous process

Capsule of
zygapophysial joint

Transverse process

Supraspinous
ligament

Interspinous
ligament

Inferior articular facet

Inferior articular process

**Vertebral ligaments of the lumbar region
(posterior oblique view)**

Anterior longitudinal ligament

Superior articular process

Ligamenta flava

Interspinous
ligament

Supraspinous
ligament

Intervertebral disc

Posterior longitudinal ligament

Inferior articular process

Ligamenta flava

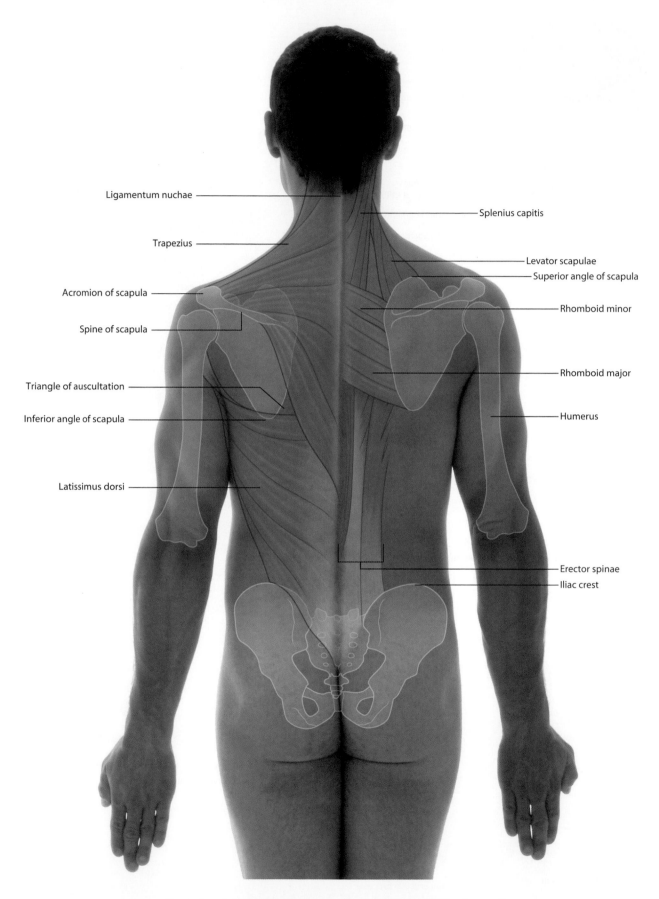

Ligamentum nuchae

Trapezius

Acromion of scapula

Spine of scapula

Triangle of auscultation

Inferior angle of scapula

Latissimus dorsi

Splenius capitis

Levator scapulae

Superior angle of scapula

Rhomboid minor

Rhomboid major

Humerus

Erector spinae

Iliac crest

Posterior view of male showing surface projections of back muscles

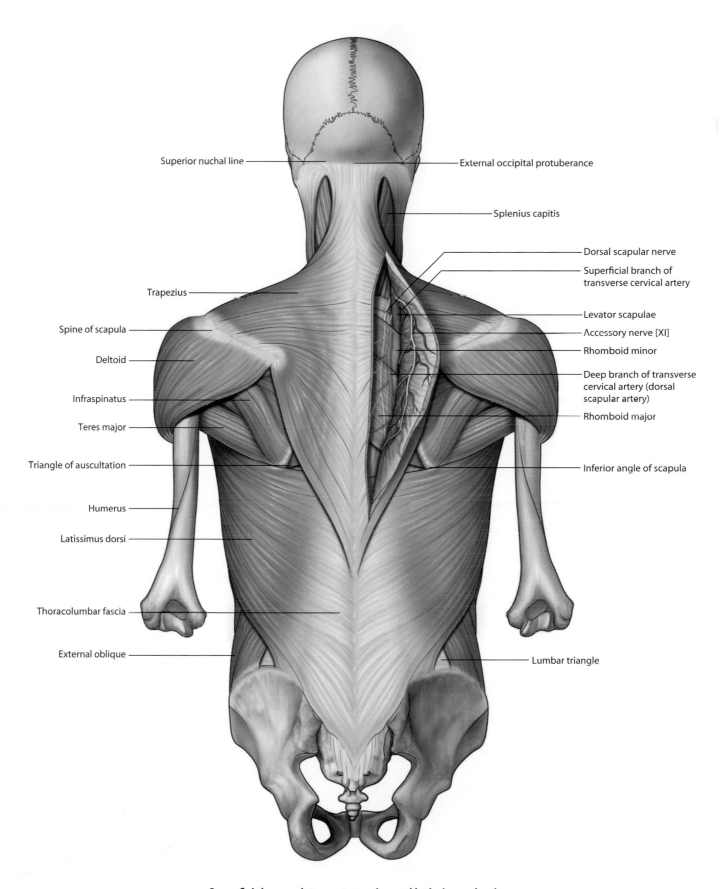

Superior nuchal line — External occipital protuberance

Splenius capitis

Dorsal scapular nerve

Superficial branch of transverse cervical artery

Trapezius

Levator scapulae

Spine of scapula

Accessory nerve [XI]

Deltoid

Rhomboid minor

Deep branch of transverse cervical artery (dorsal scapular artery)

Infraspinatus

Teres major

Rhomboid major

Triangle of auscultation

Inferior angle of scapula

Humerus

Latissimus dorsi

Thoracolumbar fascia

External oblique

Lumbar triangle

Superficial musculature – trapezius and latissimus dorsi

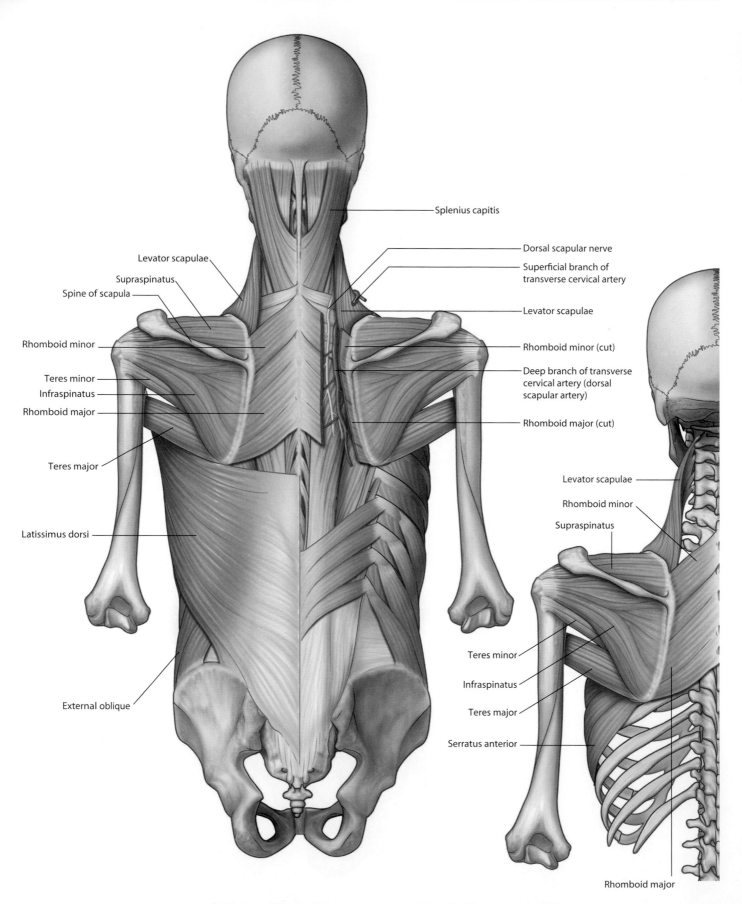

Splenius capitis

Dorsal scapular nerve

Superficial branch of transverse cervical artery

Levator scapulae

Levator scapulae

Rhomboid minor (cut)

Supraspinatus

Deep branch of transverse cervical artery (dorsal scapular artery)

Spine of scapula

Rhomboid minor

Rhomboid major (cut)

Teres minor

Infraspinatus

Rhomboid major

Teres major

Levator scapulae

Rhomboid minor

Supraspinatus

Latissimus dorsi

Teres minor

Infraspinatus

Teres major

External oblique

Serratus anterior

Rhomboid major

Superficial musculature – levator scapulae and rhomboid major and minor

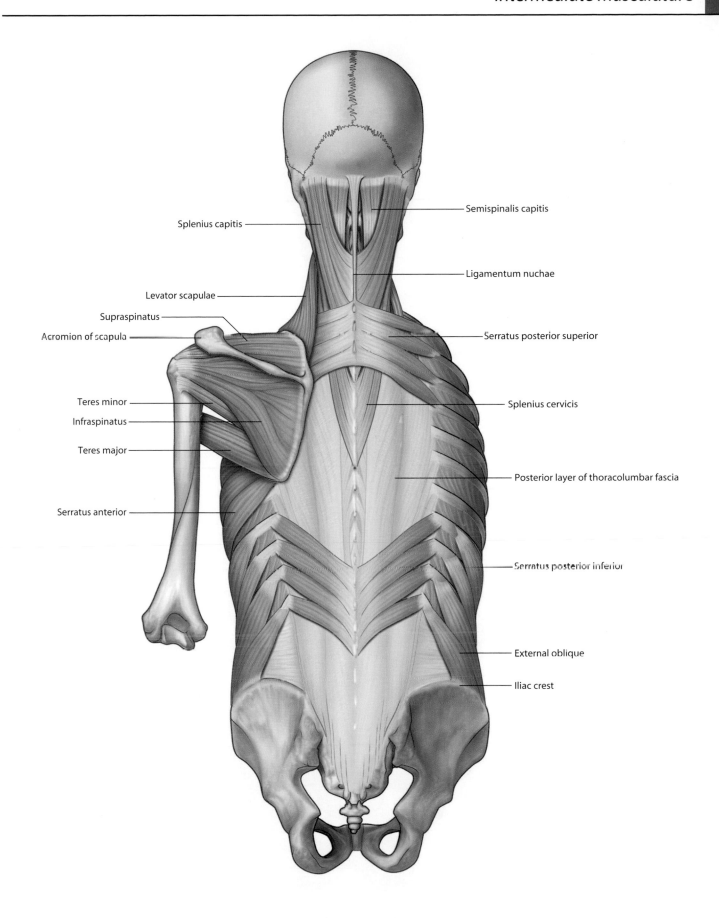

Semispinalis capitis

Splenius capitis

Ligamentum nuchae

Levator scapulae

Supraspinatus

Acromion of scapula

Serratus posterior superior

Teres minor

Infraspinatus

Splenius cervicis

Teres major

Serratus anterior

Posterior layer of thoracolumbar fascia

Serratus posterior inferior

External oblique

Iliac crest

Intermediate musculature

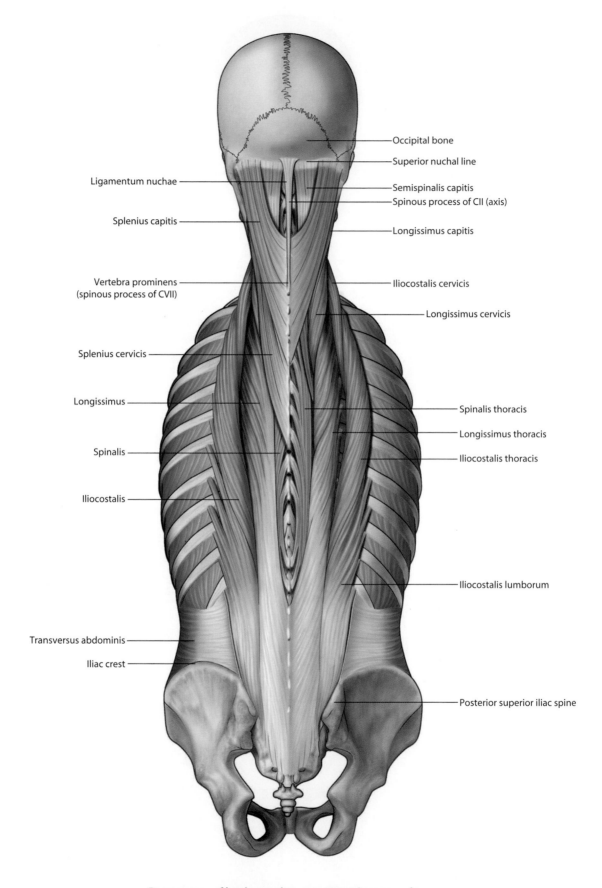

Occipital bone

Superior nuchal line

Ligamentum nuchae

Semispinalis capitis

Spinous process of CII (axis)

Splenius capitis

Longissimus capitis

Vertebra prominens
(spinous process of CVII)

Iliocostalis cervicis

Longissimus cervicis

Splenius cervicis

Longissimus

Spinalis thoracis

Longissimus thoracis

Spinalis

Iliocostalis thoracis

Iliocostalis

Iliocostalis lumborum

Transversus abdominis

Iliac crest

Posterior superior iliac spine

Deep group of back muscles – erector spinae muscles

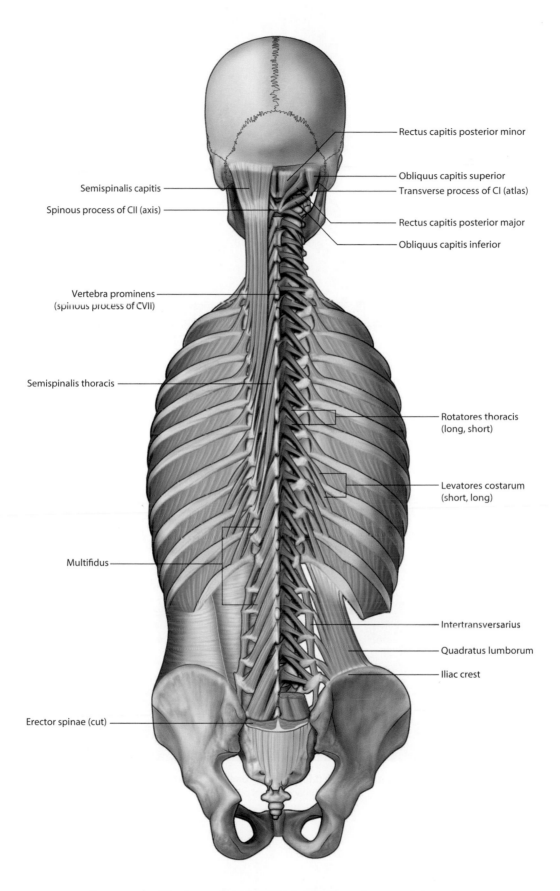

Rectus capitis posterior minor

Obliquus capitis superior

Transverse process of CI (atlas)

Rectus capitis posterior major

Obliquus capitis inferior

Semispinalis capitis

Spinous process of CII (axis)

Vertebra prominens
(spinous process of CVII)

Semispinalis thoracis

Rotatores thoracis
(long, short)

Levatores costarum
(short, long)

Multifidus

Intertransversarius

Quadratus lumborum

Iliac crest

Erector spinae (cut)

Deep group of back muscles – transversospinales and segmental muscles

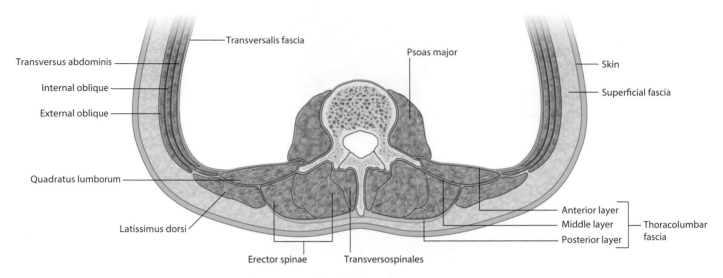

Transversalis fascia

Transversus abdominis

Internal oblique

External oblique

Psoas major

Skin

Superficial fascia

Quadratus lumborum

Latissimus dorsi

Erector spinae

Transversospinales

Anterior layer

Middle layer

Posterior layer

Thoracolumbar fascia

**Thoracolumbar fascia and the deep back muscles
(transverse section – lumbar region)**

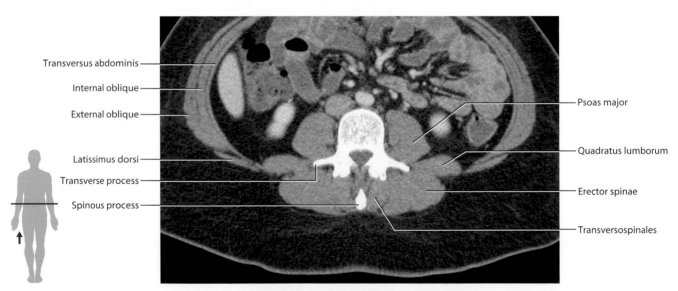

Transversus abdominis

Internal oblique

External oblique

Latissimus dorsi

Transverse process

Spinous process

Psoas major

Quadratus lumborum

Erector spinae

Transversospinales

Lumbar region (LIII) showing back musculature.
CT image in axial plane

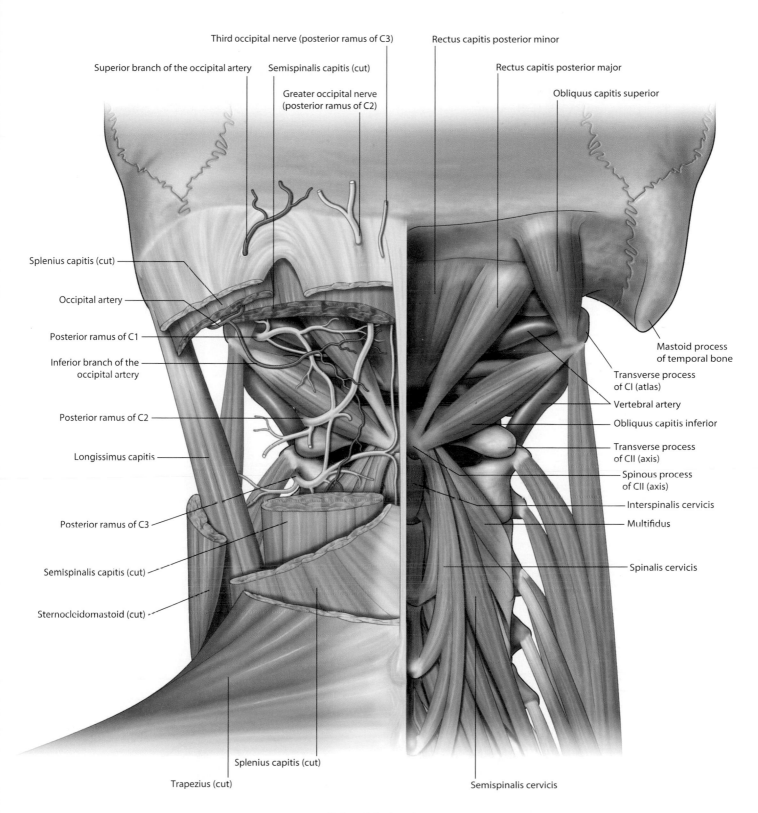

Third occipital nerve (posterior ramus of C3)

Superior branch of the occipital artery

Semispinalis capitis (cut)

Greater occipital nerve (posterior ramus of C2)

Rectus capitis posterior minor

Rectus capitis posterior major

Obliquus capitis superior

Splenius capitis (cut)

Occipital artery

Posterior ramus of C1

Inferior branch of the occipital artery

Posterior ramus of C2

Longissimus capitis

Posterior ramus of C3

Semispinalis capitis (cut)

Sternocleidomastoid (cut)

Mastoid process of temporal bone

Transverse process of CI (atlas)

Vertebral artery

Obliquus capitis inferior

Transverse process of CII (axis)

Spinous process of CII (axis)

Interspinalis cervicis

Multifidus

Spinalis cervicis

Splenius capitis (cut)

Trapezius (cut)

Semispinalis cervicis

Suboccipital region

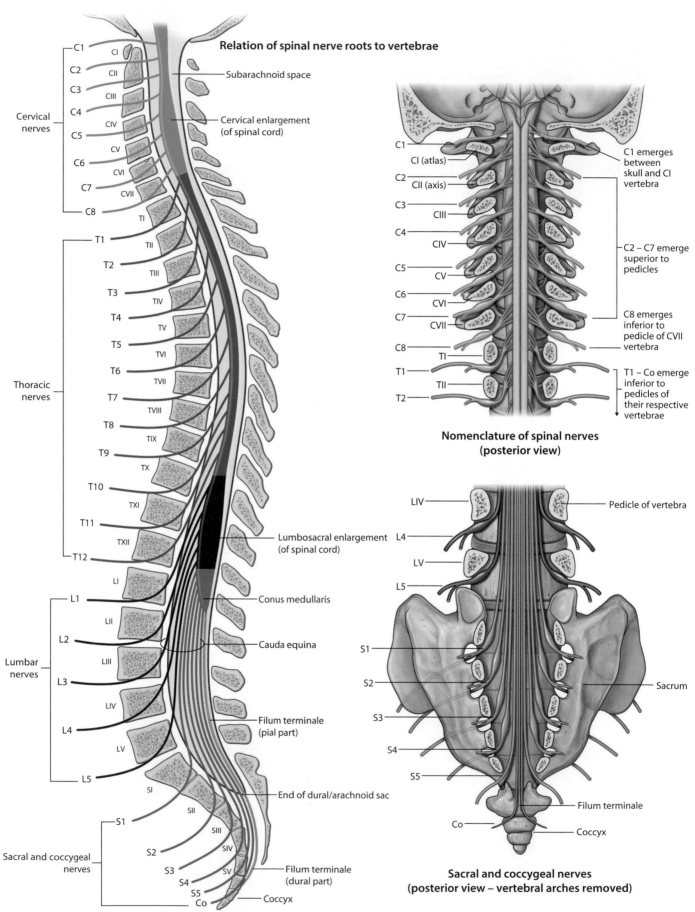

Relation of spinal nerve roots to vertebrae

Cervical nerves

- C1 — CI
- C2 — CII
- C3 — CIII
- C4 — CIV
- C5 — CV
- C6 — CVI
- C7 — CVII
- C8 — TI

Subarachnoid space

Cervical enlargement (of spinal cord)

Thoracic nerves

- T1 — TII
- T2 — TIII
- T3 — TIV
- T4 — TV
- T5 — TVI
- T6 — TVII
- T7 — TVIII
- T8 — TIX
- T9 — TX
- T10 — TXI
- T11 — TXII
- T12 — LI

Lumbar nerves

- L1 — LII
- L2 — LIII
- L3 — LIV
- L4 — LV
- L5 — SI

Sacral and coccygeal nerves

- S1 — SII
- S2 — SIII
- S3 — SIV
- S4 — SV
- S5
- Co

Lumbosacral enlargement (of spinal cord)

Conus medullaris

Cauda equina

Filum terminale (pial part)

End of dural/arachnoid sac

Filum terminale (dural part)

Coccyx

Nomenclature of spinal nerves (posterior view)

- C1 — CI (atlas) — C1 emerges between skull and CI vertebra
- C2 — CII (axis)
- C3 — CIII
- C4 — CIV — C2 – C7 emerge superior to pedicles
- C5 — CV
- C6 — CVI
- C7 — CVII — C8 emerges inferior to pedicle of CVII vertebra
- C8 — TI
- T1 — TII — T1 – Co emerge inferior to pedicles of their respective vertebrae
- T2

Sacral and coccygeal nerves (posterior view – vertebral arches removed)

- LIV — Pedicle of vertebra
- L4
- LV
- L5
- S1
- S2 — Sacrum
- S3
- S4
- S5 — Filum terminale
- Co — Coccyx

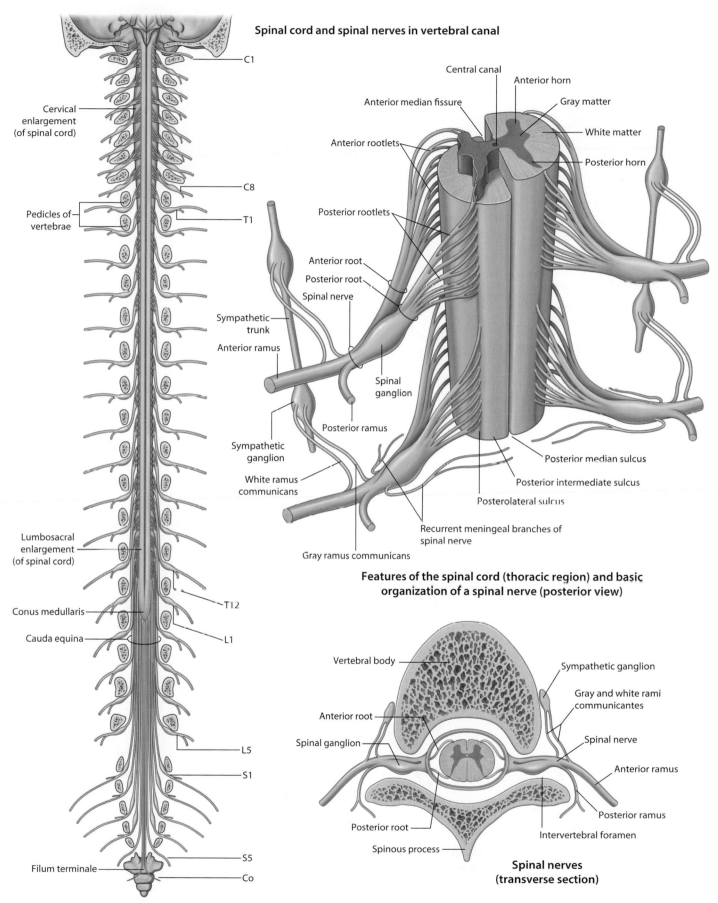

Spinal cord and spinal nerves in vertebral canal

Cervical enlargement (of spinal cord)

C1

C8

Pedicles of vertebrae

T1

Central canal

Anterior horn

Anterior median fissure

Gray matter

White matter

Anterior rootlets

Posterior horn

Posterior rootlets

Anterior root

Posterior root

Spinal nerve

Sympathetic trunk

Anterior ramus

Spinal ganglion

Posterior ramus

Sympathetic ganglion

White ramus communicans

Posterior median sulcus

Posterior intermediate sulcus

Posterolateral sulcus

Recurrent meningeal branches of spinal nerve

Gray ramus communicans

Features of the spinal cord (thoracic region) and basic organization of a spinal nerve (posterior view)

Lumbosacral enlargement (of spinal cord)

Conus medullaris

Cauda equina

T12

L1

Vertebral body

Sympathetic ganglion

Gray and white rami communicantes

Anterior root

Spinal ganglion

Spinal nerve

Anterior ramus

L5

S1

Posterior ramus

Posterior root

Intervertebral foramen

Spinous process

Spinal nerves (transverse section)

S5

Co

Filum terminale

45

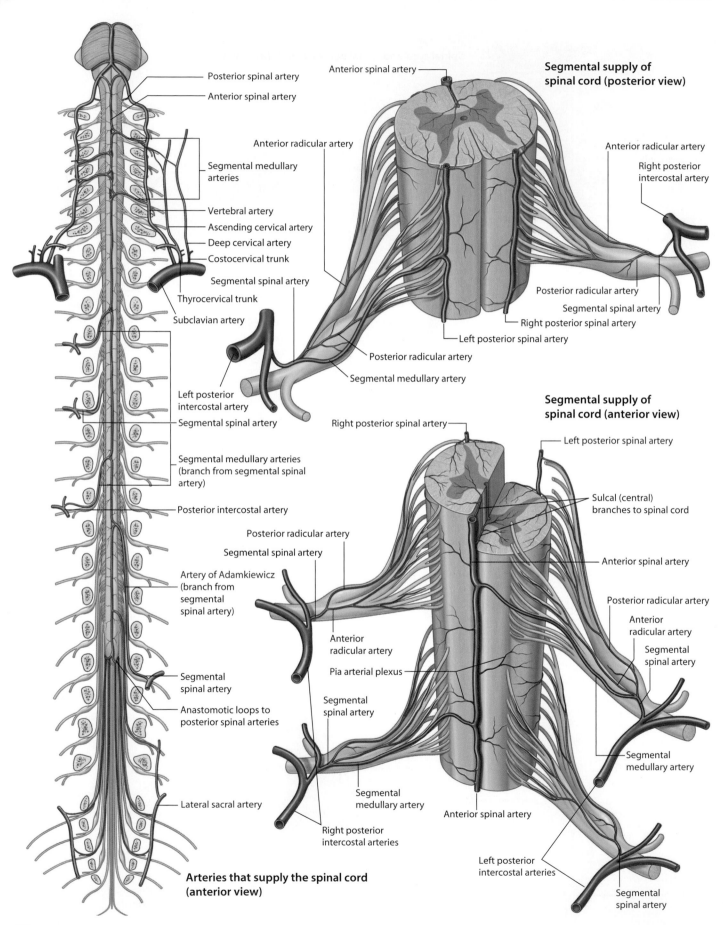

Posterior spinal artery

Anterior spinal artery

Anterior radicular artery

Segmental medullary arteries

Vertebral artery

Ascending cervical artery

Deep cervical artery

Costocervical trunk

Segmental spinal artery

Thyrocervical trunk

Subclavian artery

Left posterior intercostal artery

Segmental spinal artery

Segmental medullary arteries (branch from segmental spinal artery)

Posterior intercostal artery

Artery of Adamkiewicz (branch from segmental spinal artery)

Segmental spinal artery

Anastomotic loops to posterior spinal arteries

Lateral sacral artery

Arteries that supply the spinal cord (anterior view)

Anterior spinal artery

Segmental supply of spinal cord (posterior view)

Anterior radicular artery

Right posterior intercostal artery

Posterior radicular artery

Segmental spinal artery

Right posterior spinal artery

Left posterior spinal artery

Posterior radicular artery

Segmental medullary artery

Segmental supply of spinal cord (anterior view)

Right posterior spinal artery

Left posterior spinal artery

Sulcal (central) branches to spinal cord

Anterior spinal artery

Posterior radicular artery

Segmental spinal artery

Posterior radicular artery

Anterior radicular artery

Segmental spinal artery

Anterior radicular artery

Pia arterial plexus

Segmental spinal artery

Segmental medullary artery

Segmental medullary artery

Anterior spinal artery

Right posterior intercostal arteries

Left posterior intercostal arteries

Segmental spinal artery

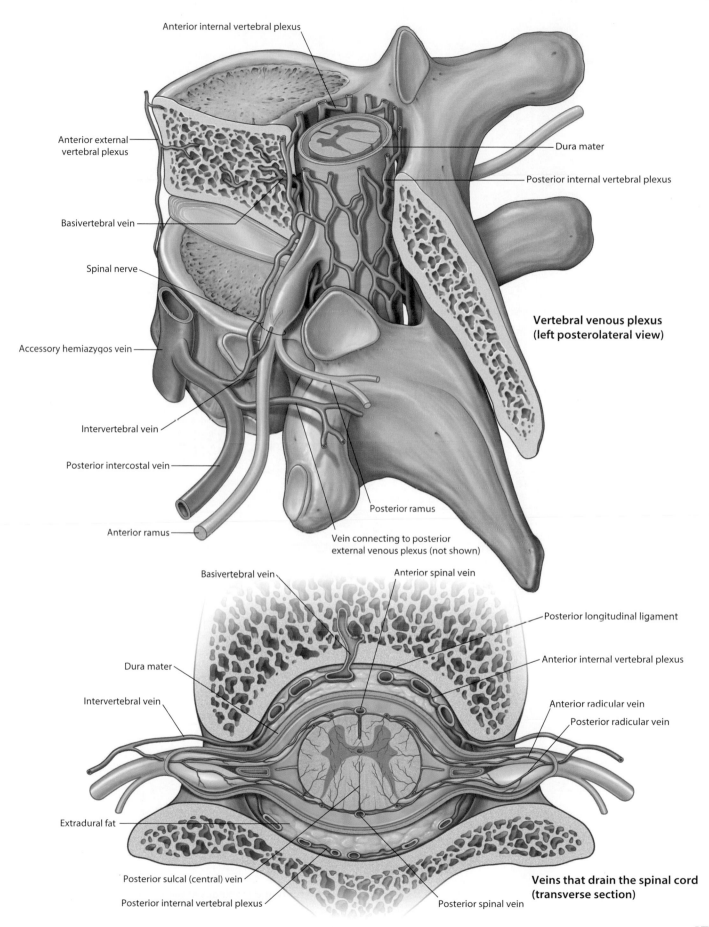

Anterior internal vertebral plexus

Anterior external vertebral plexus

Basivertebral vein

Spinal nerve

Accessory hemiazygos vein

Intervertebral vein

Posterior intercostal vein

Anterior ramus

Dura mater

Posterior internal vertebral plexus

Vertebral venous plexus (left posterolateral view)

Posterior ramus

Vein connecting to posterior external venous plexus (not shown)

Basivertebral vein

Anterior spinal vein

Dura mater

Intervertebral vein

Extradural fat

Posterior sulcal (central) vein

Posterior internal vertebral plexus

Posterior longitudinal ligament

Anterior internal vertebral plexus

Anterior radicular vein

Posterior radicular vein

Posterior spinal vein

Veins that drain the spinal cord (transverse section)

47

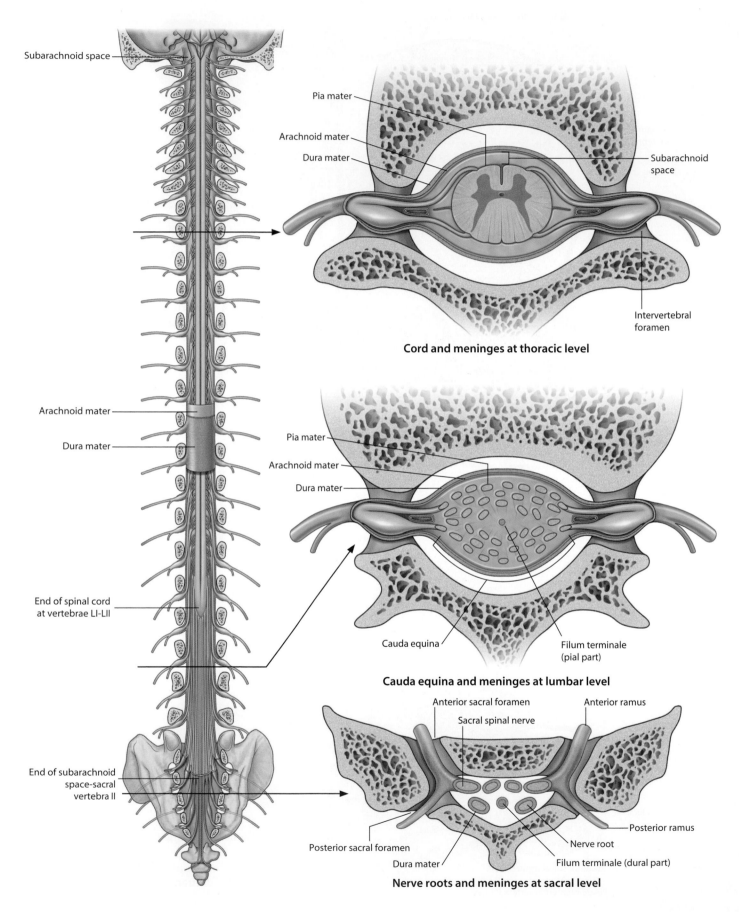

Subarachnoid space

Pia mater

Arachnoid mater

Dura mater

Subarachnoid space

Intervertebral foramen

Cord and meninges at thoracic level

Arachnoid mater

Dura mater

Pia mater

Arachnoid mater

Dura mater

End of spinal cord at vertebrae LI-LII

Cauda equina

Filum terminale (pial part)

Cauda equina and meninges at lumbar level

End of subarachnoid space-sacral vertebra II

Anterior sacral foramen

Sacral spinal nerve

Anterior ramus

Posterior ramus

Posterior sacral foramen

Dura mater

Nerve root

Filum terminale (dural part)

Nerve roots and meninges at sacral level

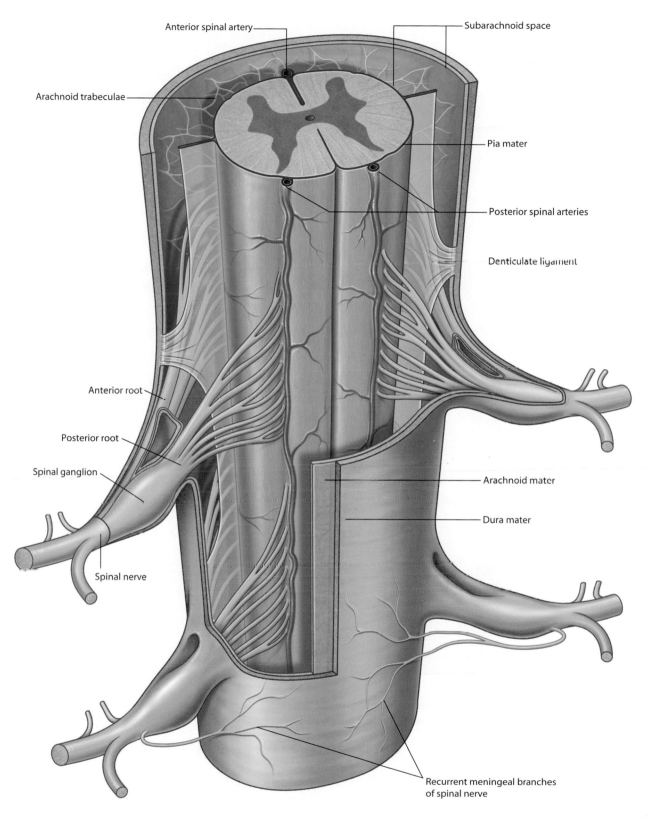

Anterior spinal artery

Subarachnoid space

Arachnoid trabeculae

Pia mater

Posterior spinal arteries

Denticulate ligament

Anterior root

Posterior root

Spinal ganglion

Arachnoid mater

Dura mater

Spinal nerve

Recurrent meningeal branches
of spinal nerve

Meninges covering parts of the thoracic region of the spinal cord (posterior view)

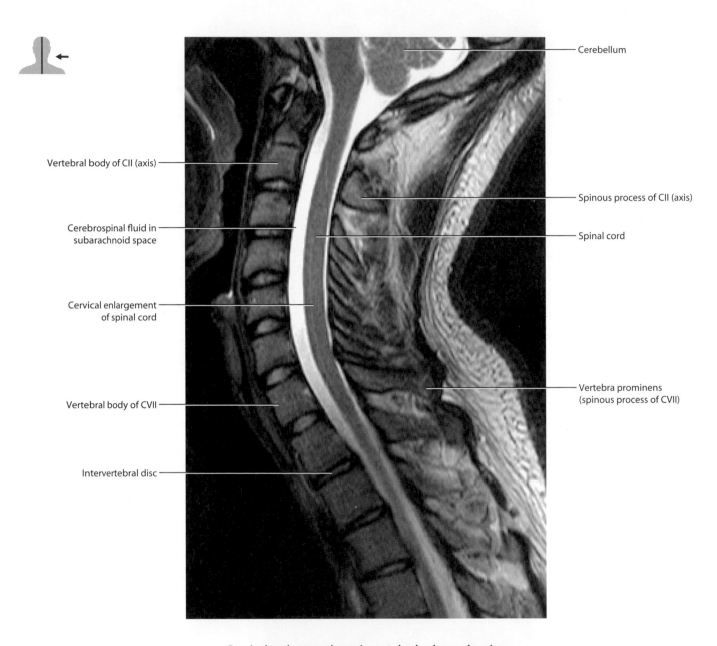

Cerebellum

Vertebral body of CII (axis)

Spinous process of CII (axis)

Cerebrospinal fluid in subarachnoid space

Spinal cord

Cervical enlargement of spinal cord

Vertebral body of CVII

Vertebra prominens (spinous process of CVII)

Intervertebral disc

Cervical and upper thoracic vertebral column showing upper and middle portions of spinal cord.
T2-weighted MR image in sagittal plane

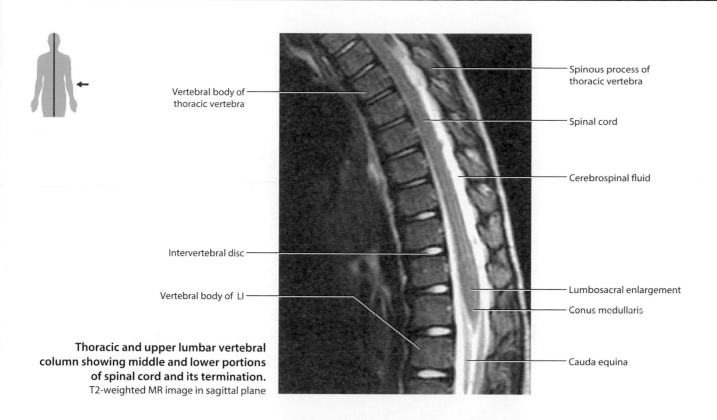

Spinous process of thoracic vertebra

Vertebral body of thoracic vertebra

Spinal cord

Cerebrospinal fluid

Intervertebral disc

Lumbosacral enlargement

Vertebral body of LI

Conus medullaris

Cauda equina

Thoracic and upper lumbar vertebral column showing middle and lower portions of spinal cord and its termination.
T2-weighted MR image in sagittal plane

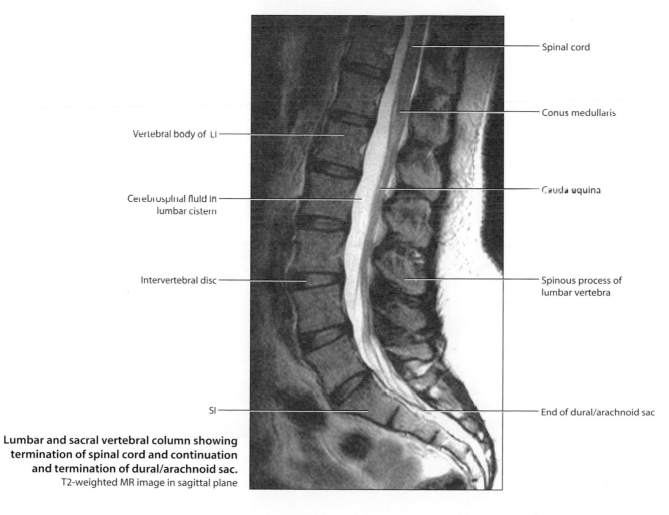

Spinal cord

Conus medullaris

Vertebral body of LI

Cerebrospinal fluid in lumbar cistern

Cauda equina

Intervertebral disc

Spinous process of lumbar vertebra

SI

End of dural/arachnoid sac

Lumbar and sacral vertebral column showing termination of spinal cord and continuation and termination of dural/arachnoid sac.
T2-weighted MR image in sagittal plane

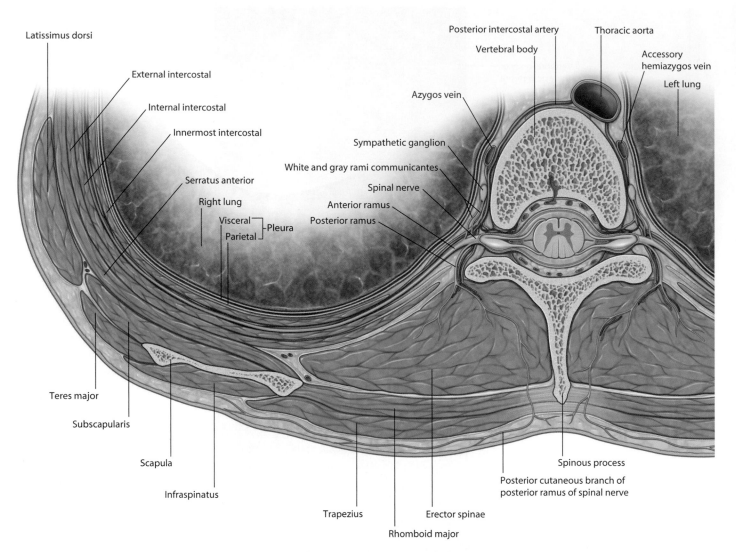

Latissimus dorsi

External intercostal

Internal intercostal

Innermost intercostal

Serratus anterior

Right lung

Visceral ⎤
Parietal ⎦ Pleura

Teres major

Subscapularis

Scapula

Infraspinatus

Trapezius

Rhomboid major

Erector spinae

Posterior intercostal artery

Vertebral body

Azygos vein

Sympathetic ganglion

White and gray rami communicantes

Spinal nerve

Anterior ramus

Posterior ramus

Thoracic aorta

Accessory hemiazygos vein

Left lung

Spinous process

Posterior cutaneous branch of posterior ramus of spinal nerve

Transverse section through thoracic region of vertebral column

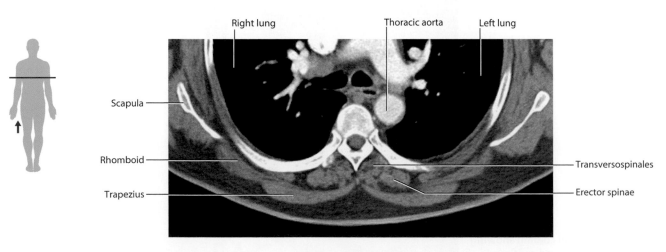

Right lung

Thoracic aorta

Left lung

Scapula

Rhomboid

Trapezius

Transversospinales

Erector spinae

Thoracic region of back.
CT image in axial plane

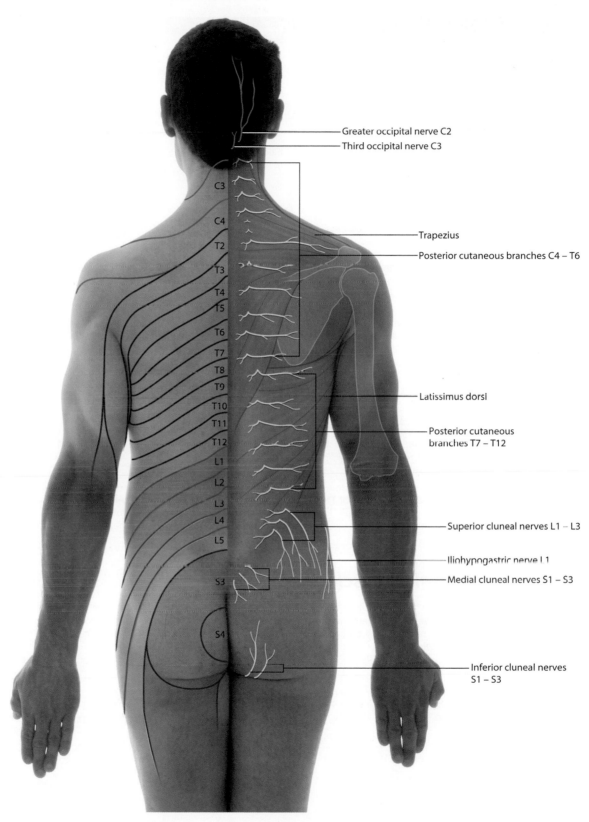

Greater occipital nerve C2

Third occipital nerve C3

Trapezius

Posterior cutaneous branches C4 – T6

Latissimus dorsl

Posterior cutaneous branches T7 – T12

Superior cluneal nerves L1 – L3

Iliohypogastric nerve L1

Medial cluneal nerves S1 – S3

Inferior cluneal nerves S1 – S3

C3
C4
T2
T3
T4
T5
T6
T7
T8
T9
T10
T11
T12
L1
L2
L3
L4
L5
S3
S4

Dermatomes and cutaneous nerves of the back

Superficial (appendicular) group of back muscles

Muscle		Origin	Insertion	Innervation	Function
Trapezius	1	Superior nuchal line, external occipital protuberance, ligamentum nuchae, spinous processes of CVII to TXII	Lateral one-third of clavicle, acromion, spine of scapula	Motor—accessory nerve [XI]; proprioception—C3 and C4	Assists in rotating the scapula during abduction of humerus above horizontal; upper fibers elevate, middle fibers adduct, and lower fibers depress scapula
Latissimus dorsi	2	Spinous processes of TVII to LV and sacrum, iliac crest, ribs X to XII	Floor of intertubercular sulcus of humerus	Thoracodorsal nerve (C6 to C8)	Extends, adducts, and medially rotates humerus
Levator scapulae	3	Transverse processes of CI to CIV	Upper portion medial border of scapula	C3 to C4 and dorsal scapular nerve (C4, C5)	Elevates scapula
Rhomboid major	4	Spinous processes of TII to TV	Medial border of scapula between spine and inferior angle	Dorsal scapular nerve (C4, C5)	Retracts (adducts) and elevates scapula
Rhomboid minor	5	Lower portion of ligamentum nuchae, spinous processes of CVII and TI	Medial border of scapula at the spine of scapula	Dorsal scapular nerve (C4, C5)	Retracts (adducts) and elevates scapula

Intermediate (respiratory) group of back muscles

Muscle		Origin	Insertion	Innervation	Function
Serratus posterior superior	6	Lower portion of ligamentum nuchae, spinous processes of CVII to TIII and supraspinous ligaments	Mastoid process, skull below lateral one-third of superior nuchal line	Anterior rami of upper thoracic nerves (T2 to T5)	Elevates ribs II to V
Serratus posterior inferior	7	Spinous processes of TXI to LIII and supraspinous ligaments	Lower border of ribs IX to XII just lateral to their angles	Anterior rami of lower thoracic nerves (T9 to T12)	Depresses ribs IX to XII and may prevent lower ribs from being elevated when the diaphragm contracts

Spinotransversales muscles

Muscle		Origin	Insertion	Innervation	Function
Splenius capitis	8	Lower half of ligamentum nuchae, spinous processes of CVII to TIV	Mastoid process, skull below lateral one-third of superior nuchal line	Posterior rami middle cervical nerves	Together—draw head backward, extending neck; individually—draw and rotate head to one side (turn face to same side)
Splenius cervicis	9	Spinous processes of TIII to TVI	Transverse processes of CI to CIII	Posterior rami lower cervical nerves	Together—extend neck; individually—draw and rotate head to one side (turn face to same side)

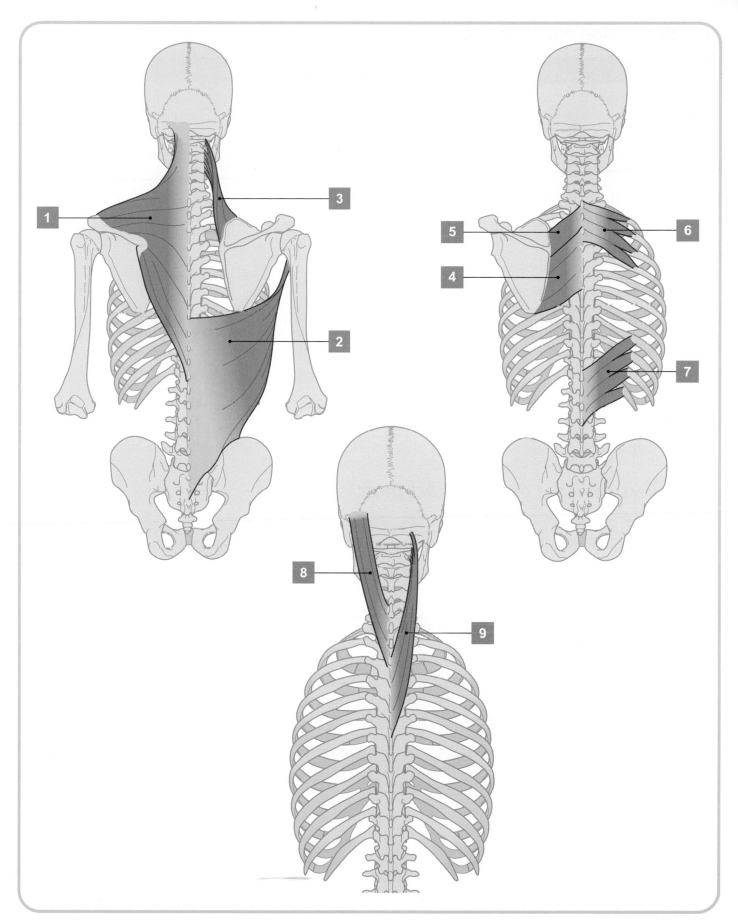

Erector spinae group of back muscles

Muscle		Origin	Insertion
Iliocostalis lumborum	1	Sacrum, spinous processes of lumbar and lower two thoracic vertebrae and their supraspinous ligaments, and the iliac crest	Angles of the lower six or seven ribs
Iliocostalis thoracis	2	Angles of the lower six ribs	Angles of the upper six ribs and the transverse process of CVII
Iliocostalis cervicis	3	Angles of ribs III to VI	Transverse processes of CIV to CVI
Longissimus thoracis	4	Blends with iliocostalis in lumbar region and is attached to transverse processes of lumbar vertebrae	Transverse processes of all thoracic vertebrae and just lateral to the tubercles of the lower nine or ten ribs
Longissimus cervicis	5	Transverse processes of upper four or five thoracic vertebrae	Transverse processes of CII to CVI
Longissimus capitis	6	Blends with iliocostalis in lumbar region and is attached to transverse processes of lumbar vertebrae	Transverse processes of all thoracic vertebrae and just lateral to the tubercles of the lower nine or ten ribs
Spinalis thoracis	7	Spinous processes of TX or TXI to LII	Spinous processes of TI to TVIII (varies)
Spinalis cervicis	8	Lower part of ligamentum nuchae and spinous process of CVII (sometimes TI to TII)	Spinous process of CII (axis)
Spinalis capitis	9	Usually blends with semispinalis capitis	With semispinalis capitis

Transversospinales group of back muscles

Muscle		Origin	Insertion
Semispinalis thoracis	10	Transverse processes of TVI to TX	Spinous processes of upper four thoracic and lower two cervical vertebrae
Semispinalis cervicis	11	Transverse processes of upper five or six thoracic vertebrae	Spinous processes of CII (axis) to CV
Semispinalis capitis	12	Transverse processes of TI to TVI (or TVII) and CVII and articular processes of CIV to CVI	Medial area between the superior and inferior nuchal lines of occipital bone
Multifidus	13	Sacrum, origin of erector spinae, posterior superior iliac spine, mammillary processes of lumbar vertebrae, transverse processes of thoracic vertebrae, and articular processes of lower four cervical vertebrae	Base of spinous processes of all vertebrae from LV to CII (axis)
Rotatores lumborum	14	Mammillary processes of lumbar vertebrae	Spinous processes of lumbar vertebrae
Rotatores thoracis	15	Transverse processes of thoracic vertebrae	Spinous processes of thoracic vertebrae
Rotatores cervicis	16	Articular processes of cervical vertebrae	Spinous processes of cervical vertebrae

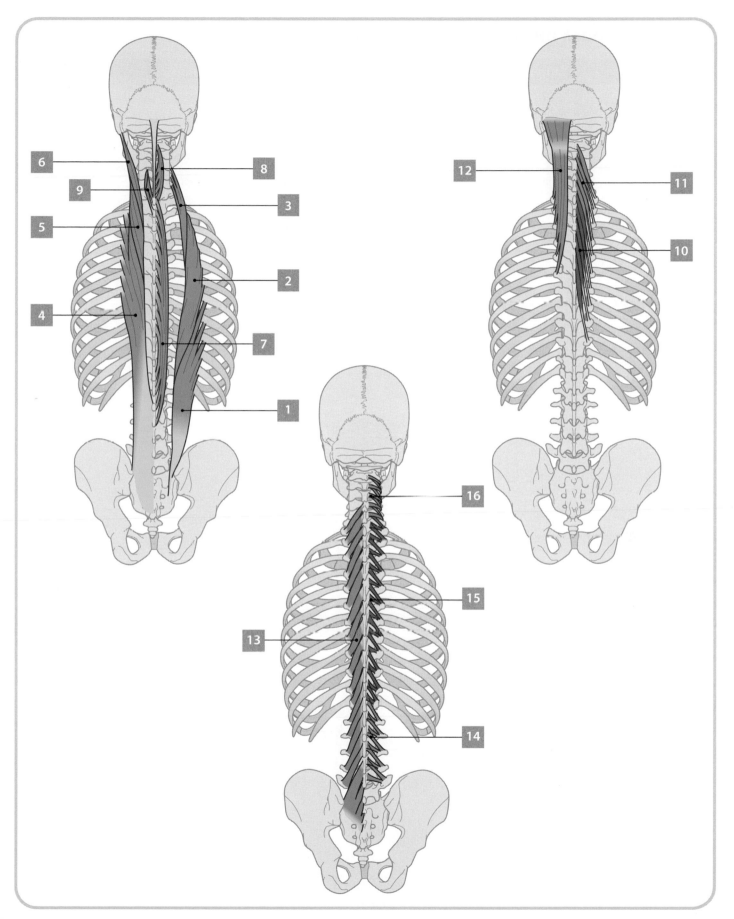

Segmental back muscles

Muscle		Origin	Insertion	Function
Levatores costarum	1	Short paired muscles arising from transverse processes of CVII to TXI	The rib below vertebra of origin near tubercle	Contraction elevates rib
Interspinales	2	Short paired muscles attached to the spinous processes of contiguous vertebrae, one on each side of the interspinous ligament		Postural muscles that stabilize adjoining vertebra during movements of vertebral column
Intertransversarii	3	Small muscles between the transverse processes of contiguous vertebrae		Postural muscles that stabilize adjoining vertebra during movements of vertebral column

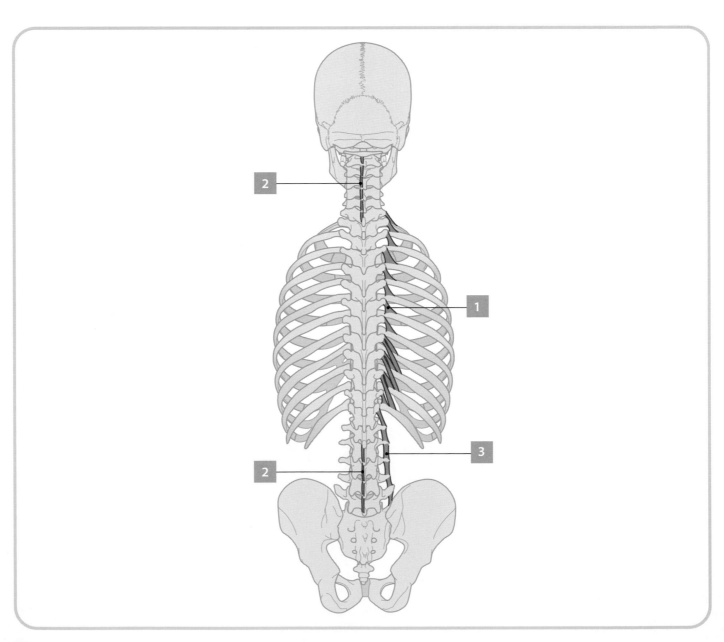

Suboccipital group of back muscles

Muscle		Origin	Insertion	Innervation	Function
Rectus capitis posterior major	1	Spinous process of axis (CII)	Lateral portion of occipital bone below inferior nuchal line	Posterior ramus of C1	Extension of head; rotation of face to same side as muscle
Rectus capitis posterior minor	2	Posterior tubercle of atlas (CI)	Medial portion of occipital bone below inferior nuchal line	Posterior ramus of C1	Extension of head
Obliquus capitis superior	3	Transverse process of atlas (CI)	Occipital bone between superior and inferior nuchal lines	Posterior ramus of C1	Extension of head and bends it to same side
Obliquus capitis inferior	4	Spinous process of axis (CII)	Transverse process of atlas (CI)	Posterior ramus of C1	Rotation of face to same side

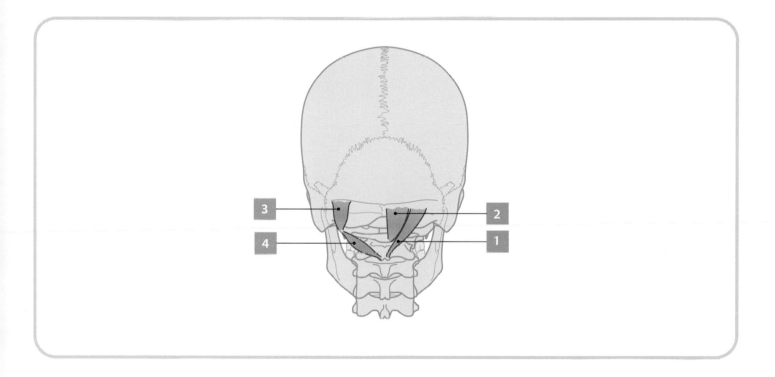

CONTENTS

3

THORAX

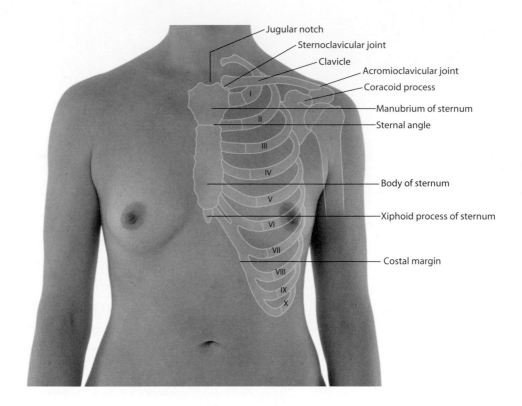

Jugular notch
Sternoclavicular joint
Clavicle
Acromioclavicular joint
Coracoid process
Manubrium of sternum
Sternal angle
Body of sternum
Xiphoid process of sternum
Costal margin

Anterior chest wall in a woman

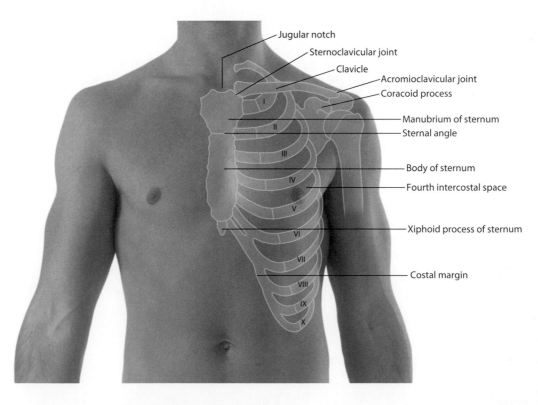

Jugular notch
Sternoclavicular joint
Clavicle
Acromioclavicular joint
Coracoid process
Manubrium of sternum
Sternal angle
Body of sternum
Fourth intercostal space
Xiphoid process of sternum
Costal margin

Anterior chest wall in a man

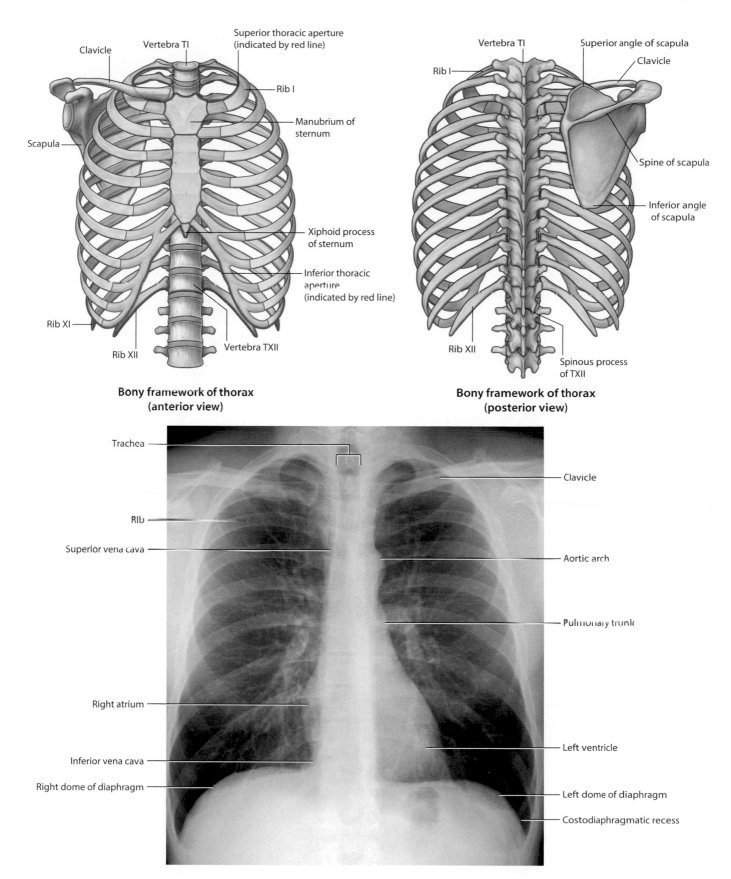

**Bony framework of thorax
(anterior view)**

Clavicle
Vertebra TI
Superior thoracic aperture (indicated by red line)
Rib I
Manubrium of sternum
Scapula
Xiphoid process of sternum
Inferior thoracic aperture (indicated by red line)
Rib XI
Rib XII
Vertebra TXII

**Bony framework of thorax
(posterior view)**

Vertebra TI
Rib I
Superior angle of scapula
Clavicle
Spine of scapula
Inferior angle of scapula
Rib XII
Spinous process of TXII

Trachea
Clavicle
Rib
Superior vena cava
Aortic arch
Pulmonary trunk
Right atrium
Inferior vena cava
Left ventricle
Right dome of diaphragm
Left dome of diaphragm
Costodiaphragmatic recess

Positioning of structures in chest.
Radiograph, AP view

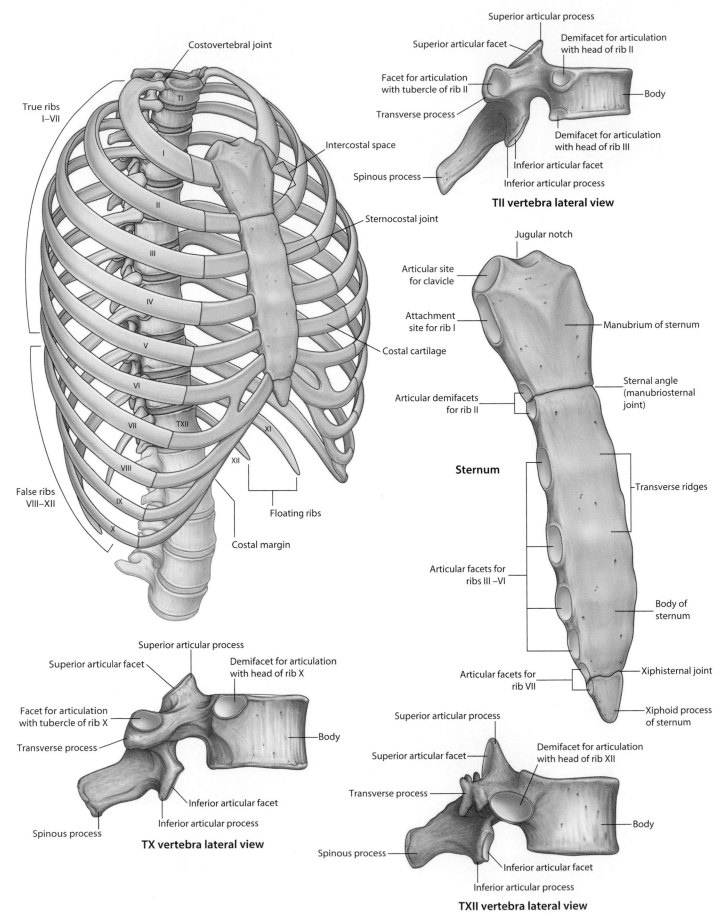

Costovertebral joint

True ribs
I–VII

TI

I

II

III

IV

V

VI

VII

TXII

VIII

IX

X

XI

XII

False ribs
VIII–XII

Intercostal space

Sternocostal joint

Costal cartilage

Floating ribs

Costal margin

Superior articular process

Superior articular facet

Facet for articulation
with tubercle of rib II

Transverse process

Spinous process

Demifacet for articulation
with head of rib II

Body

Demifacet for articulation
with head of rib III

Inferior articular facet

Inferior articular process

TII vertebra lateral view

Jugular notch

Articular site
for clavicle

Attachment
site for rib I

Articular demifacets
for rib II

Sternum

Articular facets for
ribs III –VI

Articular facets for
rib VII

Manubrium of sternum

Sternal angle
(manubriosternal
joint)

Transverse ridges

Body of
sternum

Xiphisternal joint

Xiphoid process
of sternum

Superior articular process

Superior articular facet

Facet for articulation
with tubercle of rib X

Transverse process

Spinous process

Demifacet for articulation
with head of rib X

Body

Inferior articular facet

Inferior articular process

TX vertebra lateral view

Superior articular process

Superior articular facet

Transverse process

Spinous process

Demifacet for articulation
with head of rib XII

Body

Inferior articular facet

Inferior articular process

TXII vertebra lateral view

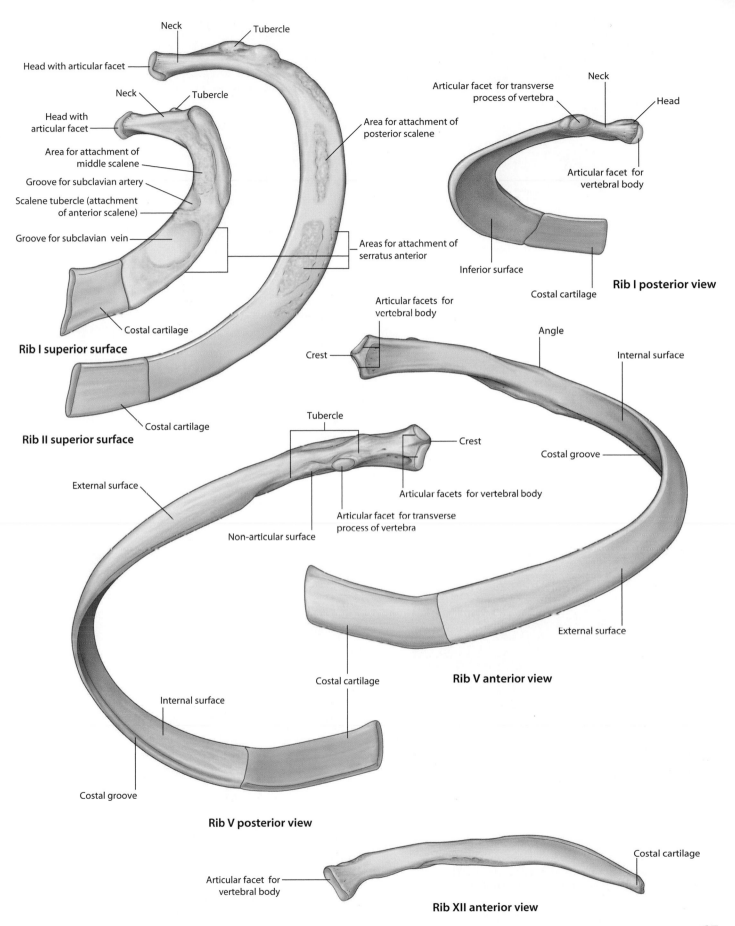

Neck

Tubercle

Head with articular facet

Neck

Tubercle

Head with articular facet

Area for attachment of middle scalene

Groove for subclavian artery

Scalene tubercle (attachment of anterior scalene)

Groove for subclavian vein

Area for attachment of posterior scalene

Costal cartilage

Areas for attachment of serratus anterior

Costal cartilage

Rib I superior surface

Rib II superior surface

Articular facet for transverse process of vertebra

Neck

Head

Articular facet for vertebral body

Inferior surface

Costal cartilage

Rib I posterior view

Articular facets for vertebral body

Crest

Angle

Internal surface

Costal groove

External surface

Tubercle

Crest

Articular facets for vertebral body

Non-articular surface

Articular facet for transverse process of vertebra

External surface

Internal surface

Costal groove

Costal cartilage

Rib V anterior view

Rib V posterior view

Articular facet for vertebral body

Costal cartilage

Rib XII anterior view

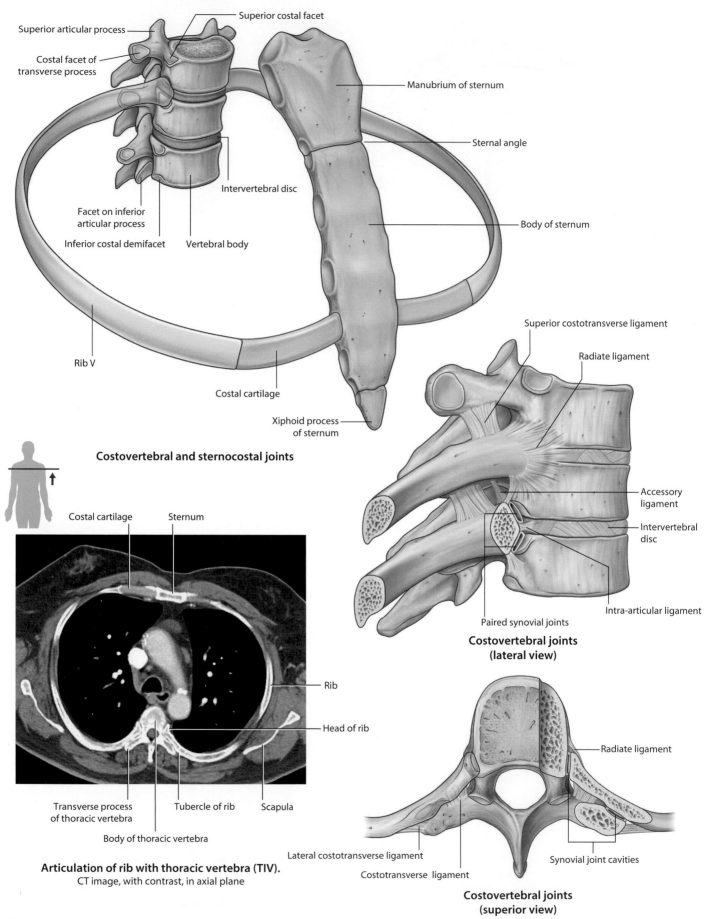

Superior articular process

Costal facet of transverse process

Superior costal facet

Manubrium of sternum

Sternal angle

Intervertebral disc

Facet on inferior articular process

Inferior costal demifacet

Vertebral body

Body of sternum

Rib V

Costal cartilage

Xiphoid process of sternum

Costovertebral and sternocostal joints

Superior costotransverse ligament

Radiate ligament

Accessory ligament

Intervertebral disc

Paired synovial joints

Intra-articular ligament

Costovertebral joints (lateral view)

Costal cartilage   Sternum

Rib

Head of rib

Transverse process of thoracic vertebra

Tubercle of rib   Scapula

Body of thoracic vertebra

Articulation of rib with thoracic vertebra (TIV).
CT image, with contrast, in axial plane

Radiate ligament

Lateral costotransverse ligament

Costotransverse ligament

Synovial joint cavities

Costovertebral joints (superior view)

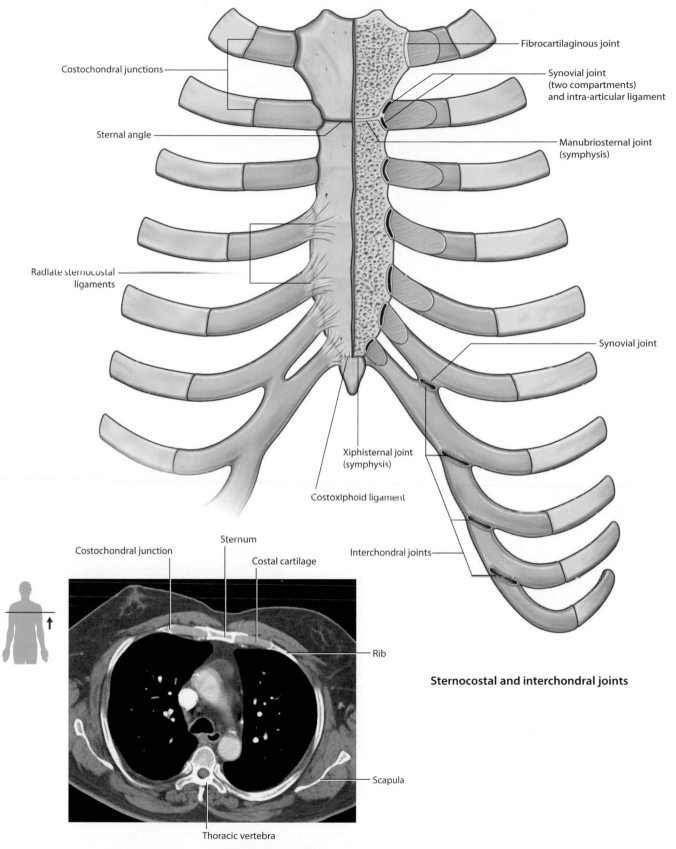

Fibrocartilaginous joint

Costochondral junctions

Synovial joint
(two compartments)
and intra-articular ligament

Sternal angle

Manubriosternal joint
(symphysis)

Radiate sternocostal
ligaments

Synovial joint

Xiphisternal joint
(symphysis)

Costoxiphoid ligament

Interchondral joints

Sternocostal and interchondral joints

Costochondral junction

Sternum

Costal cartilage

Rib

Scapula

Thoracic vertebra

Articulation of costal cartilage with sternum.
CT image, with contrast, in axial plane

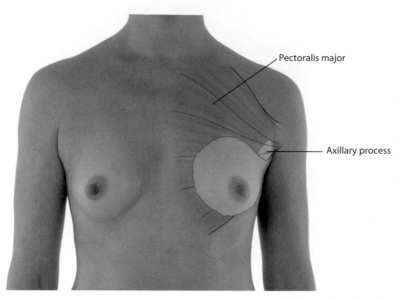

Pectoralis major

Axillary process

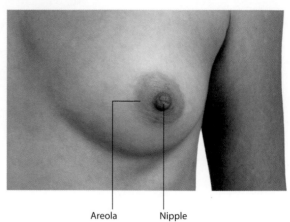

Areola　　Nipple

Anterior view

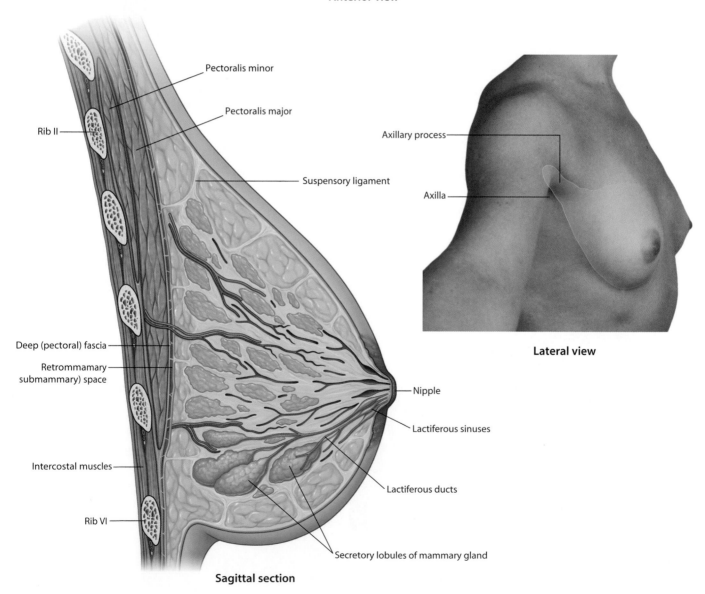

Pectoralis minor

Pectoralis major

Rib II

Suspensory ligament

Axillary process

Axilla

Deep (pectoral) fascia

Retrommamary (submammary) space

Nipple

Lactiferous sinuses

Intercostal muscles

Lactiferous ducts

Rib VI

Secretory lobules of mammary gland

Sagittal section

Lateral view

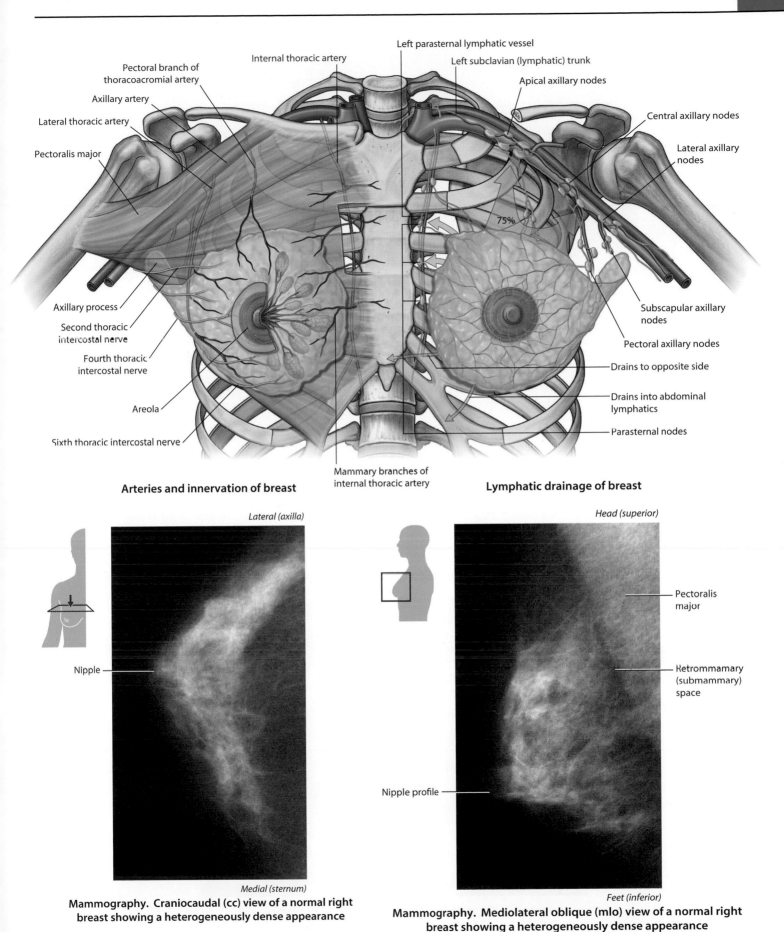

Pectoral branch of thoracoacromial artery

Axillary artery

Lateral thoracic artery

Pectoralis major

Internal thoracic artery

Left parasternal lymphatic vessel

Left subclavian (lymphatic) trunk

Apical axillary nodes

Central axillary nodes

Lateral axillary nodes

75%

Axillary process

Second thoracic intercostal nerve

Fourth thoracic intercostal nerve

Areola

Sixth thoracic intercostal nerve

Mammary branches of internal thoracic artery

Subscapular axillary nodes

Pectoral axillary nodes

Drains to opposite side

Drains into abdominal lymphatics

Parasternal nodes

Arteries and innervation of breast

Lymphatic drainage of breast

Lateral (axilla)

Nipple

Medial (sternum)

Mammography. Craniocaudal (cc) view of a normal right breast showing a heterogeneously dense appearance

Head (superior)

Pectoralis major

Retrommamary (submammary) space

Nipple profile

Feet (inferior)

Mammography. Mediolateral oblique (mlo) view of a normal right breast showing a heterogeneously dense appearance

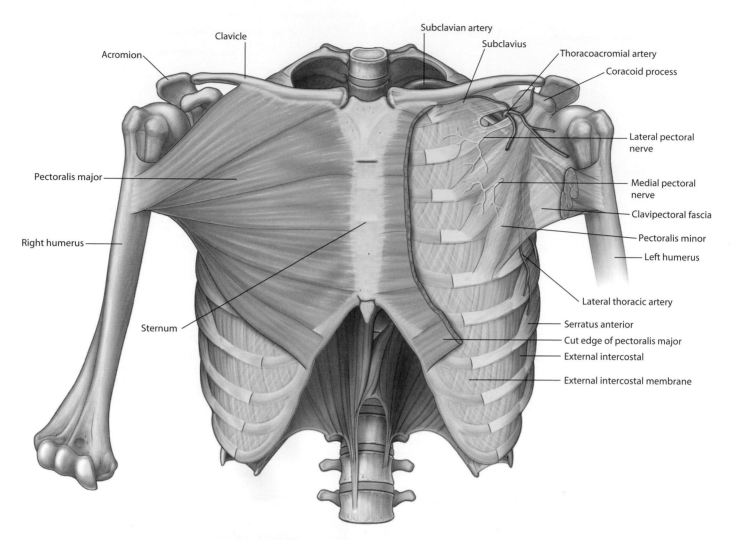

Acromion
Clavicle
Subclavian artery
Subclavius
Thoracoacromial artery
Coracoid process
Lateral pectoral nerve
Pectoralis major
Medial pectoral nerve
Clavipectoral fascia
Pectoralis minor
Right humerus
Left humerus
Sternum
Lateral thoracic artery
Serratus anterior
Cut edge of pectoralis major
External intercostal
External intercostal membrane

Pectoralis major muscle and related deep structures

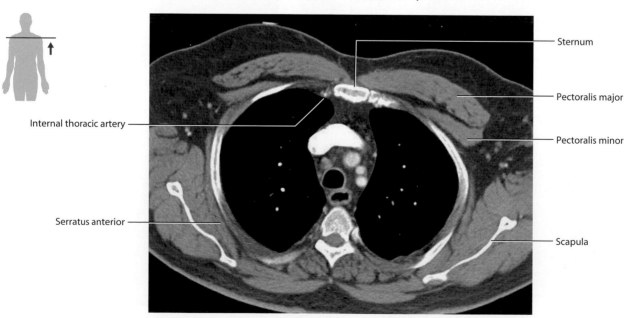

Internal thoracic artery
Serratus anterior
Sternum
Pectoralis major
Pectoralis minor
Scapula

Pectoralis major and minor muscles on anterior thoracic wall.
CT image, with contrast, in axial plane

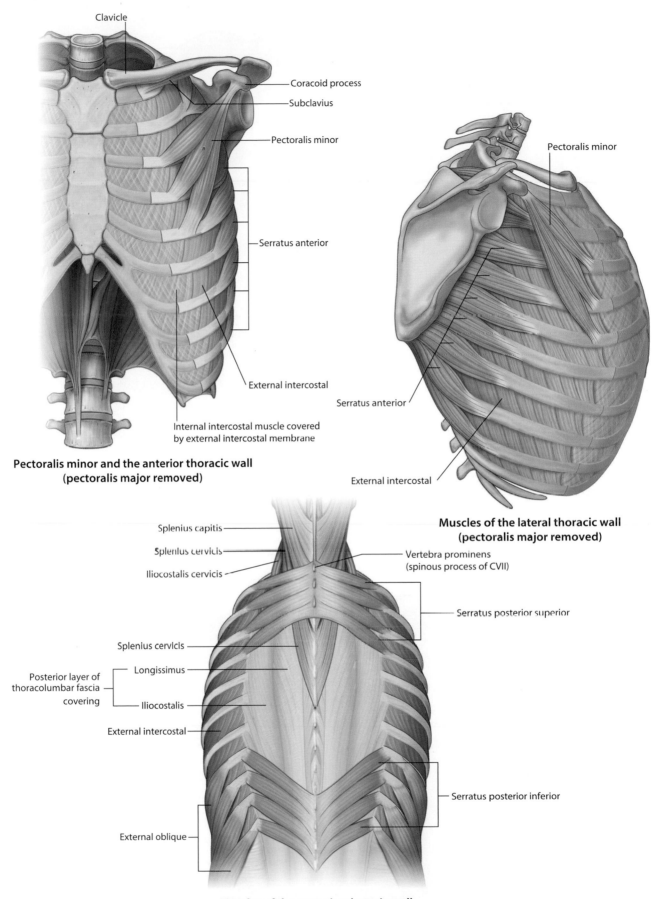

Clavicle

Coracoid process

Subclavius

Pectoralis minor

Serratus anterior

External intercostal

Internal intercostal muscle covered
by external intercostal membrane

**Pectoralis minor and the anterior thoracic wall
(pectoralis major removed)**

Pectoralis minor

Serratus anterior

External intercostal

**Muscles of the lateral thoracic wall
(pectoralis major removed)**

Splenius capitis

Splenius cervicis

Iliocostalis cervicis

Vertebra prominens
(spinous process of CVII)

Serratus posterior superior

Splenius cervicis

Longissimus

Posterior layer of
thoracolumbar fascia
covering

Iliocostalis

External intercostal

Serratus posterior inferior

External oblique

Muscles of the posterior thoracic wall

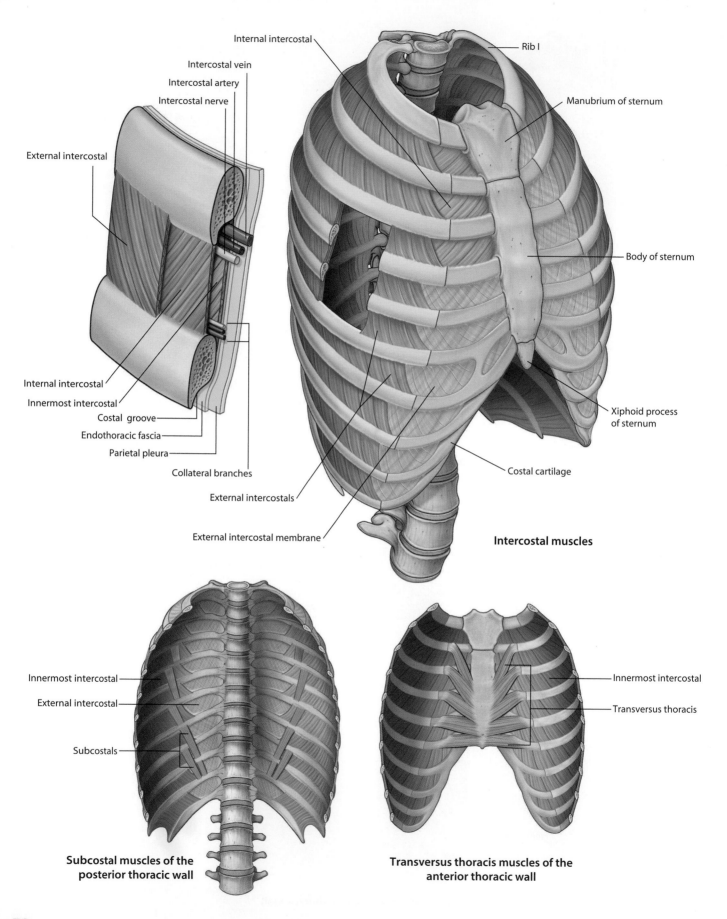

Internal intercostal

Intercostal vein

Intercostal artery

Intercostal nerve

External intercostal

Rib I

Manubrium of sternum

Body of sternum

Internal intercostal

Innermost intercostal

Costal groove

Endothoracic fascia

Parietal pleura

Collateral branches

External intercostals

External intercostal membrane

Xiphoid process of sternum

Costal cartilage

Intercostal muscles

Innermost intercostal

External intercostal

Subcostals

Innermost intercostal

Transversus thoracis

Subcostal muscles of the posterior thoracic wall

Transversus thoracis muscles of the anterior thoracic wall

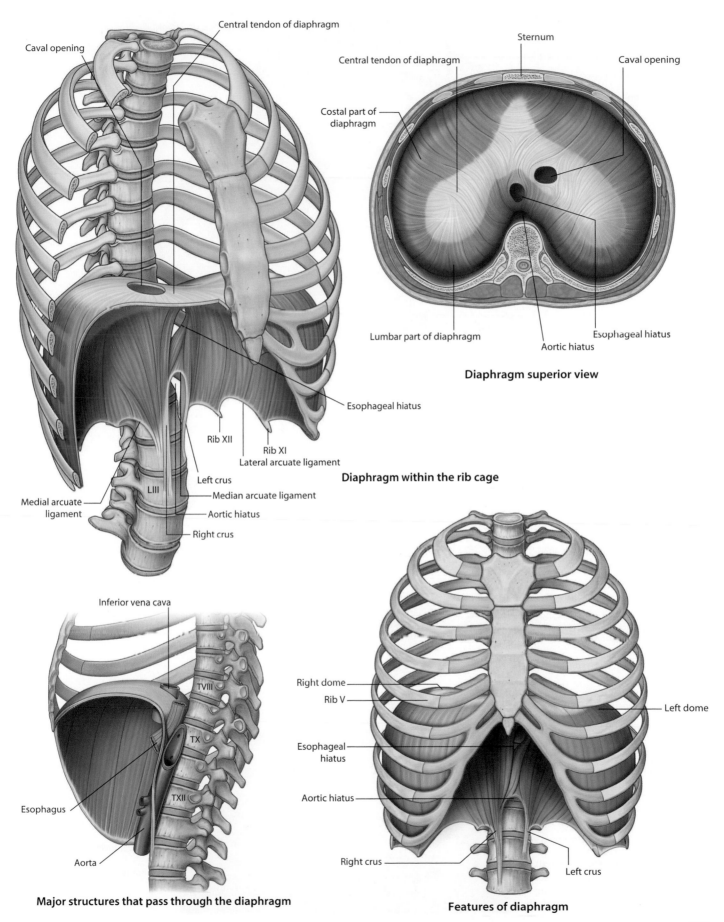

Caval opening

Central tendon of diaphragm

Sternum

Central tendon of diaphragm

Caval opening

Costal part of diaphragm

Esophageal hiatus

Lumbar part of diaphragm

Aortic hiatus

Diaphragm superior view

Esophageal hiatus

Rib XII

Rib XI

Lateral arcuate ligament

Left crus

Median arcuate ligament

LIII

Aortic hiatus

Medial arcuate ligament

Right crus

Diaphragm within the rib cage

Inferior vena cava

TVIII

TX

TXII

Esophagus

Aorta

Major structures that pass through the diaphragm

Right dome

Rib V

Esophageal hiatus

Aortic hiatus

Right crus

Left dome

Left crus

Features of diaphragm

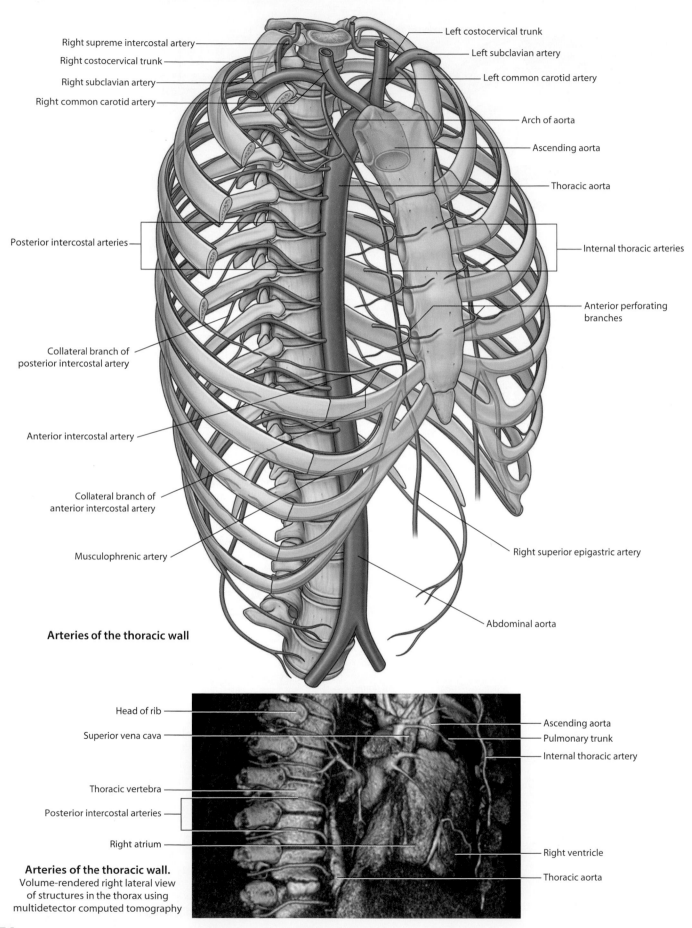

Right supreme intercostal artery

Right costocervical trunk

Right subclavian artery

Right common carotid artery

Left costocervical trunk

Left subclavian artery

Left common carotid artery

Arch of aorta

Ascending aorta

Thoracic aorta

Posterior intercostal arteries

Internal thoracic arteries

Anterior perforating branches

Collateral branch of posterior intercostal artery

Anterior intercostal artery

Collateral branch of anterior intercostal artery

Musculophrenic artery

Right superior epigastric artery

Abdominal aorta

Arteries of the thoracic wall

Head of rib

Superior vena cava

Thoracic vertebra

Posterior intercostal arteries

Right atrium

Ascending aorta

Pulmonary trunk

Internal thoracic artery

Right ventricle

Thoracic aorta

Arteries of the thoracic wall.
Volume-rendered right lateral view
of structures in the thorax using
multidetector computed tomography

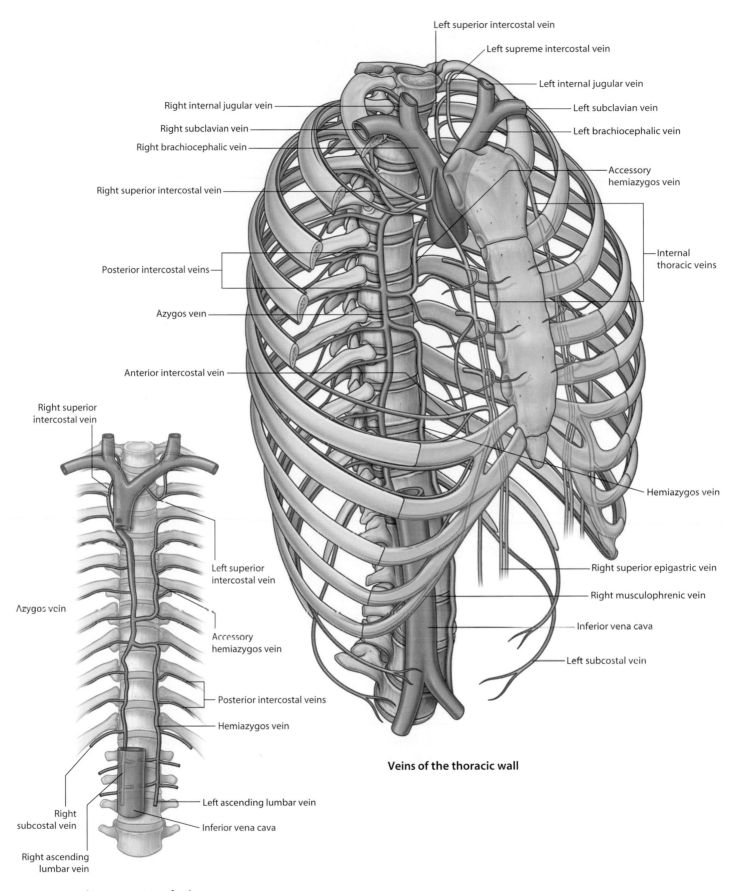

Left superior intercostal vein

Left supreme intercostal vein

Left internal jugular vein

Right internal jugular vein

Left subclavian vein

Right subclavian vein

Left brachiocephalic vein

Right brachiocephalic vein

Right superior intercostal vein

Accessory hemiazygos vein

Internal thoracic veins

Posterior intercostal veins

Azygos vein

Anterior intercostal vein

Right superior intercostal vein

Left superior intercostal vein

Azygos vein

Accessory hemiazygos vein

Posterior intercostal veins

Hemiazygos vein

Hemiazygos vein

Right superior epigastric vein

Right musculophrenic vein

Inferior vena cava

Left subcostal vein

Right subcostal vein

Left ascending lumbar vein

Inferior vena cava

Right ascending lumbar vein

Azygos system of veins

Veins of the thoracic wall

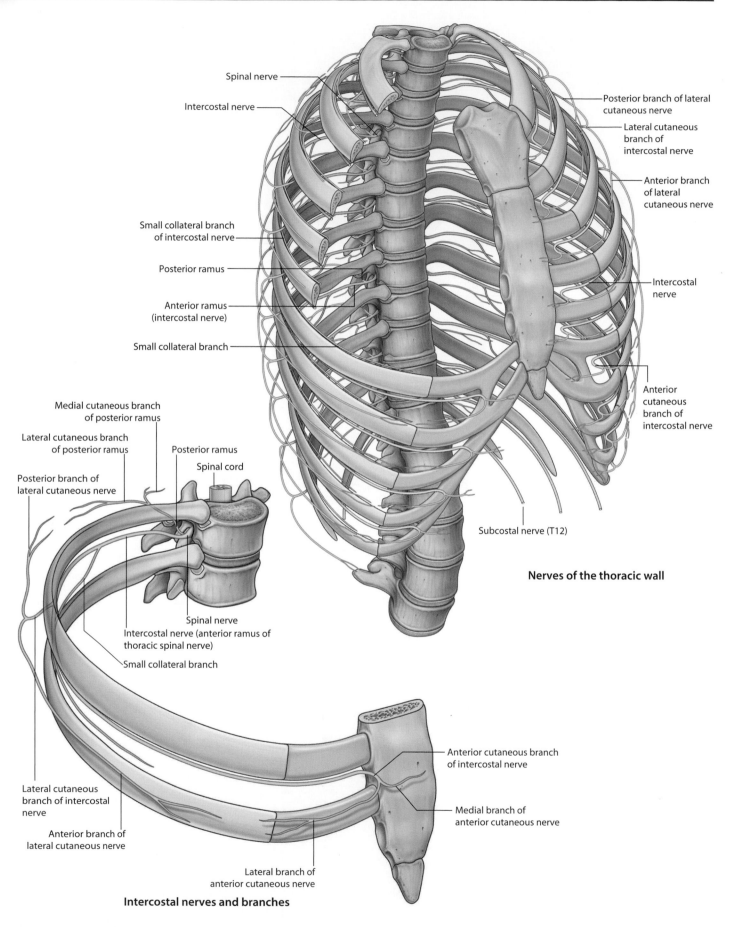

Spinal nerve

Intercostal nerve

Small collateral branch
of intercostal nerve

Posterior ramus

Anterior ramus
(intercostal nerve)

Small collateral branch

Medial cutaneous branch
of posterior ramus

Lateral cutaneous branch
of posterior ramus

Posterior branch of
lateral cutaneous nerve

Posterior ramus

Spinal cord

Spinal nerve

Intercostal nerve (anterior ramus of
thoracic spinal nerve)

Small collateral branch

Lateral cutaneous
branch of intercostal
nerve

Anterior branch of
lateral cutaneous nerve

Lateral branch of
anterior cutaneous nerve

Posterior branch of lateral
cutaneous nerve

Lateral cutaneous
branch of
intercostal nerve

Anterior branch
of lateral
cutaneous nerve

Intercostal
nerve

Anterior
cutaneous
branch of
intercostal nerve

Subcostal nerve (T12)

Anterior cutaneous branch
of intercostal nerve

Medial branch of
anterior cutaneous nerve

Nerves of the thoracic wall

Intercostal nerves and branches

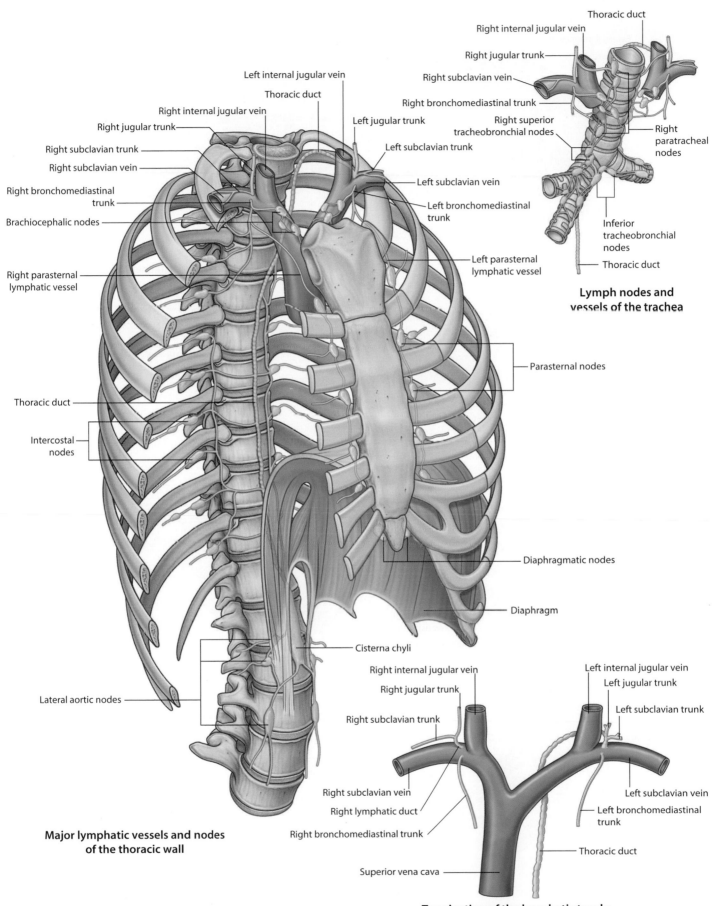

Thoracic duct

Right internal jugular vein

Right jugular trunk

Right subclavian vein

Right bronchomediastinal trunk

Right superior tracheobronchial nodes

Right paratracheal nodes

Inferior tracheobronchial nodes

Thoracic duct

Lymph nodes and vessels of the trachea

Left internal jugular vein

Thoracic duct

Right internal jugular vein

Right jugular trunk

Right subclavian trunk

Right subclavian vein

Right bronchomediastinal trunk

Brachiocephalic nodes

Left jugular trunk

Left subclavian trunk

Left subclavian vein

Left bronchomediastinal trunk

Right parasternal lymphatic vessel

Left parasternal lymphatic vessel

Parasternal nodes

Thoracic duct

Intercostal nodes

Diaphragmatic nodes

Diaphragm

Cisterna chyli

Lateral aortic nodes

Major lymphatic vessels and nodes of the thoracic wall

Right internal jugular vein

Right jugular trunk

Right subclavian trunk

Left internal jugular vein

Left jugular trunk

Left subclavian trunk

Right subclavian vein

Right lymphatic duct

Right bronchomediastinal trunk

Left subclavian vein

Left bronchomediastinal trunk

Thoracic duct

Superior vena cava

Termination of the lymphatic trunks

77

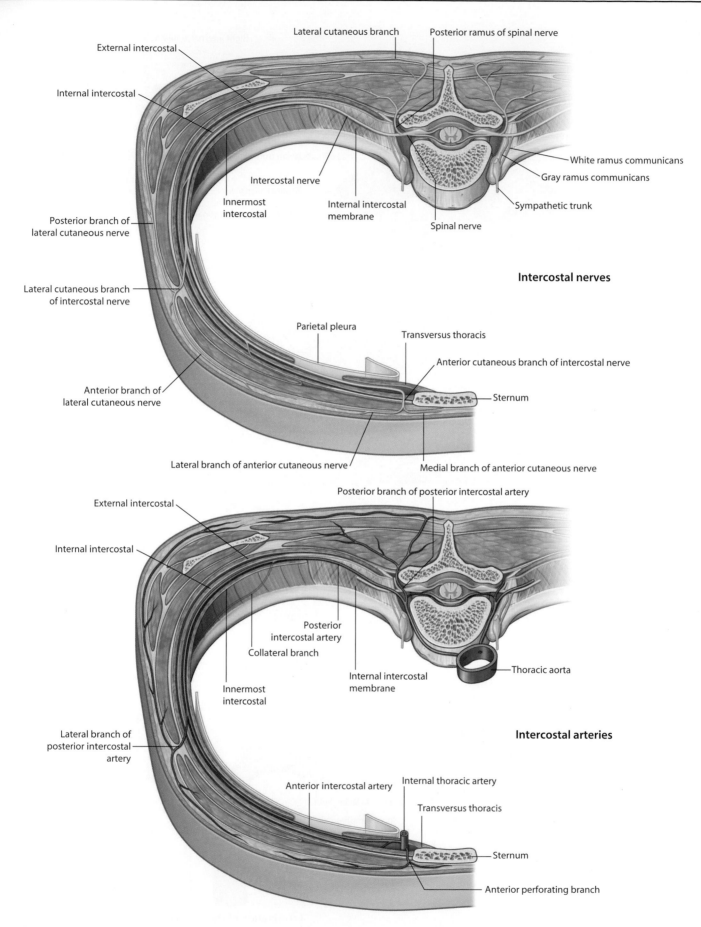

External intercostal

Internal intercostal

Lateral cutaneous branch

Posterior ramus of spinal nerve

White ramus communicans

Gray ramus communicans

Sympathetic trunk

Intercostal nerve

Innermost intercostal

Internal intercostal membrane

Spinal nerve

Posterior branch of lateral cutaneous nerve

Lateral cutaneous branch of intercostal nerve

Intercostal nerves

Parietal pleura

Transversus thoracis

Anterior cutaneous branch of intercostal nerve

Sternum

Anterior branch of lateral cutaneous nerve

Lateral branch of anterior cutaneous nerve

Medial branch of anterior cutaneous nerve

External intercostal

Internal intercostal

Posterior branch of posterior intercostal artery

Posterior intercostal artery

Collateral branch

Innermost intercostal

Internal intercostal membrane

Thoracic aorta

Intercostal arteries

Lateral branch of posterior intercostal artery

Anterior intercostal artery

Internal thoracic artery

Transversus thoracis

Sternum

Anterior perforating branch

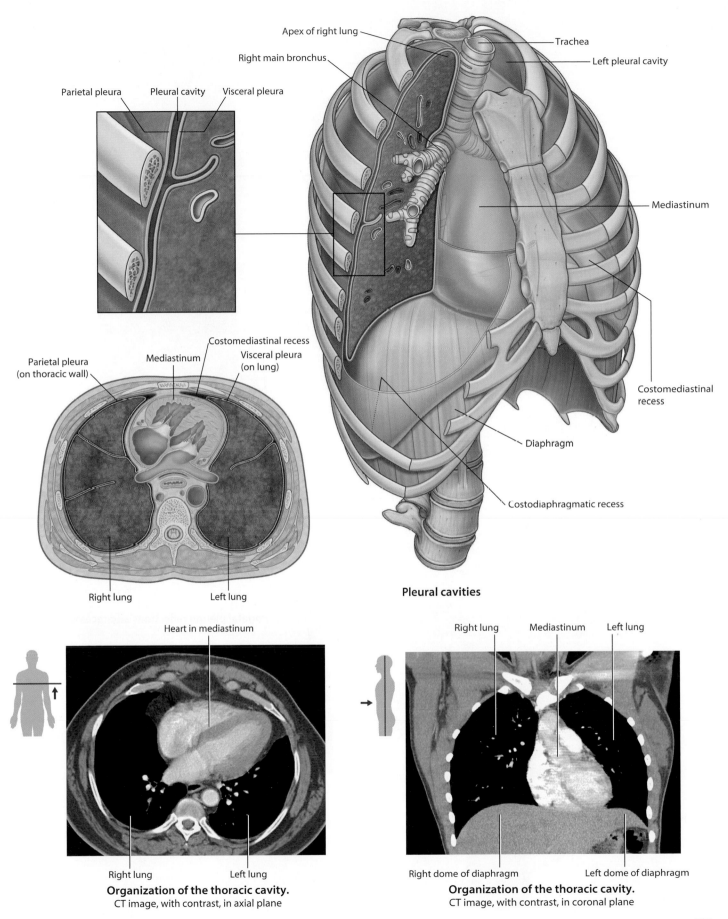

Apex of right lung

Right main bronchus

Trachea

Left pleural cavity

Parietal pleura

Pleural cavity

Visceral pleura

Mediastinum

Costomediastinal recess

Costomediastinal recess

Visceral pleura (on lung)

Parietal pleura (on thoracic wall)

Mediastinum

Diaphragm

Right lung

Left lung

Costodiaphragmatic recess

Pleural cavities

Heart in mediastinum

Right lung

Mediastinum

Left lung

Right lung

Left lung

Right dome of diaphragm

Left dome of diaphragm

Organization of the thoracic cavity.
CT image, with contrast, in axial plane

Organization of the thoracic cavity.
CT image, with contrast, in coronal plane

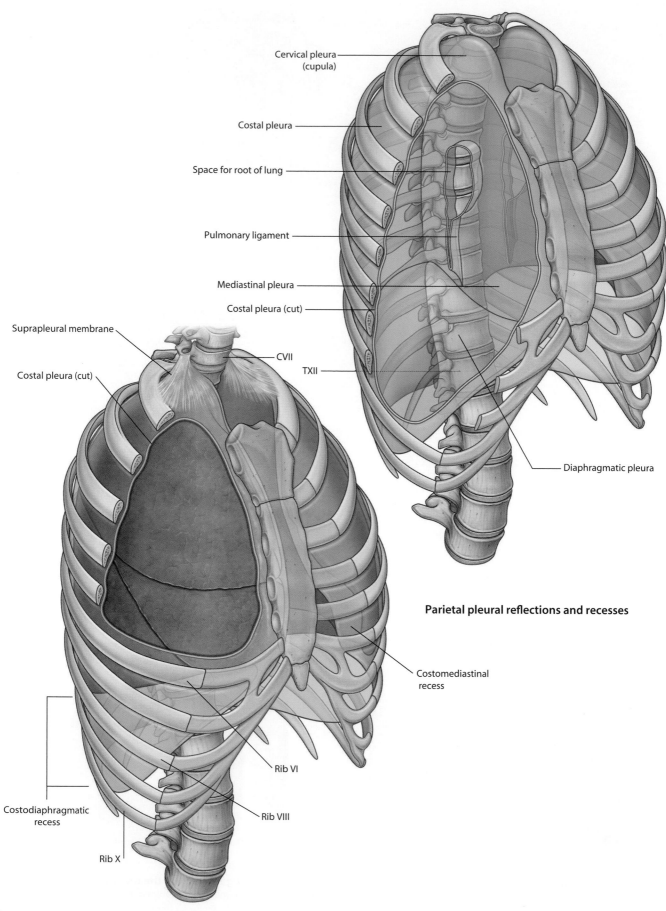

Cervical pleura
(cupula)

Costal pleura

Space for root of lung

Pulmonary ligament

Mediastinal pleura

Costal pleura (cut)

CVII

TXII

Diaphragmatic pleura

Suprapleural membrane

Costal pleura (cut)

Parietal pleural reflections and recesses

Costomediastinal
recess

Costodiaphragmatic
recess

Rib VI

Rib VIII

Rib X

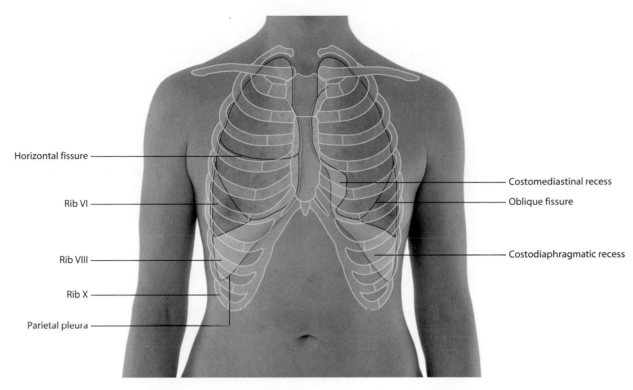

Horizontal fissure

Rib VI

Rib VIII

Rib X

Parietal pleura

Costomediastinal recess

Oblique fissure

Costodiaphragmatic recess

Surface projections of the pleura and lungs (anterior view)

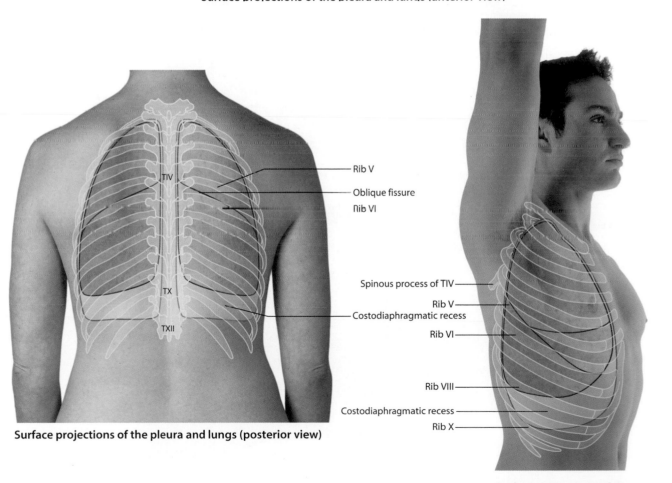

TIV

TX

TXII

Rib V

Oblique fissure

Rib VI

Surface projections of the pleura and lungs (posterior view)

Spinous process of TIV

Rib V

Costodiaphragmatic recess

Rib VI

Rib VIII

Costodiaphragmatic recess

Rib X

**Surface projections of the
pleura and right lung (lateral view)**

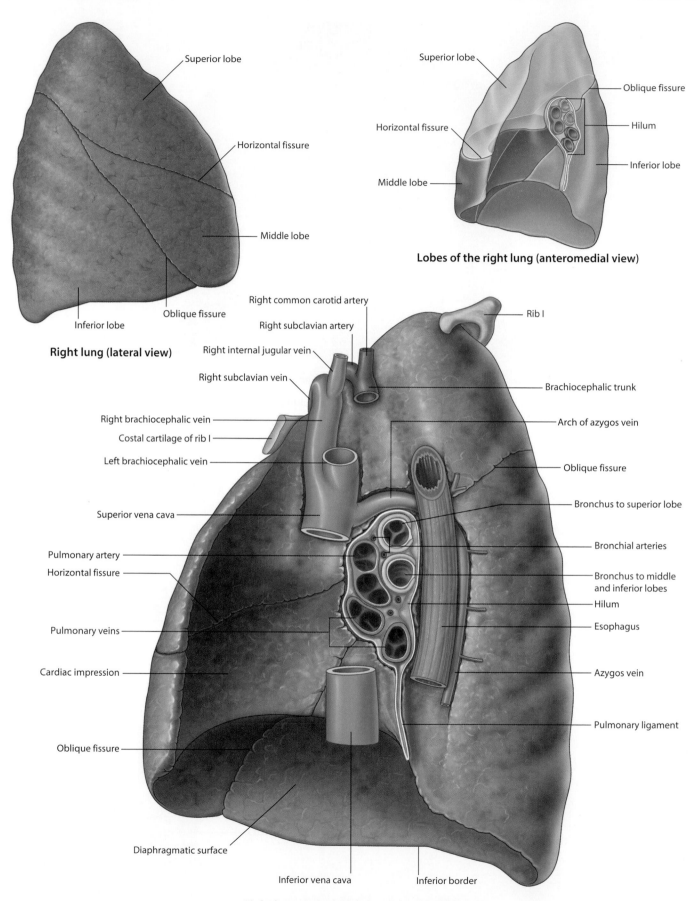

Superior lobe

Horizontal fissure

Middle lobe

Inferior lobe

Oblique fissure

Right lung (lateral view)

Superior lobe

Oblique fissure

Hilum

Horizontal fissure

Inferior lobe

Middle lobe

Lobes of the right lung (anteromedial view)

Right common carotid artery

Right subclavian artery

Right internal jugular vein

Right subclavian vein

Rib I

Right brachiocephalic vein

Costal cartilage of rib I

Left brachiocephalic vein

Brachiocephalic trunk

Arch of azygos vein

Oblique fissure

Superior vena cava

Bronchus to superior lobe

Pulmonary artery

Bronchial arteries

Horizontal fissure

Bronchus to middle and inferior lobes

Hilum

Pulmonary veins

Esophagus

Cardiac impression

Azygos vein

Oblique fissure

Pulmonary ligament

Diaphragmatic surface

Inferior vena cava

Inferior border

Right lung and related structures (medial view)

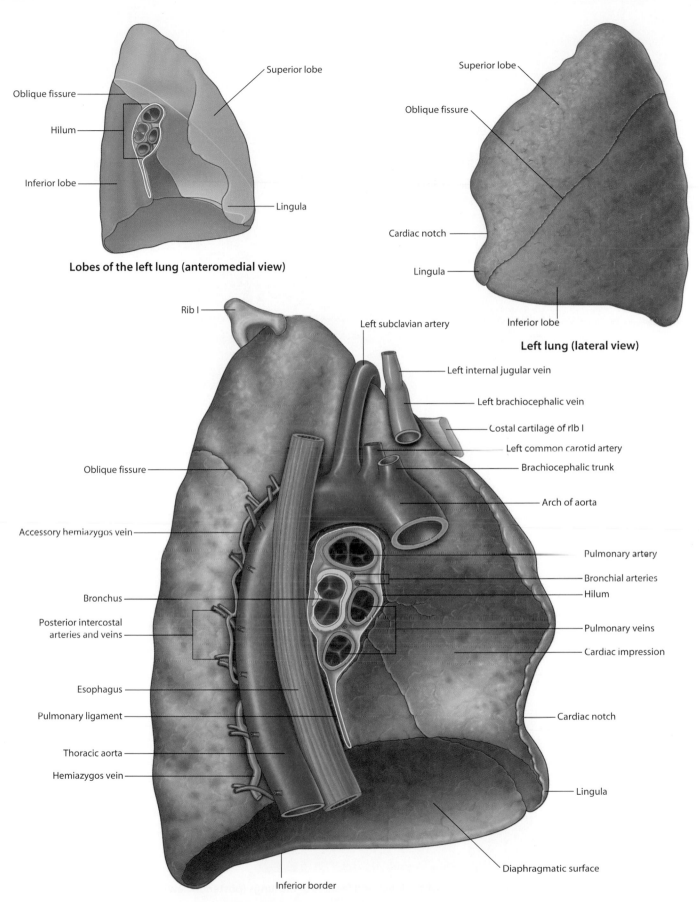

Lobes of the left lung (anteromedial view)

Oblique fissure

Hilum

Inferior lobe

Superior lobe

Lingula

Left lung (lateral view)

Superior lobe

Oblique fissure

Cardiac notch

Lingula

Inferior lobe

Left lung and related structures (medial view)

Rib I

Oblique fissure

Accessory hemiazygos vein

Bronchus

Posterior intercostal arteries and veins

Esophagus

Pulmonary ligament

Thoracic aorta

Hemiazygos vein

Inferior border

Left subclavian artery

Left internal jugular vein

Left brachiocephalic vein

Costal cartilage of rib I

Left common carotid artery

Brachiocephalic trunk

Arch of aorta

Pulmonary artery

Bronchial arteries

Hilum

Pulmonary veins

Cardiac impression

Cardiac notch

Lingula

Diaphragmatic surface

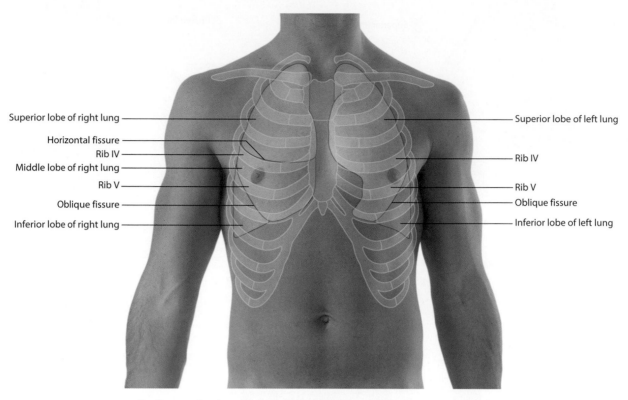

Superior lobe of right lung

Horizontal fissure

Rib IV

Middle lobe of right lung

Rib V

Oblique fissure

Inferior lobe of right lung

Superior lobe of left lung

Rib IV

Rib V

Oblique fissure

Inferior lobe of left lung

Surface projections of the lobes and fissures of the lungs (anterior view)

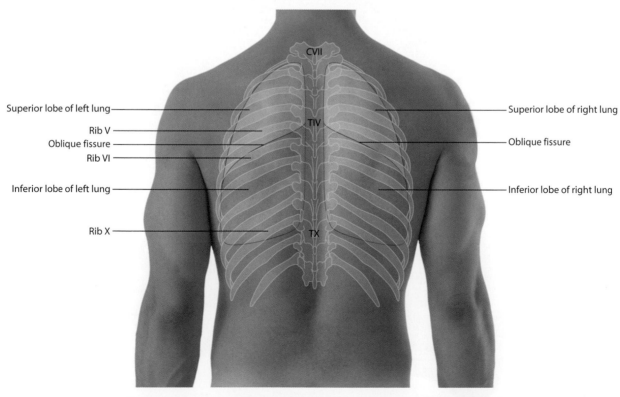

CVII

Superior lobe of left lung

Rib V

Oblique fissure

Rib VI

Inferior lobe of left lung

Rib X

TIV

TX

Superior lobe of right lung

Oblique fissure

Inferior lobe of right lung

Surface projections of the lobes and fissures of the lungs (posterior view)

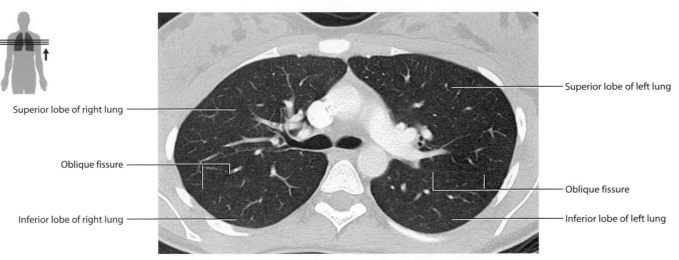

Superior lobe of right lung

Superior lobe of left lung

Oblique fissure

Oblique fissure

Inferior lobe of right lung

Inferior lobe of left lung

Right lung and left lung demonstrating superior and inferior lobes. The oblique fissures are visible
CT image, with contrast, in axial plane

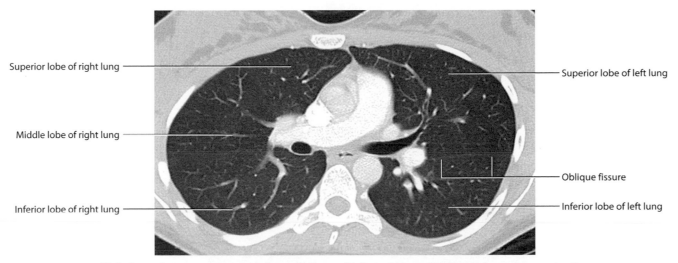

Superior lobe of right lung

Superior lobe of left lung

Middle lobe of right lung

Oblique fissure

Inferior lobe of right lung

Inferior lobe of left lung

Right lung demonstrating superior, middle, and inferior lobes and the left lung demonstrating superior and inferior lobes. The oblique fissure associated with the left lung is visible.
CT image, with contrast, in axial plane

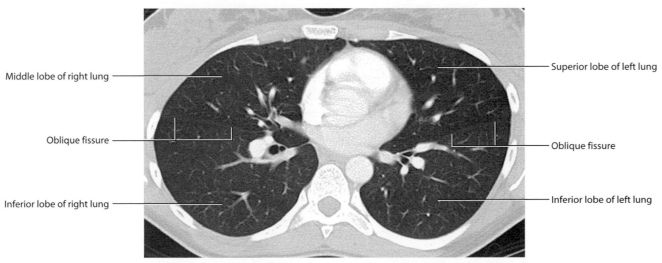

Middle lobe of right lung

Superior lobe of left lung

Oblique fissure

Oblique fissure

Inferior lobe of right lung

Inferior lobe of left lung

Right lung demonstrating middle and inferior lobes and the left lung demonstrating superior and inferior lobes. The oblique fissures are visible.
CT image, with contrast, in axial plane

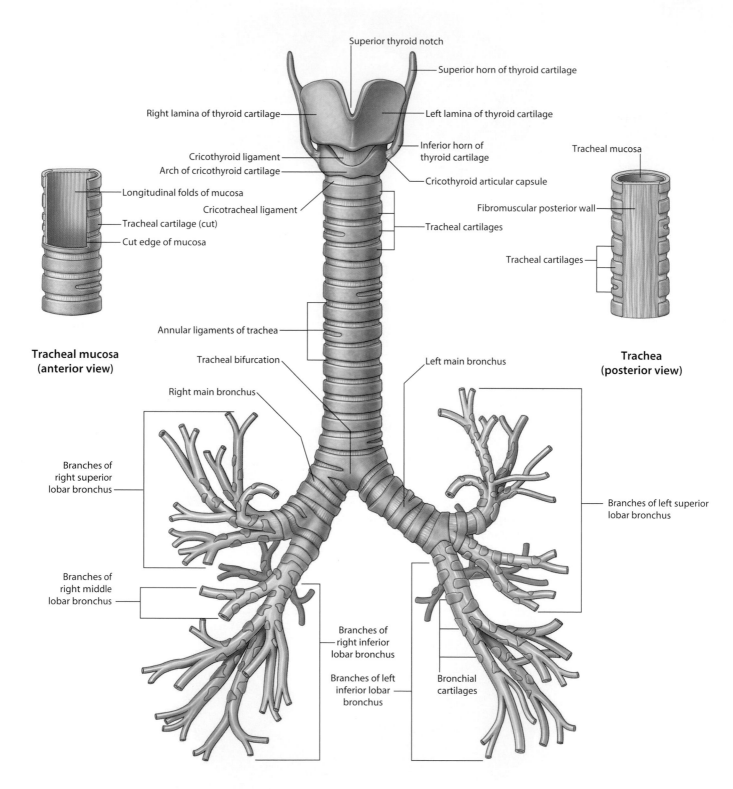

Superior thyroid notch

Superior horn of thyroid cartilage

Right lamina of thyroid cartilage

Left lamina of thyroid cartilage

Cricothyroid ligament

Inferior horn of thyroid cartilage

Arch of cricothyroid cartilage

Cricothyroid articular capsule

Tracheal mucosa

Longitudinal folds of mucosa

Tracheal cartilages

Cricotracheal ligament

Fibromuscular posterior wall

Tracheal cartilage (cut)

Cut edge of mucosa

Tracheal cartilages

Annular ligaments of trachea

Tracheal mucosa (anterior view)

Left main bronchus

Tracheal bifurcation

Trachea (posterior view)

Right main bronchus

Branches of right superior lobar bronchus

Branches of left superior lobar bronchus

Branches of right middle lobar bronchus

Branches of right inferior lobar bronchus

Branches of left inferior lobar bronchus

Bronchial cartilages

Trachea and bronchial tree

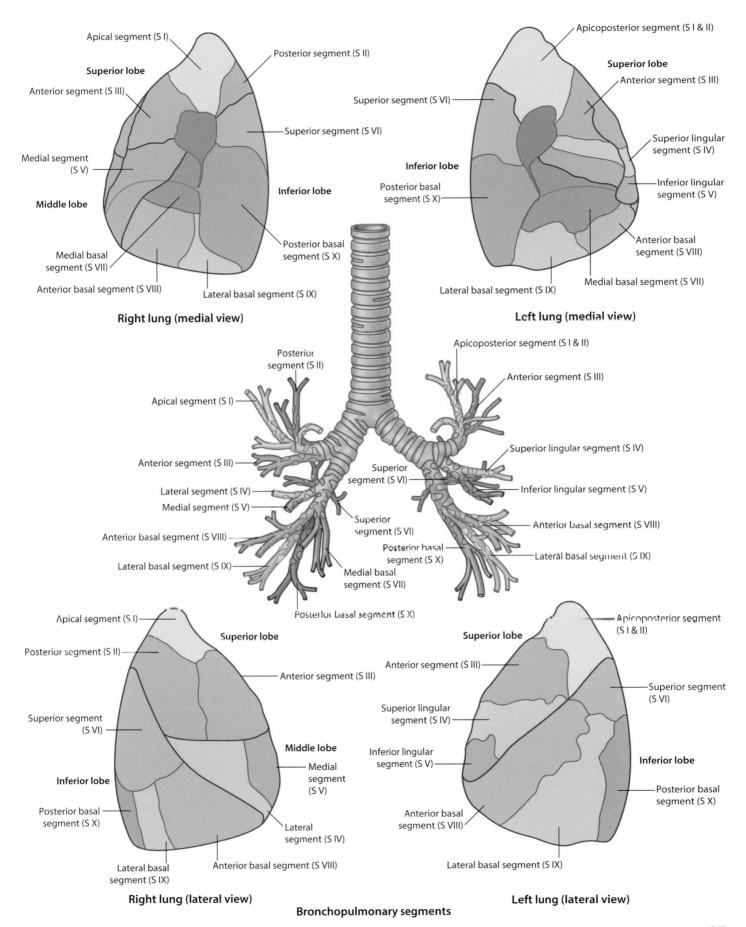

Apical segment (S I)

Posterior segment (S II)

Superior lobe

Anterior segment (S III)

Superior segment (S VI)

Medial segment (S V)

Superior segment (S VI)

Middle lobe

Inferior lobe

Medial basal segment (S VII)

Posterior basal segment (S X)

Anterior basal segment (S VIII)

Lateral basal segment (S IX)

Right lung (medial view)

Apicoposterior segment (S I & II)

Superior lobe

Anterior segment (S III)

Superior segment (S VI)

Superior lingular segment (S IV)

Inferior lobe

Inferior lingular segment (S V)

Posterior basal segment (S X)

Anterior basal segment (S VIII)

Lateral basal segment (S IX)

Medial basal segment (S VII)

Left lung (medial view)

Posterior segment (S II)

Apicoposterior segment (S I & II)

Apical segment (S I)

Anterior segment (S III)

Anterior segment (S III)

Superior lingular segment (S IV)

Lateral segment (S IV)

Medial segment (S V)

Inferior lingular segment (S V)

Superior segment (S VI)

Anterior basal segment (S VIII)

Superior segment (S VI)

Lateral basal segment (S IX)

Anterior basal segment (S VIII)

Medial basal segment (S VII)

Lateral basal segment (S IX)

Posterior basal segment (S X)

Posterior basal segment (S X)

Apical segment (S I)

Superior lobe

Apicoposterior segment (S I & II)

Posterior segment (S II)

Anterior segment (S III)

Anterior segment (S III)

Superior segment (S VI)

Superior segment (S VI)

Superior lingular segment (S IV)

Middle lobe

Medial segment (S V)

Inferior lobe

Inferior lingular segment (S V)

Inferior lobe

Posterior basal segment (S X)

Lateral segment (S IV)

Posterior basal segment (S X)

Anterior basal segment (S VIII)

Lateral basal segment (S IX)

Anterior basal segment (S VIII)

Lateral basal segment (S IX)

Right lung (lateral view)

Left lung (lateral view)

Bronchopulmonary segments

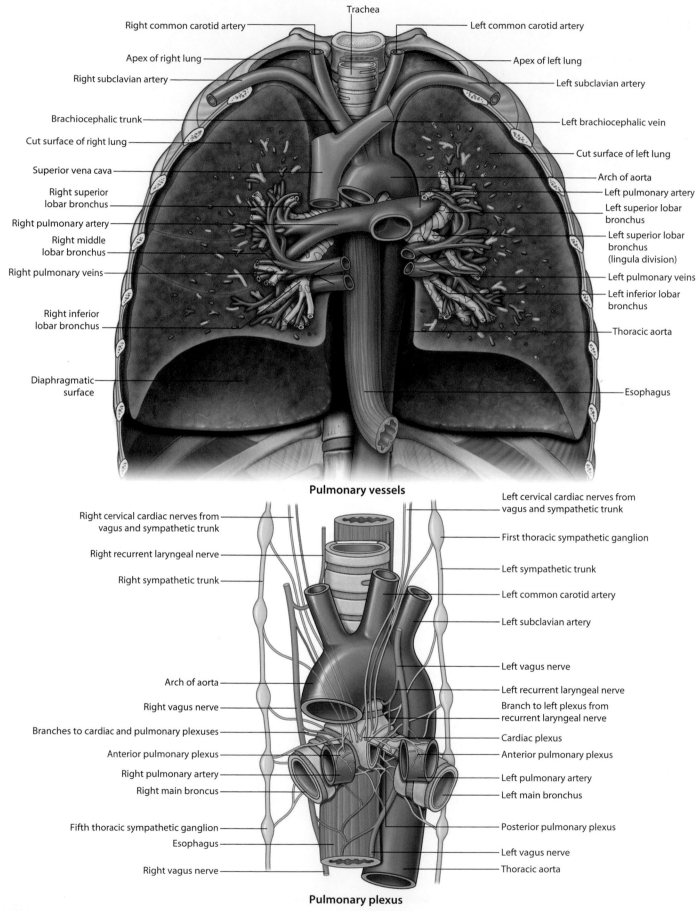

Trachea

Right common carotid artery

Apex of right lung

Right subclavian artery

Brachiocephalic trunk

Cut surface of right lung

Superior vena cava

Right superior lobar bronchus

Right pulmonary artery

Right middle lobar bronchus

Right pulmonary veins

Right inferior lobar bronchus

Diaphragmatic surface

Left common carotid artery

Apex of left lung

Left subclavian artery

Left brachiocephalic vein

Cut surface of left lung

Arch of aorta

Left pulmonary artery

Left superior lobar bronchus

Left superior lobar bronchus (lingula division)

Left pulmonary veins

Left inferior lobar bronchus

Thoracic aorta

Esophagus

Pulmonary vessels

Right cervical cardiac nerves from vagus and sympathetic trunk

Right recurrent laryngeal nerve

Right sympathetic trunk

Arch of aorta

Right vagus nerve

Branches to cardiac and pulmonary plexuses

Anterior pulmonary plexus

Right pulmonary artery

Right main broncus

Fifth thoracic sympathetic ganglion

Esophagus

Right vagus nerve

Left cervical cardiac nerves from vagus and sympathetic trunk

First thoracic sympathetic ganglion

Left sympathetic trunk

Left common carotid artery

Left subclavian artery

Left vagus nerve

Left recurrent laryngeal nerve

Branch to left plexus from recurrent laryngeal nerve

Cardiac plexus

Anterior pulmonary plexus

Left pulmonary artery

Left main bronchus

Posterior pulmonary plexus

Left vagus nerve

Thoracic aorta

Pulmonary plexus

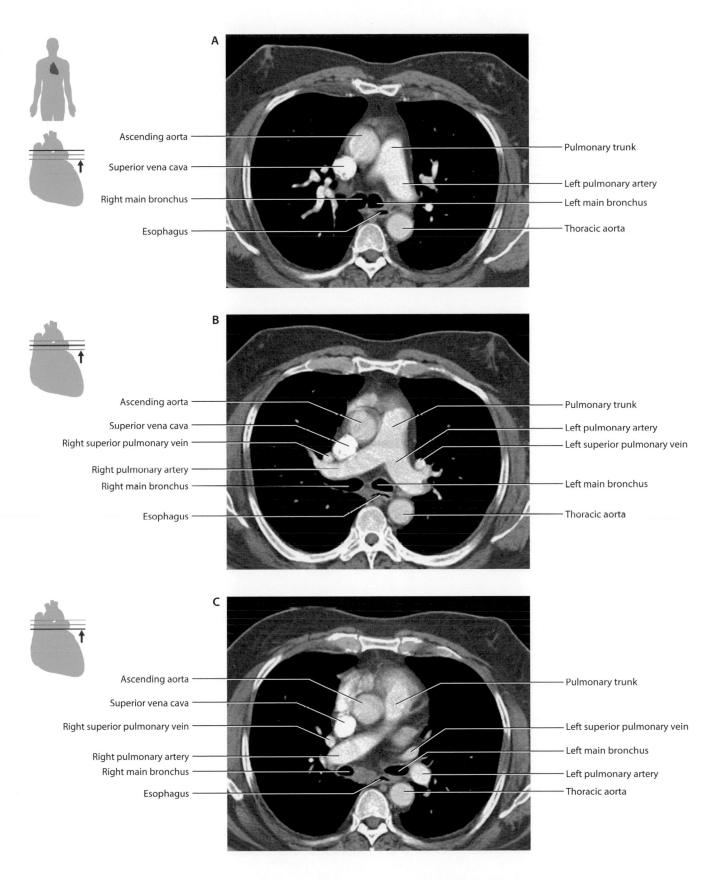

A

Ascending aorta

Superior vena cava

Right main bronchus

Esophagus

Pulmonary trunk

Left pulmonary artery

Left main bronchus

Thoracic aorta

B

Ascending aorta

Superior vena cava

Right superior pulmonary vein

Right pulmonary artery

Right main bronchus

Esophagus

Pulmonary trunk

Left pulmonary artery

Left superior pulmonary vein

Left main bronchus

Thoracic aorta

C

Ascending aorta

Superior vena cava

Right superior pulmonary vein

Right pulmonary artery

Right main bronchus

Esophagus

Pulmonary trunk

Left superior pulmonary vein

Left main bronchus

Left pulmonary artery

Thoracic aorta

A through C – Relationships of the pulmonary arteries, pulmonary veins, and bronchi in the mediastinum.
CT images, with contrast, in axial plane

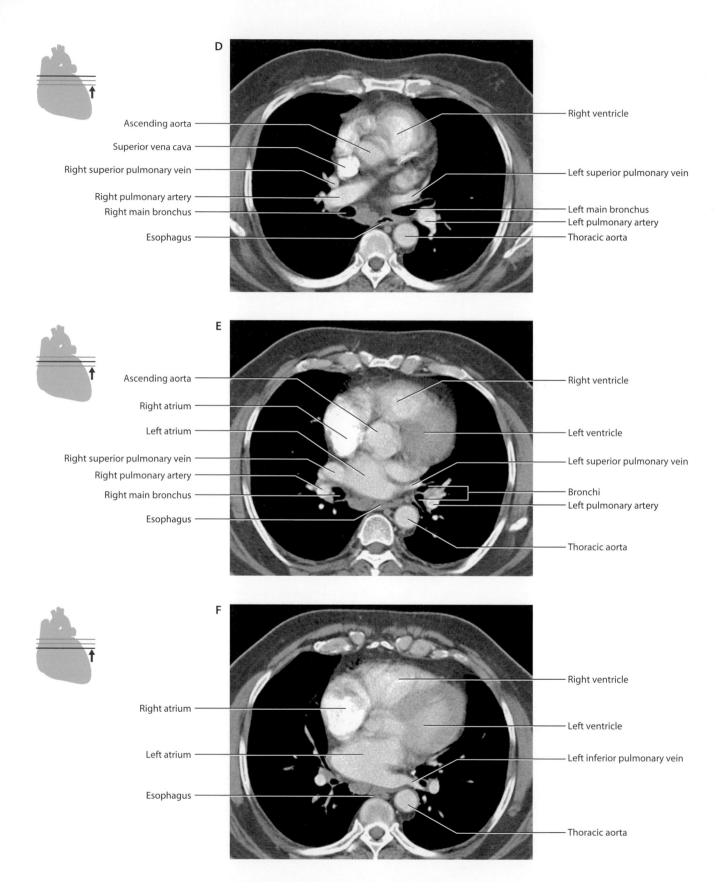

D

Ascending aorta
Superior vena cava
Right superior pulmonary vein
Right pulmonary artery
Right main bronchus
Esophagus

Right ventricle
Left superior pulmonary vein
Left main bronchus
Left pulmonary artery
Thoracic aorta

E

Ascending aorta
Right atrium
Left atrium
Right superior pulmonary vein
Right pulmonary artery
Right main bronchus
Esophagus

Right ventricle
Left ventricle
Left superior pulmonary vein
Bronchi
Left pulmonary artery
Thoracic aorta

F

Right atrium
Left atrium
Esophagus

Right ventricle
Left ventricle
Left inferior pulmonary vein
Thoracic aorta

D through F – Relationships of the pulmonary arteries, pulmonary veins, and bronchi in the mediastinum.
CT images, with contrast, in axial plane

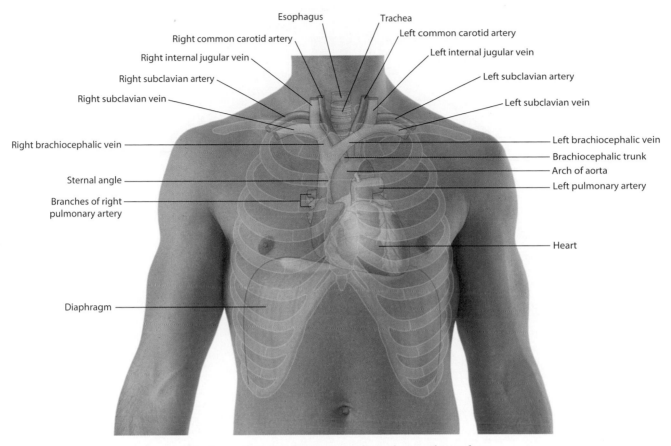

Structures of the mediastinum as they relate to the surface

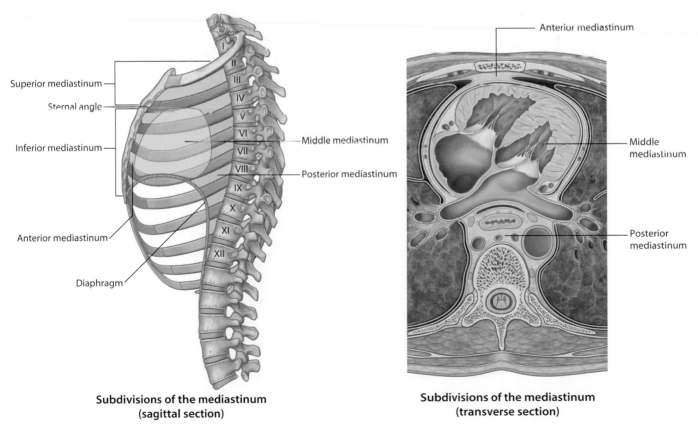

**Subdivisions of the mediastinum
(sagittal section)**

**Subdivisions of the mediastinum
(transverse section)**

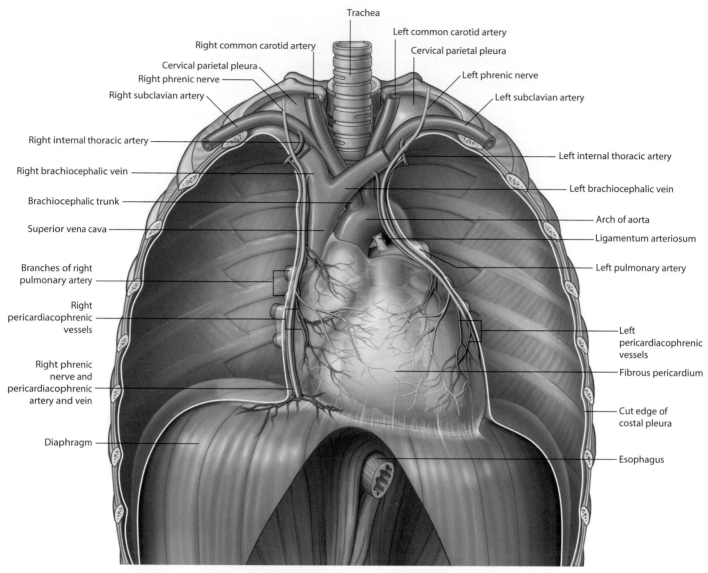

Trachea

Right common carotid artery

Left common carotid artery

Cervical parietal pleura

Cervical parietal pleura

Right phrenic nerve

Left phrenic nerve

Right subclavian artery

Left subclavian artery

Right internal thoracic artery

Left internal thoracic artery

Right brachiocephalic vein

Left brachiocephalic vein

Brachiocephalic trunk

Arch of aorta

Superior vena cava

Ligamentum arteriosum

Branches of right pulmonary artery

Left pulmonary artery

Right pericardiacophrenic vessels

Left pericardiacophrenic vessels

Right phrenic nerve and pericardiacophrenic artery and vein

Fibrous pericardium

Diaphragm

Cut edge of costal pleura

Esophagus

Pericardium with nerves and vessels

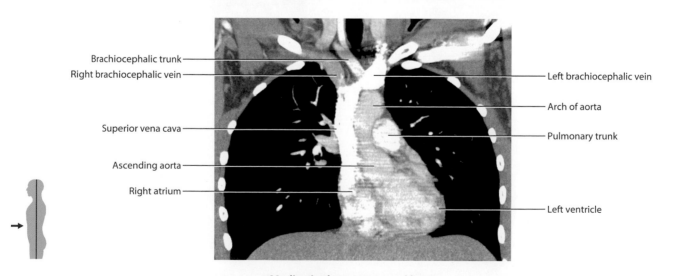

Brachiocephalic trunk

Right brachiocephalic vein

Left brachiocephalic vein

Arch of aorta

Superior vena cava

Pulmonary trunk

Ascending aorta

Right atrium

Left ventricle

Mediastinal structures and lungs.
CT image, with contrast, in coronal plane

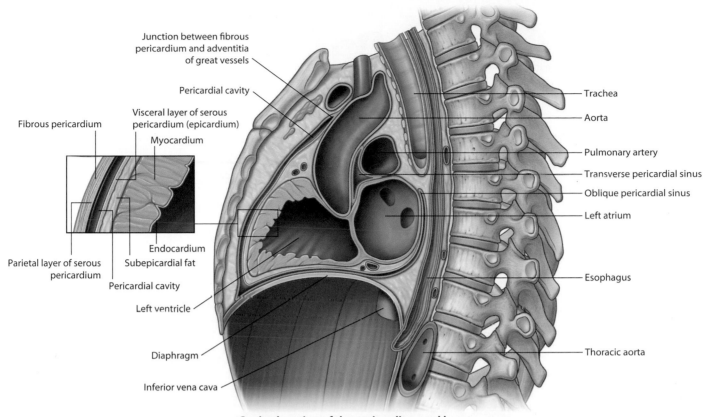

Junction between fibrous pericardium and adventitia of great vessels

Pericardial cavity

Visceral layer of serous pericardium (epicardium)

Myocardium

Fibrous pericardium

Parietal layer of serous pericardium

Subepicardial fat

Endocardium

Pericardial cavity

Left ventricle

Diaphragm

Inferior vena cava

Trachea

Aorta

Pulmonary artery

Transverse pericardial sinus

Oblique pericardial sinus

Left atrium

Esophagus

Thoracic aorta

Sagittal section of the pericardium and heart

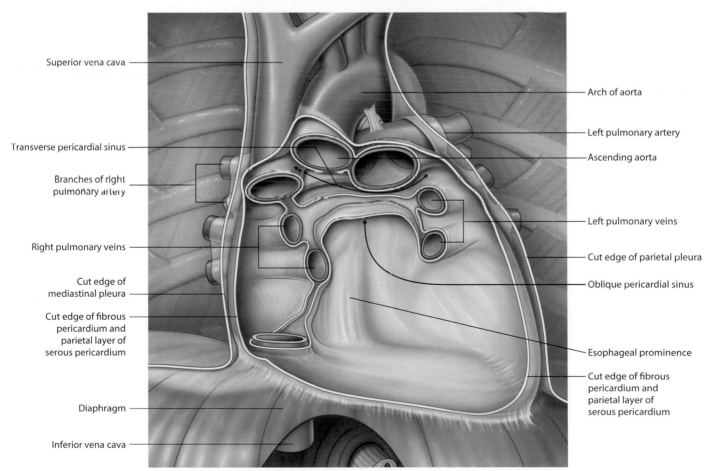

Superior vena cava

Transverse pericardial sinus

Branches of right pulmonary artery

Right pulmonary veins

Cut edge of mediastinal pleura

Cut edge of fibrous pericardium and parietal layer of serous pericardium

Diaphragm

Inferior vena cava

Arch of aorta

Left pulmonary artery

Ascending aorta

Left pulmonary veins

Cut edge of parietal pleura

Oblique pericardial sinus

Esophageal prominence

Cut edge of fibrous pericardium and parietal layer of serous pericardium

Pericardial sac with heart removed

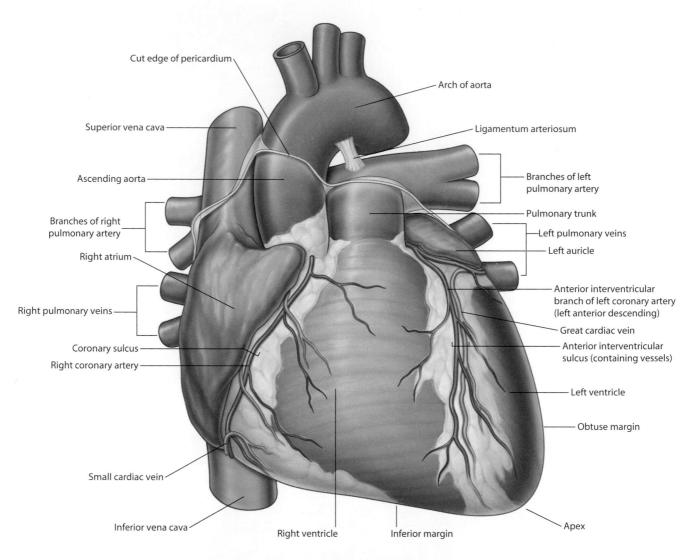

Cut edge of pericardium

Arch of aorta

Superior vena cava

Ligamentum arteriosum

Ascending aorta

Branches of left
pulmonary artery

Pulmonary trunk

Branches of right
pulmonary artery

Left pulmonary veins

Left auricle

Right atrium

Anterior interventricular
branch of left coronary artery
(left anterior descending)

Right pulmonary veins

Great cardiac vein

Coronary sulcus

Anterior interventricular
sulcus (containing vessels)

Right coronary artery

Left ventricle

Obtuse margin

Small cardiac vein

Inferior vena cava

Apex

Right ventricle

Inferior margin

Anterior surface of the heart

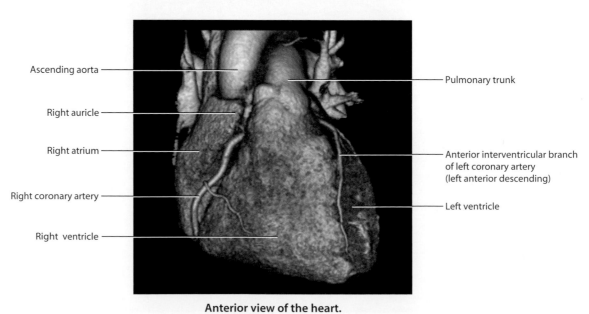

Ascending aorta

Pulmonary trunk

Right auricle

Right atrium

Anterior interventricular branch
of left coronary artery
(left anterior descending)

Right coronary artery

Left ventricle

Right ventricle

Anterior view of the heart.
Volume-rendered anterior view using multidetector computed tomography

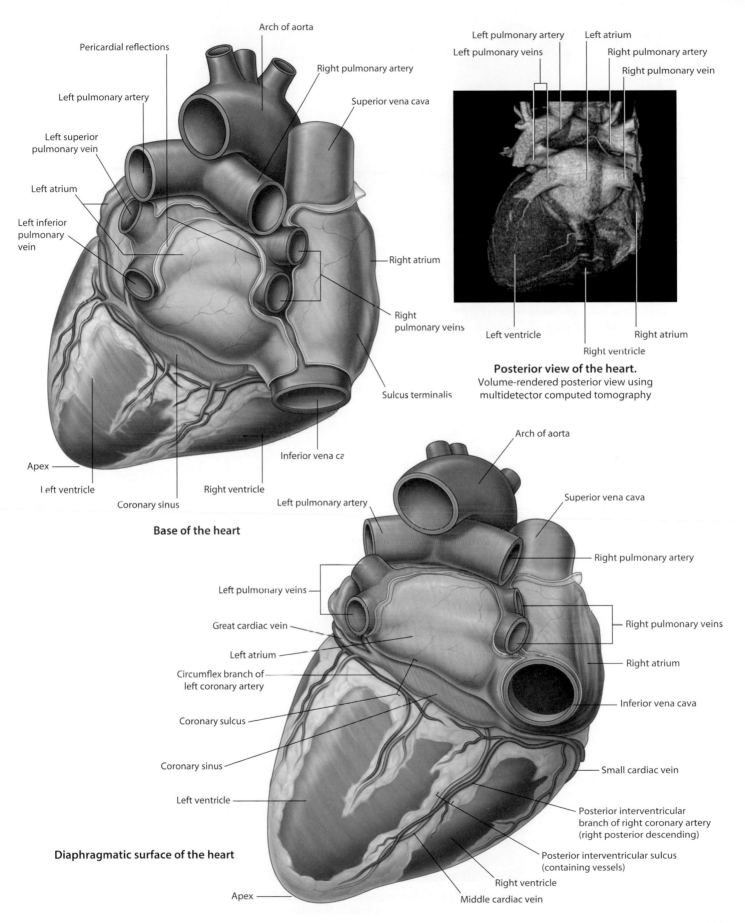

Base of the heart

Arch of aorta

Pericardial reflections

Right pulmonary artery

Left pulmonary artery

Superior vena cava

Left superior pulmonary vein

Left atrium

Left inferior pulmonary vein

Right atrium

Right pulmonary veins

Apex

Sulcus terminalis

Left ventricle

Inferior vena cava

Coronary sinus

Right ventricle

Posterior view of the heart.
Volume-rendered posterior view using multidetector computed tomography

Left pulmonary artery

Left pulmonary veins

Left atrium

Right pulmonary artery

Right pulmonary vein

Left ventricle

Right ventricle

Right atrium

Diaphragmatic surface of the heart

Arch of aorta

Left pulmonary artery

Superior vena cava

Right pulmonary artery

Left pulmonary veins

Great cardiac vein

Left atrium

Right pulmonary veins

Circumflex branch of left coronary artery

Right atrium

Coronary sulcus

Inferior vena cava

Coronary sinus

Left ventricle

Small cardiac vein

Posterior interventricular branch of right coronary artery (right posterior descending)

Posterior interventricular sulcus (containing vessels)

Apex

Right ventricle

Middle cardiac vein

95

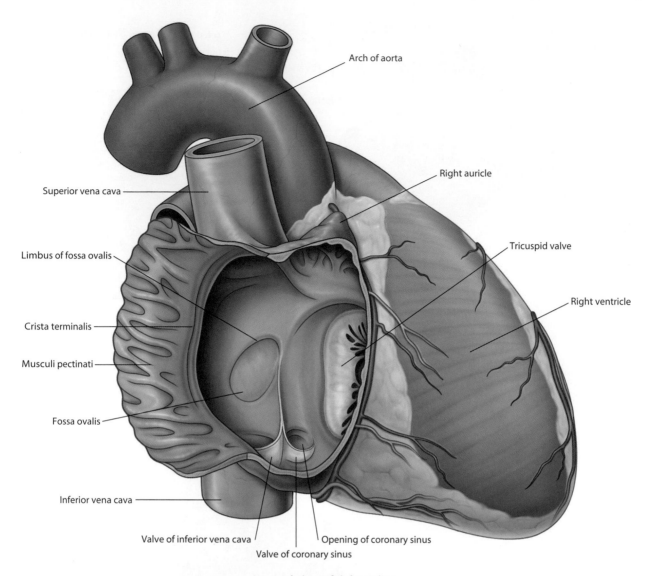

Arch of aorta

Right auricle

Superior vena cava

Tricuspid valve

Limbus of fossa ovalis

Right ventricle

Crista terminalis

Musculi pectinati

Fossa ovalis

Inferior vena cava

Valve of inferior vena cava

Opening of coronary sinus

Valve of coronary sinus

Internal view of right atrium

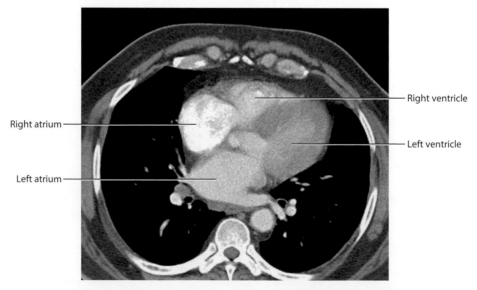

Right ventricle

Right atrium

Left ventricle

Left atrium

Positioning of right atrium in relation to other cardiac chambers.
CT image, with contrast, in axial plane

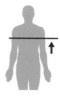

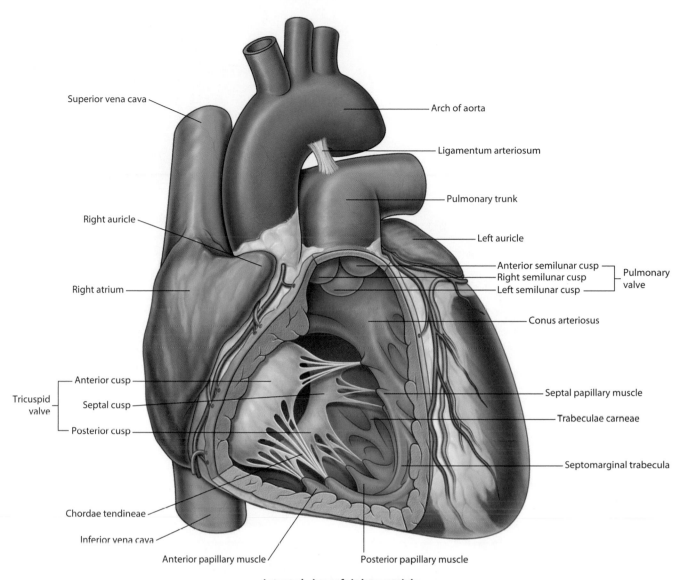

Superior vena cava

Arch of aorta

Ligamentum arteriosum

Pulmonary trunk

Right auricle

Left auricle

Anterior semilunar cusp
Right semilunar cusp } Pulmonary valve
Left semilunar cusp

Right atrium

Conus arteriosus

Anterior cusp

Septal cusp } Tricuspid valve

Posterior cusp

Septal papillary muscle

Trabeculae carneae

Septomarginal trabecula

Chordae tendineae

Inferior vena cava

Anterior papillary muscle

Posterior papillary muscle

Internal view of right ventricle

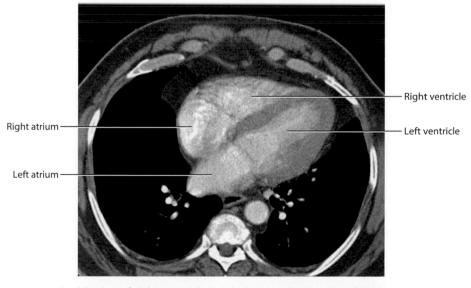

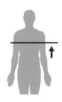

Right atrium

Right ventricle

Left ventricle

Left atrium

Positioning of right ventricle in relation to other cardiac chambers.
CT image, with contrast, in axial plane

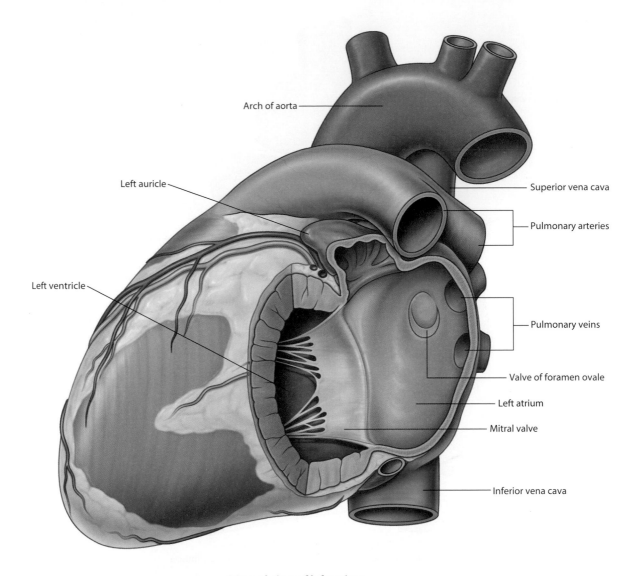

Arch of aorta

Left auricle

Left ventricle

Superior vena cava

Pulmonary arteries

Pulmonary veins

Valve of foramen ovale

Left atrium

Mitral valve

Inferior vena cava

Internal view of left atrium

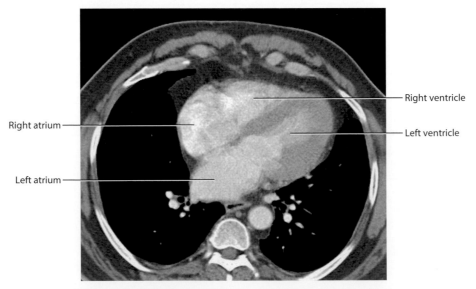

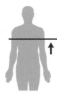

Right ventricle

Right atrium

Left ventricle

Left atrium

Positioning of left atrium in relation to other cardiac chambers.
CT image, with contrast, in axial plane

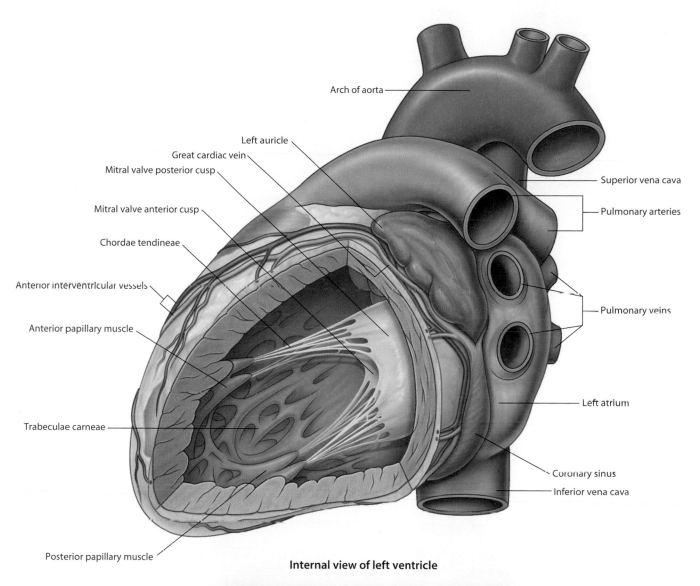

Arch of aorta

Left auricle

Great cardiac vein

Mitral valve posterior cusp

Mitral valve anterior cusp

Chordae tendineae

Anterior interventricular vessels

Anterior papillary muscle

Trabeculae carneae

Posterior papillary muscle

Superior vena cava

Pulmonary arteries

Pulmonary veins

Left atrium

Coronary sinus

Inferior vena cava

Internal view of left ventricle

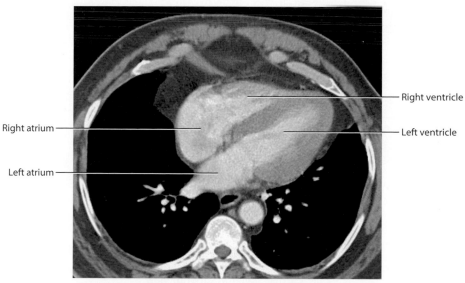

Right atrium

Left atrium

Right ventricle

Left ventricle

Positioning of left ventricle in relation to other cardiac chambers.
CT image, with contrast, in axial plane

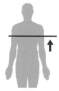

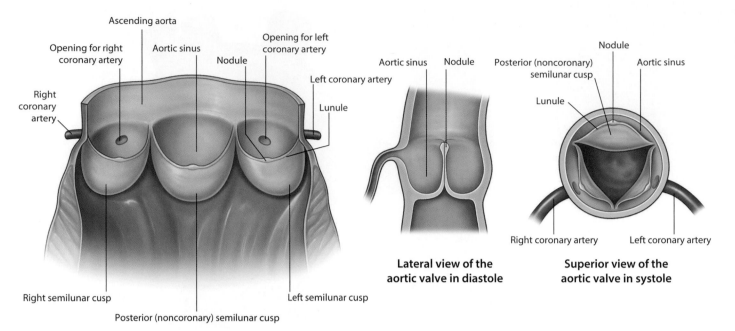

Ascending aorta

Opening for right
coronary artery

Aortic sinus

Nodule

Opening for left
coronary artery

Left coronary artery

Right
coronary
artery

Lunule

Right semilunar cusp

Left semilunar cusp

Posterior (noncoronary) semilunar cusp

**Anterior view of the aortic valve
(resected and opened out)**

Aortic sinus

Nodule

Posterior (noncoronary)
semilunar cusp

Nodule

Aortic sinus

Lunule

Right coronary artery

Left coronary artery

**Lateral view of the
aortic valve in diastole**

**Superior view of the
aortic valve in systole**

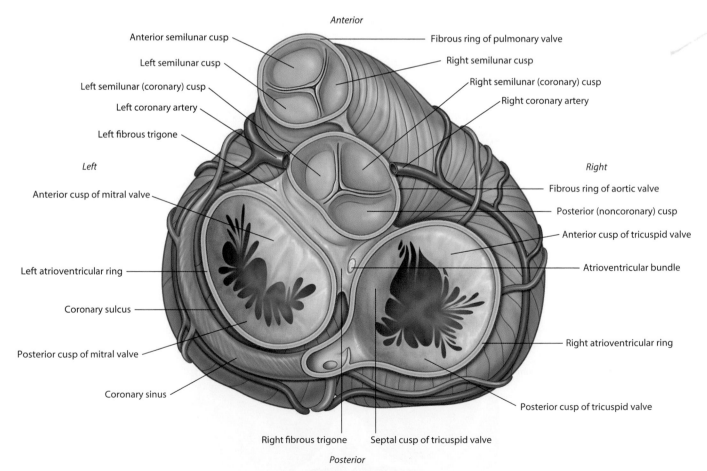

Anterior

Anterior semilunar cusp

Left semilunar cusp

Left semilunar (coronary) cusp

Left coronary artery

Left fibrous trigone

Fibrous ring of pulmonary valve

Right semilunar cusp

Right semilunar (coronary) cusp

Right coronary artery

Left

Right

Anterior cusp of mitral valve

Left atrioventricular ring

Coronary sulcus

Posterior cusp of mitral valve

Coronary sinus

Fibrous ring of aortic valve

Posterior (noncoronary) cusp

Anterior cusp of tricuspid valve

Atrioventricular bundle

Right atrioventricular ring

Posterior cusp of tricuspid valve

Right fibrous trigone

Septal cusp of tricuspid valve

Posterior

**Cardiac skeleton superior view
(atria removed)**

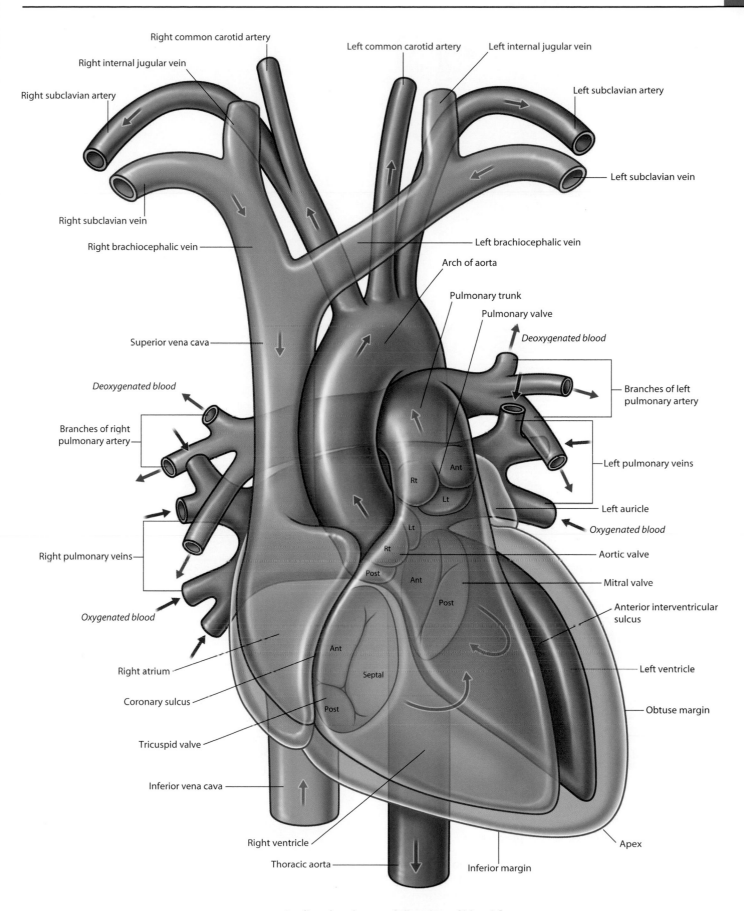

Cardiac chambers and direction of blood flow

Right common carotid artery
Right internal jugular vein
Right subclavian artery
Right subclavian vein
Right brachiocephalic vein
Superior vena cava
Deoxygenated blood
Branches of right pulmonary artery
Right pulmonary veins
Oxygenated blood
Right atrium
Coronary sulcus
Tricuspid valve
Inferior vena cava
Right ventricle
Thoracic aorta

Left common carotid artery
Left internal jugular vein
Left subclavian artery
Left subclavian vein
Left brachiocephalic vein
Arch of aorta
Pulmonary trunk
Pulmonary valve
Deoxygenated blood
Branches of left pulmonary artery
Left pulmonary veins
Left auricle
Oxygenated blood
Aortic valve
Mitral valve
Anterior interventricular sulcus
Left ventricle
Obtuse margin
Apex
Inferior margin

Ant
Rt
Lt
Lt
Rt
Post
Ant
Post
Ant
Septal
Post

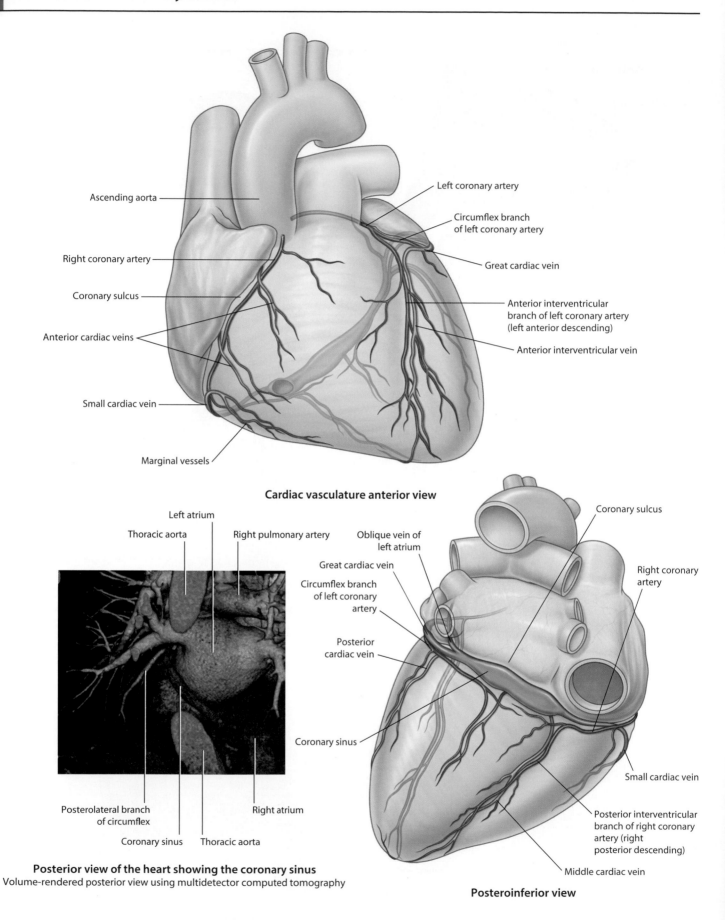

Cardiac vasculature anterior view

Ascending aorta

Right coronary artery

Coronary sulcus

Anterior cardiac veins

Small cardiac vein

Marginal vessels

Left coronary artery

Circumflex branch of left coronary artery

Great cardiac vein

Anterior interventricular branch of left coronary artery (left anterior descending)

Anterior interventricular vein

Left atrium

Thoracic aorta

Right pulmonary artery

Posterolateral branch of circumflex

Coronary sinus

Thoracic aorta

Right atrium

Posterior view of the heart showing the coronary sinus
Volume-rendered posterior view using multidetector computed tomography

Oblique vein of left atrium

Great cardiac vein

Circumflex branch of left coronary artery

Posterior cardiac vein

Coronary sinus

Coronary sulcus

Right coronary artery

Small cardiac vein

Posterior interventricular branch of right coronary artery (right posterior descending)

Middle cardiac vein

Posteroinferior view

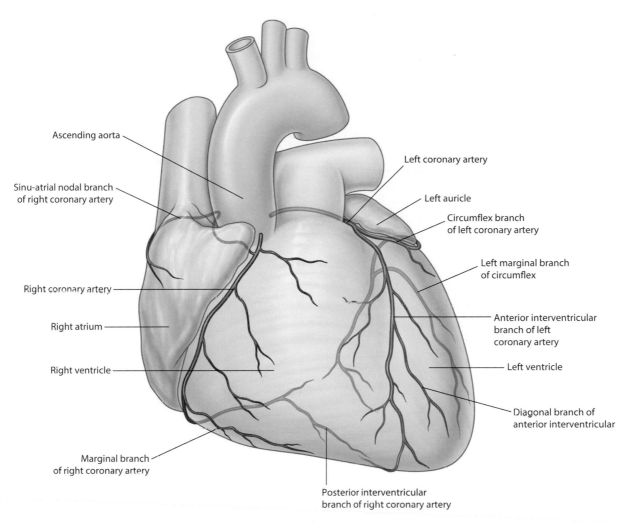

Ascending aorta

Sinu-atrial nodal branch
of right coronary artery

Right coronary artery

Right atrium

Right ventricle

Marginal branch
of right coronary artery

Left coronary artery

Left auricle

Circumflex branch
of left coronary artery

Left marginal branch
of circumflex

Anterior interventricular
branch of left
coronary artery

Left ventricle

Diagonal branch of
anterior interventricular

Posterior interventricular
branch of right coronary artery

Coronary arteries (right dominant system)

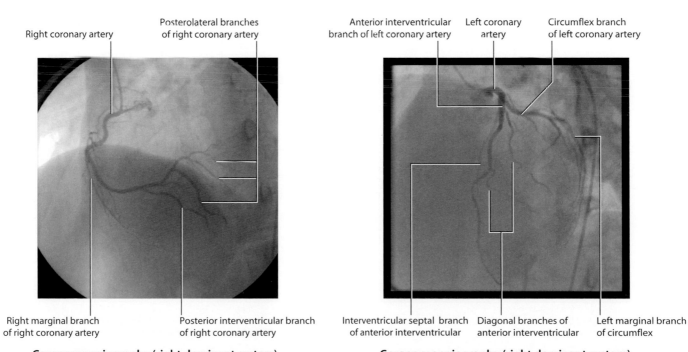

Right coronary artery

Posterolateral branches
of right coronary artery

Anterior interventricular
branch of left coronary artery

Left coronary
artery

Circumflex branch
of left coronary artery

Right marginal branch
of right coronary artery

Posterior interventricular branch
of right coronary artery

Interventricular septal branch
of anterior interventricular

Diagonal branches of
anterior interventricular

Left marginal branch
of circumflex

Coronary angiography (right dominant system).
Left anterior oblique projection, cranial angulation, of right coronary artery

Coronary angiography (right dominant system).
Left anterior oblique projection, cranial angulation, of left coronary artery

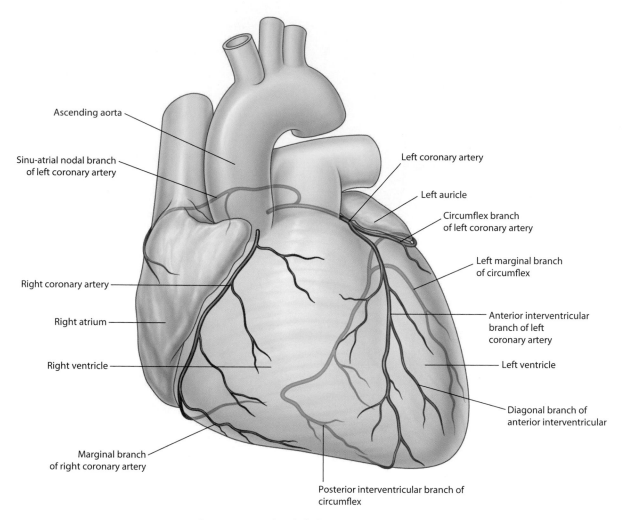

Ascending aorta

Sinu-atrial nodal branch of left coronary artery

Left coronary artery

Left auricle

Circumflex branch of left coronary artery

Left marginal branch of circumflex

Right coronary artery

Anterior interventricular branch of left coronary artery

Right atrium

Left ventricle

Right ventricle

Diagonal branch of anterior interventricular

Marginal branch of right coronary artery

Posterior interventricular branch of circumflex

Coronary arteries (left dominant system)

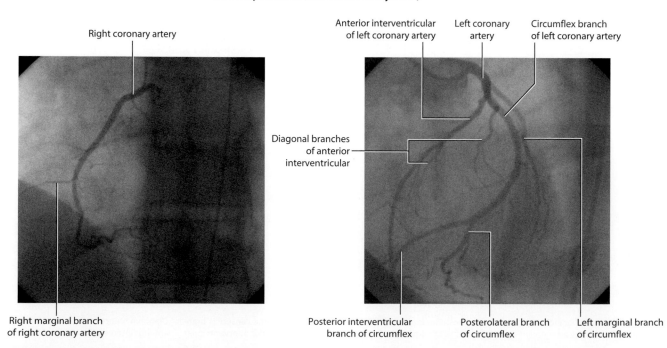

Right coronary artery

Anterior interventricular of left coronary artery

Left coronary artery

Circumflex branch of left coronary artery

Diagonal branches of anterior interventricular

Right marginal branch of right coronary artery

Posterior interventricular branch of circumflex

Posterolateral branch of circumflex

Left marginal branch of circumflex

Coronary angiography (left dominant system).
Left anterior oblique projection, cranial angulation, of right coronary artery

Coronary angiography (left dominant system).
Left anterior oblique projection, cranial angulation, of left coronary artery

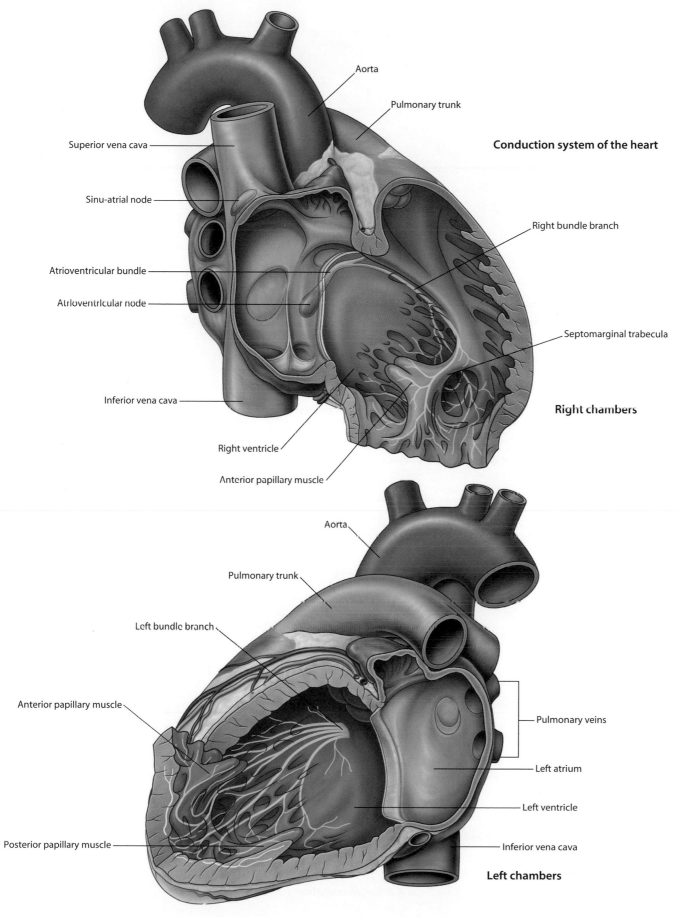

Conduction system of the heart

Aorta

Pulmonary trunk

Superior vena cava

Sinu-atrial node

Right bundle branch

Atrioventricular bundle

Atrioventricular node

Septomarginal trabecula

Inferior vena cava

Right chambers

Right ventricle

Anterior papillary muscle

Aorta

Pulmonary trunk

Left bundle branch

Anterior papillary muscle

Pulmonary veins

Left atrium

Left ventricle

Posterior papillary muscle

Inferior vena cava

Left chambers

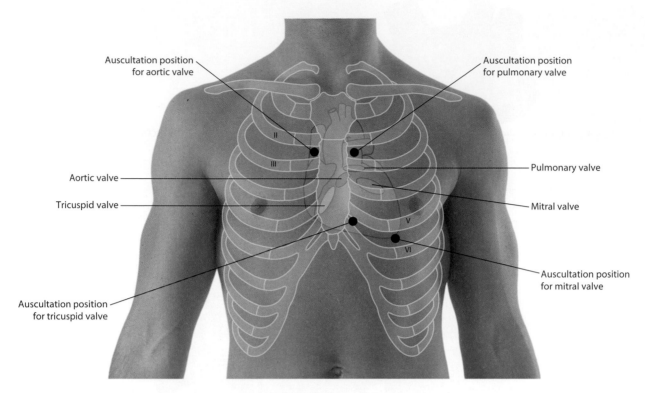

Auscultation points

Auscultation position for aortic valve

Auscultation position for pulmonary valve

Aortic valve

Pulmonary valve

Tricuspid valve

Mitral valve

Auscultation position for mitral valve

Auscultation position for tricuspid valve

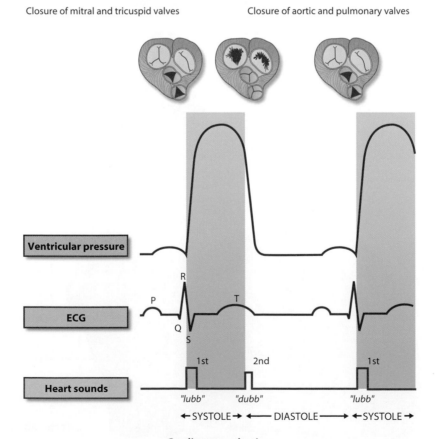

Closure of mitral and tricuspid valves

Closure of aortic and pulmonary valves

Ventricular pressure

ECG

Heart sounds

1st   2nd   1st

"lubb"   "dubb"   "lubb"

← SYSTOLE → ← DIASTOLE → ← SYSTOLE →

Cardiac auscultation

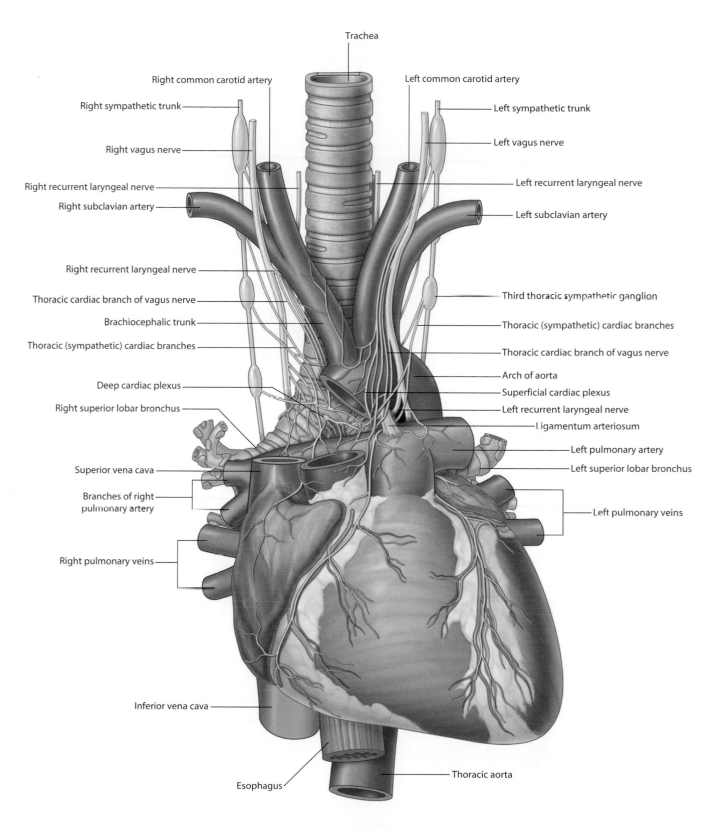

Trachea

Right common carotid artery

Right sympathetic trunk

Right vagus nerve

Right recurrent laryngeal nerve

Right subclavian artery

Right recurrent laryngeal nerve

Thoracic cardiac branch of vagus nerve

Brachiocephalic trunk

Thoracic (sympathetic) cardiac branches

Deep cardiac plexus

Right superior lobar bronchus

Superior vena cava

Branches of right pulmonary artery

Right pulmonary veins

Inferior vena cava

Esophagus

Left common carotid artery

Left sympathetic trunk

Left vagus nerve

Left recurrent laryngeal nerve

Left subclavian artery

Third thoracic sympathetic ganglion

Thoracic (sympathetic) cardiac branches

Thoracic cardiac branch of vagus nerve

Arch of aorta

Superficial cardiac plexus

Left recurrent laryngeal nerve

Ligamentum arteriosum

Left pulmonary artery

Left superior lobar bronchus

Left pulmonary veins

Thoracic aorta

Cardiac plexus and nerves of the heart

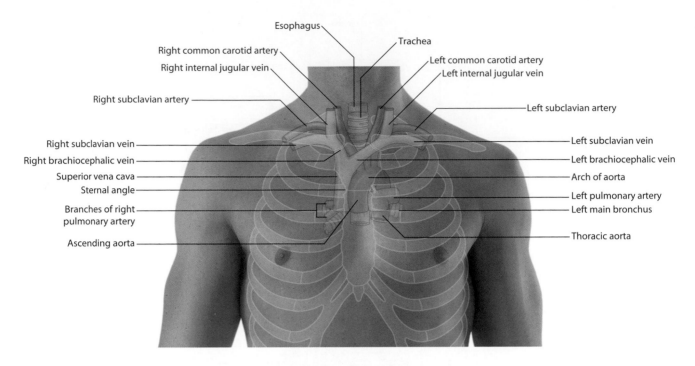

Esophagus

Trachea

Right common carotid artery

Right internal jugular vein

Left common carotid artery

Left internal jugular vein

Right subclavian artery

Left subclavian artery

Right subclavian vein

Left subclavian vein

Right brachiocephalic vein

Left brachiocephalic vein

Superior vena cava

Arch of aorta

Sternal angle

Left pulmonary artery

Branches of right pulmonary artery

Left main bronchus

Ascending aorta

Thoracic aorta

Surface projections of structures in the superior mediastinum

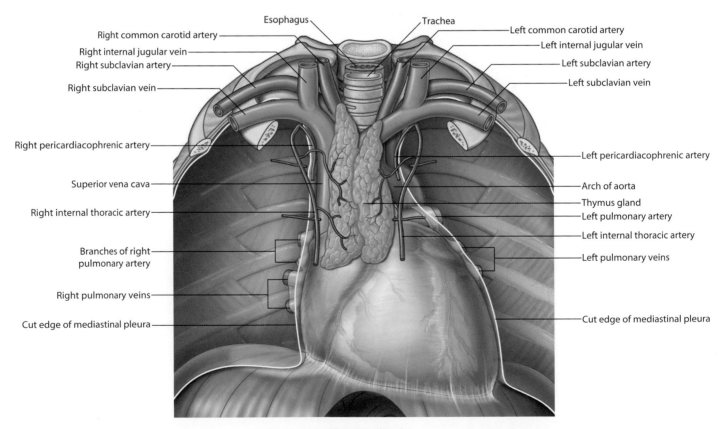

Esophagus

Trachea

Right common carotid artery

Left common carotid artery

Right internal jugular vein

Left internal jugular vein

Right subclavian artery

Left subclavian artery

Right subclavian vein

Left subclavian vein

Right pericardiacophrenic artery

Left pericardiacophrenic artery

Superior vena cava

Arch of aorta

Thymus gland

Right internal thoracic artery

Left pulmonary artery

Left internal thoracic artery

Branches of right pulmonary artery

Left pulmonary veins

Right pulmonary veins

Cut edge of mediastinal pleura

Cut edge of mediastinal pleura

Thymus gland

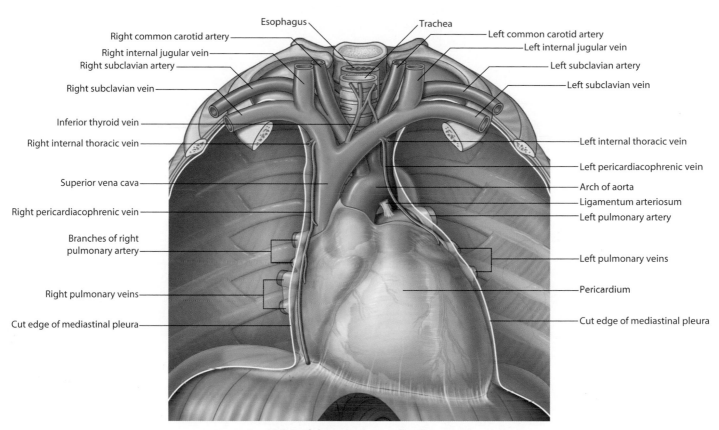

Esophagus

Right common carotid artery

Right internal jugular vein

Right subclavian artery

Right subclavian vein

Inferior thyroid vein

Right internal thoracic vein

Superior vena cava

Right pericardiacophrenic vein

Branches of right pulmonary artery

Right pulmonary veins

Cut edge of mediastinal pleura

Trachea

Left common carotid artery

Left internal jugular vein

Left subclavian artery

Left subclavian vein

Left internal thoracic vein

Left pericardiacophrenic vein

Arch of aorta

Ligamentum arteriosum

Left pulmonary artery

Left pulmonary veins

Pericardium

Cut edge of mediastinal pleura

Veins of the superior mediastinum

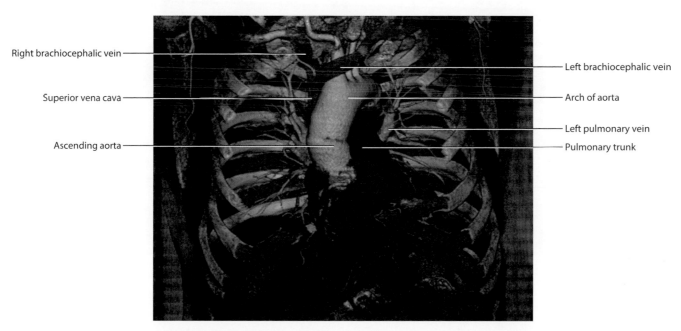

Right brachiocephalic vein

Superior vena cava

Ascending aorta

Left brachiocephalic vein

Arch of aorta

Left pulmonary vein

Pulmonary trunk

Anterior view of the superior mediastinum showing venous and arterial channels.
Volume-rendered anterior view using multidetector computed tomography

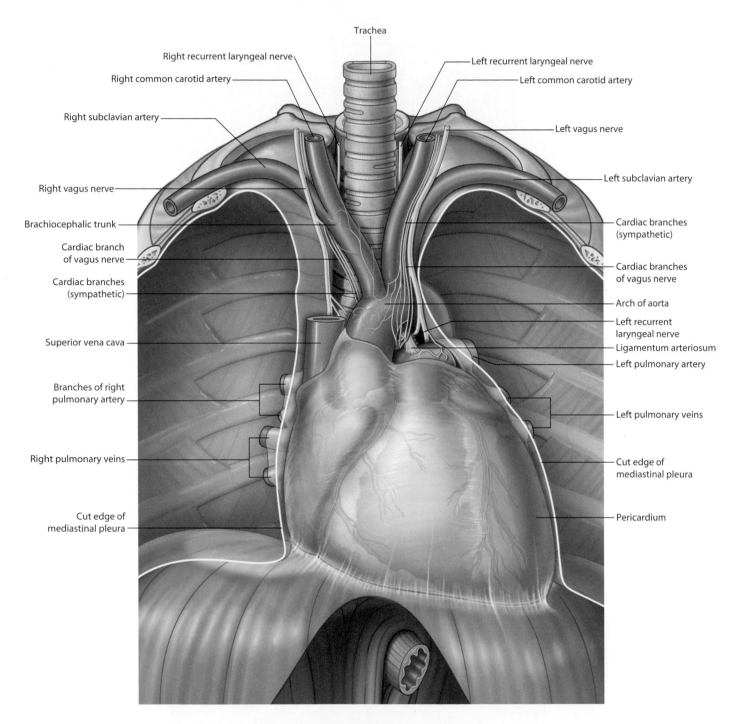

Trachea

Right recurrent laryngeal nerve

Right common carotid artery

Right subclavian artery

Right vagus nerve

Brachiocephalic trunk

Cardiac branch of vagus nerve

Cardiac branches (sympathetic)

Superior vena cava

Branches of right pulmonary artery

Right pulmonary veins

Cut edge of mediastinal pleura

Left recurrent laryngeal nerve

Left common carotid artery

Left vagus nerve

Left subclavian artery

Cardiac branches (sympathetic)

Cardiac branches of vagus nerve

Arch of aorta

Left recurrent laryngeal nerve

Ligamentum arteriosum

Left pulmonary artery

Left pulmonary veins

Cut edge of mediastinal pleura

Pericardium

Arteries and nerves of the superior mediastinum

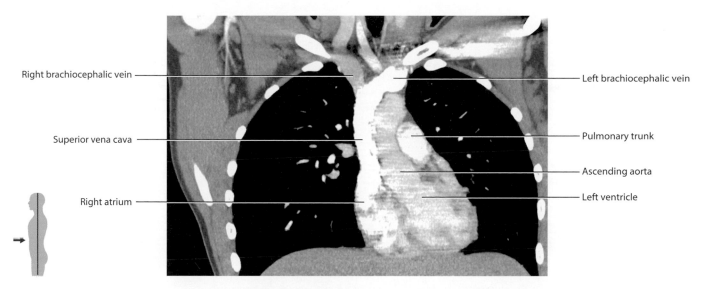

Right brachiocephalic vein

Superior vena cava

Right atrium

Left brachiocephalic vein

Pulmonary trunk

Ascending aorta

Left ventricle

Positioning of venous channels in the superior mediastinum.
CT image, with contrast, in coronal plane

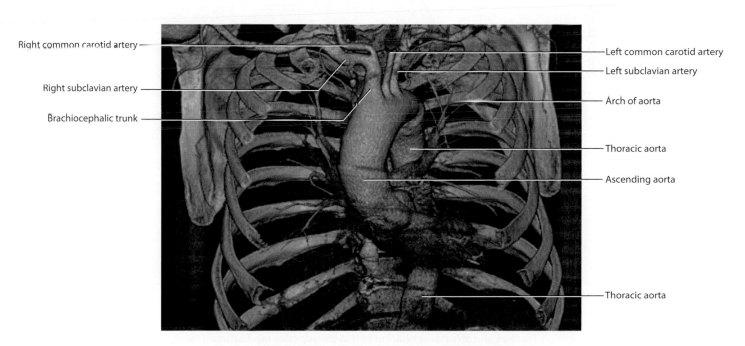

Right common carotid artery

Right subclavian artery

Brachiocephalic trunk

Left common carotid artery

Left subclavian artery

Arch of aorta

Thoracic aorta

Ascending aorta

Thoracic aorta

**Anterior view of the superior mediastinum with the venous
channels, pulmonary trunk, and heart removed.**
Volume-rendered anterior view using multidetector computed tomography

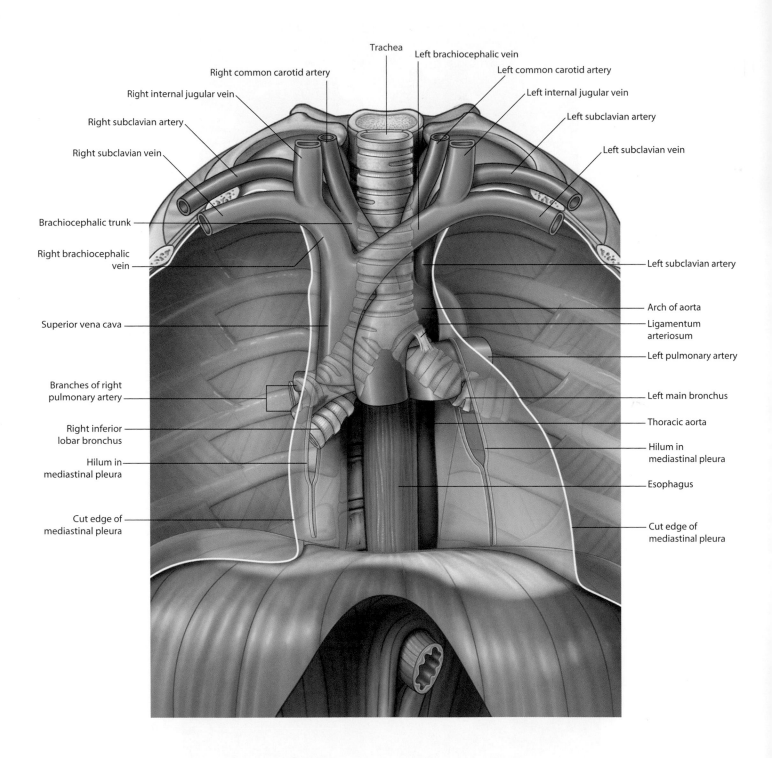

Right common carotid artery

Right internal jugular vein

Right subclavian artery

Right subclavian vein

Trachea

Left brachiocephalic vein

Left common carotid artery

Left internal jugular vein

Left subclavian artery

Left subclavian vein

Brachiocephalic trunk

Right brachiocephalic vein

Superior vena cava

Branches of right pulmonary artery

Right inferior lobar bronchus

Hilum in mediastinal pleura

Cut edge of mediastinal pleura

Left subclavian artery

Arch of aorta

Ligamentum arteriosum

Left pulmonary artery

Left main bronchus

Thoracic aorta

Hilum in mediastinal pleura

Esophagus

Cut edge of mediastinal pleura

Trachea and structures relating to it in the superior mediastinum

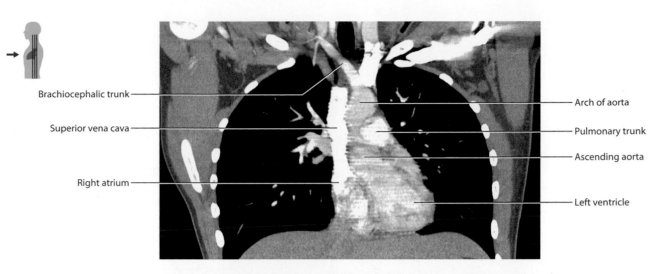

Brachiocephalic trunk

Superior vena cava

Right atrium

Arch of aorta

Pulmonary trunk

Ascending aorta

Left ventricle

Positioning of brachiocephalic trunk in relation to other structures in the superior mediastinum.
CT image, with contrast, in coronal plane

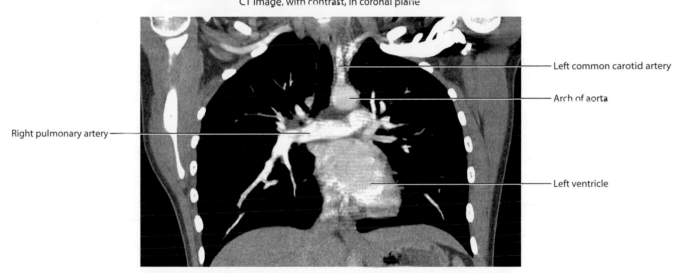

Right pulmonary artery

Left common carotid artery

Arch of aorta

Left ventricle

Positioning of left common carotid artery in relation to other structures in the superior mediastinum.
CT image, with contrast, in coronal plane

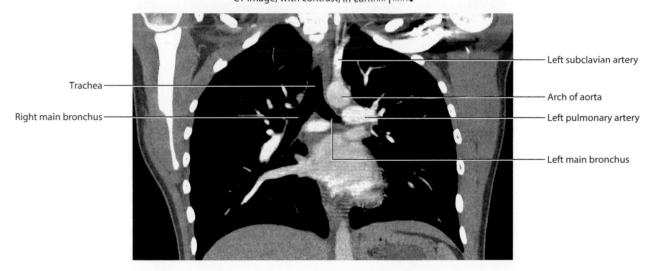

Trachea

Right main bronchus

Left subclavian artery

Arch of aorta

Left pulmonary artery

Left main bronchus

Positioning of left subclavian artery and the bifurcation of the trachea in relation to other structures in the superior mediastinum.
CT image, with contrast, in coronal plane

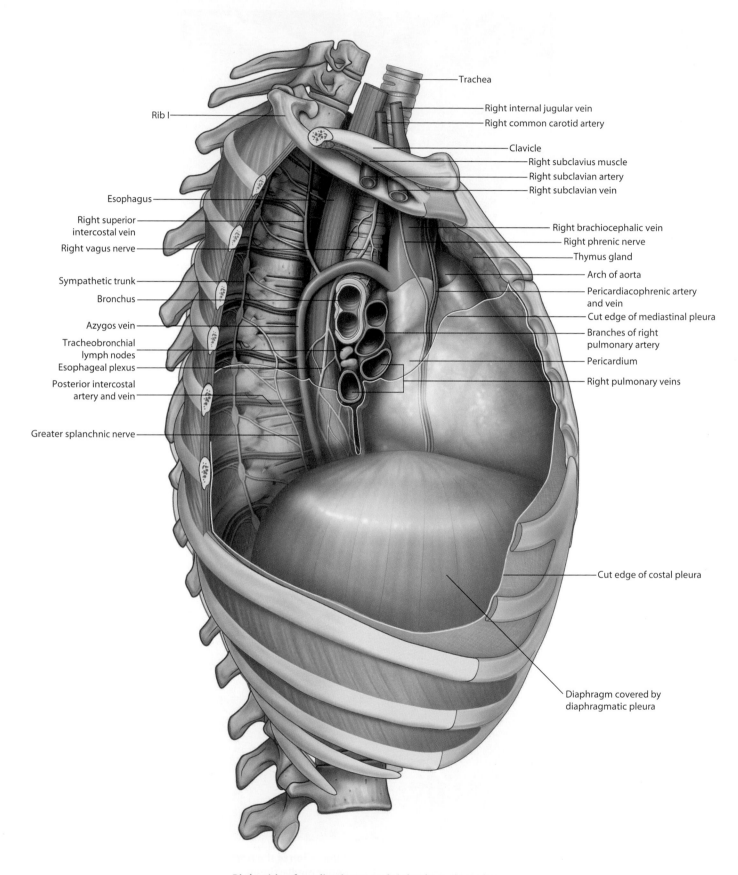

Trachea

Right internal jugular vein

Right common carotid artery

Rib I

Clavicle

Right subclavius muscle

Right subclavian artery

Right subclavian vein

Esophagus

Right superior intercostal vein

Right vagus nerve

Right brachiocephalic vein

Right phrenic nerve

Thymus gland

Sympathetic trunk

Arch of aorta

Bronchus

Pericardiacophrenic artery and vein

Azygos vein

Cut edge of mediastinal pleura

Tracheobronchial lymph nodes

Branches of right pulmonary artery

Esophageal plexus

Pericardium

Posterior intercostal artery and vein

Right pulmonary veins

Greater splanchnic nerve

Cut edge of costal pleura

Diaphragm covered by diaphragmatic pleura

Right side of mediastinum and right thoracic cavity

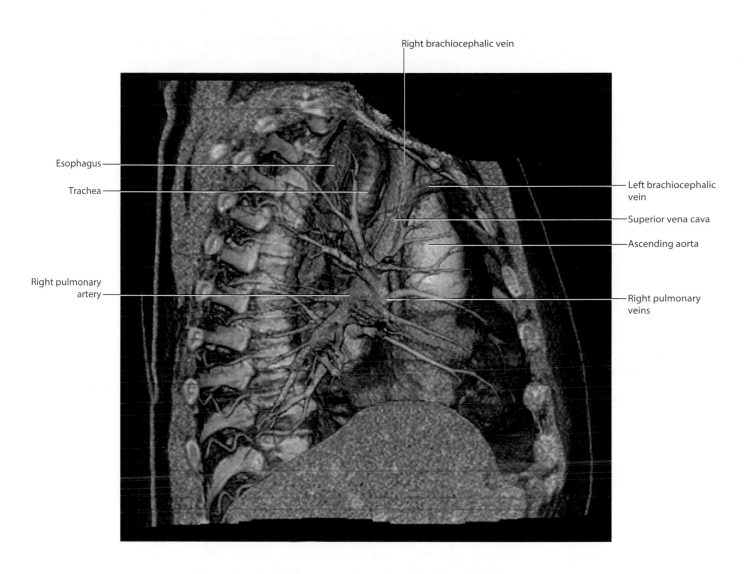

Right brachiocephalic vein

Esophagus

Trachea

Left brachiocephalic vein

Superior vena cava

Ascending aorta

Right pulmonary artery

Right pulmonary veins

View of mediastinal structures from the right side of the thorax.
Volume-rendered lateral view from the right side using multidetector computed tomography

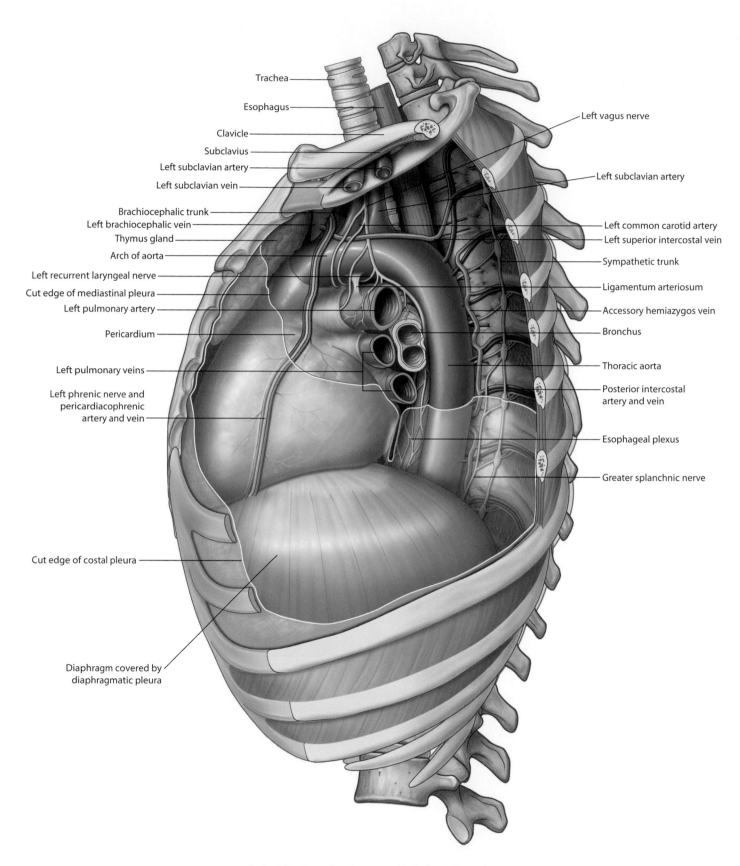

Trachea

Esophagus

Clavicle

Subclavius

Left subclavian artery

Left subclavian vein

Brachiocephalic trunk

Left brachiocephalic vein

Thymus gland

Arch of aorta

Left recurrent laryngeal nerve

Cut edge of mediastinal pleura

Left pulmonary artery

Pericardium

Left pulmonary veins

Left phrenic nerve and pericardiacophrenic artery and vein

Cut edge of costal pleura

Diaphragm covered by diaphragmatic pleura

Left vagus nerve

Left subclavian artery

Left common carotid artery

Left superior intercostal vein

Sympathetic trunk

Ligamentum arteriosum

Accessory hemiazygos vein

Bronchus

Thoracic aorta

Posterior intercostal artery and vein

Esophageal plexus

Greater splanchnic nerve

Left side of mediastinum and left thoracic cavity

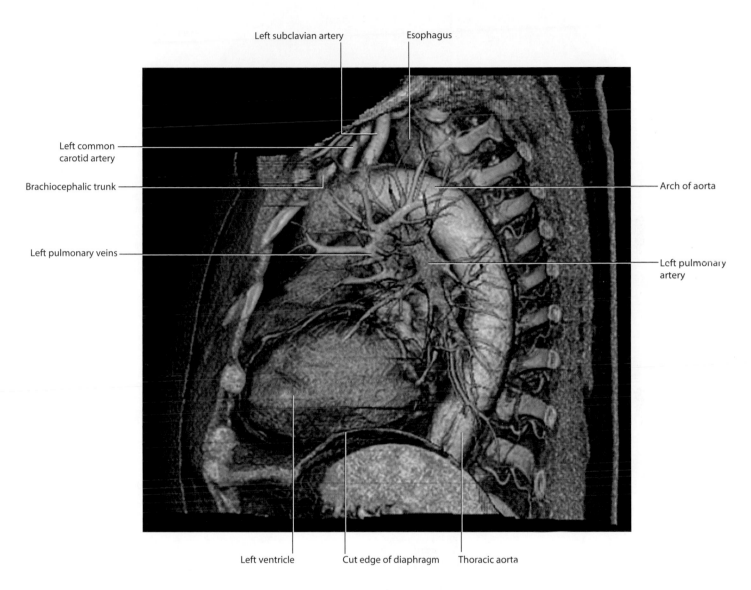

Left subclavian artery   Esophagus

Left common carotid artery

Brachiocephalic trunk

Left pulmonary veins

Arch of aorta

Left pulmonary artery

Left ventricle   Cut edge of diaphragm   Thoracic aorta

View of mediastinal structures from the left side of the thorax.
Volume-rendered lateral view from the left side using multidetector computed tomography

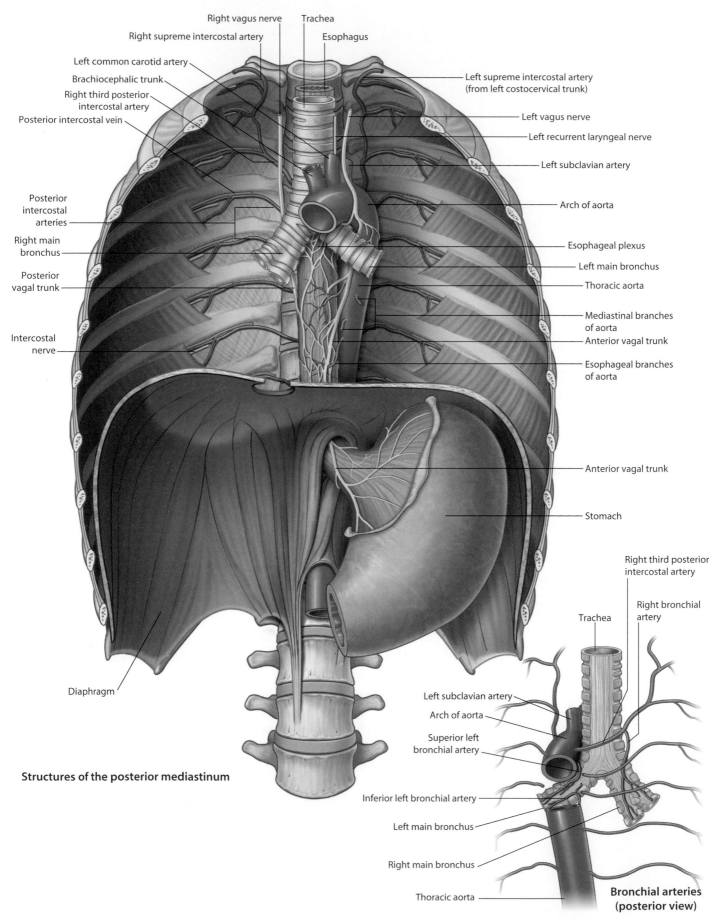

Right vagus nerve

Right supreme intercostal artery

Trachea

Esophagus

Left common carotid artery

Brachiocephalic trunk

Right third posterior intercostal artery

Posterior intercostal vein

Left supreme intercostal artery (from left costocervical trunk)

Left vagus nerve

Left recurrent laryngeal nerve

Left subclavian artery

Posterior intercostal arteries

Right main bronchus

Posterior vagal trunk

Arch of aorta

Esophageal plexus

Left main bronchus

Thoracic aorta

Mediastinal branches of aorta

Anterior vagal trunk

Esophageal branches of aorta

Intercostal nerve

Anterior vagal trunk

Stomach

Diaphragm

Structures of the posterior mediastinum

Right third posterior intercostal artery

Right bronchial artery

Trachea

Left subclavian artery

Arch of aorta

Superior left bronchial artery

Inferior left bronchial artery

Left main bronchus

Right main bronchus

Thoracic aorta

Bronchial arteries (posterior view)

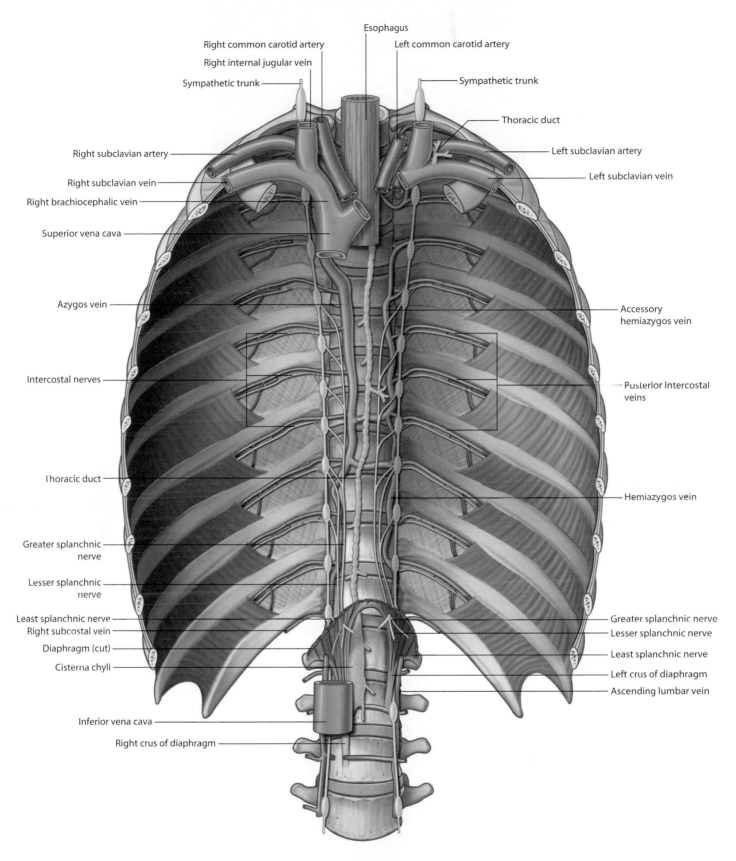

Esophagus

Right common carotid artery

Left common carotid artery

Right internal jugular vein

Sympathetic trunk

Sympathetic trunk

Thoracic duct

Right subclavian artery

Left subclavian artery

Right subclavian vein

Left subclavian vein

Right brachiocephalic vein

Superior vena cava

Azygos vein

Accessory hemiazygos vein

Posterior intercostal veins

Intercostal nerves

Thoracic duct

Hemiazygos vein

Greater splanchnic nerve

Lesser splanchnic nerve

Least splanchnic nerve

Greater splanchnic nerve

Right subcostal vein

Lesser splanchnic nerve

Diaphragm (cut)

Least splanchnic nerve

Cisterna chyli

Left crus of diaphragm

Ascending lumbar vein

Inferior vena cava

Right crus of diaphragm

**Structures of the posterior mediastinum
(thoracic aorta and esophagus removed)**

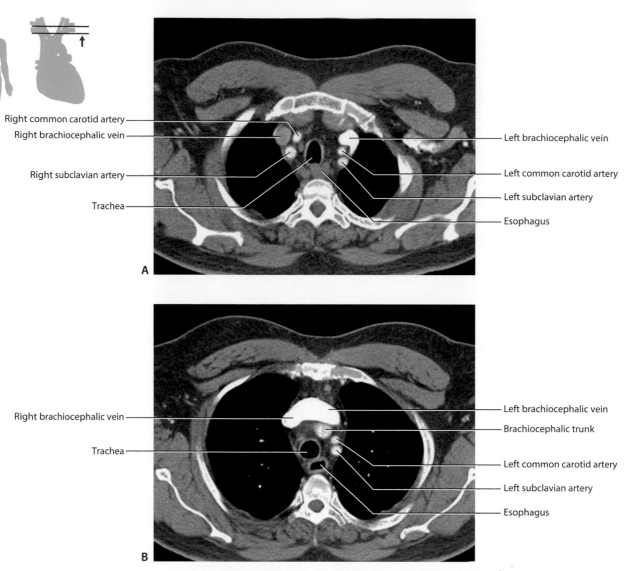

Right common carotid artery
Right brachiocephalic vein
Right subclavian artery
Trachea

Left brachiocephalic vein
Left common carotid artery
Left subclavian artery
Esophagus

A

Right brachiocephalic vein
Trachea

Left brachiocephalic vein
Brachiocephalic trunk
Left common carotid artery
Left subclavian artery
Esophagus

B

A through I – This is a series of images that pass through the thorax from superior to inferior showing the various mediastinal structures and their relationships with each other.
CT images, with contrast, in axial plane

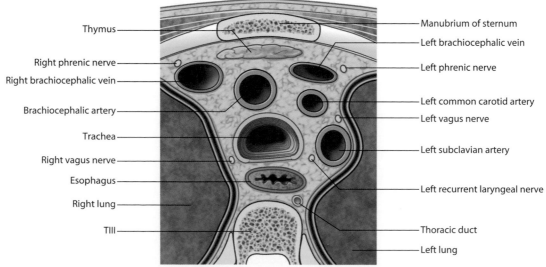

Thymus
Right phrenic nerve
Right brachiocephalic vein
Brachiocephalic artery
Trachea
Right vagus nerve
Esophagus
Right lung
TIII

Manubrium of sternum
Left brachiocephalic vein
Left phrenic nerve
Left common carotid artery
Left vagus nerve
Left subclavian artery
Left recurrent laryngeal nerve
Thoracic duct
Left lung

Transverse section through the superior mediastinum at the level of vertebra TIII

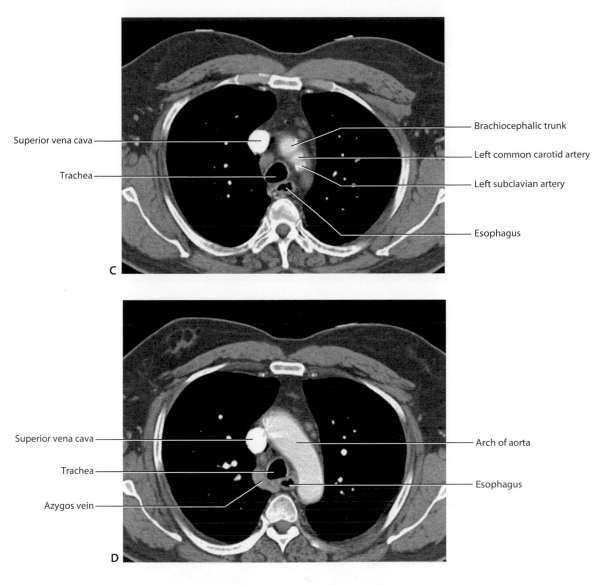

C

- Superior vena cava
- Trachea
- Brachiocephalic trunk
- Left common carotid artery
- Left subclavian artery
- Esophagus

D

- Superior vena cava
- Trachea
- Azygos vein
- Arch of aorta
- Esophagus

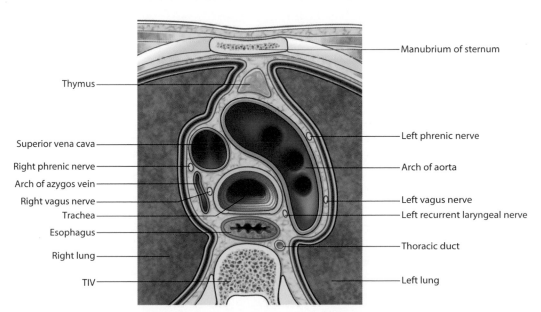

- Manubrium of sternum
- Thymus
- Superior vena cava
- Right phrenic nerve
- Arch of azygos vein
- Right vagus nerve
- Trachea
- Esophagus
- Right lung
- TIV
- Left phrenic nerve
- Arch of aorta
- Left vagus nerve
- Left recurrent laryngeal nerve
- Thoracic duct
- Left lung

Transverse section through the superior mediastinum at the level of vertebra TIV

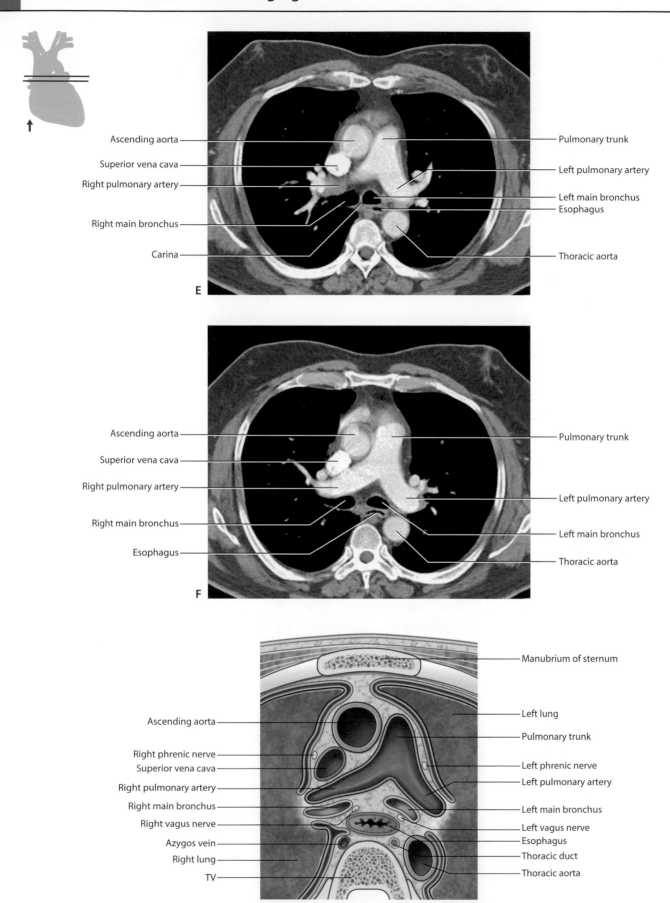

Ascending aorta — Pulmonary trunk
Superior vena cava — Left pulmonary artery
Right pulmonary artery — Left main bronchus
— Esophagus
Right main bronchus —
Carina — Thoracic aorta

E

Ascending aorta — Pulmonary trunk
Superior vena cava —
Right pulmonary artery — Left pulmonary artery
Right main bronchus — Left main bronchus
Esophagus — Thoracic aorta

F

Manubrium of sternum
Ascending aorta — Left lung
— Pulmonary trunk
Right phrenic nerve — Left phrenic nerve
Superior vena cava —
Right pulmonary artery — Left pulmonary artery
Right main bronchus — Left main bronchus
Right vagus nerve — Left vagus nerve
Azygos vein — Esophagus
Right lung — Thoracic duct
TV — Thoracic aorta

Transverse section through the superior mediastinum at the level of vertebra TV

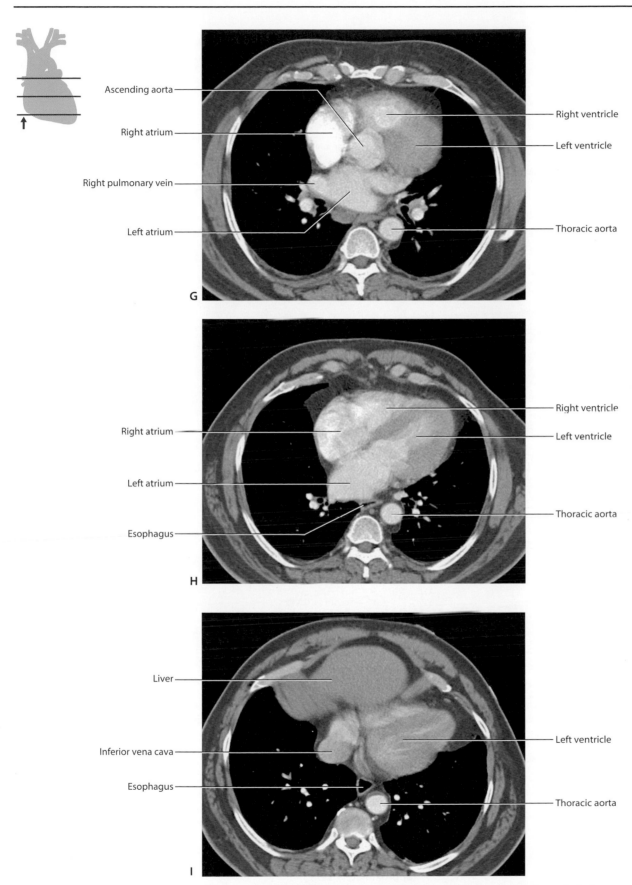

Ascending aorta

Right atrium

Right pulmonary vein

Left atrium

Right ventricle

Left ventricle

Thoracic aorta

G

Right atrium

Left atrium

Esophagus

Right ventricle

Left ventricle

Thoracic aorta

H

Liver

Inferior vena cava

Esophagus

Left ventricle

Thoracic aorta

I

A through I – This is a series of images that pass through the thorax from superior to inferior showing the various mediastinal structures and their relationships with each other.
CT images, with contrast, in axial plane

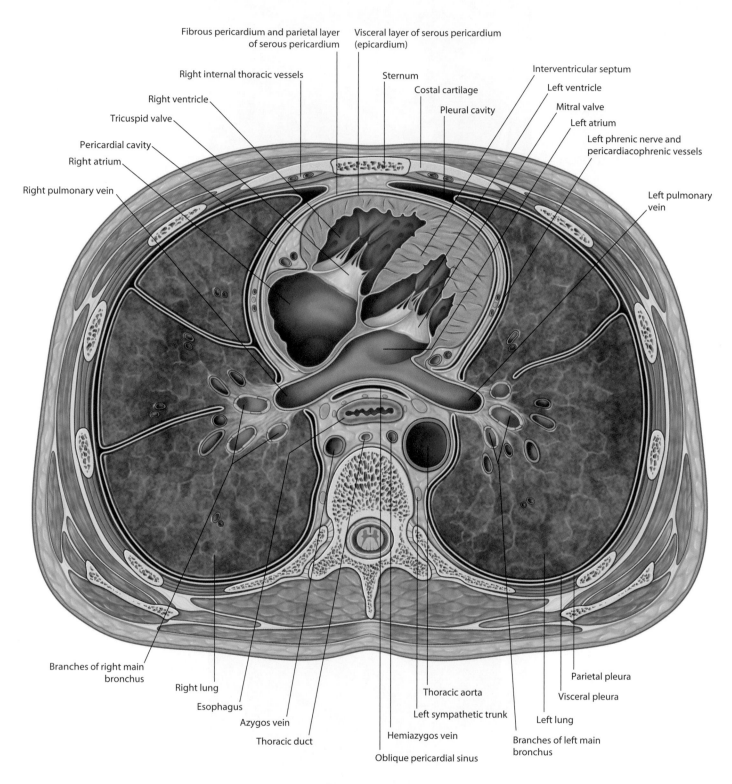

Fibrous pericardium and parietal layer of serous pericardium

Visceral layer of serous pericardium (epicardium)

Right internal thoracic vessels

Sternum

Interventricular septum

Right ventricle

Costal cartilage

Left ventricle

Tricuspid valve

Pleural cavity

Mitral valve

Pericardial cavity

Left atrium

Right atrium

Left phrenic nerve and pericardiacophrenic vessels

Right pulmonary vein

Left pulmonary vein

Branches of right main bronchus

Right lung

Esophagus

Azygos vein

Thoracic duct

Oblique pericardial sinus

Hemiazygos vein

Left sympathetic trunk

Thoracic aorta

Branches of left main bronchus

Left lung

Visceral pleura

Parietal pleura

**Transverse section through thorax
(approximately TVII)**

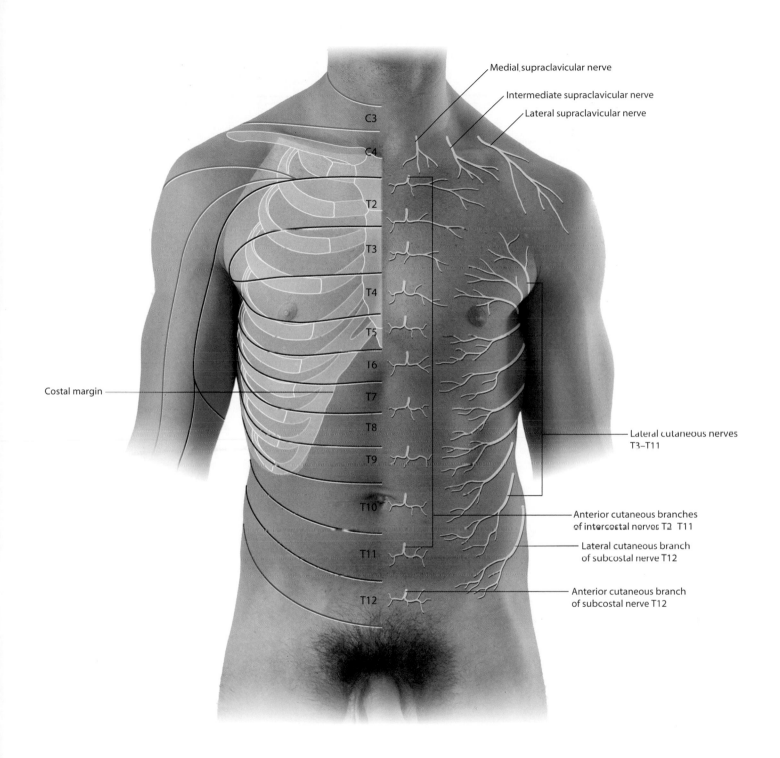

Medial supraclavicular nerve

Intermediate supraclavicular nerve

Lateral supraclavicular nerve

C3

C4

T2

T3

T4

T5

I6

T7

T8

T9

T10

T11

T12

Costal margin

Lateral cutaneous nerves T3–T11

Anterior cutaneous branches of intercostal nerves T2–T11

Lateral cutaneous branch of subcostal nerve T12

Anterior cutaneous branch of subcostal nerve T12

Dermatomes and cutaneous nerves of the thoracic region

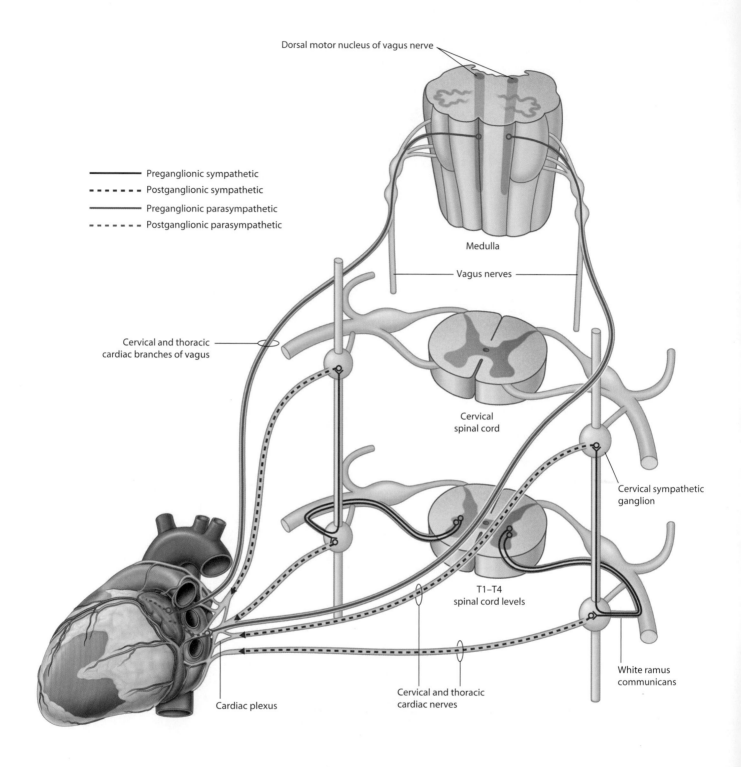

Dorsal motor nucleus of vagus nerve

Preganglionic sympathetic
Postganglionic sympathetic
Preganglionic parasympathetic
Postganglionic parasympathetic

Medulla

Vagus nerves

Cervical and thoracic
cardiac branches of vagus

Cervical
spinal cord

Cervical sympathetic
ganglion

T1–T4
spinal cord levels

White ramus
communicans

Cardiac plexus

Cervical and thoracic
cardiac nerves

**Visceral efferent (motor) innervation of the heart
(sympathetic and parasympathetic)**

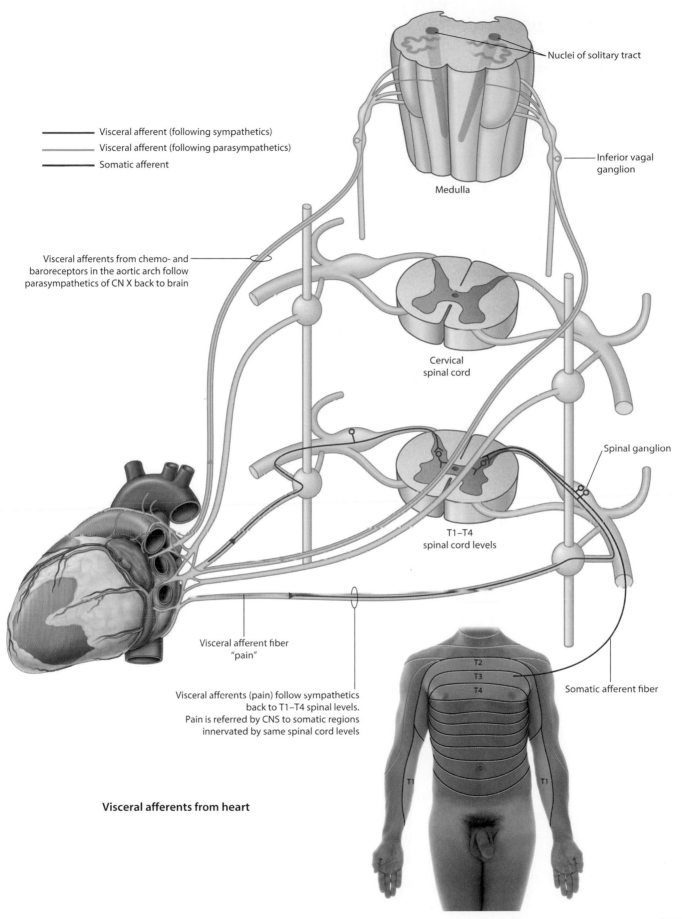

Nuclei of solitary tract

Visceral afferent (following sympathetics)
Visceral afferent (following parasympathetics)
Somatic afferent

Inferior vagal ganglion

Medulla

Visceral afferents from chemo- and baroreceptors in the aortic arch follow parasympathetics of CN X back to brain

Cervical spinal cord

Spinal ganglion

T1–T4 spinal cord levels

Visceral afferent fiber "pain"

Visceral afferents (pain) follow sympathetics back to T1–T4 spinal levels. Pain is referred by CNS to somatic regions innervated by same spinal cord levels

Somatic afferent fiber

T2
T3
T4
T1   T1

Visceral afferents from heart

Muscles of the pectoral region

Muscle		Origin	Insertion	Innervation	Function
Pectoralis major	1	Medial half of clavicle and anterior surface of sternum, first seven costal cartilages, aponeurosis of external oblique	Lateral lip of intertubercular sulcus of humerus	Medial and lateral pectoral nerves	Adduction, medial rotation, and flexion of the humerus at the shoulder joint
Subclavius	2	Rib I at junction between rib and costal cartilage	Groove on inferior surface of middle third of clavicle	Nerve to subclavius	Pulls clavicle medially to stabilize sternoclavicular joint; depresses tip of shoulder
Pectoralis minor	3	Anterior surfaces of the third, fourth and fifth ribs, and deep fascia overlying the related intercostal spaces	Coracoid process of scapula	Medial pectoral nerves	Depresses tip of shoulder; protracts scapula

Muscles of the thoracic wall

Muscle		Origin	Insertion	Innervation	Function
External intercostal	4	Inferior margin of rib above	Superior margin of rib below	Intercostal nerves; T1–T11	Most active during inspiration; supports intercostal space; moves ribs superiorly
Internal intercostal	5	Lateral edge of costal groove of rib above	Superior margin of rib below deep to the attachment of the related external intercostal	Intercostal nerves; T1–T11	Most active during expiration; supports intercostal space; moves ribs inferiorly
Innermost intercostal	6	Medial edge of costal groove of rib above	Internal aspect of superior margin of rib below	Intercostal nerves; T1–T11	Acts with internal intercostal muscles
Subcostales	7	Internal surface (near angle) of lower ribs	Internal surface of second or third rib below	Related intercostal nerves	May depress ribs
Transversus thoracis	8	Inferior margins and internal surfaces of costal cartilages of second to sixth ribs	Inferior aspect of deep surface of body of sternum, xiphoid process and costal cartilages ribs IV–VII	Related intercostal nerves	Depresses costal cartilages

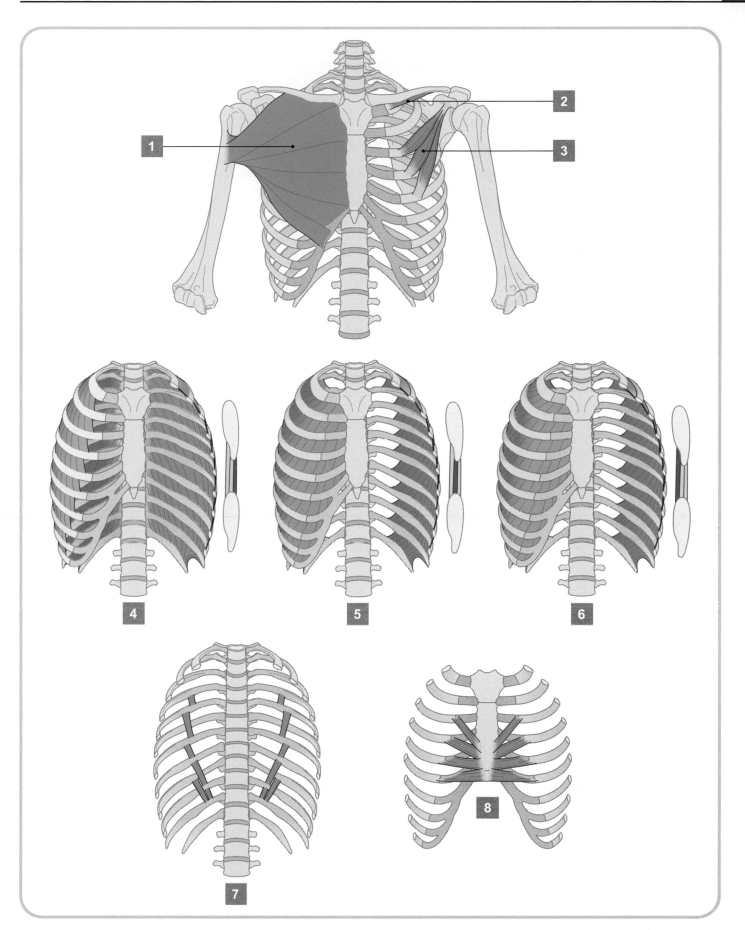

Branches of the thoracic aorta

Branches		Origin and course
Pericardial branches	1	A few small vessels to the posterior surface of the pericardial sac
Bronchial branches	2	Vary in number, size, and origin—usually, two left bronchial arteries from the thoracic aorta and one right bronchial artery from the third posterior intercostal artery or the superior left bronchial artery
Esophageal branches	3	Four or five vessels from the anterior aspect of the thoracic aorta, which form a continuous anastomotic chain—anastomotic connections include esophageal branches of the inferior thyroid artery superiorly, and esophageal branches of the left inferior phrenic and the left gastric arteries inferiorly
Mediastinal branches	4	Several small branches supplying lymph nodes, vessels, nerves, and areolar tissue in the posterior mediastinum
Posterior intercostal arteries	5	Usually nine pairs of vessels branching from the posterior surface of the thoracic aorta—usually supply lower nine intercostal spaces (first two spaces are supplied by the supreme intercostal artery—a branch of the costocervical trunk)
Superior phrenic arteries	6	Small vessels from the lower part of the thoracic aorta supplying the posterior part of the superior surface of the diaphragm—they anastomose with the musculophrenic and pericardiacophrenic arteries
Subcostal artery	7	The lowest pair of branches from the thoracic aorta located inferior to rib XII

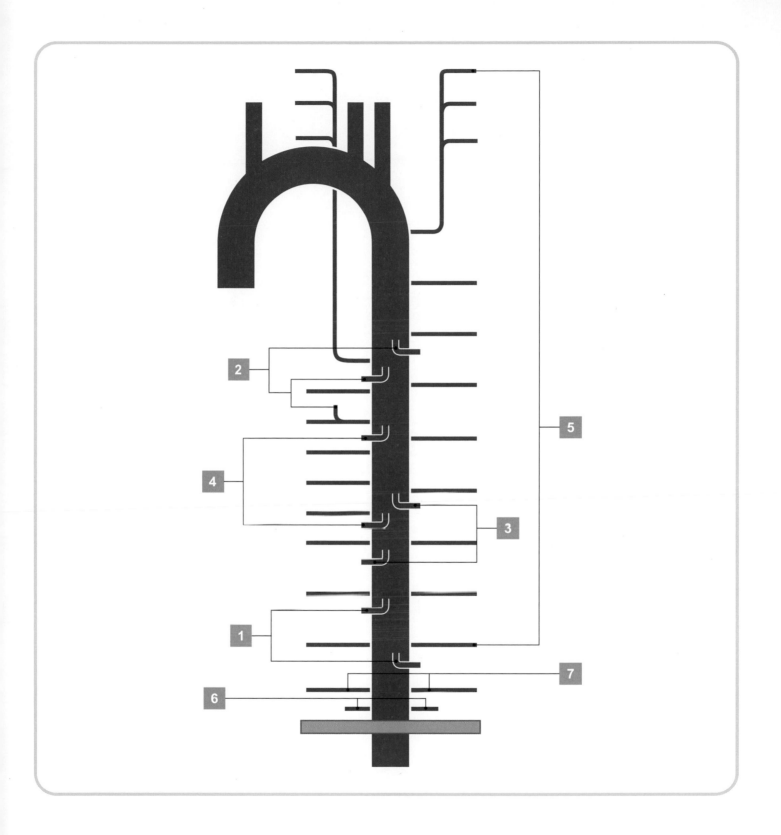

4 ABDOMEN

CONTENTS

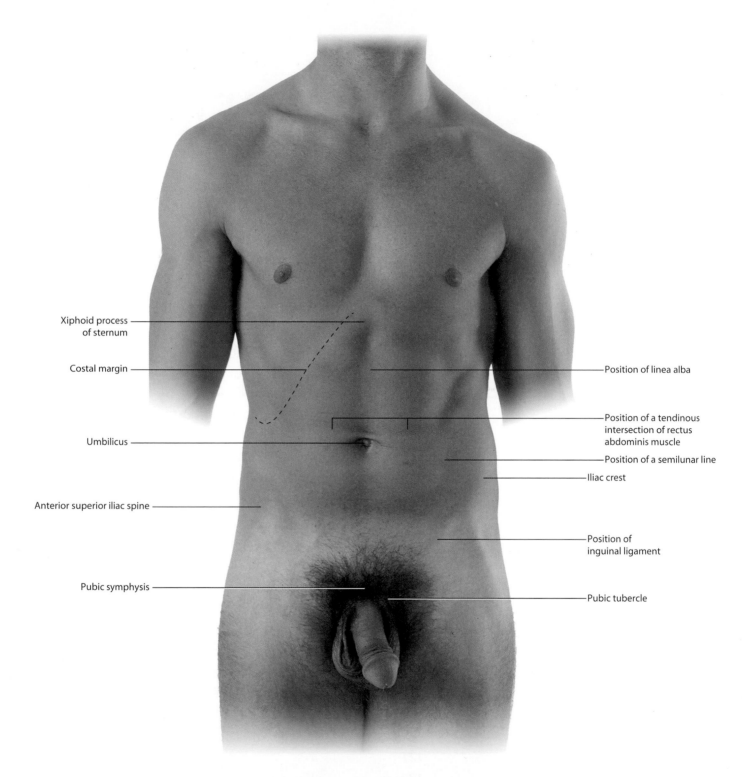

Xiphoid process
of sternum

Costal margin

Umbilicus

Anterior superior iliac spine

Pubic symphysis

Position of linea alba

Position of a tendinous
intersection of rectus
abdominis muscle

Position of a semilunar line

Iliac crest

Position of
inguinal ligament

Pubic tubercle

Anterior abdominal wall surface anatomy

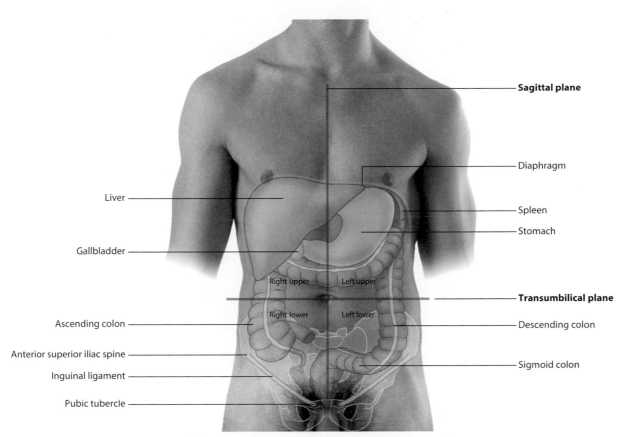

Sagittal plane

Diaphragm

Liver

Spleen

Stomach

Gallbladder

Right upper | Left upper

Transumbilical plane

Ascending colon

Right lower | Left lower

Descending colon

Anterior superior iliac spine

Inguinal ligament

Sigmoid colon

Pubic tubercle

Abdominal quadrants and the positions of major viscera

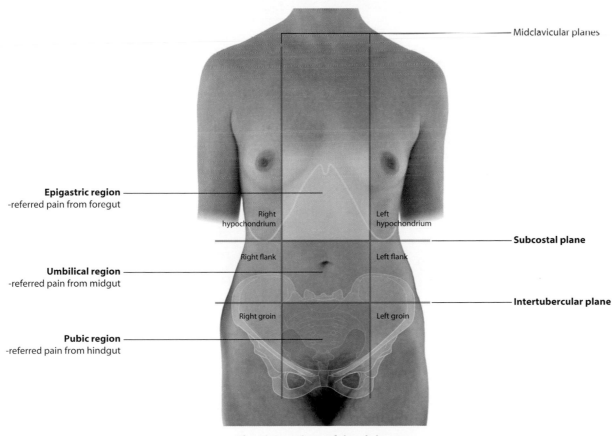

Midclavicular planes

Epigastric region
-referred pain from foregut

Right
hypochondrium

Left
hypochondrium

Subcostal plane

Right flank | Left flank

Umbilical region
-referred pain from midgut

Intertubercular plane

Right groin | Left groin

Pubic region
-referred pain from hindgut

The nine regions of the abdomen

135

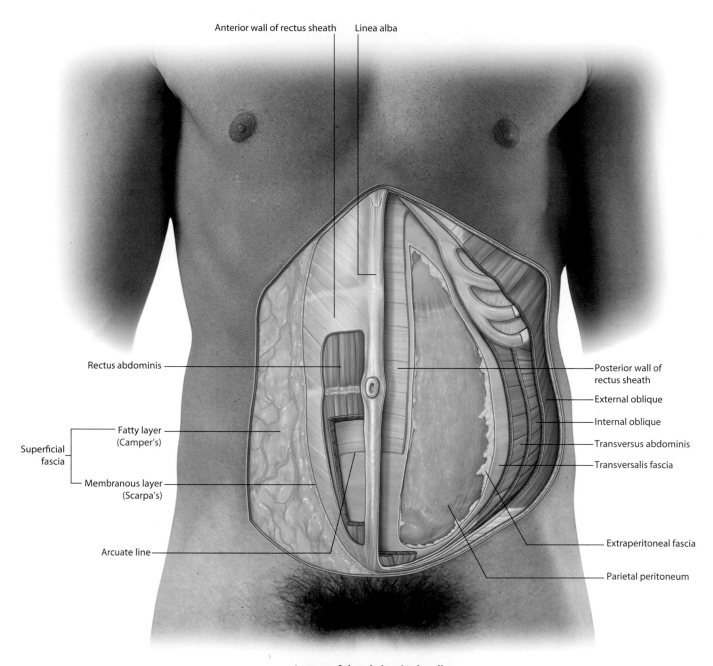

Anterior wall of rectus sheath

Linea alba

Rectus abdominis

Posterior wall of rectus sheath

External oblique

Internal oblique

Transversus abdominis

Transversalis fascia

Superficial fascia

Fatty layer (Camper's)

Membranous layer (Scarpa's)

Arcuate line

Extraperitoneal fascia

Parietal peritoneum

Layers of the abdominal wall

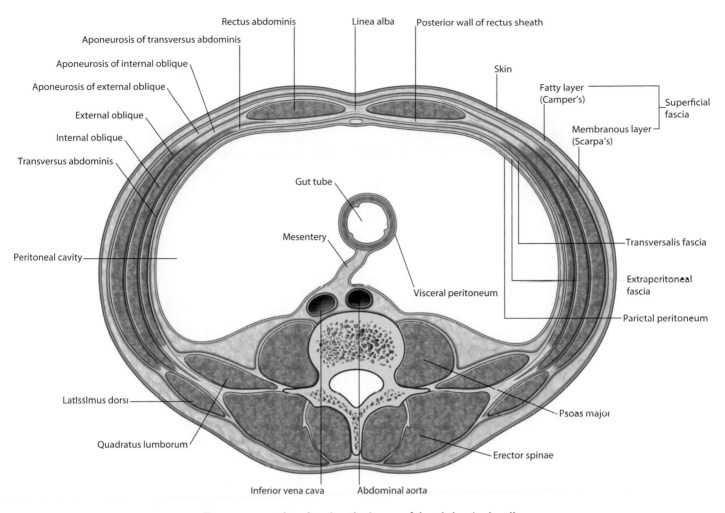

Rectus abdominis
Aponeurosis of transversus abdominis
Aponeurosis of internal oblique
Aponeurosis of external oblique
External oblique
Internal oblique
Transversus abdominis
Peritoneal cavity
Latissimus dorsi
Quadratus lumborum
Inferior vena cava
Abdominal aorta
Erector spinae
Psoas major
Parietal peritoneum
Extraperitoneal fascia
Transversalis fascia
Visceral peritoneum
Mesentery
Gut tube
Membranous layer (Scarpa's)
Superficial fascia
Fatty layer (Camper's)
Skin
Posterior wall of rectus sheath
Linea alba

Transverse section showing the layers of the abdominal wall (above umbilicus)

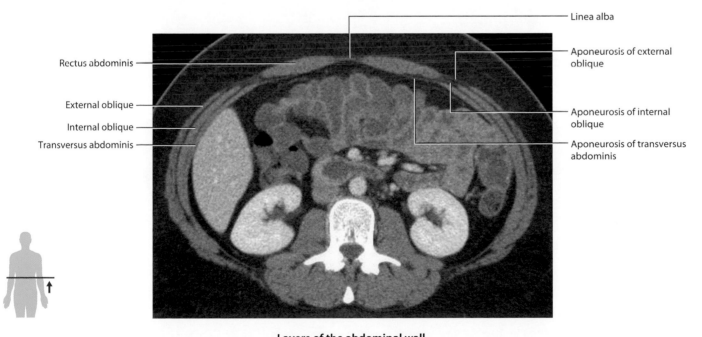

Linea alba
Rectus abdominis
External oblique
Internal oblique
Transversus abdominis
Aponeurosis of external oblique
Aponeurosis of internal oblique
Aponeurosis of transversus abdominis

Layers of the abdominal wall.
CT image, with contrast, in axial plane

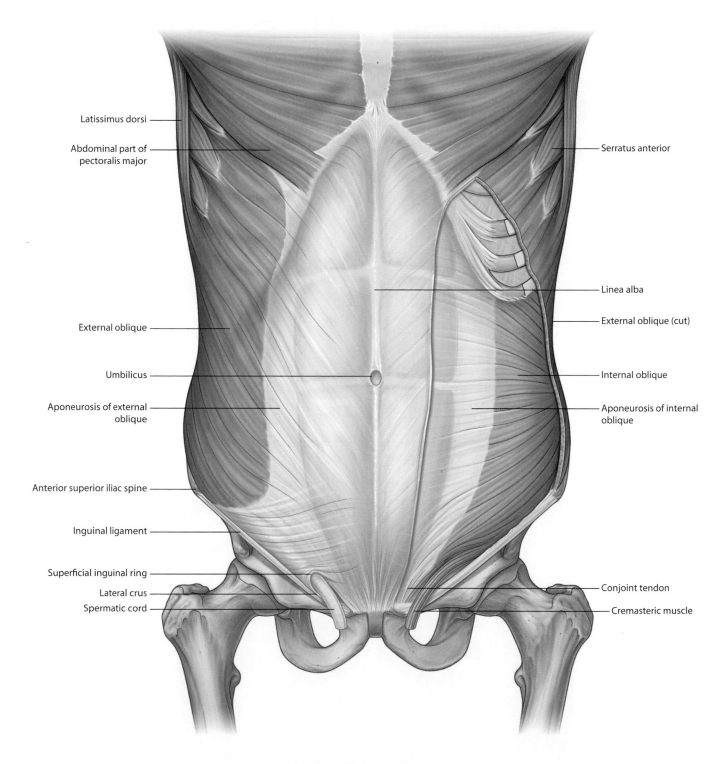

Latissimus dorsi

Abdominal part of pectoralis major

Serratus anterior

Linea alba

External oblique

External oblique (cut)

Umbilicus

Internal oblique

Aponeurosis of external oblique

Aponeurosis of internal oblique

Anterior superior iliac spine

Inguinal ligament

Superficial inguinal ring

Conjoint tendon

Lateral crus

Spermatic cord

Cremasteric muscle

External and internal oblique muscles

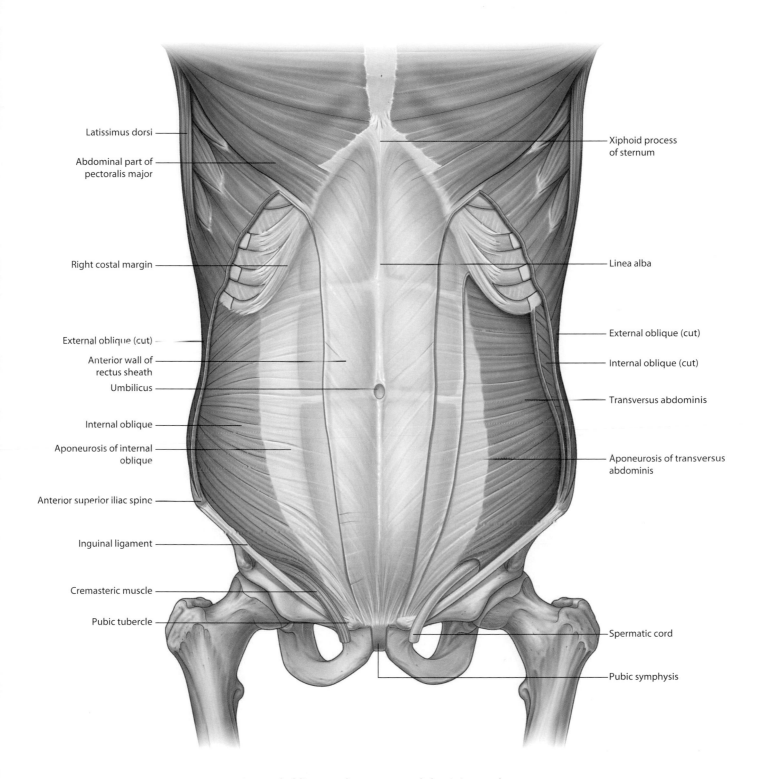

Internal oblique and transversus abdominis muscles

Latissimus dorsi

Abdominal part of pectoralis major

Right costal margin

External oblique (cut)

Anterior wall of rectus sheath

Umbilicus

Internal oblique

Aponeurosis of internal oblique

Anterior superior iliac spine

Inguinal ligament

Cremasteric muscle

Pubic tubercle

Xiphoid process of sternum

Linea alba

External oblique (cut)

Internal oblique (cut)

Transversus abdominis

Aponeurosis of transversus abdominis

Spermatic cord

Pubic symphysis

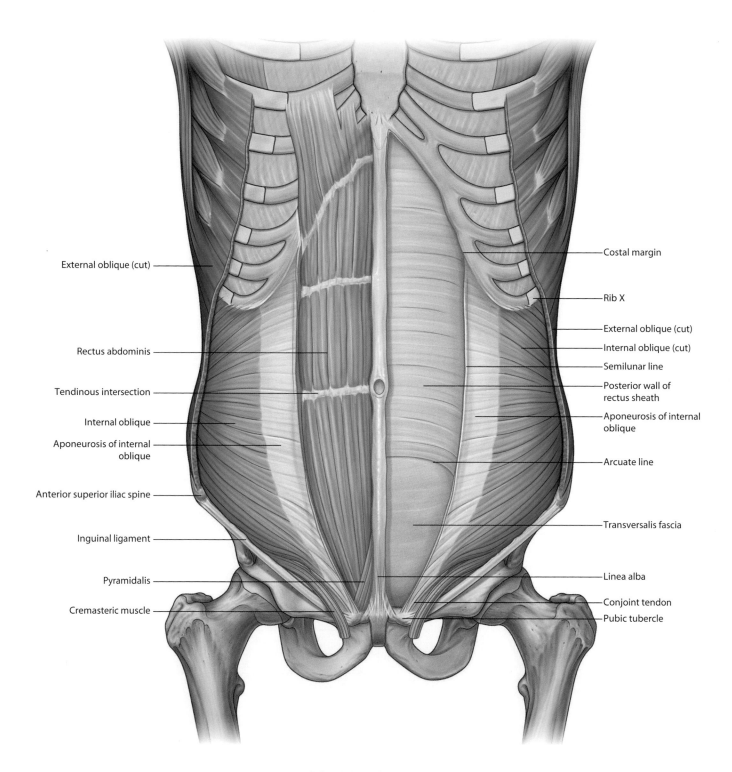

External oblique (cut)

Rectus abdominis

Tendinous intersection

Internal oblique

Aponeurosis of internal oblique

Anterior superior iliac spine

Inguinal ligament

Pyramidalis

Cremasteric muscle

Costal margin

Rib X

External oblique (cut)

Internal oblique (cut)

Semilunar line

Posterior wall of rectus sheath

Aponeurosis of internal oblique

Arcuate line

Transversalis fascia

Linea alba

Conjoint tendon

Pubic tubercle

Rectus abdominis and pyramidalis muscles

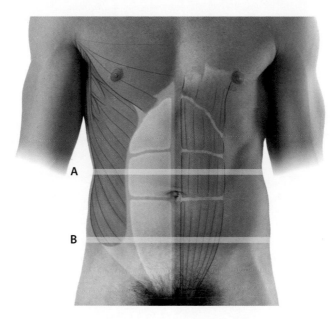

Organization of the rectus sheath.
A. Transverse section through the upper three quarters of the rectus sheath
B. Transverse section through the lower one quarter of the rectus sheath

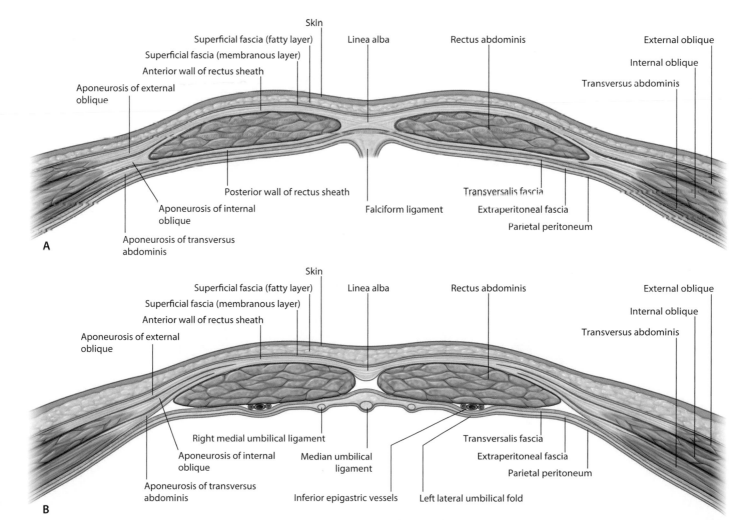

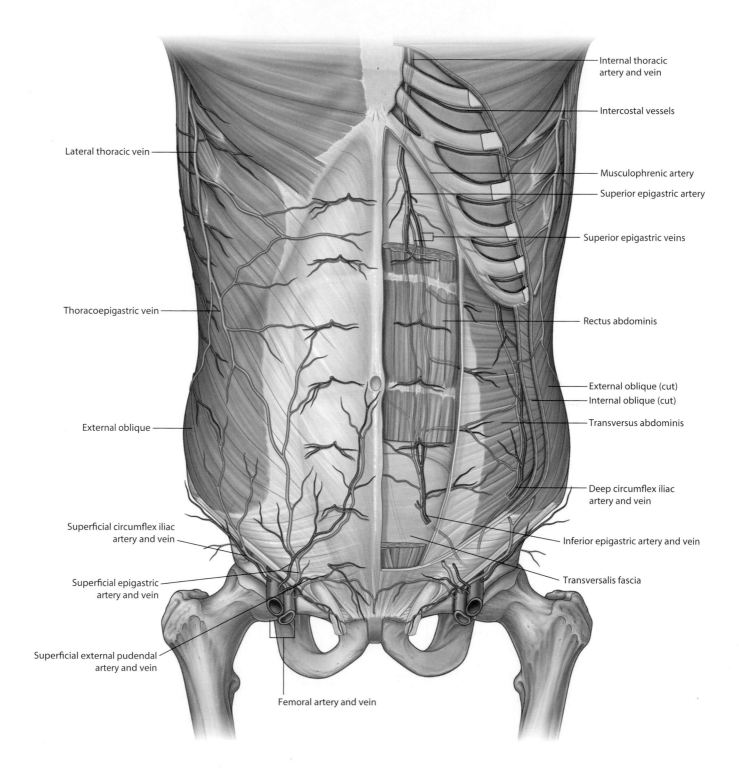

Internal thoracic artery and vein

Intercostal vessels

Musculophrenic artery

Superior epigastric artery

Superior epigastric veins

Rectus abdominis

External oblique (cut)

Internal oblique (cut)

Transversus abdominis

Deep circumflex iliac artery and vein

Inferior epigastric artery and vein

Transversalis fascia

Lateral thoracic vein

Thoracoepigastric vein

External oblique

Superficial circumflex iliac artery and vein

Superficial epigastric artery and vein

Superficial external pudendal artery and vein

Femoral artery and vein

Vasculature of the anterior abdominal wall

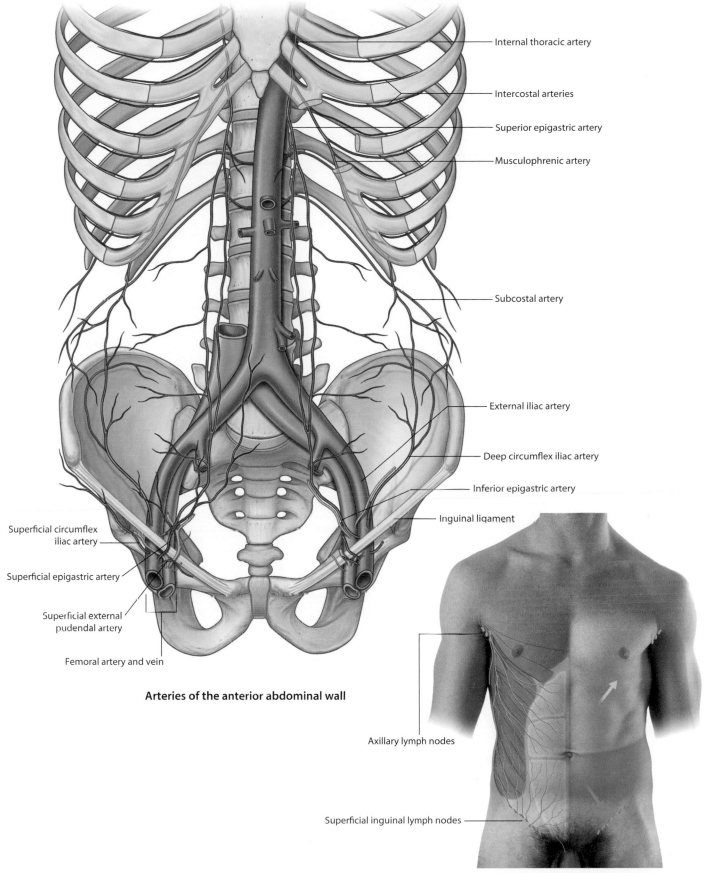

Internal thoracic artery

Intercostal arteries

Superior epigastric artery

Musculophrenic artery

Subcostal artery

External iliac artery

Deep circumflex iliac artery

Inferior epigastric artery

Inguinal ligament

Superficial circumflex iliac artery

Superficial epigastric artery

Superficial external pudendal artery

Femoral artery and vein

Arteries of the anterior abdominal wall

Axillary lymph nodes

Superficial inguinal lymph nodes

Superficial lymphatic drainage of the anterolateral abdominal wall

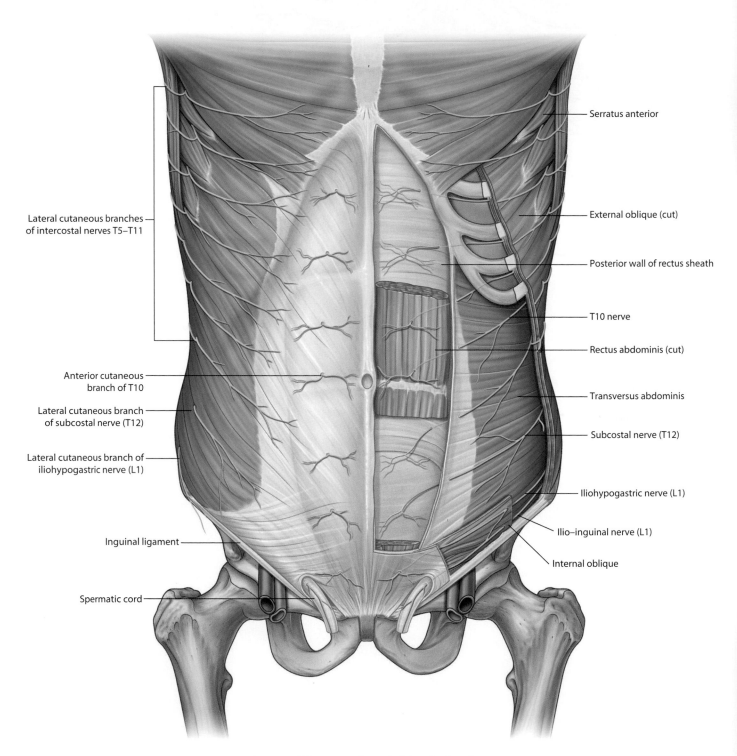

Lateral cutaneous branches
of intercostal nerves T5–T11

Anterior cutaneous
branch of T10

Lateral cutaneous branch
of subcostal nerve (T12)

Lateral cutaneous branch of
iliohypogastric nerve (L1)

Inguinal ligament

Spermatic cord

Serratus anterior

External oblique (cut)

Posterior wall of rectus sheath

T10 nerve

Rectus abdominis (cut)

Transversus abdominis

Subcostal nerve (T12)

Iliohypogastric nerve (L1)

Ilio–inguinal nerve (L1)

Internal oblique

Nerves of the anterolateral abdominal wall

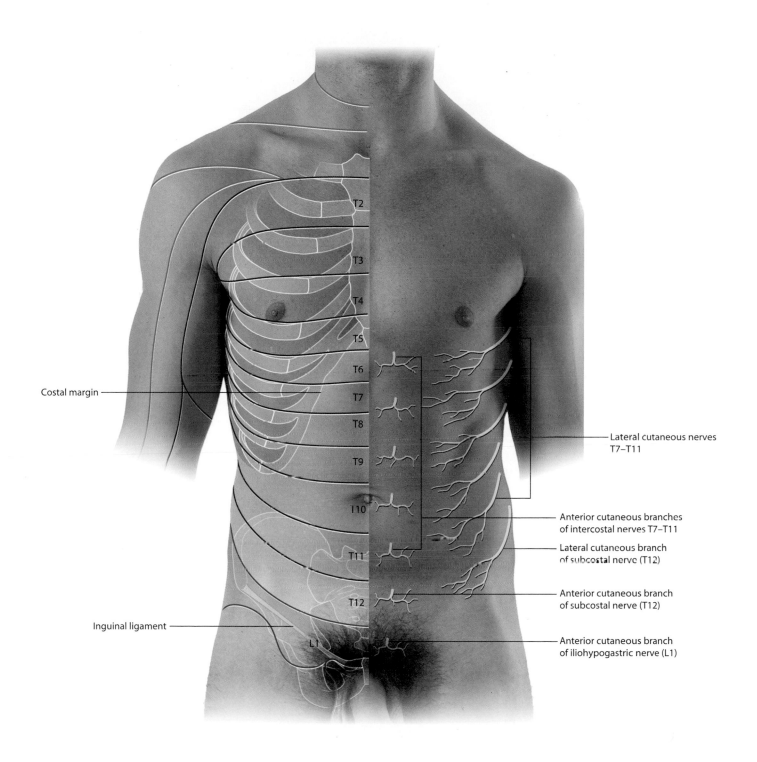

T2

T3

T4

T5

T6

Costal margin

T7

T8

T9

I10

T11

T12

Inguinal ligament

L1

Lateral cutaneous nerves
T7–T11

Anterior cutaneous branches
of intercostal nerves T7–T11

Lateral cutaneous branch
of subcostal nerve (T12)

Anterior cutaneous branch
of subcostal nerve (T12)

Anterior cutaneous branch
of iliohypogastric nerve (L1)

Dermatomes and cutaneous nerves of the anterolateral abdominal wall

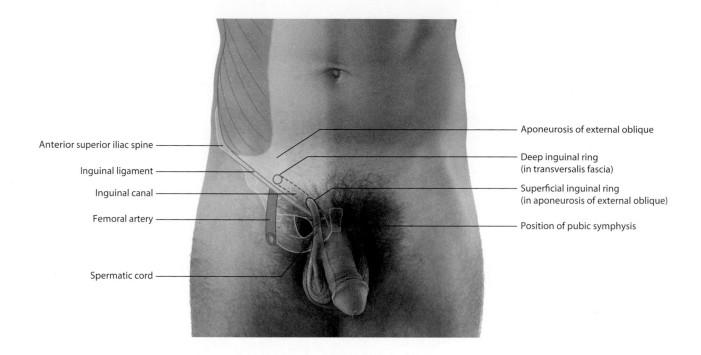

Anterior superior iliac spine

Inguinal ligament

Inguinal canal

Femoral artery

Spermatic cord

Aponeurosis of external oblique

Deep inguinal ring
(in transversalis fascia)

Superficial inguinal ring
(in aponeurosis of external oblique)

Position of pubic symphysis

Inguinal region in a man

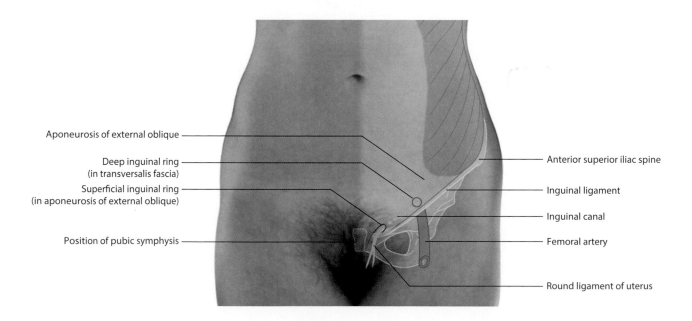

Aponeurosis of external oblique

Deep inguinal ring
(in transversalis fascia)

Superficial inguinal ring
(in aponeurosis of external oblique)

Position of pubic symphysis

Anterior superior iliac spine

Inguinal ligament

Inguinal canal

Femoral artery

Round ligament of uterus

Inguinal region in a woman

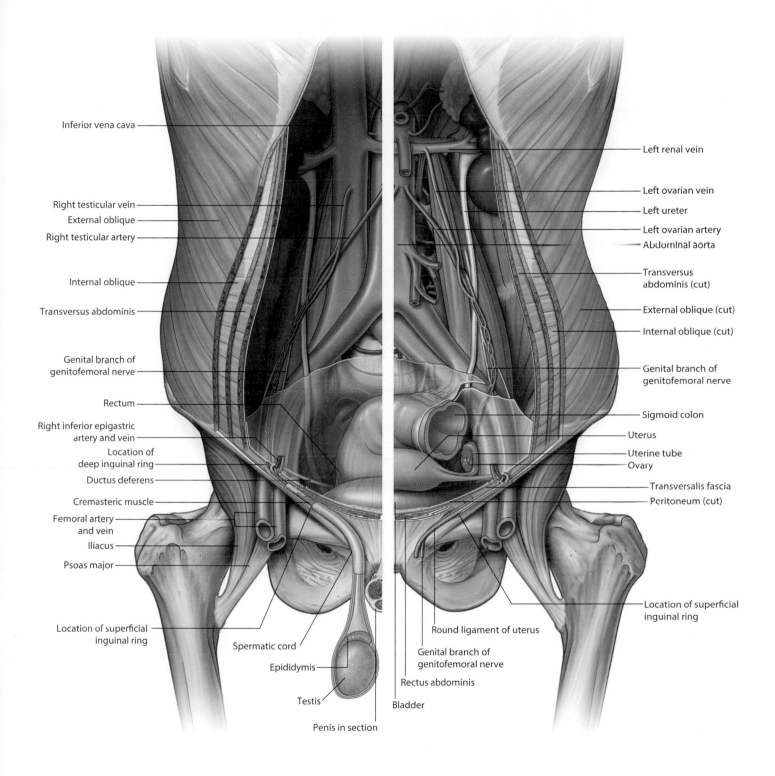

Inferior vena cava

Right testicular vein
External oblique
Right testicular artery

Internal oblique

Transversus abdominis

Genital branch of
genitofemoral nerve

Rectum

Right inferior epigastric
artery and vein

Location of
deep inguinal ring

Ductus deferens

Cremasteric muscle

Femoral artery
and vein

Iliacus

Psoas major

Location of superficial
inguinal ring

Spermatic cord

Epididymis

Testis

Penis in section

Bladder

Rectus abdominis

Genital branch of
genitofemoral nerve

Round ligament of uterus

Left renal vein

Left ovarian vein
Left ureter
Left ovarian artery
Abdominal aorta

Transversus
abdominis (cut)

External oblique (cut)
Internal oblique (cut)

Genital branch of
genitofemoral nerve

Sigmoid colon

Uterus

Uterine tube
Ovary

Transversalis fascia
Peritoneum (cut)

Location of superficial
inguinal ring

Inguinal region in men

Inguinal region in women

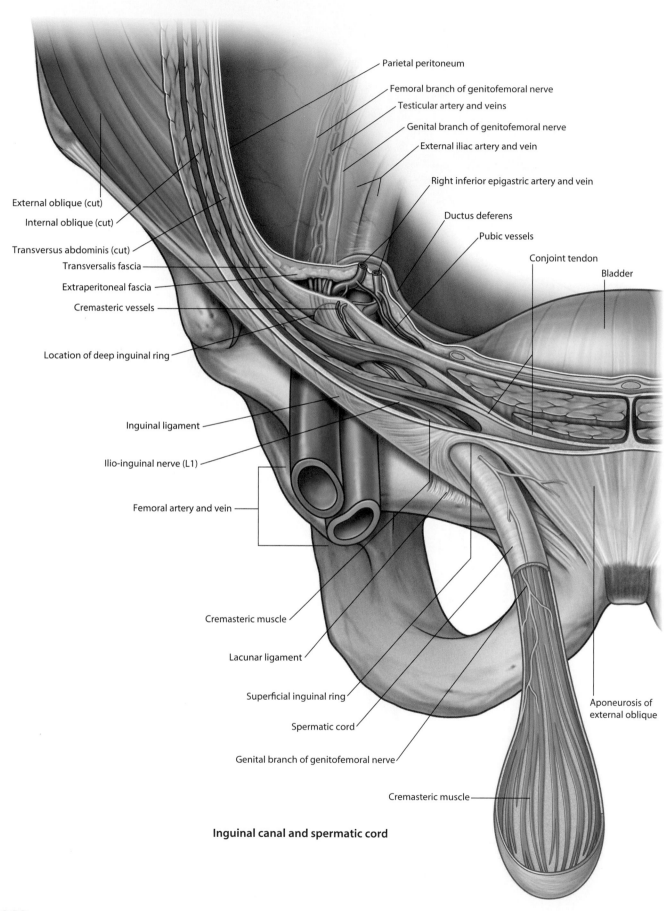

Parietal peritoneum

Femoral branch of genitofemoral nerve

Testicular artery and veins

Genital branch of genitofemoral nerve

External iliac artery and vein

Right inferior epigastric artery and vein

External oblique (cut)

Internal oblique (cut)

Transversus abdominis (cut)

Transversalis fascia

Extraperitoneal fascia

Cremasteric vessels

Location of deep inguinal ring

Ductus deferens

Pubic vessels

Conjoint tendon

Bladder

Inguinal ligament

Ilio-inguinal nerve (L1)

Femoral artery and vein

Cremasteric muscle

Lacunar ligament

Superficial inguinal ring

Spermatic cord

Genital branch of genitofemoral nerve

Cremasteric muscle

Aponeurosis of external oblique

Inguinal canal and spermatic cord

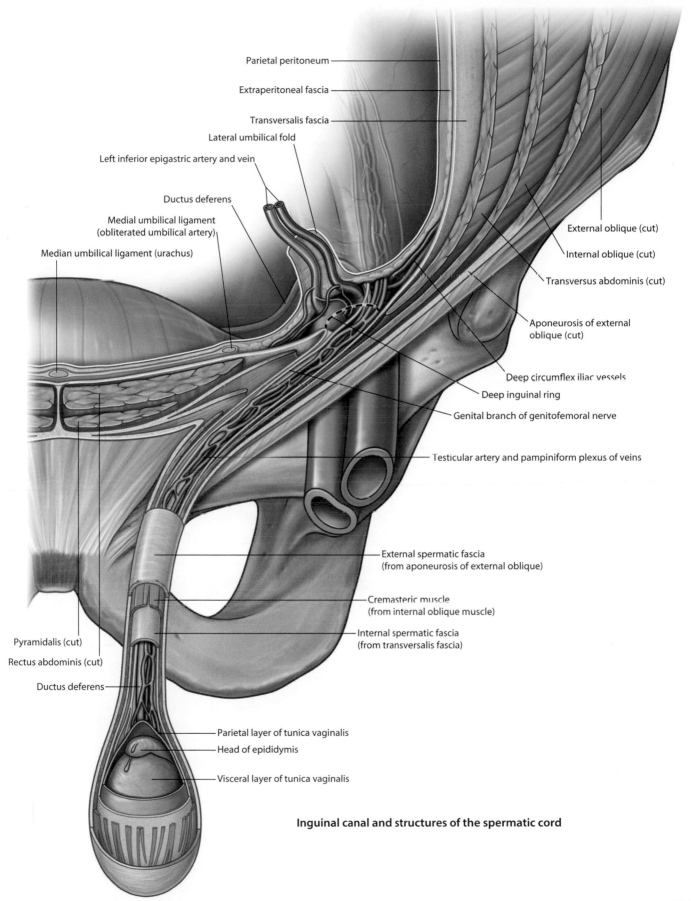

Parietal peritoneum

Extraperitoneal fascia

Transversalis fascia

Lateral umbilical fold

Left inferior epigastric artery and vein

Ductus deferens

Medial umbilical ligament
(obliterated umbilical artery)

Median umbilical ligament (urachus)

External oblique (cut)

Internal oblique (cut)

Transversus abdominis (cut)

Aponeurosis of external
oblique (cut)

Deep circumflex iliac vessels

Deep inguinal ring

Genital branch of genitofemoral nerve

Testicular artery and pampiniform plexus of veins

External spermatic fascia
(from aponeurosis of external oblique)

Cremasteric muscle
(from internal oblique muscle)

Internal spermatic fascia
(from transversalis fascia)

Pyramidalis (cut)

Rectus abdominis (cut)

Ductus deferens

Parietal layer of tunica vaginalis

Head of epididymis

Visceral layer of tunica vaginalis

Inguinal canal and structures of the spermatic cord

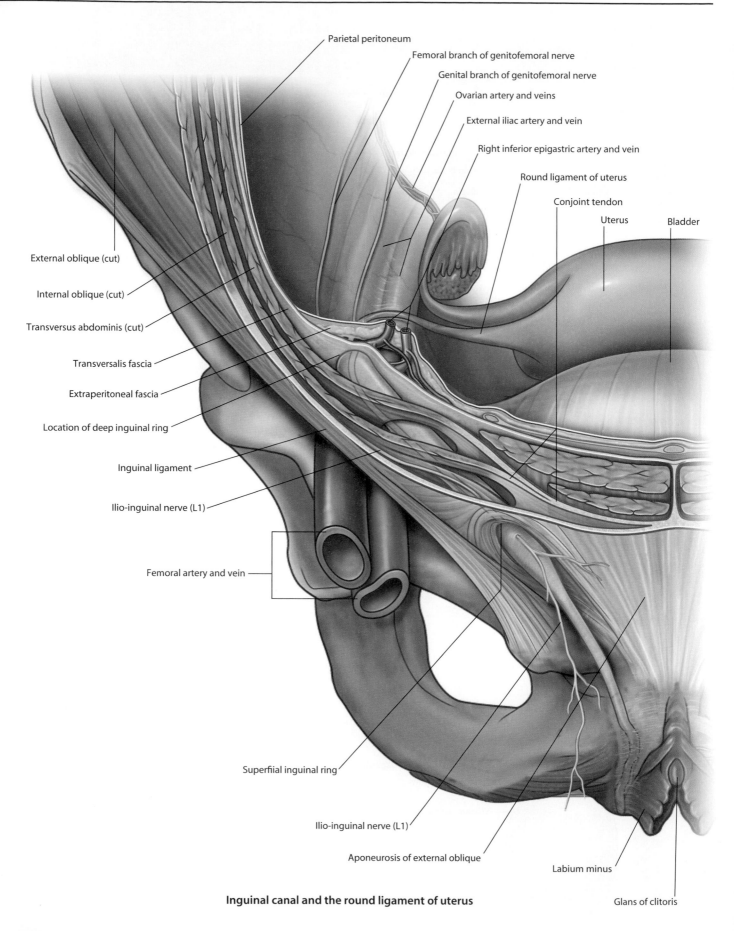

Parietal peritoneum

Femoral branch of genitofemoral nerve

Genital branch of genitofemoral nerve

Ovarian artery and veins

External iliac artery and vein

Right inferior epigastric artery and vein

Round ligament of uterus

Conjoint tendon

Uterus

Bladder

External oblique (cut)

Internal oblique (cut)

Transversus abdominis (cut)

Transversalis fascia

Extraperitoneal fascia

Location of deep inguinal ring

Inguinal ligament

Ilio-inguinal nerve (L1)

Femoral artery and vein

Superfiial inguinal ring

Ilio-inguinal nerve (L1)

Aponeurosis of external oblique

Labium minus

Glans of clitoris

Inguinal canal and the round ligament of uterus

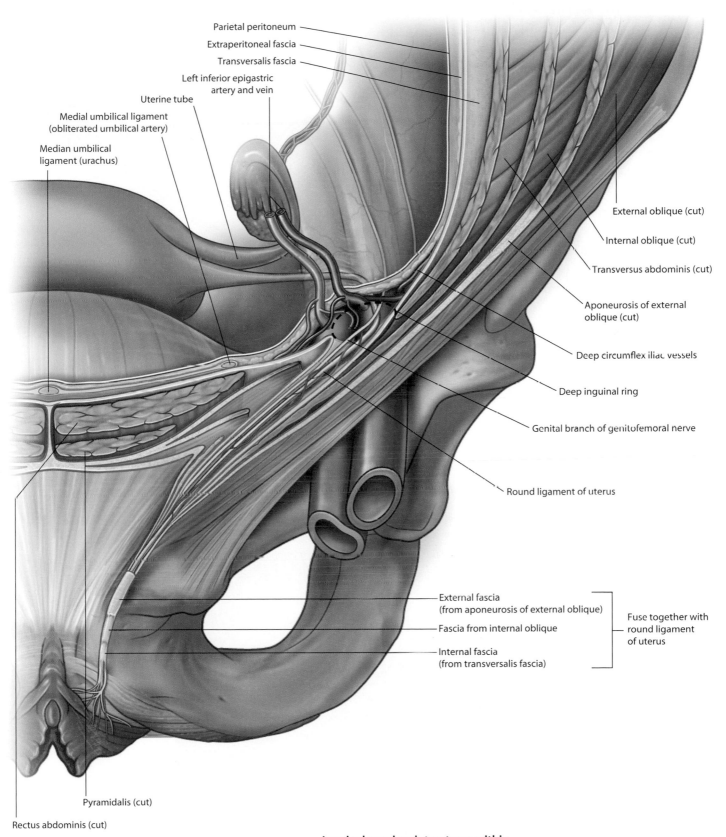

Parietal peritoneum

Extraperitoneal fascia

Transversalis fascia

Left inferior epigastric artery and vein

Uterine tube

Medial umbilical ligament (obliterated umbilical artery)

Median umbilical ligament (urachus)

External oblique (cut)

Internal oblique (cut)

Transversus abdominis (cut)

Aponeurosis of external oblique (cut)

Deep circumflex iliac vessels

Deep inguinal ring

Genital branch of genitofemoral nerve

Round ligament of uterus

External fascia (from aponeurosis of external oblique)

Fascia from internal oblique

Internal fascia (from transversalis fascia)

Fuse together with round ligament of uterus

Pyramidalis (cut)

Rectus abdominis (cut)

Inguinal canal and structures within

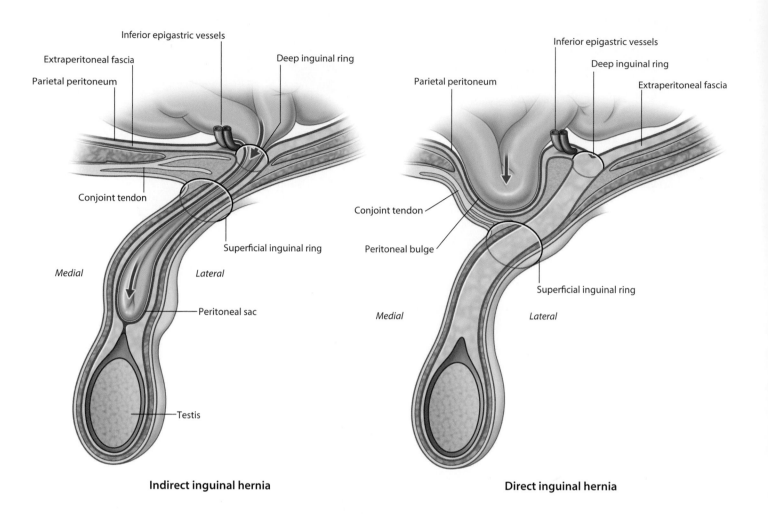

Indirect inguinal hernia

Inferior epigastric vessels

Extraperitoneal fascia

Parietal peritoneum

Deep inguinal ring

Conjoint tendon

Superficial inguinal ring

Medial

Lateral

Peritoneal sac

Testis

Direct inguinal hernia

Inferior epigastric vessels

Deep inguinal ring

Extraperitoneal fascia

Parietal peritoneum

Conjoint tendon

Peritoneal bulge

Superficial inguinal ring

Medial

Lateral

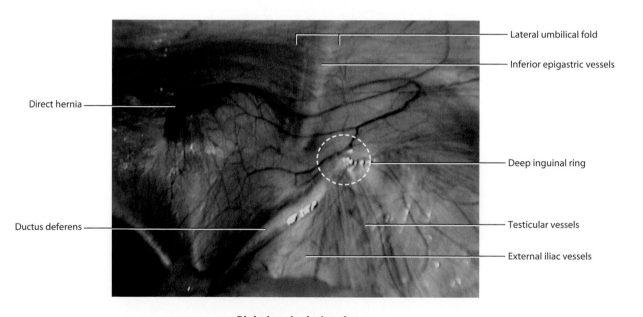

Direct hernia

Ductus deferens

Lateral umbilical fold

Inferior epigastric vessels

Deep inguinal ring

Testicular vessels

External iliac vessels

Right inguinal triangle.
Laparoscopic view showing the parietal peritoneum still covering the area
(inside the peritoneal cavity looking anteroinferior)

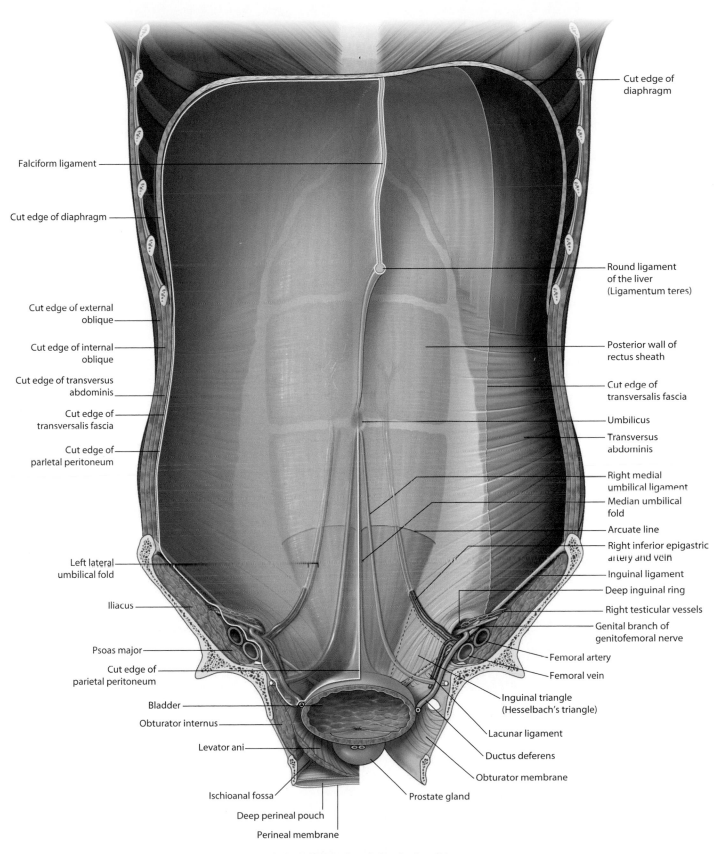

Cut edge of diaphragm

Falciform ligament

Cut edge of diaphragm

Cut edge of external oblique

Cut edge of internal oblique

Cut edge of transversus abdominis

Cut edge of transversalis fascia

Cut edge of parietal peritoneum

Left lateral umbilical fold

Iliacus

Psoas major

Cut edge of parietal peritoneum

Bladder

Obturator internus

Levator ani

Ischioanal fossa

Deep perineal pouch

Perineal membrane

Round ligament of the liver (Ligamentum teres)

Posterior wall of rectus sheath

Cut edge of transversalis fascia

Umbilicus

Transversus abdominis

Right medial umbilical ligament

Median umbilical fold

Arcuate line

Right inferior epigastric artery and vein

Inguinal ligament

Deep inguinal ring

Right testicular vessels

Genital branch of genitofemoral nerve

Femoral artery

Femoral vein

Inguinal triangle (Hesselbach's triangle)

Lacunar ligament

Ductus deferens

Obturator membrane

Prostate gland

Internal view of anterior abdominal wall in men

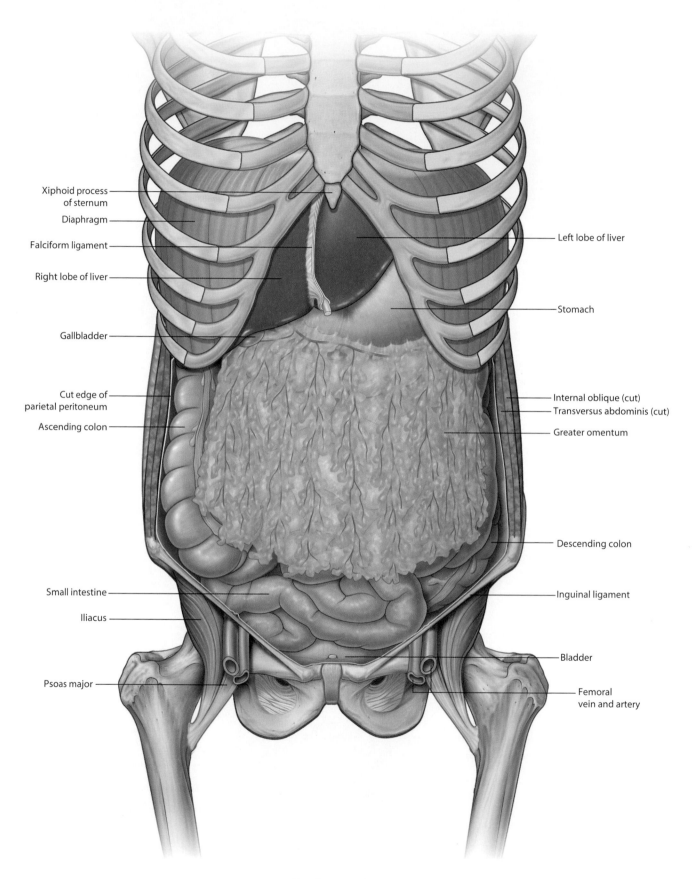

Xiphoid process
of sternum

Diaphragm

Falciform ligament

Right lobe of liver

Gallbladder

Cut edge of
parietal peritoneum

Ascending colon

Small intestine

Iliacus

Psoas major

Left lobe of liver

Stomach

Internal oblique (cut)

Transversus abdominis (cut)

Greater omentum

Descending colon

Inguinal ligament

Bladder

Femoral
vein and artery

Greater omentum

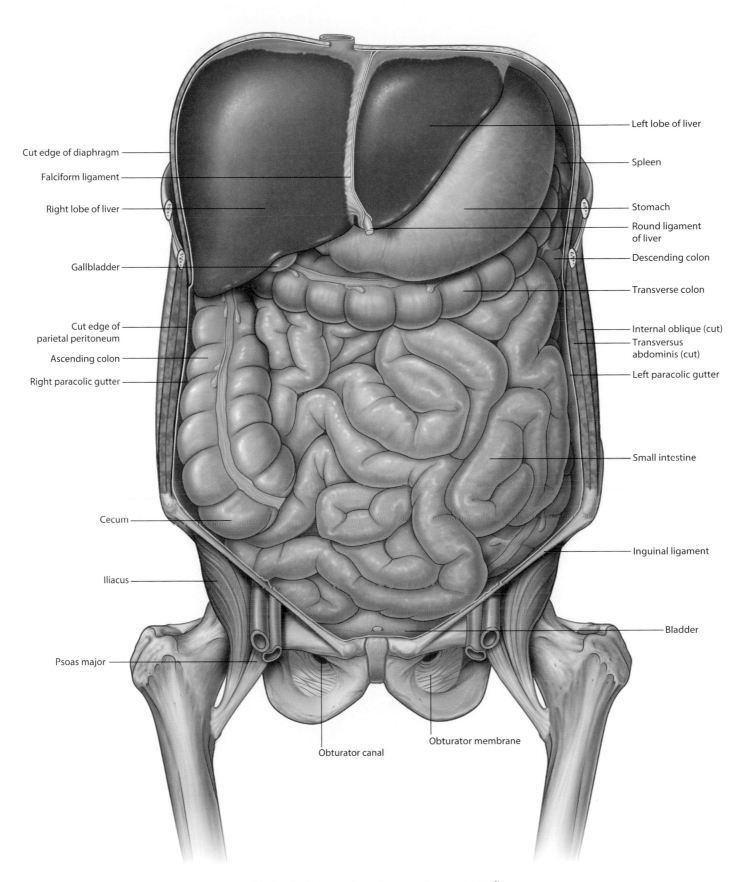

Left lobe of liver

Cut edge of diaphragm

Falciform ligament

Right lobe of liver

Gallbladder

Cut edge of
parietal peritoneum

Ascending colon

Right paracolic gutter

Cecum

Iliacus

Psoas major

Spleen

Stomach

Round ligament
of liver

Descending colon

Transverse colon

Internal oblique (cut)

Transversus
abdominis (cut)

Left paracolic gutter

Small intestine

Inguinal ligament

Bladder

Obturator membrane

Obturator canal

Abdominal viscera (greater omentum removed)

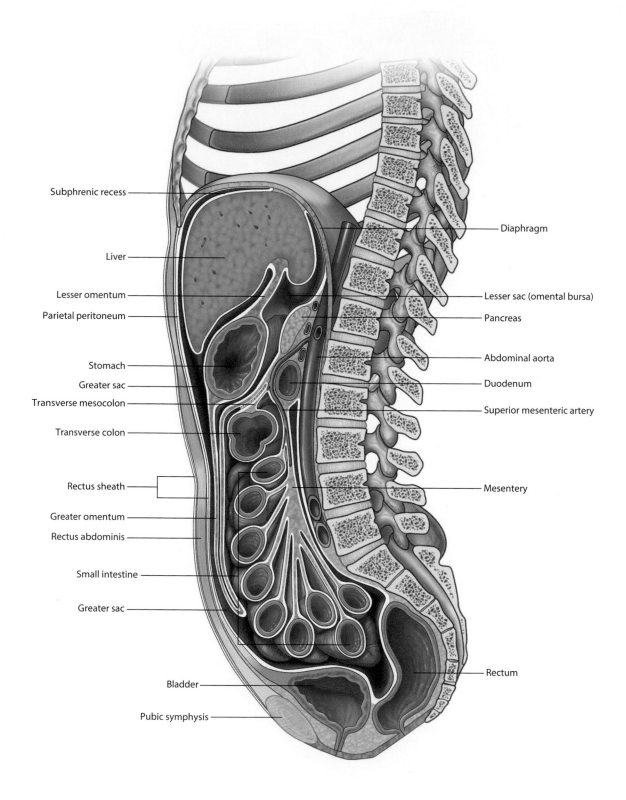

Subphrenic recess

Liver

Lesser omentum

Parietal peritoneum

Stomach

Greater sac

Transverse mesocolon

Transverse colon

Rectus sheath

Greater omentum

Rectus abdominis

Small intestine

Greater sac

Bladder

Pubic symphysis

Diaphragm

Lesser sac (omental bursa)

Pancreas

Abdominal aorta

Duodenum

Superior mesenteric artery

Mesentery

Rectum

Greater and lesser sacs of the peritoneal cavity

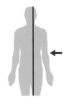

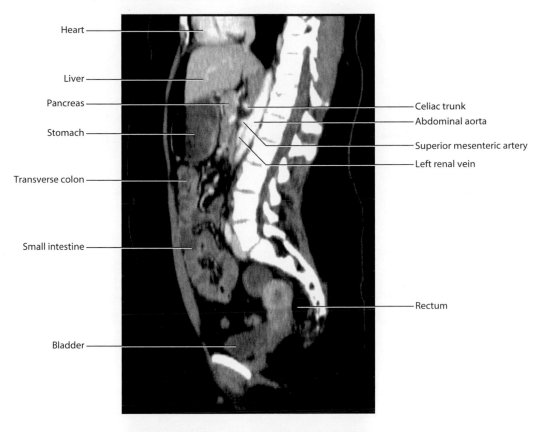

Heart

Liver

Pancreas — Celiac trunk
— Abdominal aorta

Stomach — Superior mesenteric artery
— Left renal vein

Transverse colon

Small intestine

Rectum

Bladder

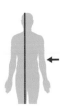

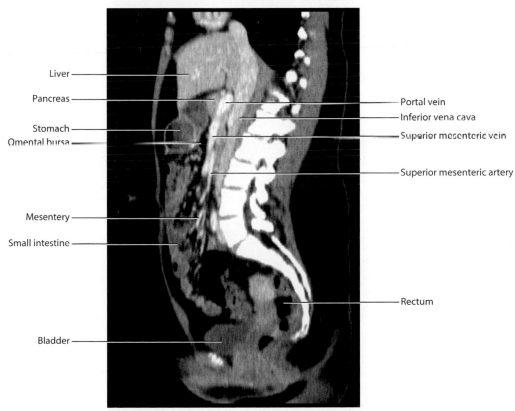

Liver

Pancreas — Portal vein
— Inferior vena cava

Stomach — Superior mesenteric vein
Omental bursa

Superior mesenteric artery

Mesentery

Small intestine

Rectum

Bladder

Arrangement of abdominal contents in peritoneal cavity.
CT images with contrast, in sagittal plane

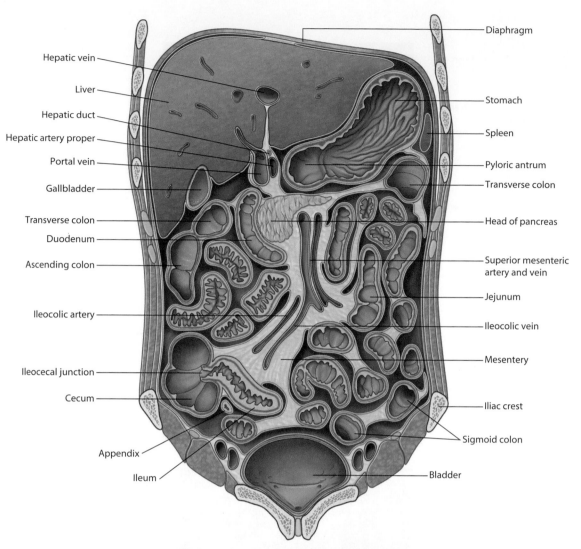

Hepatic vein

Liver

Hepatic duct

Hepatic artery proper

Portal vein

Gallbladder

Transverse colon

Duodenum

Ascending colon

Ileocolic artery

Ileocecal junction

Cecum

Appendix

Ileum

Diaphragm

Stomach

Spleen

Pyloric antrum

Transverse colon

Head of pancreas

Superior mesenteric artery and vein

Jejunum

Ileocolic vein

Mesentery

Iliac crest

Sigmoid colon

Bladder

Coronal section

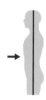

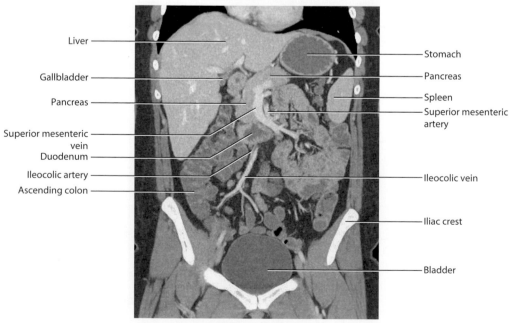

Liver

Gallbladder

Pancreas

Superior mesenteric vein

Duodenum

Ileocolic artery

Ascending colon

Stomach

Pancreas

Spleen

Superior mesenteric artery

Ileocolic vein

Iliac crest

Bladder

Coronal section.
CT image with contrast, in coronal plane

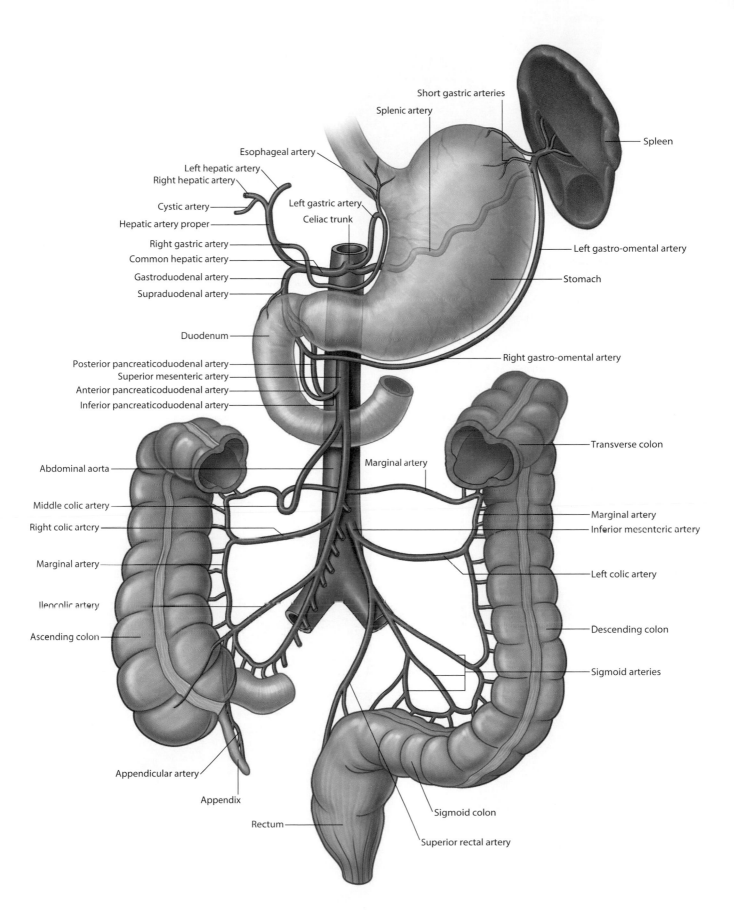

Short gastric arteries

Splenic artery

Esophageal artery

Left hepatic artery

Right hepatic artery

Cystic artery

Hepatic artery proper

Right gastric artery

Common hepatic artery

Gastroduodenal artery

Supraduodenal artery

Left gastric artery

Celiac trunk

Spleen

Left gastro-omental artery

Stomach

Duodenum

Posterior pancreaticoduodenal artery

Superior mesenteric artery

Anterior pancreaticoduodenal artery

Inferior pancreaticoduodenal artery

Right gastro-omental artery

Transverse colon

Abdominal aorta

Middle colic artery

Right colic artery

Marginal artery

Ileocolic artery

Ascending colon

Marginal artery

Marginal artery

Inferior mesenteric artery

Left colic artery

Descending colon

Sigmoid arteries

Appendicular artery

Appendix

Rectum

Sigmoid colon

Superior rectal artery

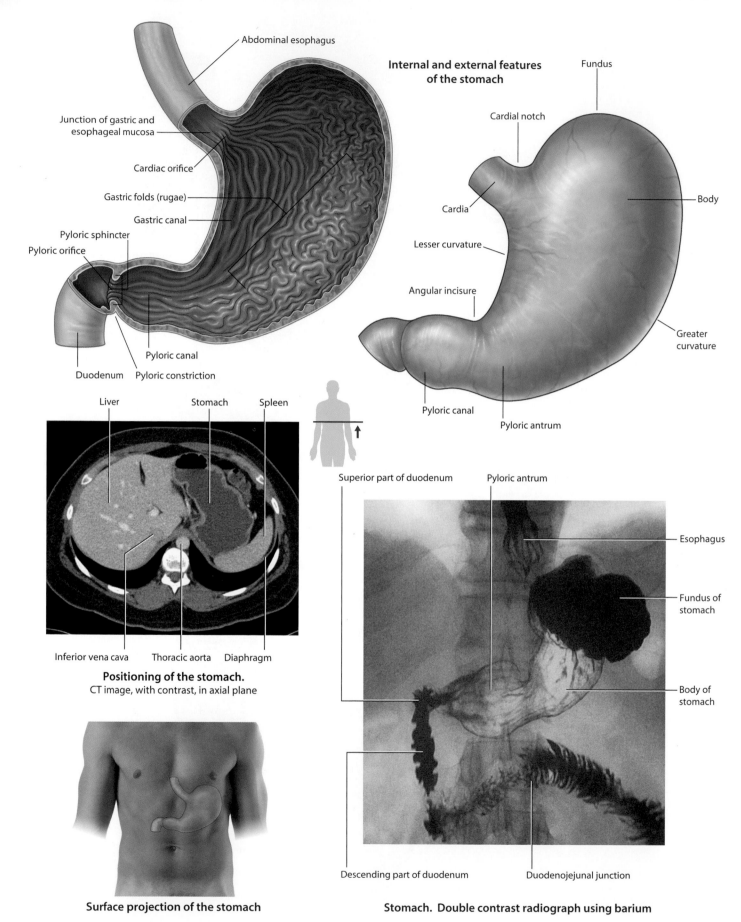

Abdominal esophagus

Internal and external features of the stomach

Fundus

Cardial notch

Junction of gastric and esophageal mucosa

Cardia

Body

Cardiac orifice

Gastric folds (rugae)

Lesser curvature

Gastric canal

Angular incisure

Pyloric sphincter

Pyloric orifice

Greater curvature

Duodenum   Pyloric constriction

Pyloric canal

Pyloric canal   Pyloric antrum

Liver   Stomach   Spleen

Inferior vena cava   Thoracic aorta   Diaphragm

Positioning of the stomach.
CT image, with contrast, in axial plane

Superior part of duodenum   Pyloric antrum

Esophagus

Fundus of stomach

Body of stomach

Descending part of duodenum   Duodenojejunal junction

Surface projection of the stomach

Stomach. Double contrast radiograph using barium

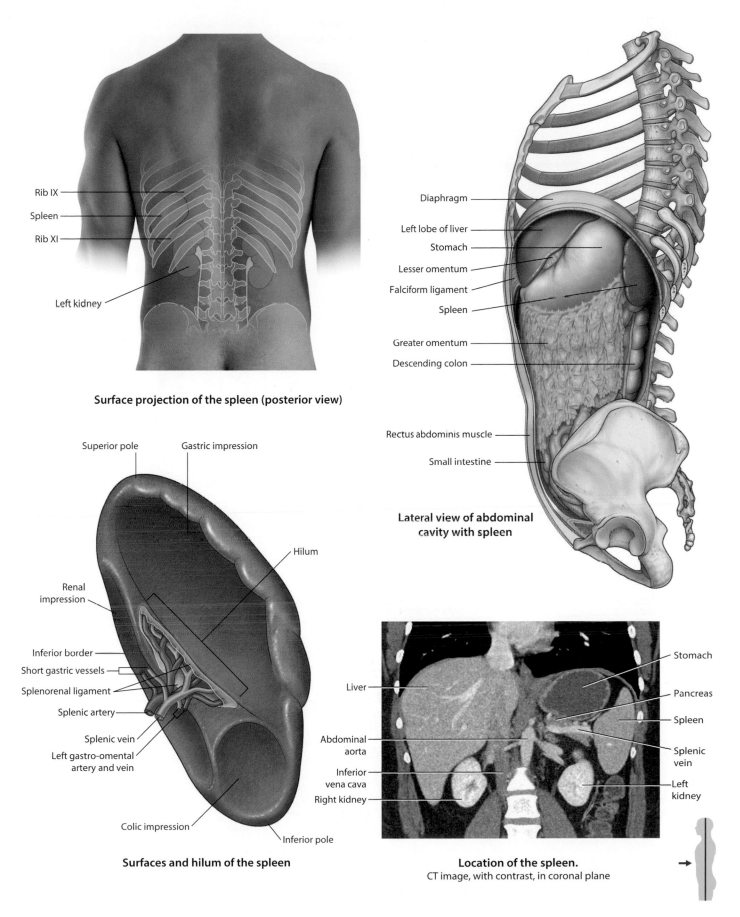

Rib IX

Spleen

Rib XI

Left kidney

Surface projection of the spleen (posterior view)

Diaphragm

Left lobe of liver

Stomach

Lesser omentum

Falciform ligament

Spleen

Greater omentum

Descending colon

Rectus abdominis muscle

Small intestine

Lateral view of abdominal cavity with spleen

Superior pole

Gastric impression

Hilum

Renal impression

Inferior border

Short gastric vessels

Splenorenal ligament

Splenic artery

Splenic vein

Left gastro-omental artery and vein

Colic impression

Inferior pole

Surfaces and hilum of the spleen

Liver

Abdominal aorta

Inferior vena cava

Right kidney

Stomach

Pancreas

Spleen

Splenic vein

Left kidney

Location of the spleen.
CT image, with contrast, in coronal plane

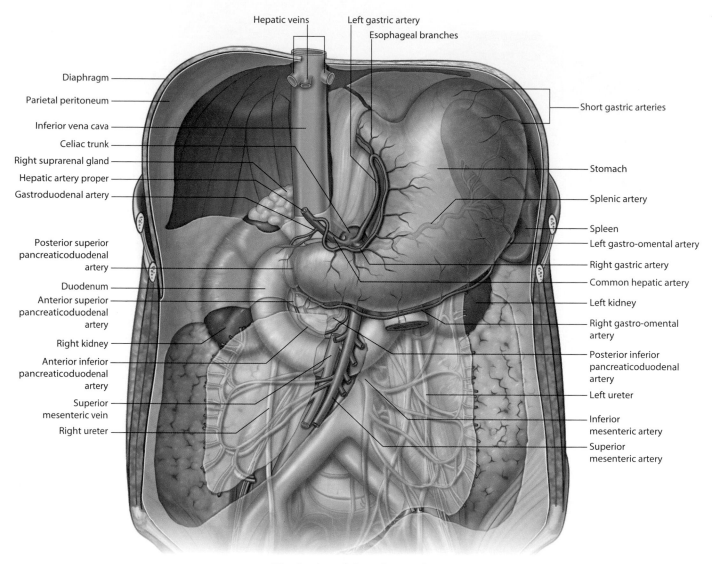

Hepatic veins

Left gastric artery

Esophageal branches

Diaphragm

Parietal peritoneum

Inferior vena cava

Celiac trunk

Right suprarenal gland

Hepatic artery proper

Gastroduodenal artery

Posterior superior pancreaticoduodenal artery

Duodenum

Anterior superior pancreaticoduodenal artery

Right kidney

Anterior inferior pancreaticoduodenal artery

Superior mesenteric vein

Right ureter

Short gastric arteries

Stomach

Splenic artery

Spleen

Left gastro-omental artery

Right gastric artery

Common hepatic artery

Left kidney

Right gastro-omental artery

Posterior inferior pancreaticoduodenal artery

Left ureter

Inferior mesenteric artery

Superior mesenteric artery

Distribution of the celiac trunk

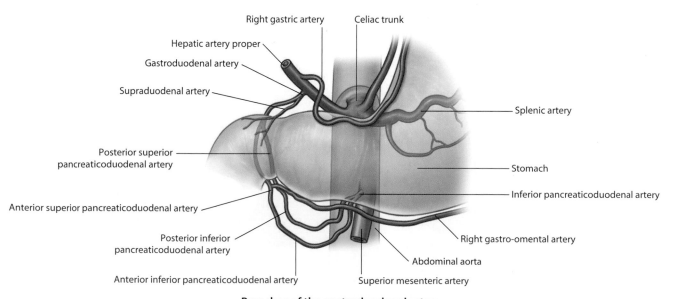

Right gastric artery

Celiac trunk

Hepatic artery proper

Gastroduodenal artery

Supraduodenal artery

Posterior superior pancreaticoduodenal artery

Anterior superior pancreaticoduodenal artery

Posterior inferior pancreaticoduodenal artery

Anterior inferior pancreaticoduodenal artery

Splenic artery

Stomach

Inferior pancreaticoduodenal artery

Right gastro-omental artery

Abdominal aorta

Superior mesenteric artery

Branches of the gastroduodenal artery

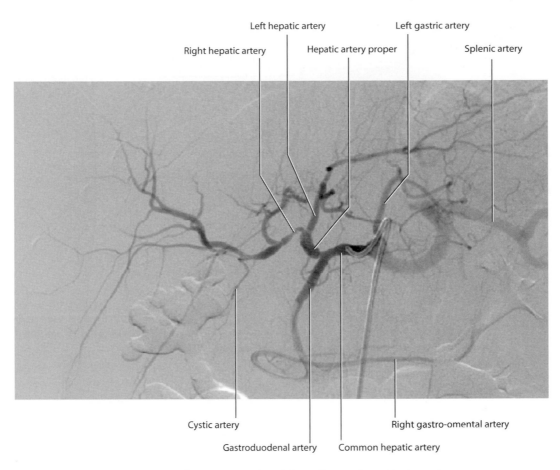

Left hepatic artery
Right hepatic artery
Hepatic artery proper
Left gastric artery
Splenic artery

Cystic artery
Gastroduodenal artery
Common hepatic artery
Right gastro-omental artery

Digital subtraction angiography of the celiac trunk and its branches

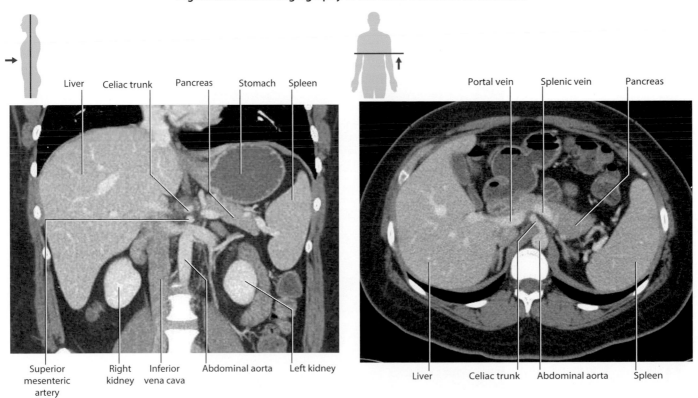

Liver Celiac trunk Pancreas Stomach Spleen

Portal vein Splenic vein Pancreas

Superior mesenteric artery Right kidney Inferior vena cava Abdominal aorta Left kidney

Liver Celiac trunk Abdominal aorta Spleen

Positioning of the celiac trunk in relation to other structures.
CT image, with contrast, in coronal plane

Branching of the celiac trunk from the abdominal aorta.
CT image, with contrast, in axial plane

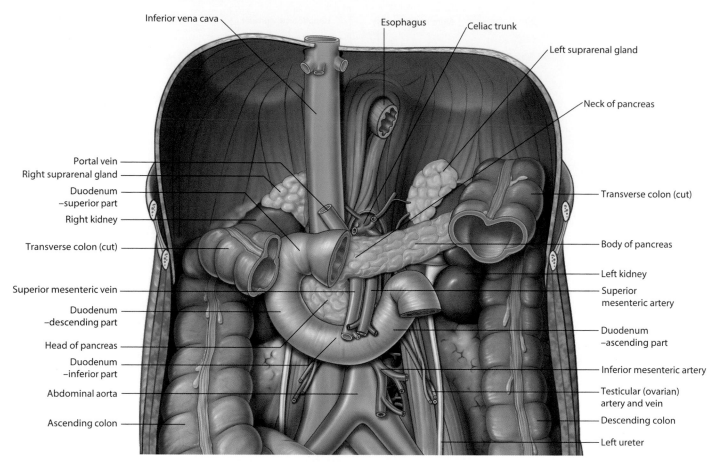

Inferior vena cava

Esophagus

Celiac trunk

Left suprarenal gland

Neck of pancreas

Portal vein

Right suprarenal gland

Duodenum –superior part

Right kidney

Transverse colon (cut)

Superior mesenteric vein

Duodenum –descending part

Head of pancreas

Duodenum –inferior part

Abdominal aorta

Ascending colon

Transverse colon (cut)

Body of pancreas

Left kidney

Superior mesenteric artery

Duodenum –ascending part

Inferior mesenteric artery

Testicular (ovarian) artery and vein

Descending colon

Left ureter

Duodenum in situ

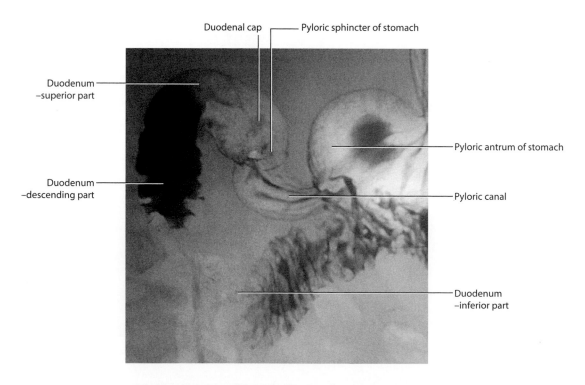

Duodenal cap

Pyloric sphincter of stomach

Duodenum –superior part

Duodenum –descending part

Pyloric antrum of stomach

Pyloric canal

Duodenum –inferior part

Double contrast radiograph showing the duodenal cap

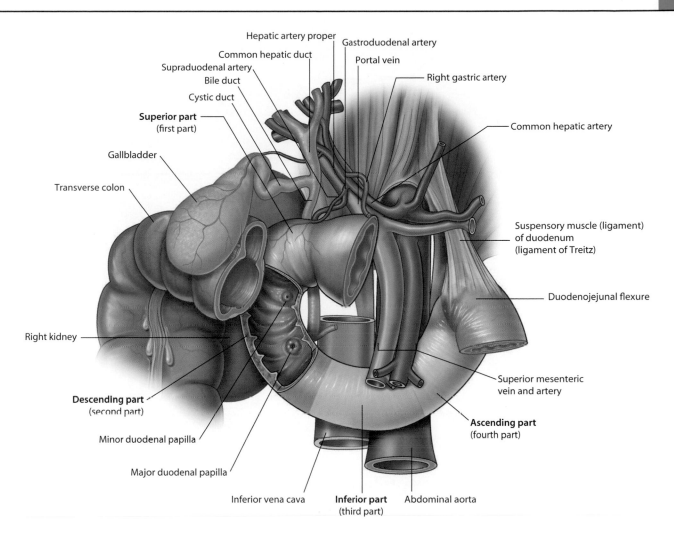

Hepatic artery proper

Common hepatic duct

Gastroduodenal artery

Supraduodenal artery

Portal vein

Bile duct

Cystic duct

Right gastric artery

Superior part
(first part)

Common hepatic artery

Gallblander

Transverse colon

Suspensory muscle (ligament)
of duodenum
(ligament of Treitz)

Duodenojejunal flexure

Right kidney

Superior mesenteric
vein and artery

Descending part
(second part)

Ascending part
(fourth part)

Minor duodenal papilla

Major duodenal papilla

Inferior vena cava

Inferior part
(third part)

Abdominal aorta

Parts of the duodenum and related structures

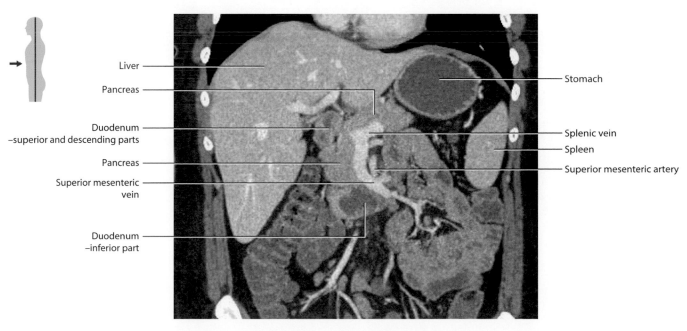

Liver

Stomach

Pancreas

Duodenum
–superior and descending parts

Splenic vein

Spleen

Pancreas

Superior mesenteric artery

Superior mesenteric
vein

Duodenum
–inferior part

Relationship of duodenum to structures in the vicinity.
CT image, with contrast, in coronal plane

165

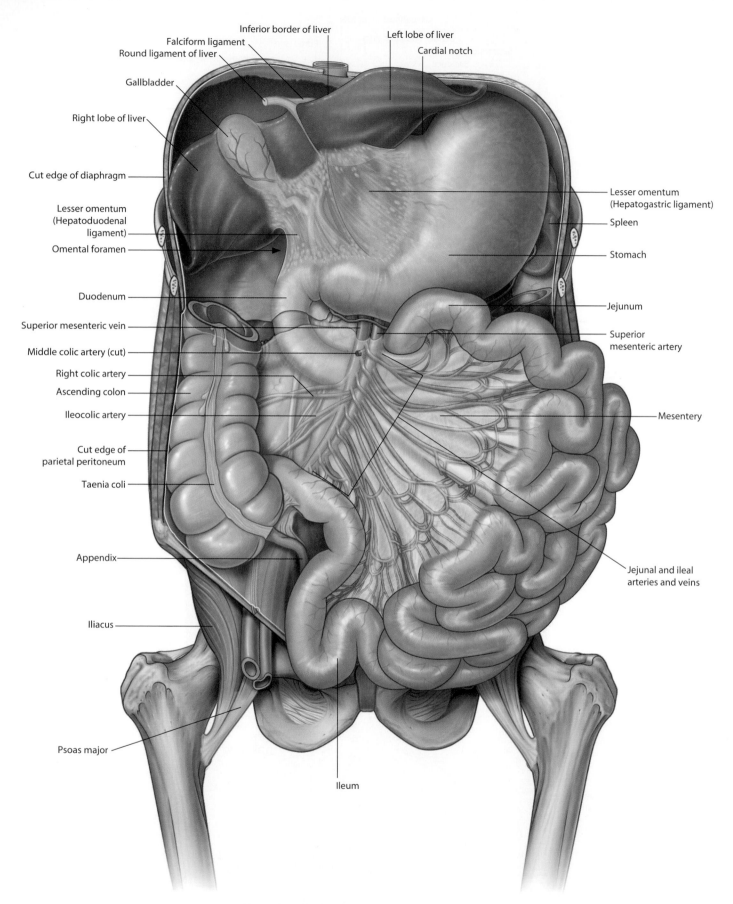

Inferior border of liver

Falciform ligament

Round ligament of liver

Gallbladder

Right lobe of liver

Cut edge of diaphragm

Lesser omentum (Hepatoduodenal ligament)

Omental foramen

Duodenum

Superior mesenteric vein

Middle colic artery (cut)

Right colic artery

Ascending colon

Ileocolic artery

Cut edge of parietal peritoneum

Taenia coli

Appendix

Iliacus

Psoas major

Left lobe of liver

Cardial notch

Lesser omentum (Hepatogastric ligament)

Spleen

Stomach

Jejunum

Superior mesenteric artery

Mesentery

Jejunal and ileal arteries and veins

Ileum

Small intestine displaced to show superior mesenteric vessels

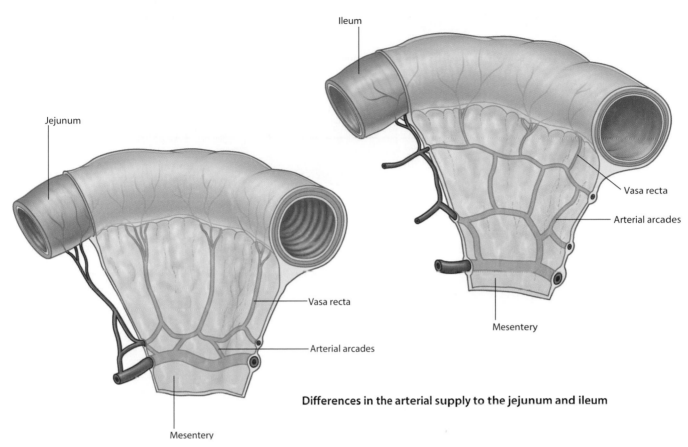

Differences in the arterial supply to the jejunum and ileum

Jejunum

Vasa recta

Arterial arcades

Mesentery

Ileum

Vasa recta

Arterial arcades

Mesentery

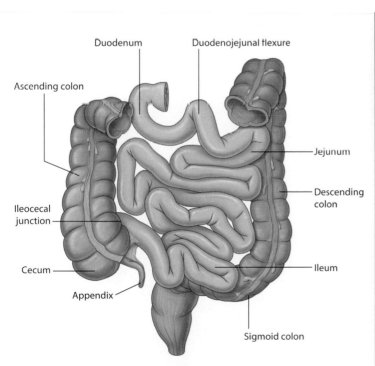

Duodenum

Duodenojejunal flexure

Ascending colon

Ileocecal junction

Cecum

Appendix

Jejunum

Descending colon

Ileum

Sigmoid colon

Jejunum and ileum

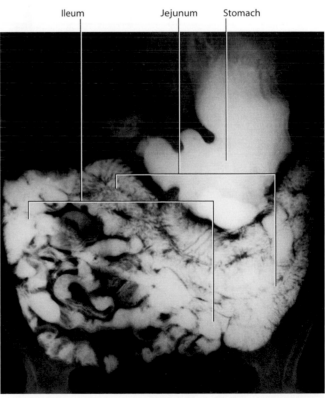

Ileum

Jejunum

Stomach

Radiograph using barium, showing jejunum and ileum

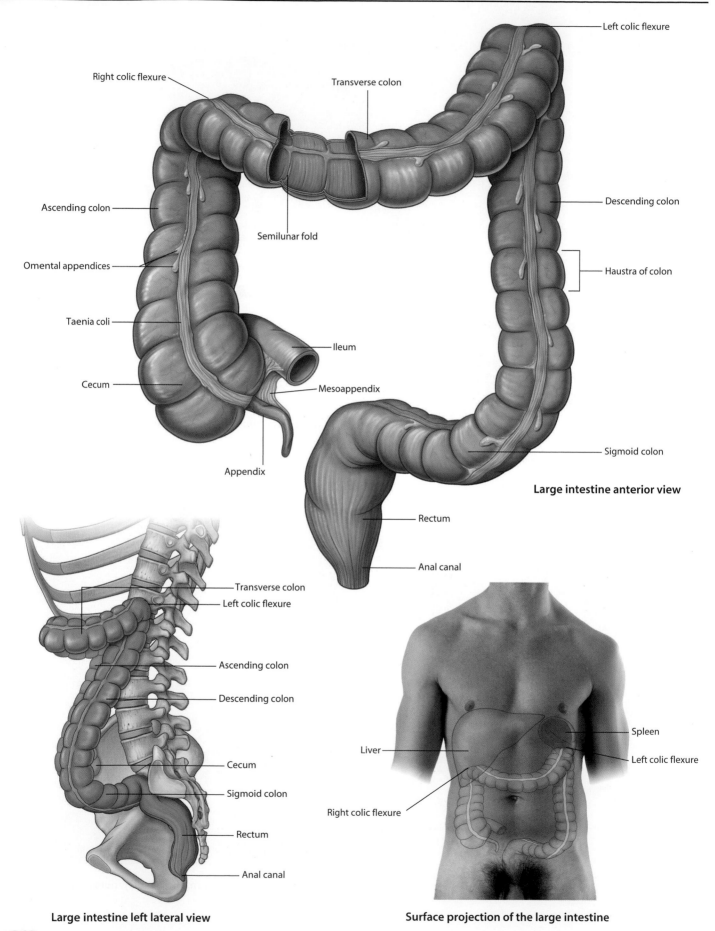

Left colic flexure

Right colic flexure

Transverse colon

Descending colon

Ascending colon

Semilunar fold

Haustra of colon

Omental appendices

Taenia coli

Ileum

Cecum

Mesoappendix

Sigmoid colon

Appendix

Large intestine anterior view

Rectum

Anal canal

Transverse colon

Left colic flexure

Ascending colon

Descending colon

Cecum

Sigmoid colon

Rectum

Anal canal

Liver

Spleen

Left colic flexure

Right colic flexure

Large intestine left lateral view

Surface projection of the large intestine

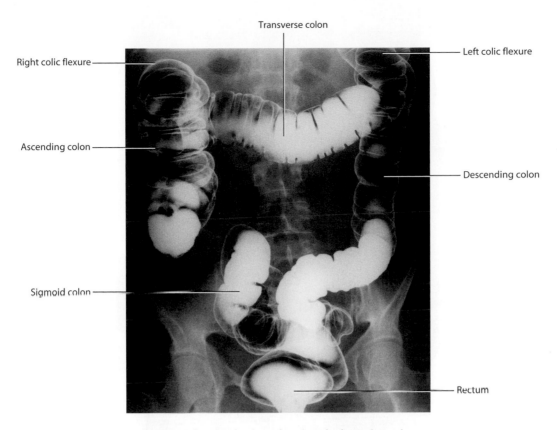

Transverse colon

Right colic flexure

Left colic flexure

Ascending colon

Descending colon

Sigmoid colon

Rectum

Radiograph using barium showing the large intestine

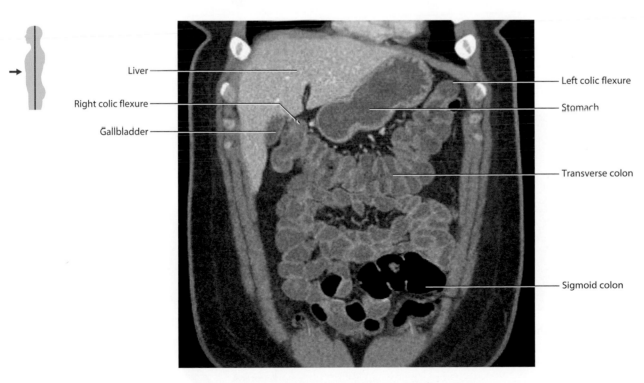

Liver

Left colic flexure

Right colic flexure

Stomach

Gallbladder

Transverse colon

Sigmoid colon

Transverse colon showing right and left colic flexures.
CT image, with contrast, in coronal plane

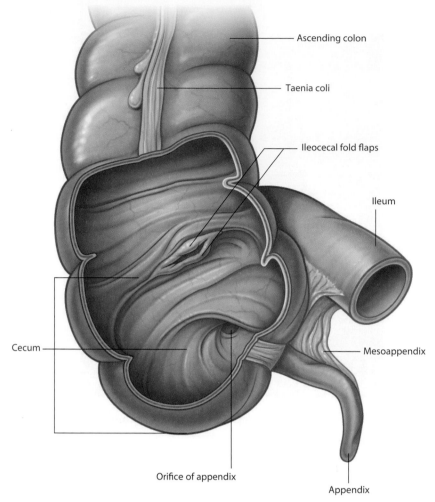

Ascending colon

Taenia coli

Ileocecal fold flaps

Ileum

Cecum

Mesoappendix

Orifice of appendix

Appendix

Ileocecal junction

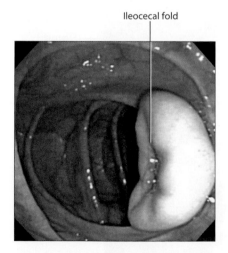

Ileocecal fold

Colonoscopy showing ileocecal fold

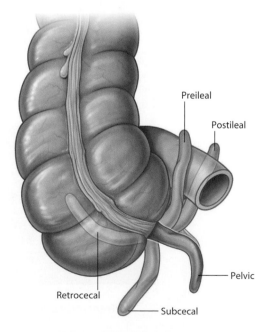

Preileal

Postileal

Pelvic

Retrocecal

Subcecal

Positions of the appendix

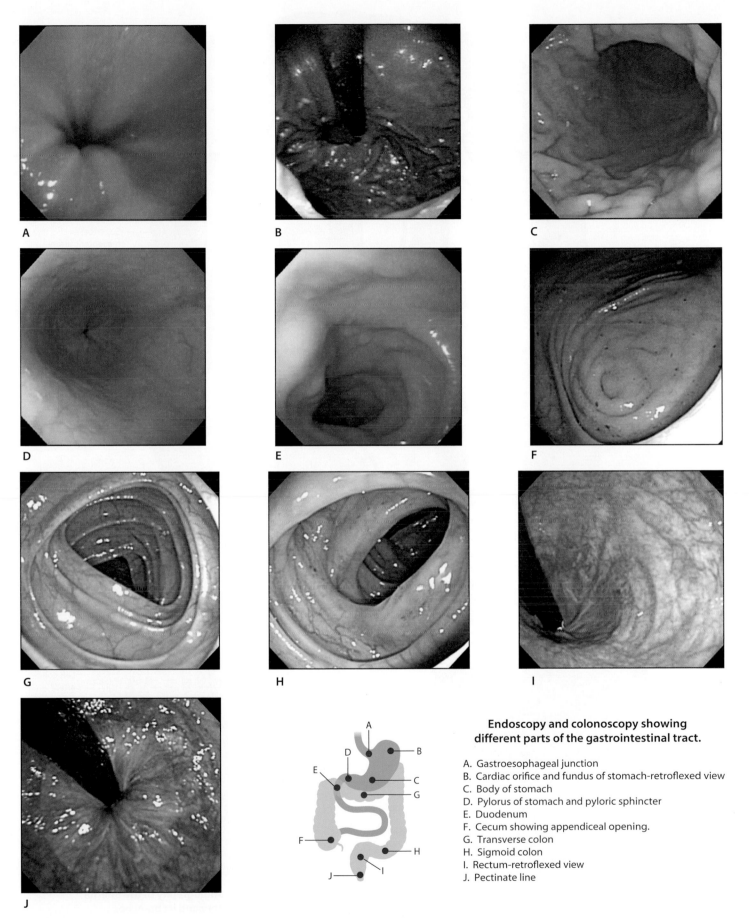

Endoscopy and colonoscopy showing different parts of the gastrointestinal tract.

A. Gastroesophageal junction
B. Cardiac orifice and fundus of stomach-retroflexed view
C. Body of stomach
D. Pylorus of stomach and pyloric sphincter
E. Duodenum
F. Cecum showing appendiceal opening.
G. Transverse colon
H. Sigmoid colon
I. Rectum-retroflexed view
J. Pectinate line

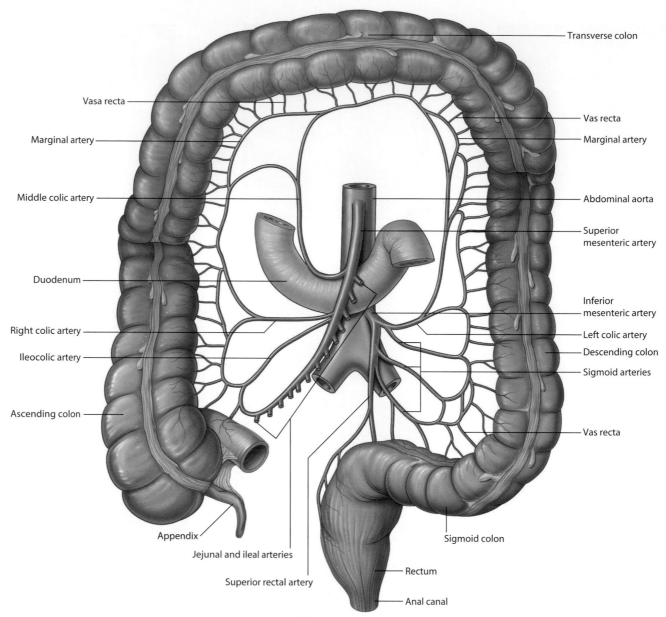

Transverse colon

Vasa recta

Marginal artery

Middle colic artery

Duodenum

Right colic artery

Ileocolic artery

Ascending colon

Vas recta

Marginal artery

Abdominal aorta

Superior mesenteric artery

Inferior mesenteric artery

Left colic artery

Descending colon

Sigmoid arteries

Vas recta

Appendix

Jejunal and ileal arteries

Superior rectal artery

Sigmoid colon

Rectum

Anal canal

Superior and inferior mesenteric arteries

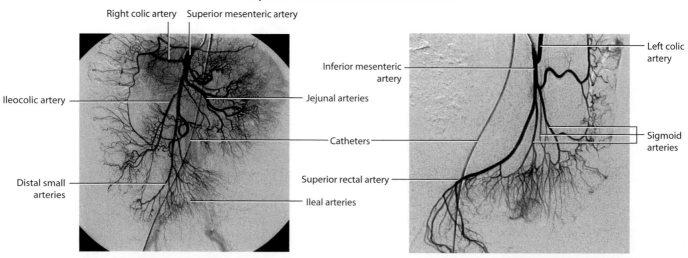

Right colic artery   Superior mesenteric artery

Ileocolic artery

Distal small arteries

Inferior mesenteric artery

Jejunal arteries

Catheters

Superior rectal artery

Ileal arteries

Left colic artery

Sigmoid arteries

Digital subtraction angiography of the superior mesenteric artery and its branches

Digital subtraction angiography of the inferior mesenteric artery and its branches

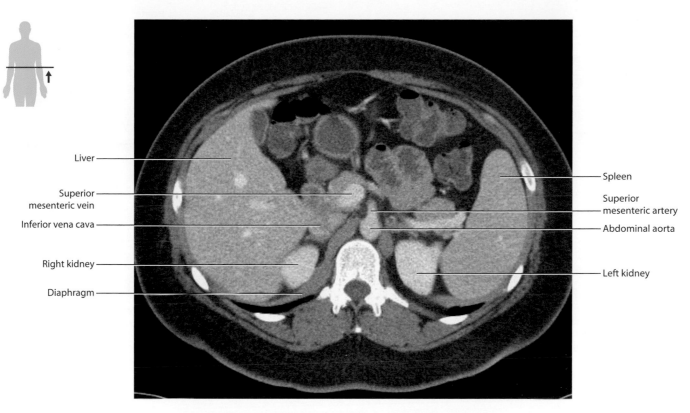

Liver

Superior
mesenteric vein

Inferior vena cava

Right kidney

Diaphragm

Spleen

Superior
mesenteric artery

Abdominal aorta

Left kidney

Branching of the superior mesenteric artery from the abdominal aorta.
CT image, with contrast, in axial plane

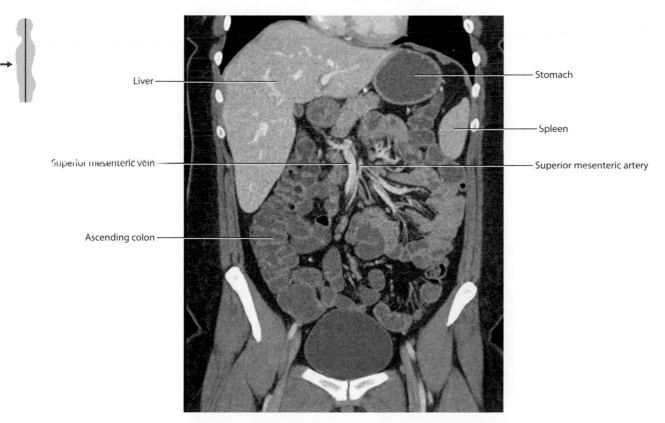

Liver

Superior mesenteric vein

Ascending colon

Stomach

Spleen

Superior mesenteric artery

Positioning of the superior mesenteric artery in relation to other structures.
CT image, with contrast, in coronal plane

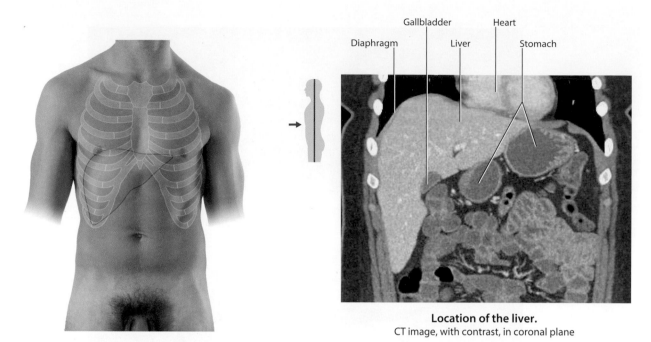

Surface projection of the liver anterior view

Location of the liver.
CT image, with contrast, in coronal plane

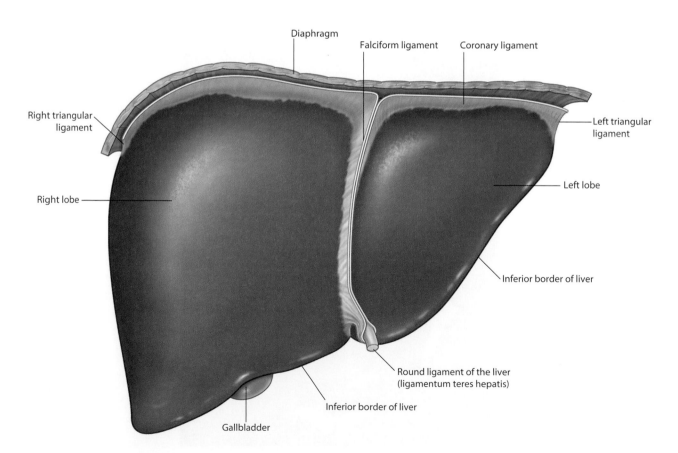

Anterior surface of liver

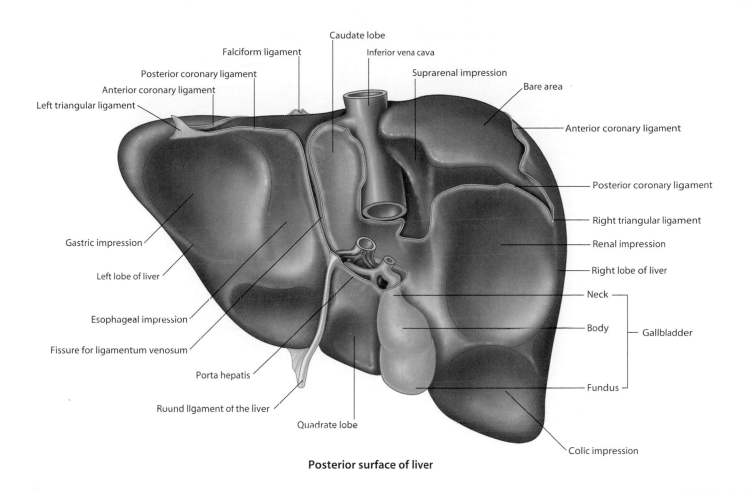

Caudate lobe

Falciform ligament

Inferior vena cava

Posterior coronary ligament

Suprarenal impression

Anterior coronary ligament

Bare area

Left triangular ligament

Anterior coronary ligament

Posterior coronary ligament

Gastric impression

Right triangular ligament

Renal impression

Left lobe of liver

Right lobe of liver

Esophageal impression

Neck

Body

Gallbladder

Fissure for ligamentum venosum

Porta hepatis

Fundus

Round ligament of the liver

Quadrate lobe

Colic impression

Posterior surface of liver

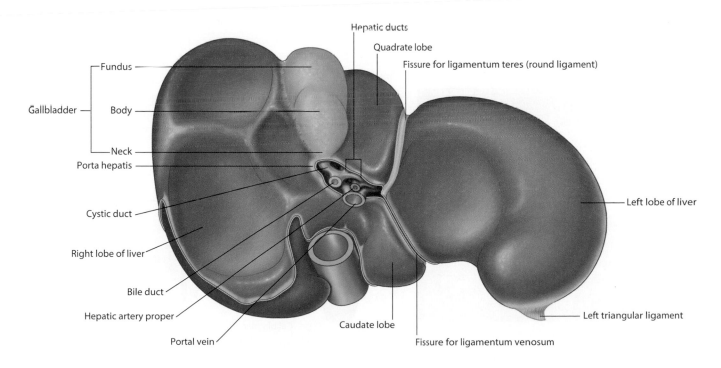

Hepatic ducts

Quadrate lobe

Fundus

Fissure for ligamentum teres (round ligament)

Gallbladder

Body

Neck

Porta hepatis

Left lobe of liver

Cystic duct

Right lobe of liver

Bile duct

Left triangular ligament

Hepatic artery proper

Caudate lobe

Portal vein

Fissure for ligamentum venosum

Visceral surface of liver

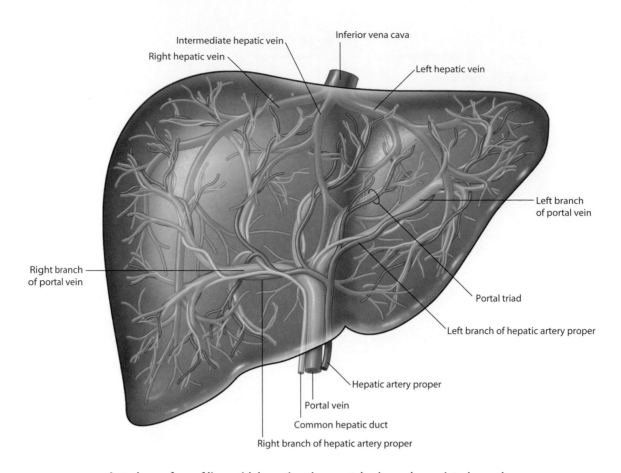

Intermediate hepatic vein

Right hepatic vein

Inferior vena cava

Left hepatic vein

Left branch of portal vein

Right branch of portal vein

Portal triad

Left branch of hepatic artery proper

Hepatic artery proper

Portal vein

Common hepatic duct

Right branch of hepatic artery proper

Anterior surface of liver with hepatic veins, portal vein, and associated vessels

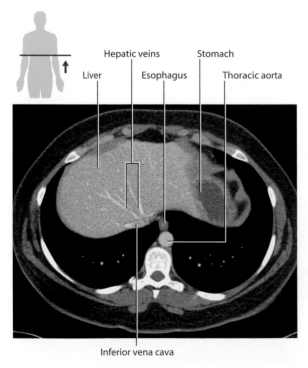

Liver

Hepatic veins

Esophagus

Stomach

Thoracic aorta

Inferior vena cava

Hepatic veins entering the inferior vena cava in the substance of the liver.
CT image, with contrast, in axial plane

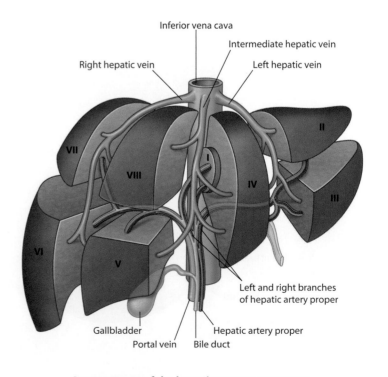

Inferior vena cava

Right hepatic vein

Intermediate hepatic vein

Left hepatic vein

VII

VIII

I

II

IV

III

VI

V

Gallbladder

Portal vein

Bile duct

Hepatic artery proper

Left and right branches of hepatic artery proper

Arrangement of the hepatic venous segments

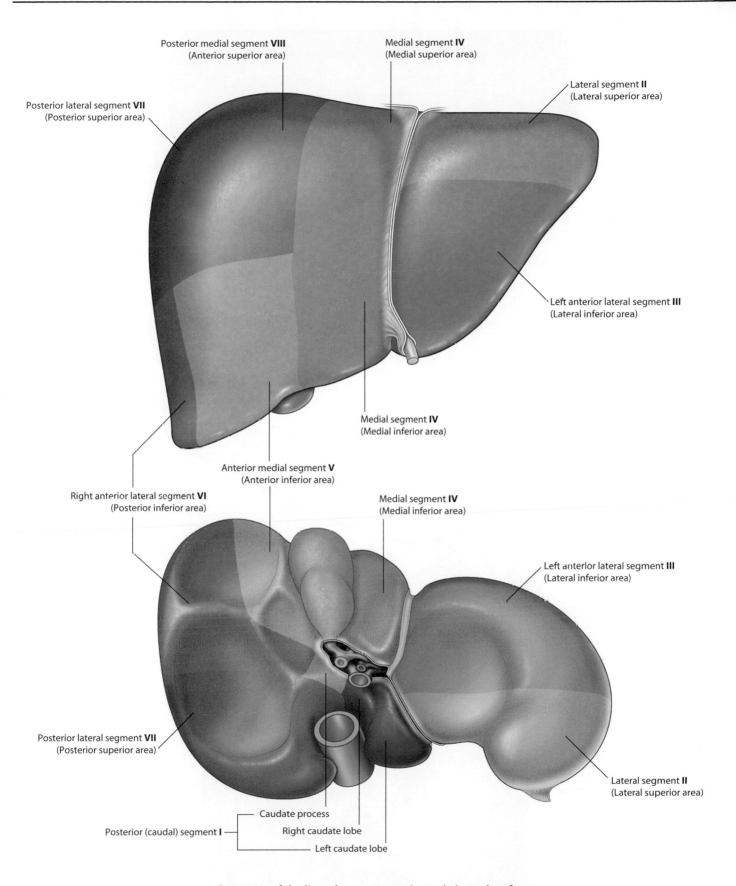

Posterior medial segment **VIII**
(Anterior superior area)

Medial segment **IV**
(Medial superior area)

Lateral segment **II**
(Lateral superior area)

Posterior lateral segment **VII**
(Posterior superior area)

Left anterior lateral segment **III**
(Lateral inferior area)

Medial segment **IV**
(Medial inferior area)

Anterior medial segment **V**
(Anterior inferior area)

Right anterior lateral segment **VI**
(Posterior inferior area)

Medial segment **IV**
(Medial inferior area)

Left anterior lateral segment **III**
(Lateral inferior area)

Posterior lateral segment **VII**
(Posterior superior area)

Caudate process

Posterior (caudal) segment **I**

Right caudate lobe

Left caudate lobe

Lateral segment **II**
(Lateral superior area)

Segments of the liver shown on anterior and visceral surfaces

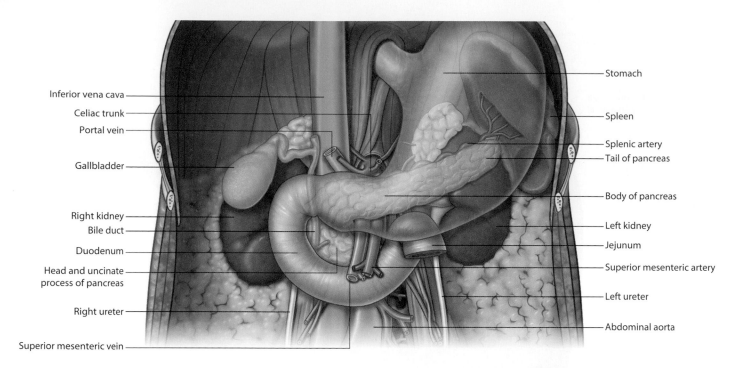

Inferior vena cava
Celiac trunk
Portal vein
Gallbladder
Right kidney
Bile duct
Duodenum
Head and uncinate process of pancreas
Right ureter
Superior mesenteric vein

Stomach
Spleen
Splenic artery
Tail of pancreas
Body of pancreas
Left kidney
Jejunum
Superior mesenteric artery
Left ureter
Abdominal aorta

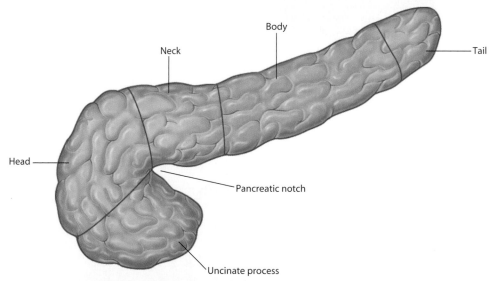

Neck
Body
Tail
Head
Pancreatic notch
Uncinate process

Anterior surface of the pancreas

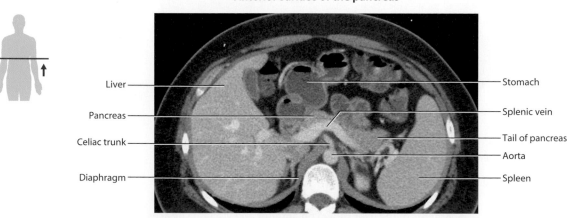

Liver
Pancreas
Celiac trunk
Diaphragm

Stomach
Splenic vein
Tail of pancreas
Aorta
Spleen

Pancreas.
CT image, with contrast, in axial plane

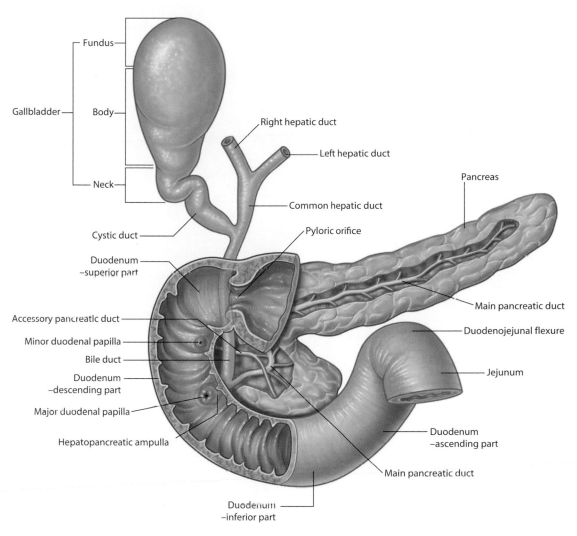

Fundus

Gallbladder | **Body**

Neck

Right hepatic duct

Left hepatic duct

Pancreas

Common hepatic duct

Cystic duct

Pyloric orifice

Duodenum
–superior part

Accessory pancreatic duct

Minor duodenal papilla

Bile duct

Duodenum
–descending part

Major duodenal papilla

Hepatopancreatic ampulla

Main pancreatic duct

Duodenojejunal flexure

Jejunum

Duodenum
–ascending part

Main pancreatic duct

Duodenum
–inferior part

Bile and pancreatic ducts

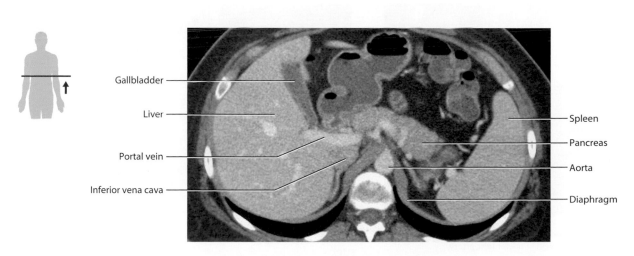

Gallbladder

Liver

Portal vein

Inferior vena cava

Spleen

Pancreas

Aorta

Diaphragm

Positioning of the gallbladder in relation to other structures.
CT image, with contrast, in axial plane

179

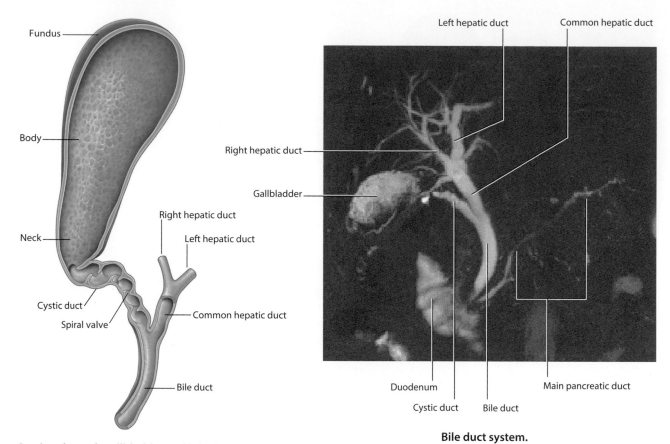

Fundus

Body

Neck

Cystic duct

Spiral valve

Right hepatic duct

Left hepatic duct

Common hepatic duct

Bile duct

Section through gallbladder and bile ducts

Left hepatic duct

Common hepatic duct

Right hepatic duct

Gallbladder

Duodenum

Cystic duct

Bile duct

Main pancreatic duct

Bile duct system.
Percutaneous transhepatic cholangiogram

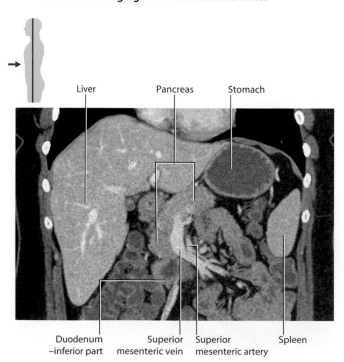

Liver

Pancreas

Stomach

Duodenum
–inferior part

Superior
mesenteric vein

Superior
mesenteric artery

Spleen

Positioning of the pancreas in relation to other structures.
CT image, with contrast, in coronal plane

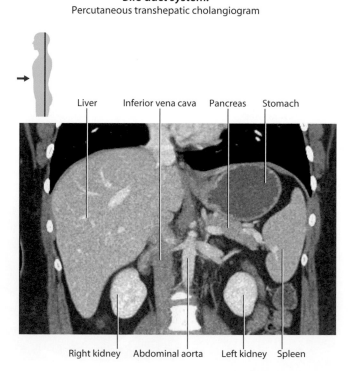

Liver

Inferior vena cava

Pancreas

Stomach

Right kidney

Abdominal aorta

Left kidney

Spleen

Relationship of pancreas to the stomach and spleen.
CT image, with contrast, in coronal plane

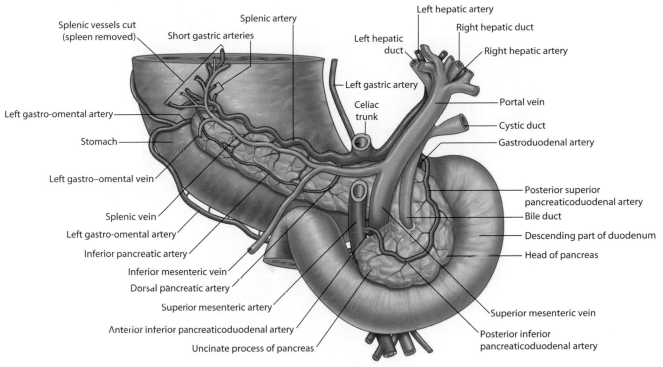

Splenic vessels cut (spleen removed)

Short gastric arteries

Splenic artery

Left hepatic artery

Right hepatic duct

Left hepatic duct

Right hepatic artery

Left gastric artery

Celiac trunk

Portal vein

Cystic duct

Gastroduodenal artery

Left gastro-omental artery

Stomach

Left gastro–omental vein

Splenic vein

Left gastro-omental artery

Inferior pancreatic artery

Inferior mesenteric vein

Dorsal pancreatic artery

Superior mesenteric artery

Anterior inferior pancreaticoduodenal artery

Uncinate process of pancreas

Posterior superior pancreaticoduodenal artery

Bile duct

Descending part of duodenum

Head of pancreas

Superior mesenteric vein

Posterior inferior pancreaticoduodenal artery

Vasculature of the pancreas posterior view

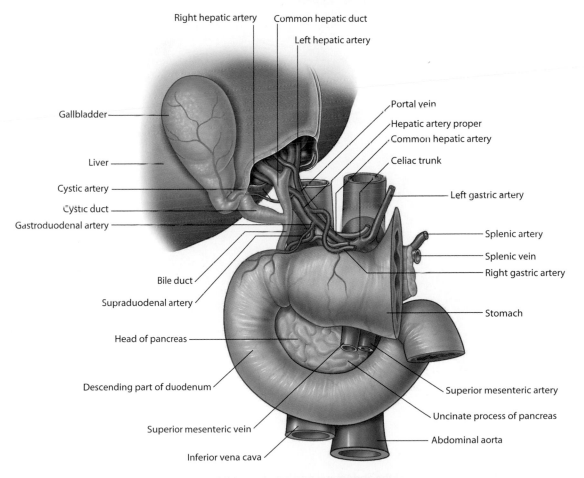

Right hepatic artery

Common hepatic duct

Left hepatic artery

Gallbladder

Liver

Cystic artery

Cystic duct

Gastroduodenal artery

Bile duct

Supraduodenal artery

Head of pancreas

Descending part of duodenum

Superior mesenteric vein

Inferior vena cava

Portal vein

Hepatic artery proper

Common hepatic artery

Celiac trunk

Left gastric artery

Splenic artery

Splenic vein

Right gastric artery

Stomach

Superior mesenteric artery

Uncinate process of pancreas

Abdominal aorta

Distribution of the common hepatic artery

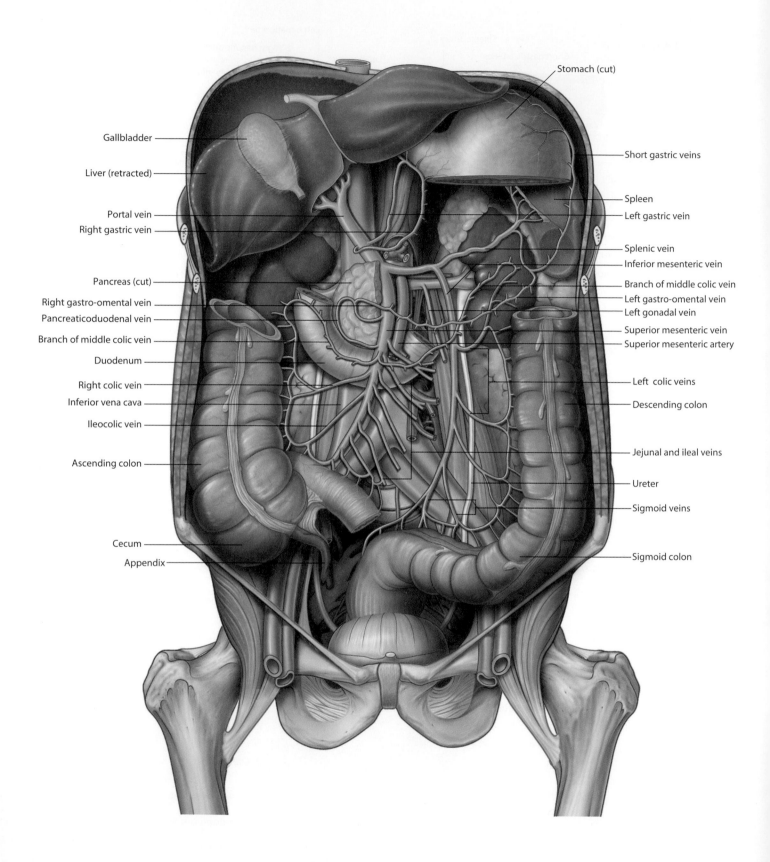

Gallbladder

Liver (retracted)

Portal vein
Right gastric vein

Pancreas (cut)
Right gastro-omental vein
Pancreaticoduodenal vein
Branch of middle colic vein
Duodenum
Right colic vein
Inferior vena cava
Ileocolic vein

Ascending colon

Cecum
Appendix

Stomach (cut)

Short gastric veins

Spleen
Left gastric vein

Splenic vein
Inferior mesenteric vein
Branch of middle colic vein
Left gastro-omental vein
Left gonadal vein
Superior mesenteric vein
Superior mesenteric artery

Left colic veins

Descending colon

Jejunal and ileal veins

Ureter

Sigmoid veins

Sigmoid colon

Venous drainage of the abdominal portion of the gastrointestinal tract in situ

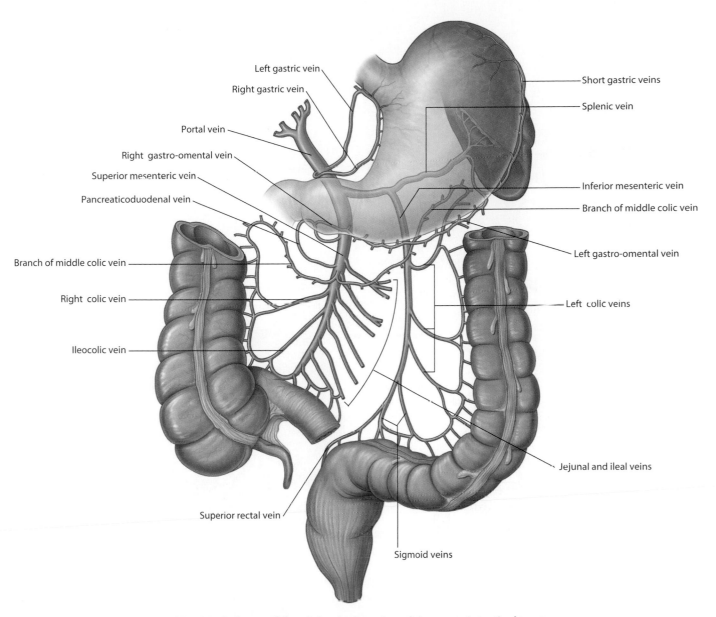

Left gastric vein

Right gastric vein

Portal vein

Right gastro-omental vein

Superior mesenteric vein

Pancreaticoduodenal vein

Branch of middle colic vein

Right colic vein

Ileocolic vein

Superior rectal vein

Short gastric veins

Splenic vein

Inferior mesenteric vein

Branch of middle colic vein

Left gastro-omental vein

Left colic veins

Jejunal and ileal veins

Sigmoid veins

Venous drainage of the abdominal portion of the gastrointestinal tract

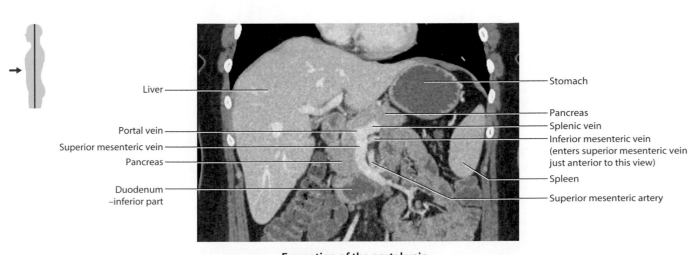

Liver

Portal vein

Superior mesenteric vein

Pancreas

Duodenum
–inferior part

Stomach

Pancreas

Splenic vein

Inferior mesenteric vein
(enters superior mesenteric vein
just anterior to this view)

Spleen

Superior mesenteric artery

Formation of the portal vein.
CT image, with contrast, in coronal plane

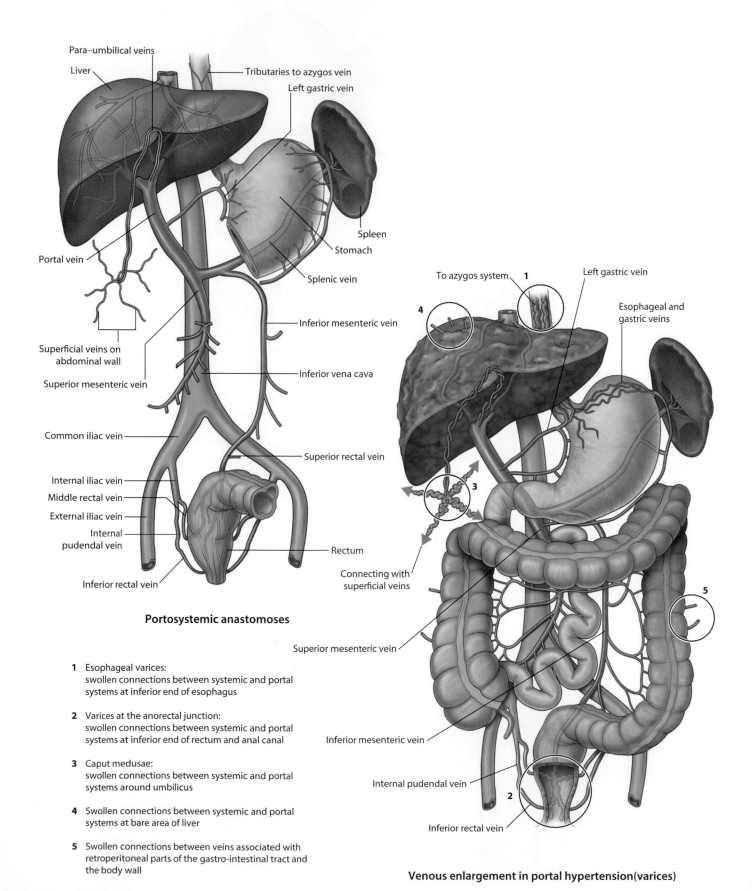

Portosystemic anastomoses

1 Esophageal varices:
   swollen connections between systemic and portal
   systems at inferior end of esophagus

2 Varices at the anorectal junction:
   swollen connections between systemic and portal
   systems at inferior end of rectum and anal canal

3 Caput medusae:
   swollen connections between systemic and portal
   systems around umbilicus

4 Swollen connections between systemic and portal
   systems at bare area of liver

5 Swollen connections between veins associated with
   retroperitoneal parts of the gastro-intestinal tract and
   the body wall

Venous enlargement in portal hypertension(varices)

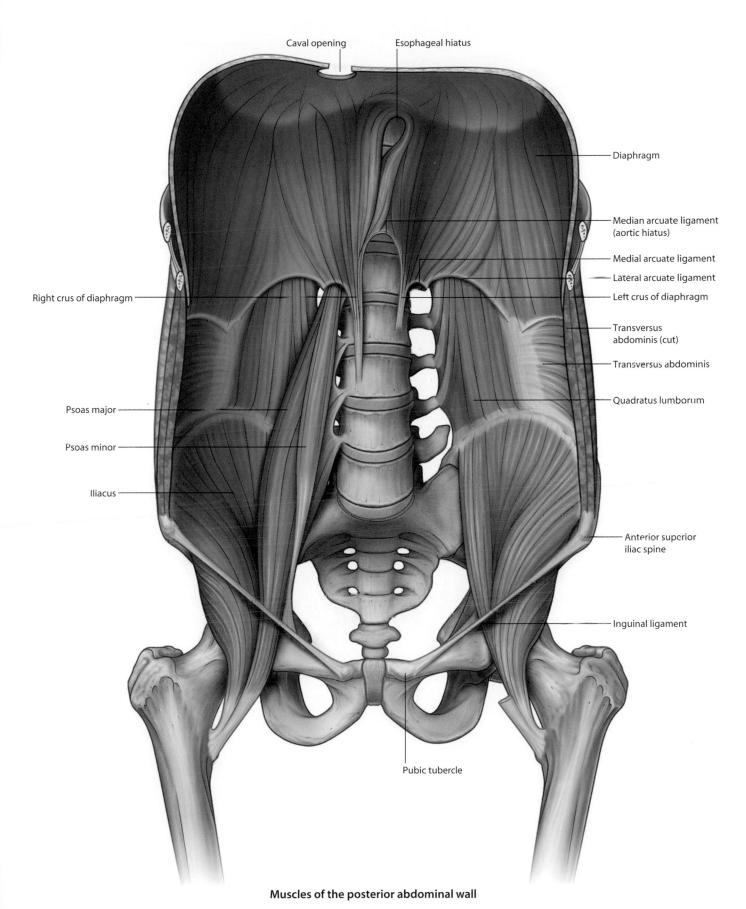

Caval opening

Esophageal hiatus

Diaphragm

Median arcuate ligament (aortic hiatus)

Medial arcuate ligament

Lateral arcuate ligament

Right crus of diaphragm

Left crus of diaphragm

Transversus abdominis (cut)

Transversus abdominis

Quadratus lumborum

Psoas major

Psoas minor

Iliacus

Anterior superior iliac spine

Inguinal ligament

Pubic tubercle

Muscles of the posterior abdominal wall

185

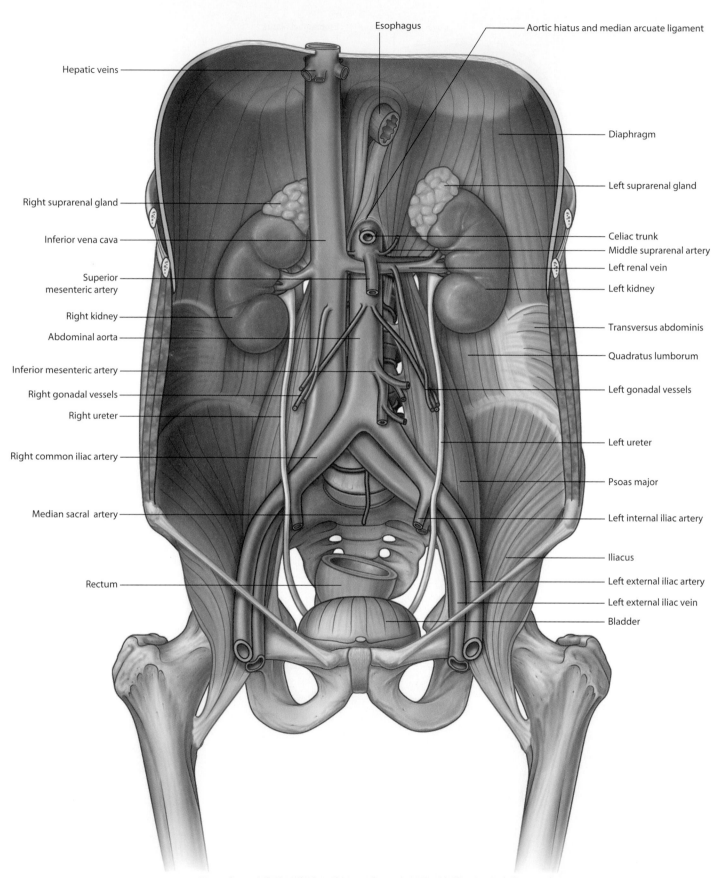

Esophagus

Aortic hiatus and median arcuate ligament

Hepatic veins

Diaphragm

Right suprarenal gland

Left suprarenal gland

Inferior vena cava

Celiac trunk

Middle suprarenal artery

Left renal vein

Superior mesenteric artery

Left kidney

Right kidney

Transversus abdominis

Abdominal aorta

Quadratus lumborum

Inferior mesenteric artery

Left gonadal vessels

Right gonadal vessels

Left ureter

Right ureter

Right common iliac artery

Psoas major

Median sacral artery

Left internal iliac artery

Iliacus

Left external iliac artery

Rectum

Left external iliac vein

Bladder

Vessels and their relationship to the posterior abdominal wall

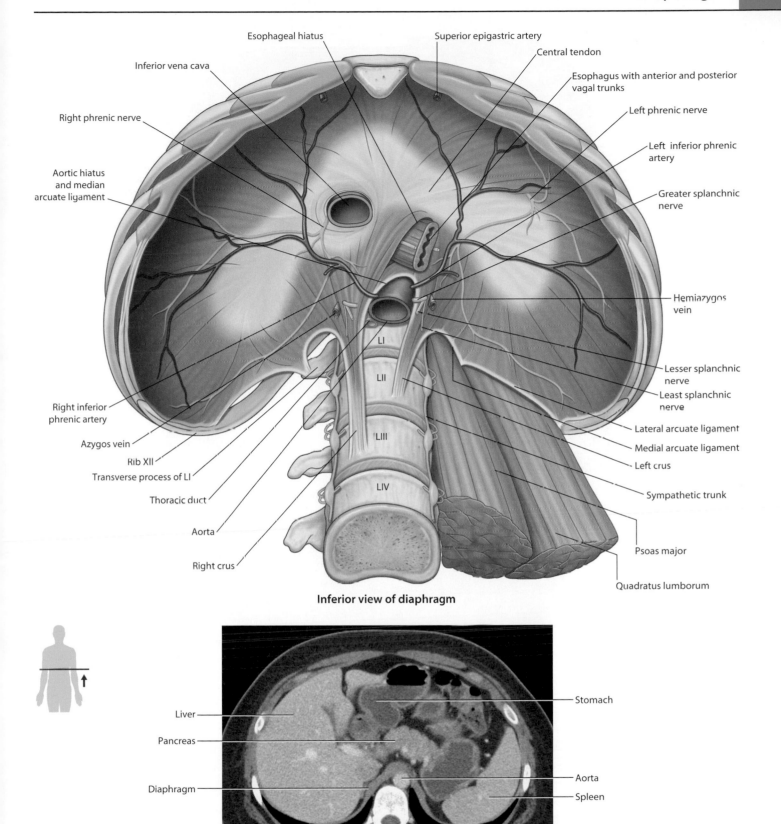

Inferior view of diaphragm

Positioning of the diaphragm in relation to other structures.
CT image, with contrast, in axial plane

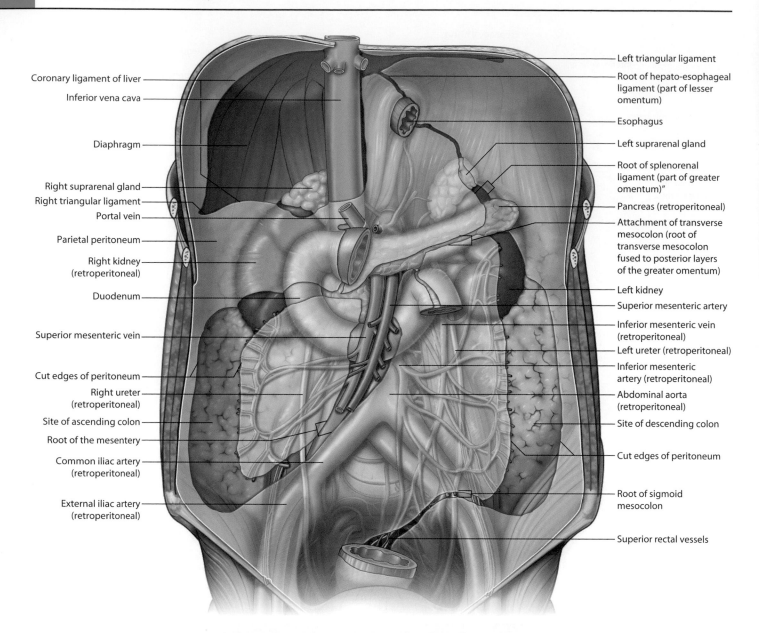

Coronary ligament of liver

Inferior vena cava

Diaphragm

Right suprarenal gland

Right triangular ligament

Portal vein

Parietal peritoneum

Right kidney (retroperitoneal)

Duodenum

Superior mesenteric vein

Cut edges of peritoneum

Right ureter (retroperitoneal)

Site of ascending colon

Root of the mesentery

Common iliac artery (retroperitoneal)

External iliac artery (retroperitoneal)

Left triangular ligament

Root of hepato-esophageal ligament (part of lesser omentum)

Esophagus

Left suprarenal gland

Root of splenorenal ligament (part of greater omentum)"

Pancreas (retroperitoneal)

Attachment of transverse mesocolon (root of transverse mesocolon fused to posterior layers of the greater omentum)

Left kidney

Superior mesenteric artery

Inferior mesenteric vein (retroperitoneal)

Left ureter (retroperitoneal)

Inferior mesenteric artery (retroperitoneal)

Abdominal aorta (retroperitoneal)

Site of descending colon

Cut edges of peritoneum

Root of sigmoid mesocolon

Superior rectal vessels

Peritoneum and the retroperitoneal position of the kidneys

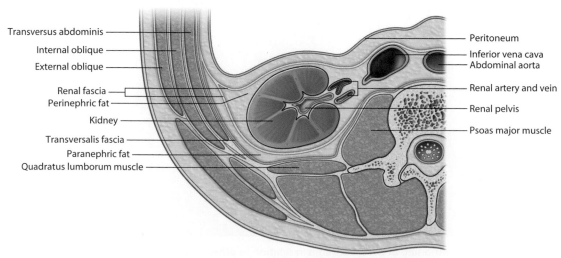

Transversus abdominis

Internal oblique

External oblique

Renal fascia

Perinephric fat

Kidney

Transversalis fascia

Paranephric fat

Quadratus lumborum muscle

Peritoneum

Inferior vena cava

Abdominal aorta

Renal artery and vein

Renal pelvis

Psoas major muscle

Organization of fat and fascia surrounding the kidneys

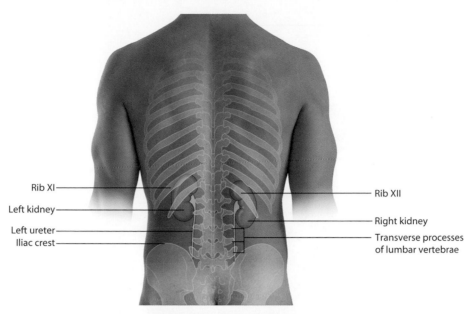

Surface projection of the kidneys and ureters (posterior view)

Rib XI — Left kidney — Left ureter — Iliac crest

Rib XII — Right kidney — Transverse processes of lumbar vertebrae

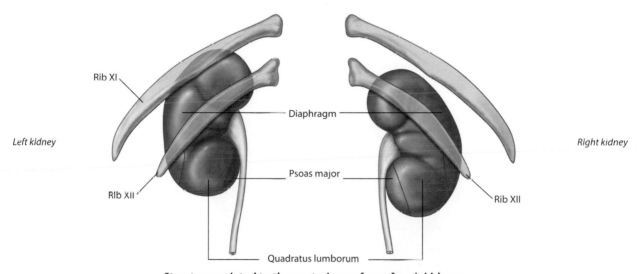

Left kidney

Rib XI — Diaphragm — Psoas major — Rib XII — Quadratus lumborum

Right kidney

Rib XII

Structures related to the posterior surface of each kidney

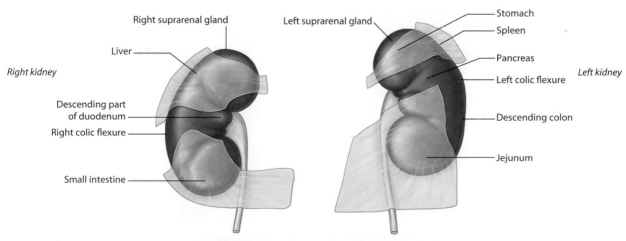

Right kidney

Right suprarenal gland — Liver — Descending part of duodenum — Right colic flexure — Small intestine

Left suprarenal gland — Stomach — Spleen — Pancreas — Left colic flexure — Descending colon — Jejunum

Left kidney

Structures related to the anterior surface of each kidney

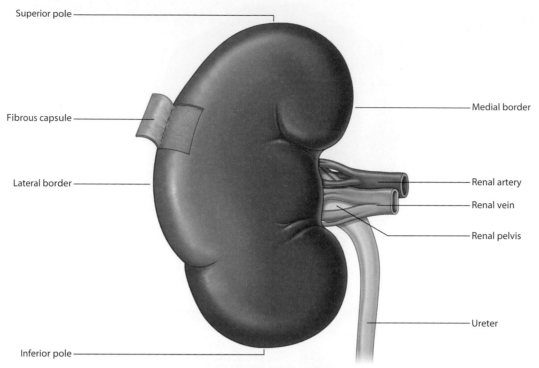

Superior pole

Fibrous capsule

Lateral border

Inferior pole

Medial border

Renal artery

Renal vein

Renal pelvis

Ureter

Anterior surface of right kidney

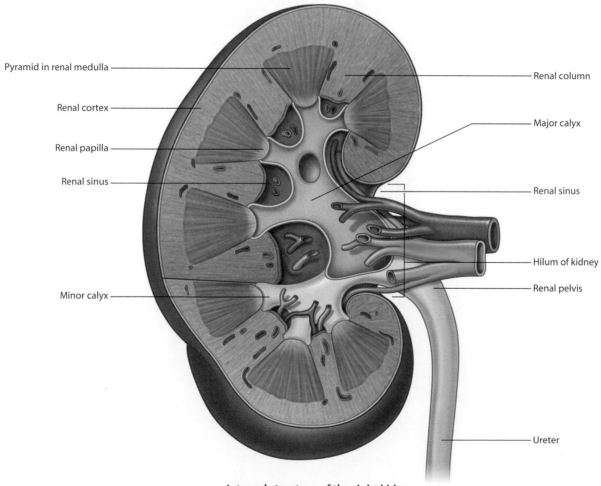

Pyramid in renal medulla

Renal cortex

Renal papilla

Renal sinus

Minor calyx

Renal column

Major calyx

Renal sinus

Hilum of kidney

Renal pelvis

Ureter

Internal structure of the right kidney

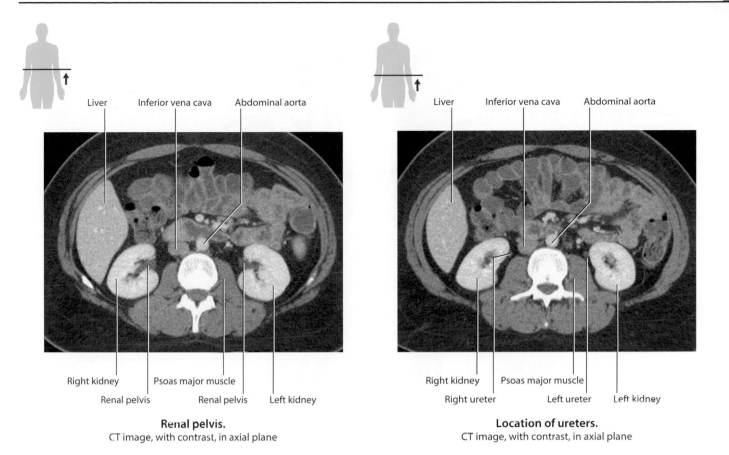

Liver | Inferior vena cava | Abdominal aorta

Right kidney | Psoas major muscle
Renal pelvis | Renal pelvis | Left kidney

Renal pelvis.
CT image, with contrast, in axial plane

Liver | Inferior vena cava | Abdominal aorta

Right kidney | Psoas major muscle
Right ureter | Left ureter | Left kidney

Location of ureters.
CT image, with contrast, in axial plane

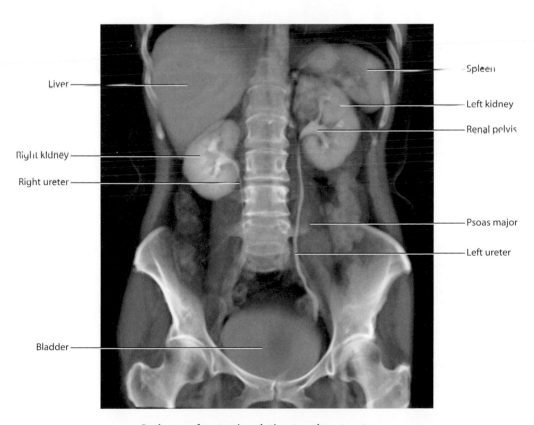

Liver

Spleen

Left kidney

Renal pelvis

Right kidney

Right ureter

Psoas major

Left ureter

Bladder

Pathway of ureter in relation to other structures.
Coronal view of 3-D urogram using multidetector computed tomography

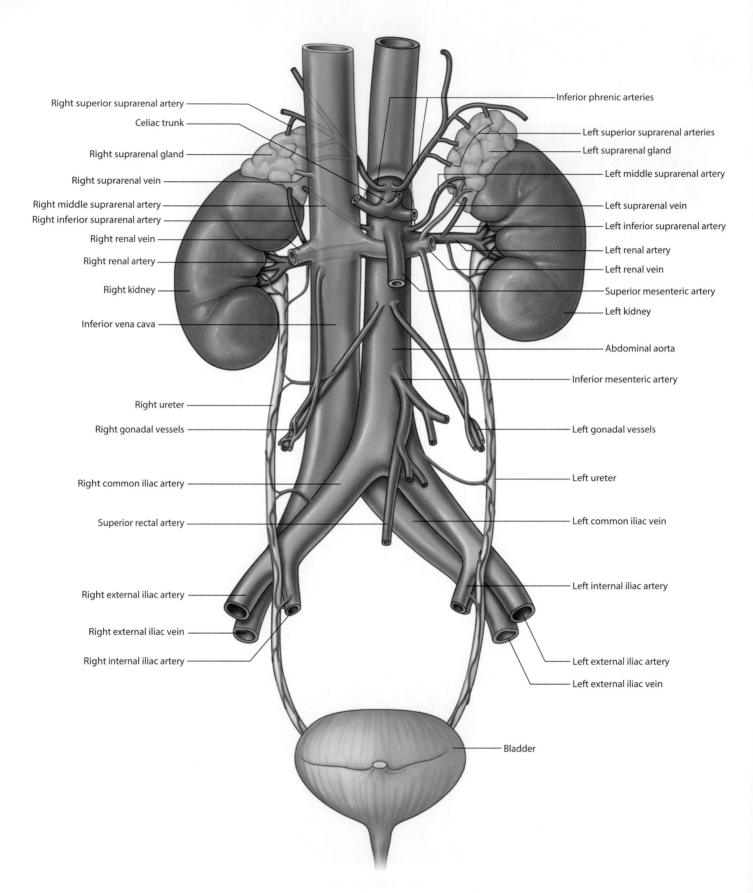

Right superior suprarenal artery

Celiac trunk

Right suprarenal gland

Right suprarenal vein

Right middle suprarenal artery

Right inferior suprarenal artery

Right renal vein

Right renal artery

Right kidney

Inferior vena cava

Right ureter

Right gonadal vessels

Right common iliac artery

Superior rectal artery

Right external iliac artery

Right external iliac vein

Right internal iliac artery

Inferior phrenic arteries

Left superior suprarenal arteries

Left suprarenal gland

Left middle suprarenal artery

Left suprarenal vein

Left inferior suprarenal artery

Left renal artery

Left renal vein

Superior mesenteric artery

Left kidney

Abdominal aorta

Inferior mesenteric artery

Left gonadal vessels

Left ureter

Left common iliac vein

Left internal iliac artery

Left external iliac artery

Left external iliac vein

Bladder

Vasculature relating to kidneys, suprarenal glands, and ureters

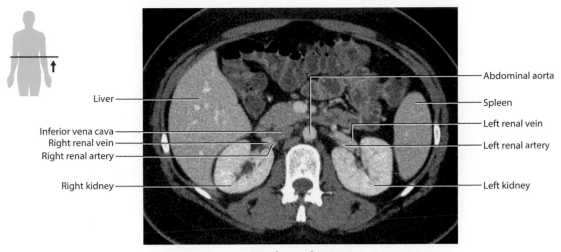

Liver

Inferior vena cava
Right renal vein
Right renal artery

Right kidney

Abdominal aorta

Spleen

Left renal vein

Left renal artery

Left kidney

Renal vasculature.
CT image, with contrast, in axial plane

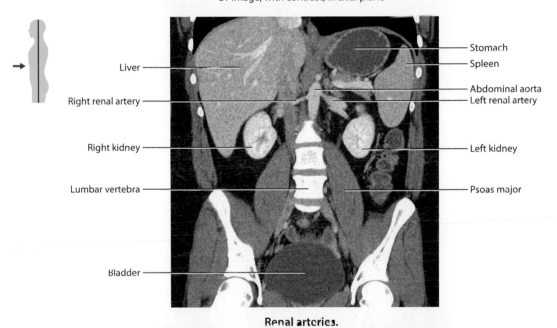

Liver

Right renal artery

Right kidney

Lumbar vertebra

Bladder

Stomach
Spleen

Abdominal aorta
Left renal artery

Left kidney

Psoas major

Renal arteries.
CT image, with contrast, in coronal plane

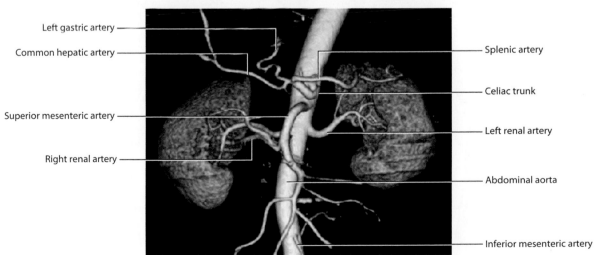

Left gastric artery

Common hepatic artery

Superior mesenteric artery

Right renal artery

Splenic artery

Celiac trunk

Left renal artery

Abdominal aorta

Inferior mesenteric artery

Renal arteries.
Volume-rendered anterior view using multidetector computer tomography

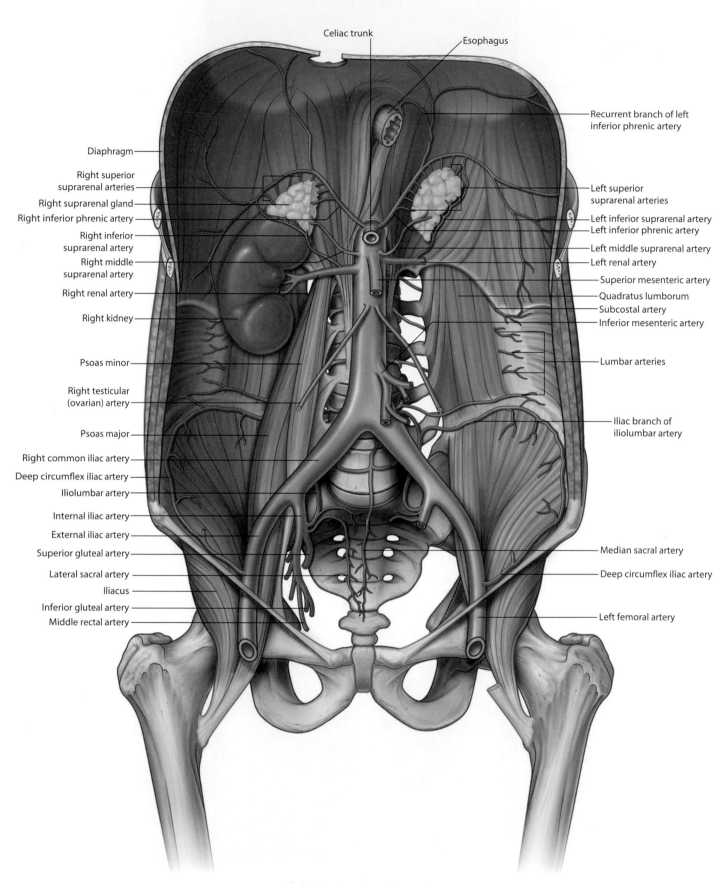

Celiac trunk

Esophagus

Recurrent branch of left inferior phrenic artery

Diaphragm

Right superior suprarenal arteries

Right suprarenal gland

Right inferior phrenic artery

Right inferior suprarenal artery

Right middle suprarenal artery

Right renal artery

Right kidney

Psoas minor

Right testicular (ovarian) artery

Psoas major

Right common iliac artery

Deep circumflex iliac artery

Iliolumbar artery

Internal iliac artery

External iliac artery

Superior gluteal artery

Lateral sacral artery

Iliacus

Inferior gluteal artery

Middle rectal artery

Left superior suprarenal arteries

Left inferior suprarenal artery

Left inferior phrenic artery

Left middle suprarenal artery

Left renal artery

Superior mesenteric artery

Quadratus lumborum

Subcostal artery

Inferior mesenteric artery

Lumbar arteries

Iliac branch of iliolumbar artery

Median sacral artery

Deep circumflex iliac artery

Left femoral artery

Abdominal aorta and branches

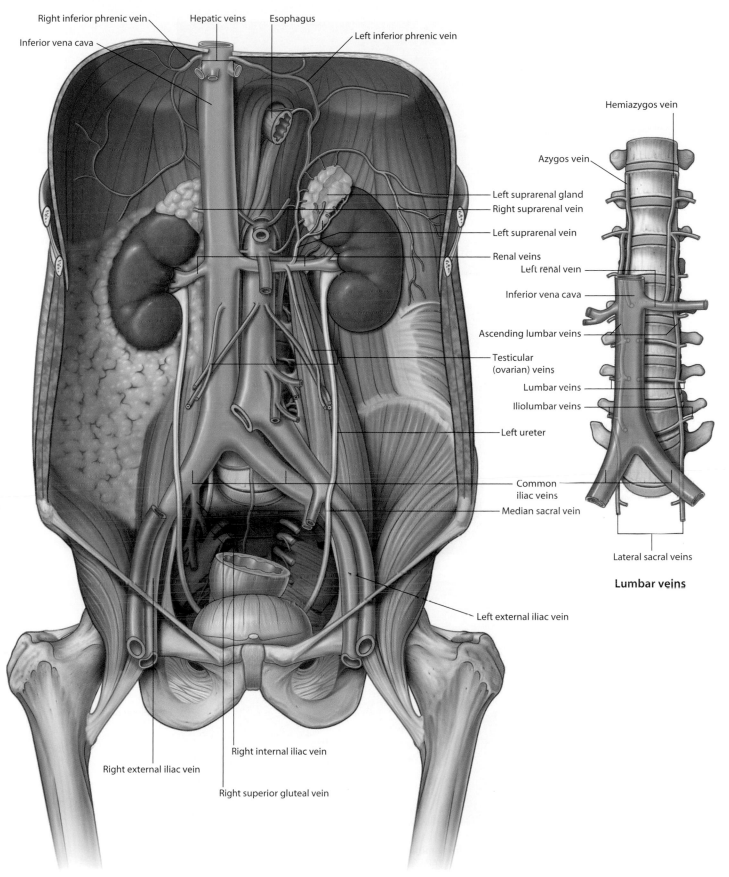

Right inferior phrenic vein

Hepatic veins

Esophagus

Left inferior phrenic vein

Inferior vena cava

Hemiazygos vein

Azygos vein

Left suprarenal gland

Right suprarenal vein

Left suprarenal vein

Renal veins

Left renal vein

Inferior vena cava

Ascending lumbar veins

Testicular (ovarian) veins

Lumbar veins

Iliolumbar veins

Left ureter

Common iliac veins

Median sacral vein

Lateral sacral veins

Lumbar veins

Left external iliac vein

Right external iliac vein

Right internal iliac vein

Right superior gluteal vein

Inferior vena cava and tributaries

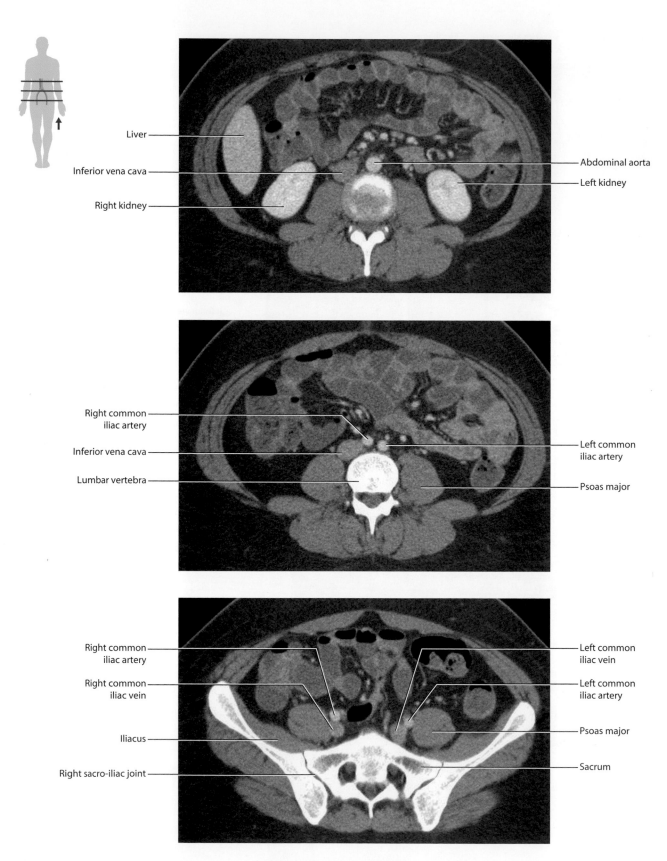

Liver

Inferior vena cava

Right kidney

Abdominal aorta

Left kidney

Right common iliac artery

Inferior vena cava

Lumbar vertebra

Left common iliac artery

Psoas major

Right common iliac artery

Right common iliac vein

Iliacus

Right sacro-iliac joint

Left common iliac vein

Left common iliac artery

Psoas major

Sacrum

Abdominal aorta and inferior vena cava.
CT images, with contrast, in axial plane

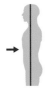

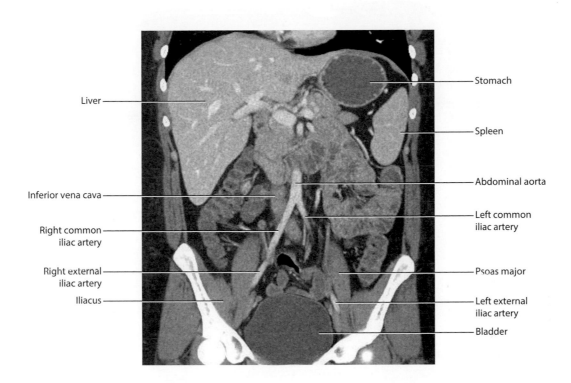

Liver

Stomach

Spleen

Abdominal aorta

Inferior vena cava

Left common
iliac artery

Right common
iliac artery

Psoas major

Right external
iliac artery

Left external
iliac artery

Iliacus

Bladder

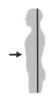

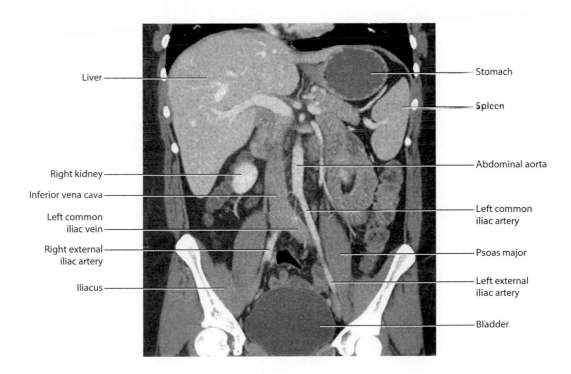

Liver

Stomach

Spleen

Abdominal aorta

Right kidney

Inferior vena cava

Left common
iliac artery

Left common
iliac vein

Right external
iliac artery

Psoas major

Left external
iliac artery

Iliacus

Bladder

Positioning of the abdominal aorta and inferior vena cava in relation to other structures.
CT images, with contrast, in coronal plane

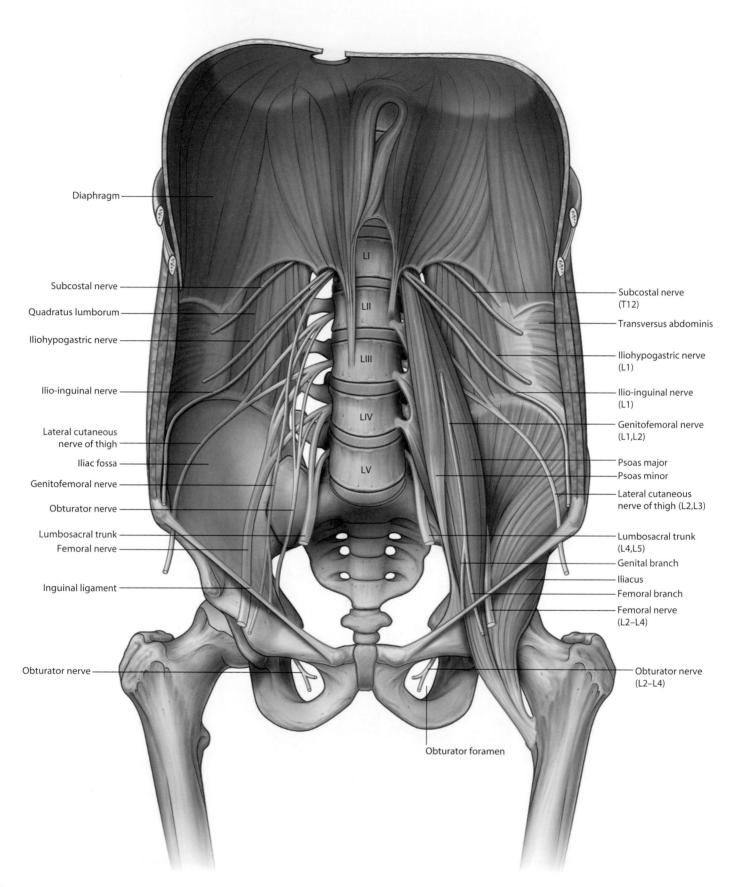

Diaphragm

Subcostal nerve

Quadratus lumborum

Iliohypogastric nerve

Ilio-inguinal nerve

Lateral cutaneous
nerve of thigh

Iliac fossa

Genitofemoral nerve

Obturator nerve

Lumbosacral trunk

Femoral nerve

Inguinal ligament

Obturator nerve

LI

LII

LIII

LIV

LV

Subcostal nerve
(T12)

Transversus abdominis

Iliohypogastric nerve
(L1)

Ilio-inguinal nerve
(L1)

Genitofemoral nerve
(L1,L2)

Psoas major

Psoas minor

Lateral cutaneous
nerve of thigh (L2,L3)

Lumbosacral trunk
(L4,L5)

Genital branch

Iliacus

Femoral branch

Femoral nerve
(L2–L4)

Obturator nerve
(L2–L4)

Obturator foramen

Lumbar plexus

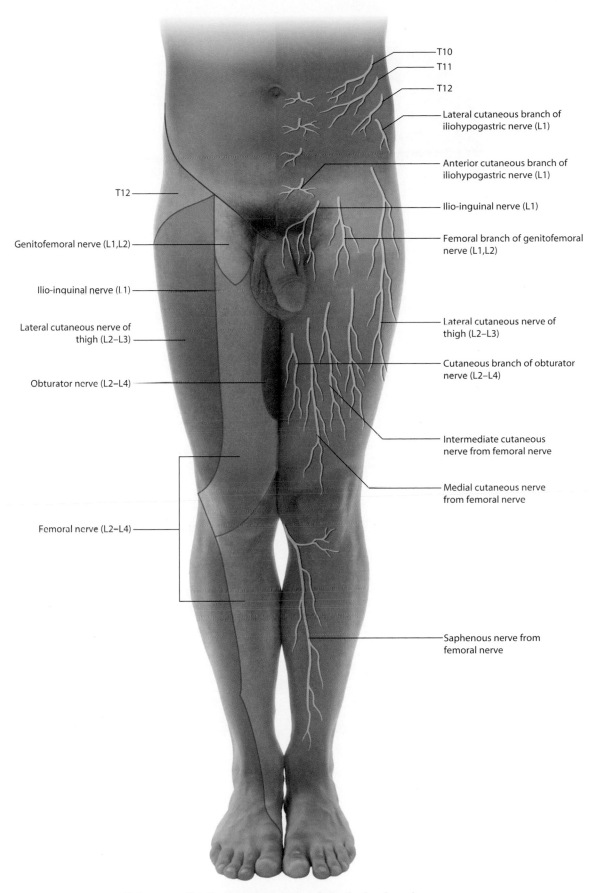

T10
T11
T12
Lateral cutaneous branch of iliohypogastric nerve (L1)
Anterior cutaneous branch of iliohypogastric nerve (L1)
Ilio-inguinal nerve (L1)
Femoral branch of genitofemoral nerve (L1,L2)
Lateral cutaneous nerve of thigh (L2–L3)
Cutaneous branch of obturator nerve (L2–L4)
Intermediate cutaneous nerve from femoral nerve
Medial cutaneous nerve from femoral nerve
Saphenous nerve from femoral nerve

T12
Genitofemoral nerve (L1,L2)
Ilio-inguinal nerve (L1)
Lateral cutaneous nerve of thigh (L2–L3)
Obturator nerve (L2–L4)
Femoral nerve (L2–L4)

Cutaneous distribution of the nerves from the lumbar plexus

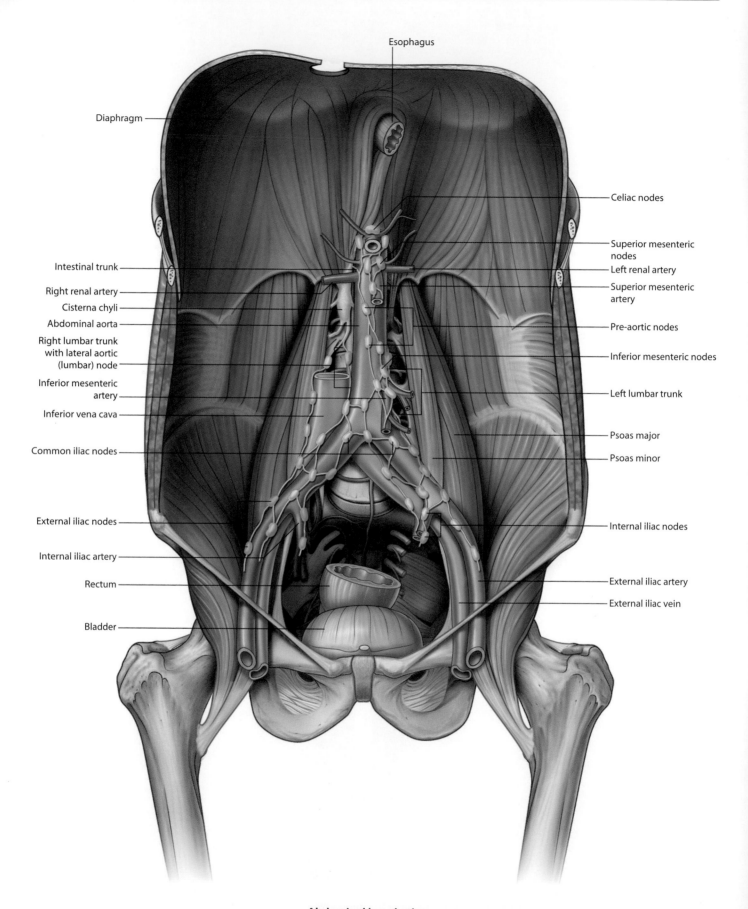

Esophagus

Diaphragm

Celiac nodes

Superior mesenteric nodes

Intestinal trunk

Left renal artery

Right renal artery

Superior mesenteric artery

Cisterna chyli

Abdominal aorta

Pre-aortic nodes

Right lumbar trunk with lateral aortic (lumbar) node

Inferior mesenteric nodes

Inferior mesenteric artery

Left lumbar trunk

Inferior vena cava

Psoas major

Common iliac nodes

Psoas minor

External iliac nodes

Internal iliac nodes

Internal iliac artery

Rectum

External iliac artery

External iliac vein

Bladder

Abdominal lymphatics

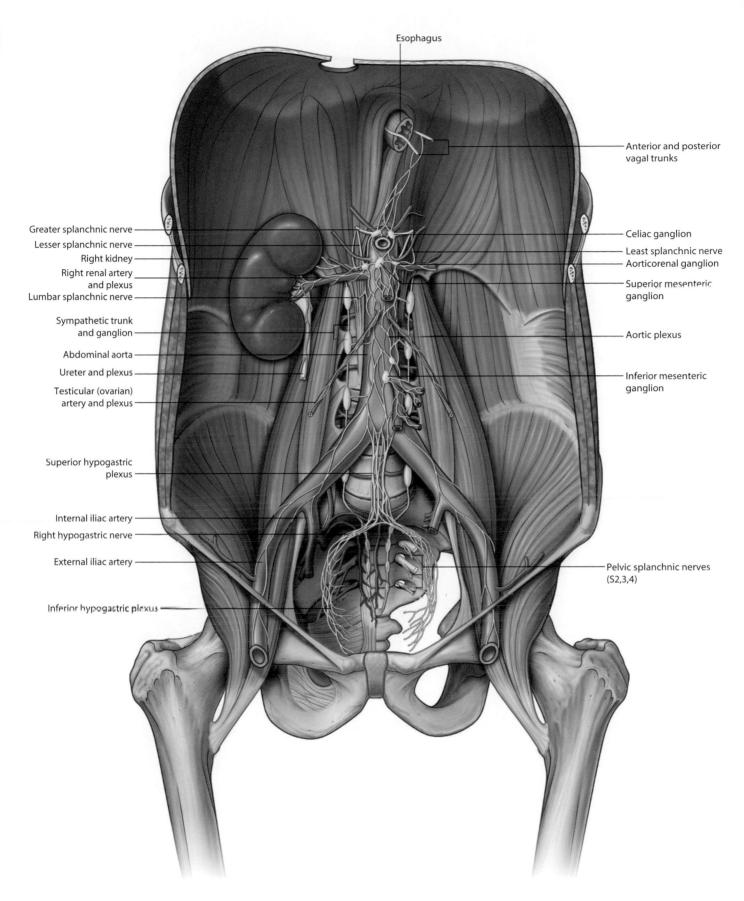

Esophagus

Anterior and posterior vagal trunks

Greater splanchnic nerve

Lesser splanchnic nerve

Right kidney

Right renal artery and plexus

Lumbar splanchnic nerve

Sympathetic trunk and ganglion

Abdominal aorta

Ureter and plexus

Testicular (ovarian) artery and plexus

Superior hypogastric plexus

Internal iliac artery

Right hypogastric nerve

External iliac artery

Inferior hypogastric plexus

Celiac ganglion

Least splanchnic nerve

Aorticorenal ganglion

Superior mesenteric ganglion

Aortic plexus

Inferior mesenteric ganglion

Pelvic splanchnic nerves (S2,3,4)

Prevertebral plexuses and ganglia with sympathetic trunks

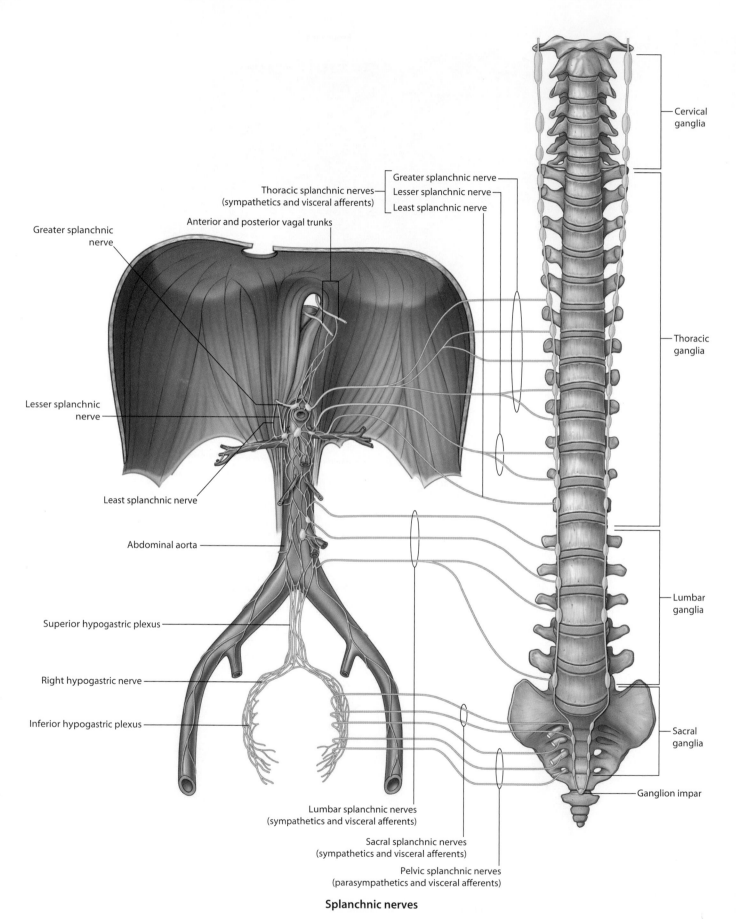

Greater splanchnic nerve

Thoracic splanchnic nerves (sympathetics and visceral afferents)

Anterior and posterior vagal trunks

Greater splanchnic nerve

Lesser splanchnic nerve

Least splanchnic nerve

Cervical ganglia

Thoracic ganglia

Lesser splanchnic nerve

Least splanchnic nerve

Abdominal aorta

Superior hypogastric plexus

Right hypogastric nerve

Inferior hypogastric plexus

Lumbar ganglia

Sacral ganglia

Ganglion impar

Lumbar splanchnic nerves (sympathetics and visceral afferents)

Sacral splanchnic nerves (sympathetics and visceral afferents)

Pelvic splanchnic nerves (parasympathetics and visceral afferents)

Splanchnic nerves

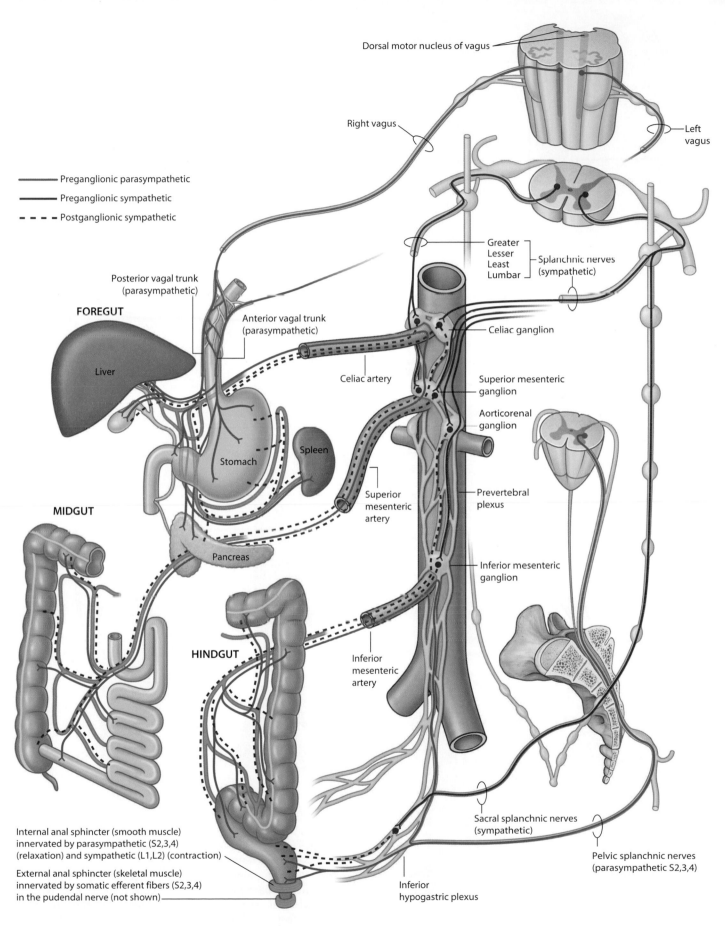

Dorsal motor nucleus of vagus

Right vagus

Left vagus

Preganglionic parasympathetic
Preganglionic sympathetic
Postganglionic sympathetic

Greater
Lesser
Least — Splanchnic nerves
Lumbar (sympathetic)

Posterior vagal trunk
(parasympathetic)

FOREGUT

Anterior vagal trunk
(parasympathetic)

Celiac ganglion

Liver

Celiac artery

Superior mesenteric
ganglion

Aorticorenal
ganglion

Stomach

Spleen

Prevertebral
plexus

MIDGUT

Superior
mesenteric
artery

Pancreas

Inferior mesenteric
ganglion

HINDGUT

Inferior
mesenteric
artery

Internal anal sphincter (smooth muscle)
innervated by parasympathetic (S2,3,4)
(relaxation) and sympathetic (L1,L2) (contraction)

External anal sphincter (skeletal muscle)
innervated by somatic efferent fibers (S2,3,4)
in the pudendal nerve (not shown)

Sacral splanchnic nerves
(sympathetic)

Pelvic splanchnic nerves
(parasympathetic S2,3,4)

Inferior
hypogastric plexus

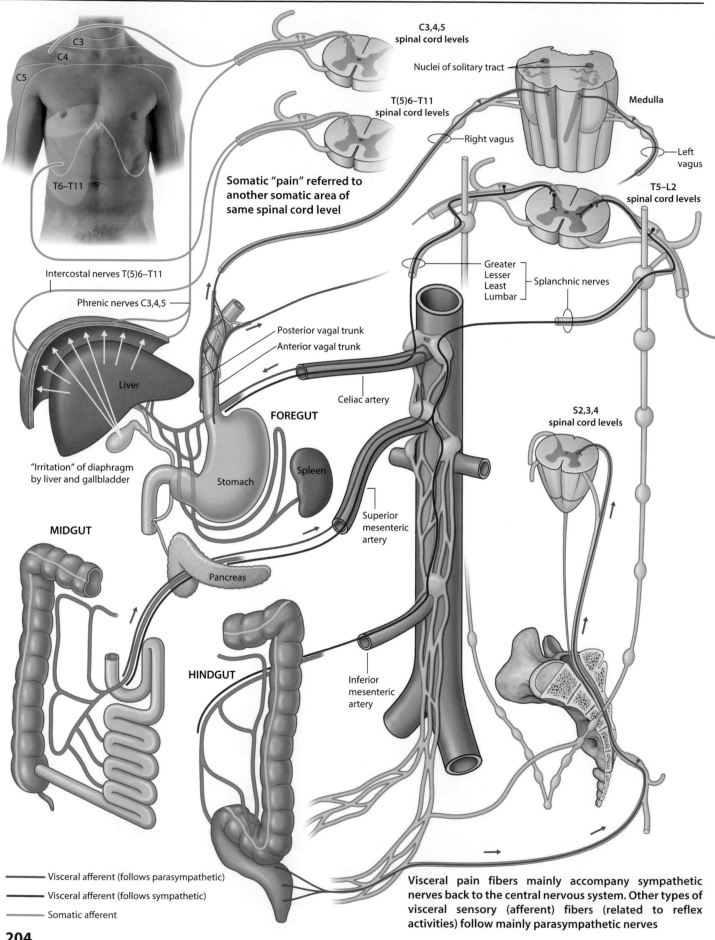

C3,4,5
spinal cord levels

Nuclei of solitary tract

Medulla

T(5)6–T11
spinal cord levels

Right vagus

Left vagus

T5–L2
spinal cord levels

C3

C4

C5

T6–T11

Somatic "pain" referred to
another somatic area of
same spinal cord level

Intercostal nerves T(5)6–T11

Phrenic nerves C3,4,5

Greater
Lesser
Least
Lumbar — Splanchnic nerves

Posterior vagal trunk

Anterior vagal trunk

Celiac artery

FOREGUT

Liver

"Irritation" of diaphragm
by liver and gallbladder

Stomach

Spleen

S2,3,4
spinal cord levels

MIDGUT

Superior
mesenteric
artery

Pancreas

HINDGUT

Inferior
mesenteric
artery

— Visceral afferent (follows parasympathetic)

— Visceral afferent (follows sympathetic)

— Somatic afferent

Visceral pain fibers mainly accompany sympathetic
nerves back to the central nervous system. Other types of
visceral sensory (afferent) fibers (related to reflex
activities) follow mainly parasympathetic nerves

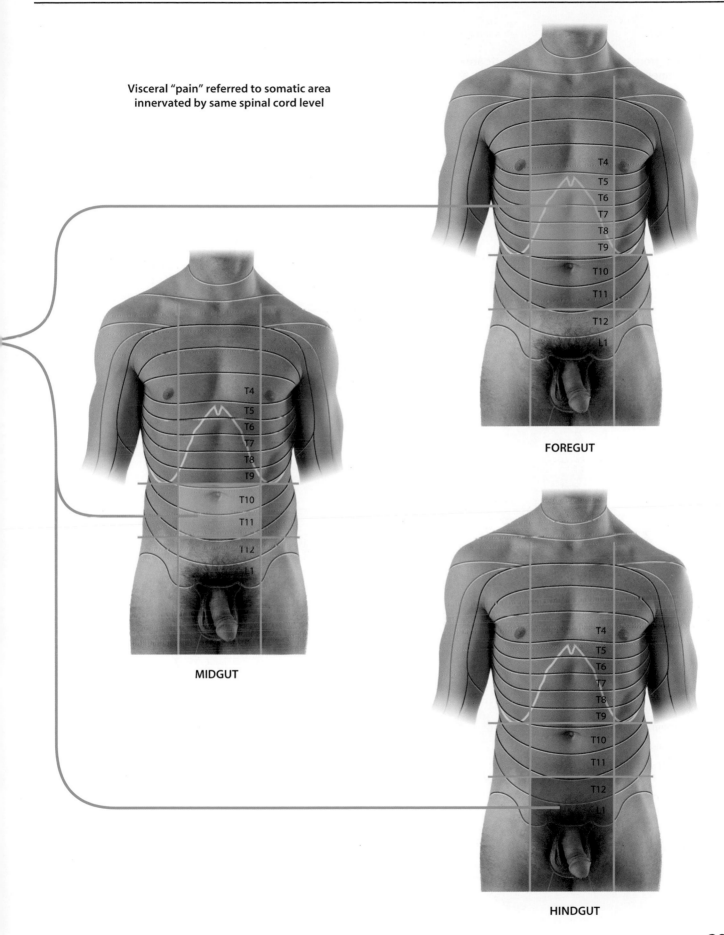

Visceral "pain" referred to somatic area
innervated by same spinal cord level

FOREGUT

MIDGUT

HINDGUT

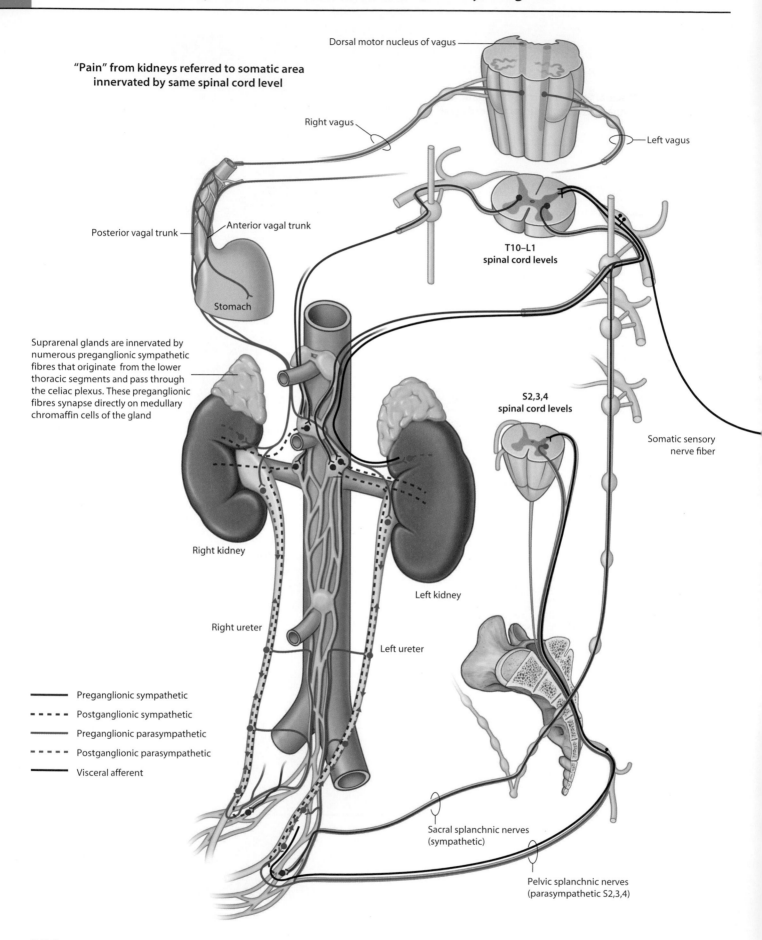

"Pain" from kidneys referred to somatic area innervated by same spinal cord level

Dorsal motor nucleus of vagus

Right vagus

Left vagus

Posterior vagal trunk

Anterior vagal trunk

T10–L1 spinal cord levels

Stomach

Suprarenal glands are innervated by numerous preganglionic sympathetic fibres that originate from the lower thoracic segments and pass through the celiac plexus. These preganglionic fibres synapse directly on medullary chromaffin cells of the gland

S2,3,4 spinal cord levels

Somatic sensory nerve fiber

Right kidney

Left kidney

Right ureter

Left ureter

——— Preganglionic sympathetic

- - - - Postganglionic sympathetic

——— Preganglionic parasympathetic

- - - - Postganglionic parasympathetic

——— Visceral afferent

Sacral splanchnic nerves (sympathetic)

Pelvic splanchnic nerves (parasympathetic S2,3,4)

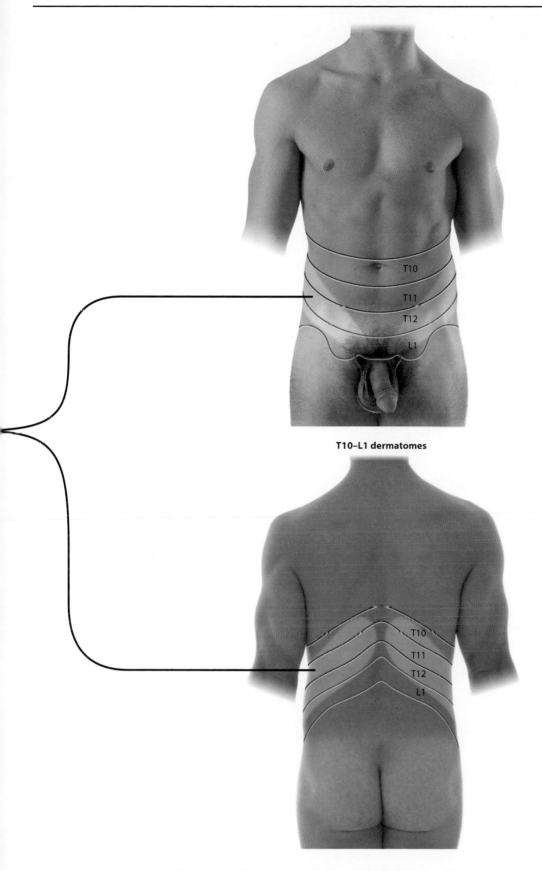

T10–L1 dermatomes

Pain fibers mainly follow sympathetic nerves to the central nervous system (CNS). This pain is 'referred' by the CNS to the somatic area innervated by the same spinal levels. Other types of visceral afferent (sensory) fibers (related to reflex activities) follow mainly parasympathetic nerves

Abdominal wall muscles

Muscle		Origin	Insertion	Innervation	Function
External oblique	1	Muscular slips from the outer surfaces of the lower eight ribs (ribs V to XII)	Lateral lip of iliac crest; aponeurosis ending in midline raphe (linea alba)	Anterior rami of lower six thoracic spinal nerves (T7 to T12)	Compress abdominal contents; both muscles flex trunk; each muscle bends trunk to same side, turning anterior part of abdomen to opposite side
Internal oblique	2	Thoracolumbar fascia; iliac crest between origins of external and transversus; lateral two-thirds of inguinal ligament	Inferior border of the lower three or four ribs; aponeurosis ending in linea alba; pubic crest and pectineal line	Anterior rami of lower six thoracic spinal nerves (T7 to T12) and L1	Compress abdominal contents; both muscles flex trunk; each muscle bends trunk and turns anterior part of abdomen to same side
Transversus abdominis	3	Thoracolumbar fascia; medial lip of iliac crest; lateral one-third of inguinal ligament; costal cartilages lower six ribs (ribs VII to XII)	Aponeurosis ending in linea alba; pubic crest and pectineal line	Anterior rami of lower six thoracic spinal nerves (T7 to T12) and L1	Compress abdominal contents
Rectus abdominis	4	Pubic crest, pubic tubercle, and pubic symphysis	Costal cartilages of ribs V to VII; xiphoid process	Anterior rami of lower seven thoracic spinal nerves (T7 to T12)	Compress abdominal contents; flex vertebral column; tense abdominal wall
Pyramidalis	5	Front of pubis and pubic symphysis	Into linea alba	Anterior ramus of T12	Tenses the linea alba

Posterior abdominal wall muscles

Muscle		Origin	Insertion	Innervation	Function
Psoas major	6	Lateral surface of bodies of TXII and LI to LV vertebrae, transverse processes of the lumbar vertebrae, and the intervertebral discs between TXII and LI to LV vertebrae	Lesser trochanter of the femur	Anterior rami of L1 to L3	Flexion of thigh at hip joint
Psoas minor	7	Lateral surface of bodies of TXII and LI vertebrae and intervening intervertebral disc	Pectineal line of the pelvic brim and iliopubic eminence	Anterior rami of L1	Weak flexion of lumbar vertebral column
Quadratus lumborum	8	Transverse process of LV vertebra, iliolumbar ligament, and iliac crest	Transverse processes of LI to LIV vertebrae and inferior border of rib XII	Anterior rami of T12 and L1 to L4	Depress and stabilize rib XII and some lateral bending of trunk
Iliacus	9	Upper two-thirds of iliac fossa, anterior sacro-iliac and iliolumbar ligaments, and upper lateral surface of sacrum	Lesser trochanter of femur	Femoral nerve (L2 to L4)	Flexion of thigh at hip joint

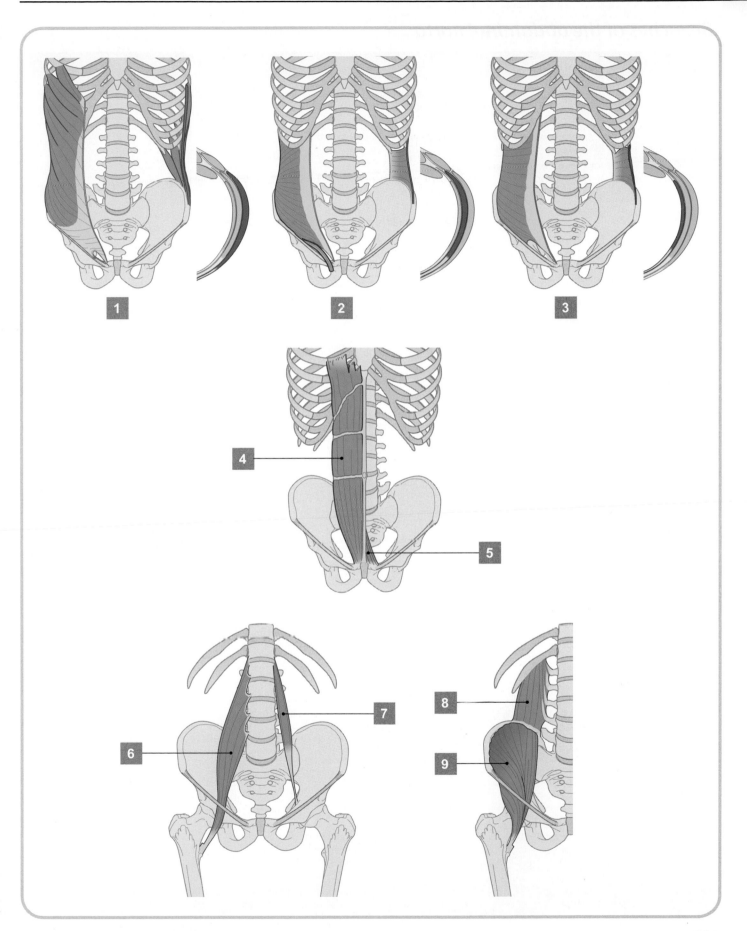

Branches of the abdominal aorta

Artery		Branch	Origin	Parts supplied
Celiac trunk	1	Anterior	Immediately inferior to the aortic hiatus of the diaphragm	Abdominal foregut
Superior mesenteric artery	2	Anterior	Immediately inferior to the celiac trunk	Abdominal midgut
Inferior mesenteric artery	3	Anterior	Inferior to the renal arteries	Abdominal hindgut
Middle suprarenal arteries	4	Lateral	Immediately superior to the renal arteries	Suprarenal glands
Renal arteries	5	Lateral	Immediately inferior to the superior mesenteric artery	Kidneys
Testicular or ovarian arteries	6	Paired anterior	Inferior to the renal arteries	Testes in male and ovaries in female
Inferior phrenic arteries	7	Lateral	Immediately inferior to the aortic hiatus	Diaphragm
Lumbar arteries	8	Posterior	Usually four pairs	Posterior abdominal wall and spinal cord
Median sacral artery	9	Posterior	Just superior to the aortic bifurcation, passes inferiorly across lumbar vertebrae, sacrum, and coccyx	
Common iliac arteries	10	Terminal	Bifurcation usually occurs at the level of LIV vertebra	

Branches of the lumbar plexus

Branch		Origin	Spinal segments	Function: motor	Function: sensory
Iliohypogastric	1	Anterior ramus L1	L1	Internal oblique and transversus abdominis	Posterolateral gluteal skin and skin in pubic region
Ilio-inguinal	2	Anterior ramus L1	L1	Internal oblique and transversus abdominis	Skin in the upper medial thigh, and either the skin over the root of the penis and anterior scrotum or the mons pubis and labium majus
Genitofemoral	3	Anterior rami L1 and L2	L1, L2	Genital branch—male cremasteric muscle	Genital branch—skin of anterior scrotum or skin of mons pubis and labium majus; femoral branch—skin of upper anterior thigh
Lateral cutaneous nerve of thigh	4	Anterior rami L2 and L3	L2, L3		Skin on anterior and lateral thigh to the knee
Obturator	5	Anterior rami L2 to L4	L2 to L4	Obturator externus, pectineus, and muscles in medial compartment of thigh	Skin on medial aspect of the thigh
Femoral	6	Anterior rami L2 to L4	L2 to L4	Iliacus, pectineus, and muscles in anterior compartment of thigh	Skin on anterior thigh and medial surface of leg

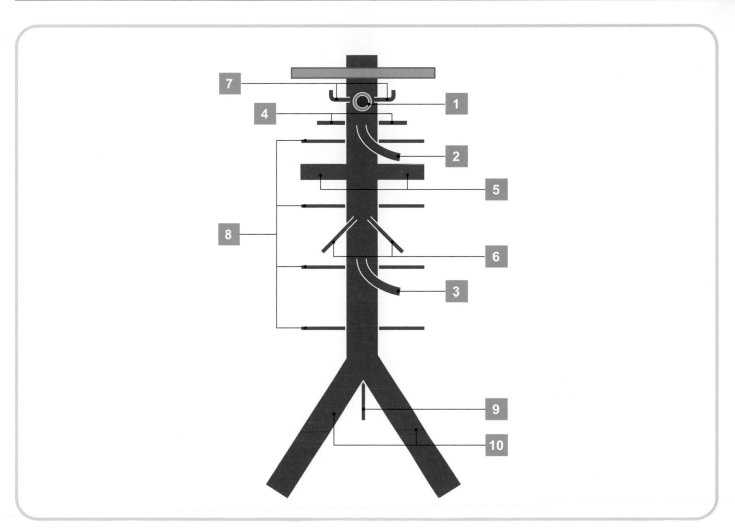

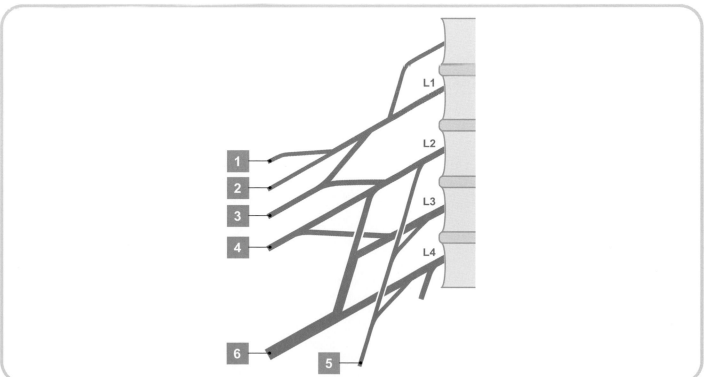

5

PELVIS AND PERINEUM

CONTENTS

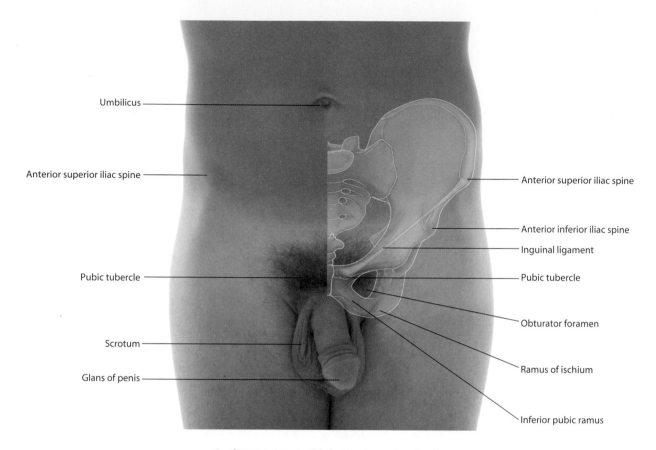

Umbilicus

Anterior superior iliac spine

Anterior superior iliac spine

Anterior inferior iliac spine

Inguinal ligament

Pubic tubercle

Pubic tubercle

Obturator foramen

Scrotum

Ramus of ischium

Glans of penis

Inferior pubic ramus

Surface anatomy with bones (anterior view)

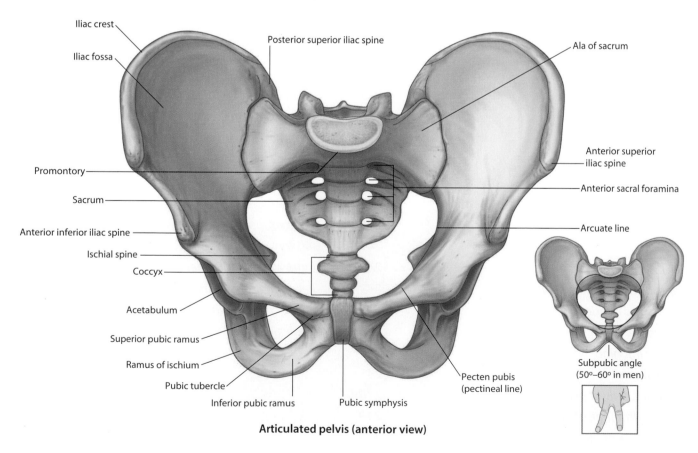

Iliac crest

Iliac fossa

Posterior superior iliac spine

Ala of sacrum

Promontory

Anterior superior
iliac spine

Sacrum

Anterior sacral foramina

Anterior inferior iliac spine

Arcuate line

Ischial spine

Coccyx

Acetabulum

Superior pubic ramus

Ramus of ischium

Pubic tubercle

Pecten pubis
(pectineal line)

Inferior pubic ramus

Pubic symphysis

Subpubic angle
(50°–60° in men)

Articulated pelvis (anterior view)

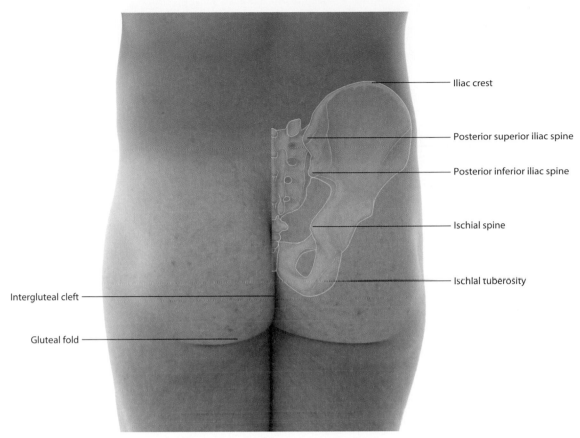

Surface anatomy with bones (posterior view)

Iliac crest

Posterior superior iliac spine

Posterior inferior iliac spine

Ischial spine

Ischial tuberosity

Intergluteal cleft

Gluteal fold

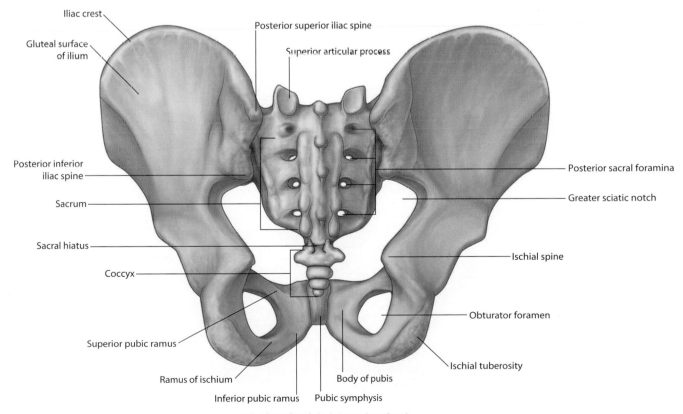

Articulated pelvis (posterior view)

Iliac crest

Gluteal surface of ilium

Posterior superior iliac spine

Superior articular process

Posterior inferior iliac spine

Sacrum

Sacral hiatus

Coccyx

Superior pubic ramus

Ramus of ischium

Inferior pubic ramus

Pubic symphysis

Body of pubis

Posterior sacral foramina

Greater sciatic notch

Ischial spine

Obturator foramen

Ischial tuberosity

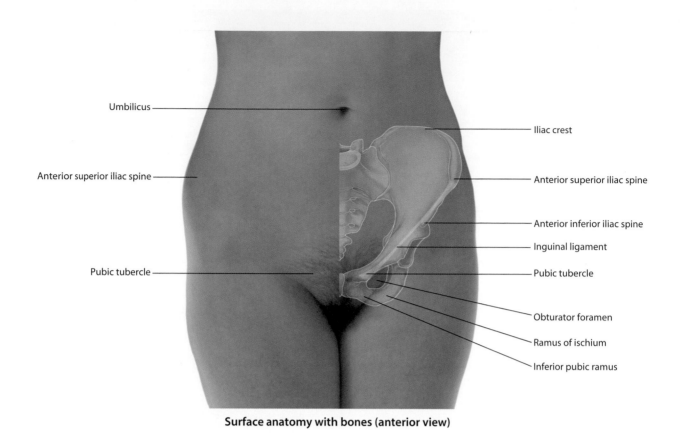

Umbilicus

Anterior superior iliac spine

Pubic tubercle

Iliac crest

Anterior superior iliac spine

Anterior inferior iliac spine

Inguinal ligament

Pubic tubercle

Obturator foramen

Ramus of ischium

Inferior pubic ramus

Surface anatomy with bones (anterior view)

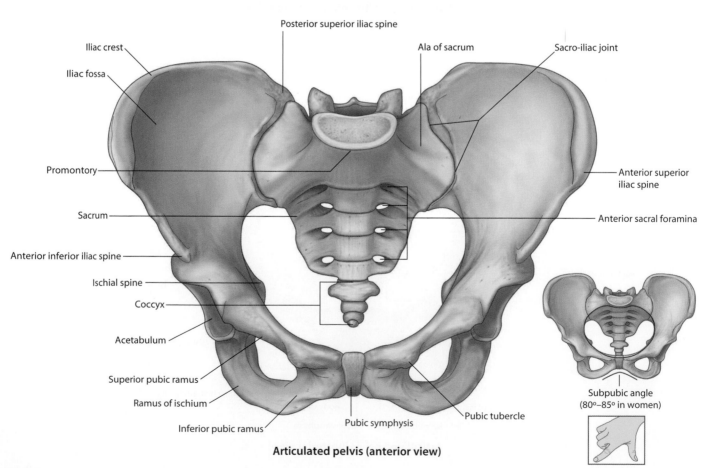

Posterior superior iliac spine

Ala of sacrum

Sacro-iliac joint

Iliac crest

Iliac fossa

Promontory

Sacrum

Anterior inferior iliac spine

Ischial spine

Coccyx

Acetabulum

Superior pubic ramus

Ramus of ischium

Inferior pubic ramus

Pubic symphysis

Pubic tubercle

Anterior superior iliac spine

Anterior sacral foramina

Subpubic angle
(80°–85° in women)

Articulated pelvis (anterior view)

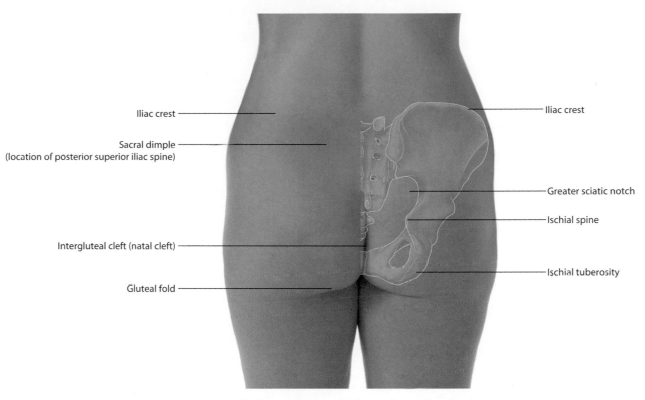

Surface anatomy with bones (posterior view)

Iliac crest

Sacral dimple
(location of posterior superior iliac spine)

Intergluteal cleft (natal cleft)

Gluteal fold

Iliac crest

Greater sciatic notch

Ischial spine

Ischial tuberosity

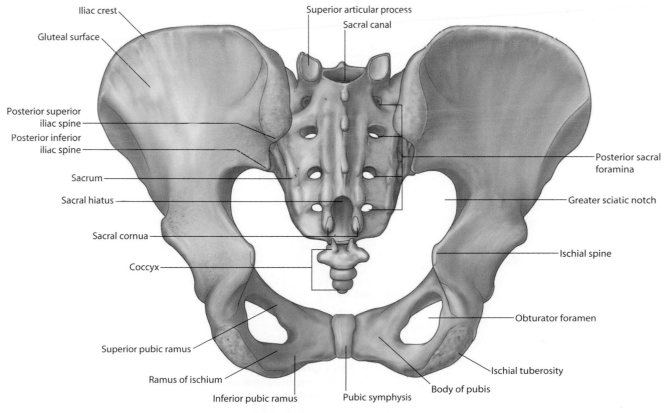

Articulated pelvis (posterior view)

Iliac crest

Gluteal surface

Posterior superior
iliac spine

Posterior inferior
iliac spine

Sacrum

Sacral hiatus

Sacral cornua

Coccyx

Superior pubic ramus

Ramus of ischium

Inferior pubic ramus

Superior articular process

Sacral canal

Posterior sacral
foramina

Greater sciatic notch

Ischial spine

Obturator foramen

Ischial tuberosity

Body of pubis

Pubic symphysis

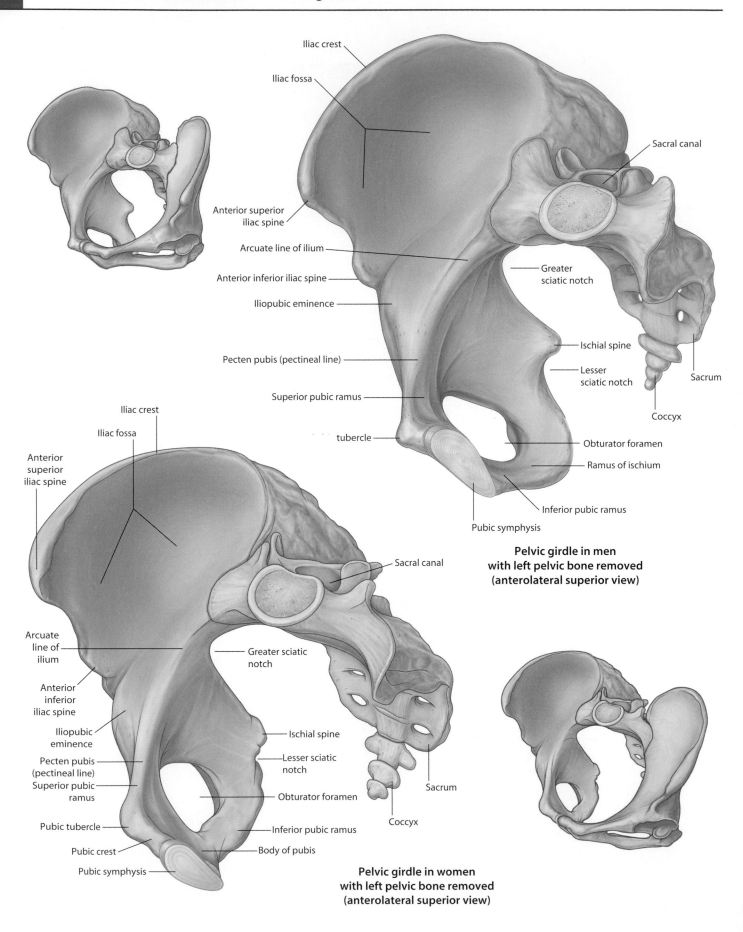

Iliac crest

Iliac fossa

Sacral canal

Anterior superior
iliac spine

Arcuate line of ilium

Greater
sciatic notch

Anterior inferior iliac spine

Iliopubic eminence

Ischial spine

Pecten pubis (pectineal line)

Lesser
sciatic notch

Sacrum

Superior pubic ramus

Coccyx

tubercle

Obturator foramen

Ramus of ischium

Inferior pubic ramus

Pubic symphysis

**Pelvic girdle in men
with left pelvic bone removed
(anterolateral superior view)**

Iliac crest

Iliac fossa

Anterior
superior
iliac spine

Sacral canal

Arcuate
line of
ilium

Greater sciatic
notch

Anterior
inferior
iliac spine

Iliopubic
eminence

Ischial spine

Pecten pubis
(pectineal line)

Lesser sciatic
notch

Superior pubic
ramus

Obturator foramen

Pubic tubercle

Inferior pubic ramus

Sacrum

Pubic crest

Body of pubis

Coccyx

Pubic symphysis

**Pelvic girdle in women
with left pelvic bone removed
(anterolateral superior view)**

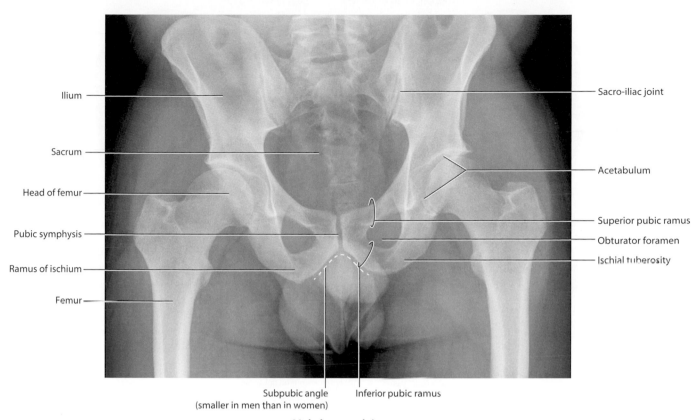

Ilium

Sacrum

Head of femur

Pubic symphysis

Ramus of ischium

Femur

Sacro-iliac joint

Acetabulum

Superior pubic ramus

Obturator foramen

Ischial tuberosity

Subpubic angle
(smaller in men than in women)

Inferior pubic ramus

Male bony pelvis.
Radiograph, anterior-posterior view

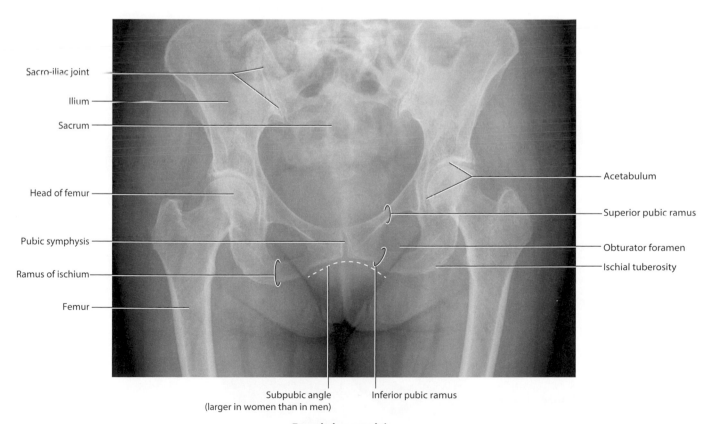

Sacro-iliac joint

Ilium

Sacrum

Head of femur

Pubic symphysis

Ramus of ischium

Femur

Acetabulum

Superior pubic ramus

Obturator foramen

Ischial tuberosity

Subpubic angle
(larger in women than in men)

Inferior pubic ramus

Female bony pelvis.
Radiograph, anterior-posterior view

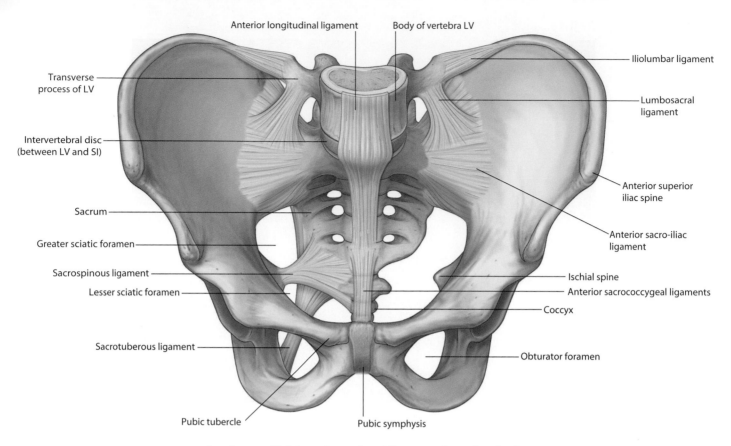

Anterior longitudinal ligament

Body of vertebra LV

Iliolumbar ligament

Transverse process of LV

Lumbosacral ligament

Intervertebral disc (between LV and SI)

Anterior superior iliac spine

Sacrum

Anterior sacro-iliac ligament

Greater sciatic foramen

Sacrospinous ligament

Ischial spine

Lesser sciatic foramen

Anterior sacrococcygeal ligaments

Coccyx

Sacrotuberous ligament

Obturator foramen

Pubic tubercle

Pubic symphysis

Lumbosacral joints and associated ligaments (anterior view)

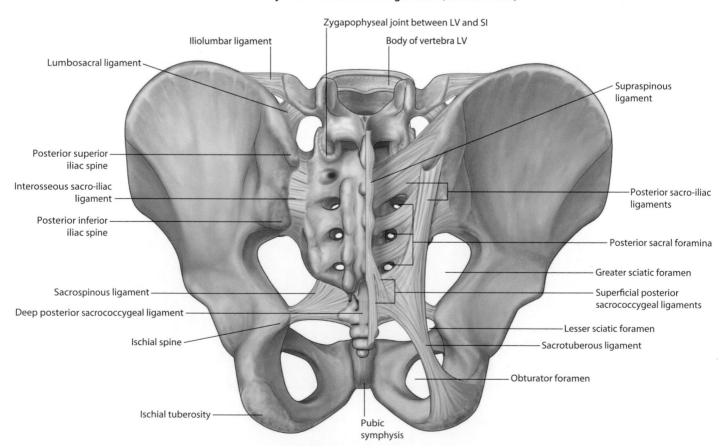

Zygapophyseal joint between LV and SI

Iliolumbar ligament

Body of vertebra LV

Lumbosacral ligament

Supraspinous ligament

Posterior superior iliac spine

Interosseous sacro-iliac ligament

Posterior sacro-iliac ligaments

Posterior inferior iliac spine

Posterior sacral foramina

Greater sciatic foramen

Sacrospinous ligament

Superficial posterior sacrococcygeal ligaments

Deep posterior sacrococcygeal ligament

Ischial spine

Lesser sciatic foramen

Sacrotuberous ligament

Obturator foramen

Ischial tuberosity

Pubic symphysis

Lumbosacral joints and associated ligaments (posterior view)

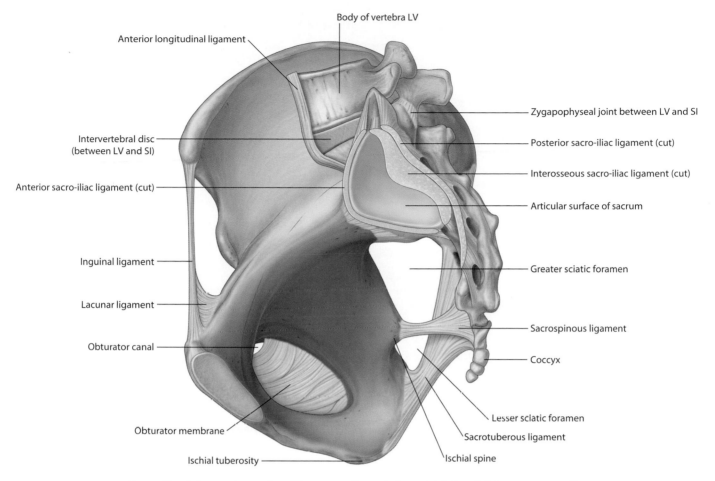

Body of vertebra LV

Anterior longitudinal ligament

Intervertebral disc
(between LV and SI)

Anterior sacro-iliac ligament (cut)

Inguinal ligament

Lacunar ligament

Obturator canal

Obturator membrane

Ischial tuberosity

Zygapophyseal joint between LV and SI

Posterior sacro-iliac ligament (cut)

Interosseous sacro-iliac ligament (cut)

Articular surface of sacrum

Greater sciatic foramen

Sacrospinous ligament

Coccyx

Lesser sciatic foramen

Sacrotuberous ligament

Ischial spine

Sacro-iliac joints and associated ligaments (lateral view with left pelvic bone removed)

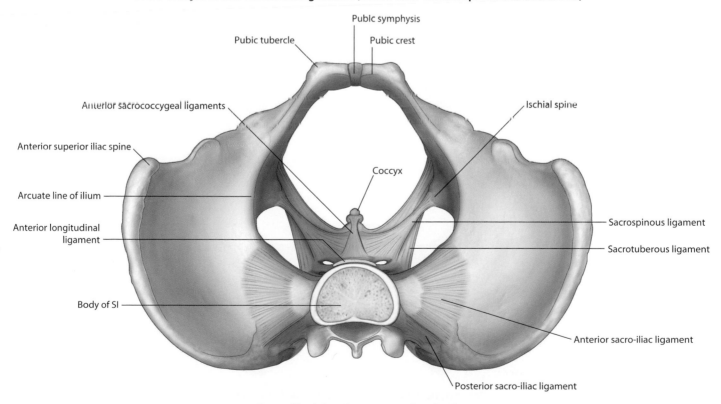

Pubic symphysis

Pubic tubercle

Pubic crest

Anterior sacrococcygeal ligaments

Anterior superior iliac spine

Arcuate line of ilium

Anterior longitudinal
ligament

Body of SI

Coccyx

Ischial spine

Sacrospinous ligament

Sacrotuberous ligament

Anterior sacro-iliac ligament

Posterior sacro-iliac ligament

Sacro-iliac joints (anterosuperior view)

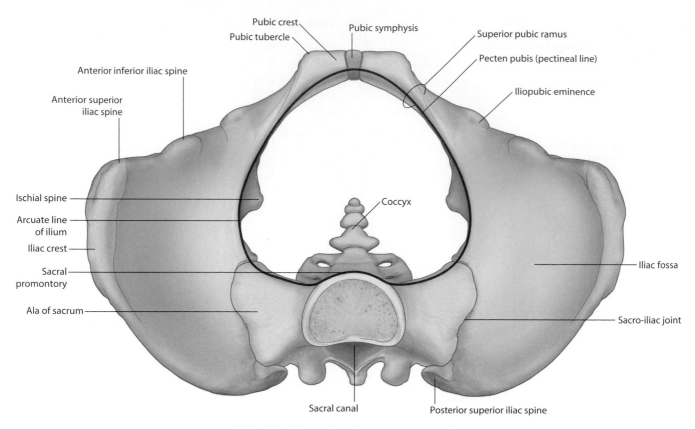

Pubic crest

Pubic tubercle

Pubic symphysis

Superior pubic ramus

Pecten pubis (pectineal line)

Anterior inferior iliac spine

Iliopubic eminence

Anterior superior iliac spine

Ischial spine

Arcuate line of ilium

Iliac crest

Sacral promontory

Ala of sacrum

Coccyx

Iliac fossa

Sacro-iliac joint

Sacral canal

Posterior superior iliac spine

Pelvic inlet (shown in red; anterosuperior view)

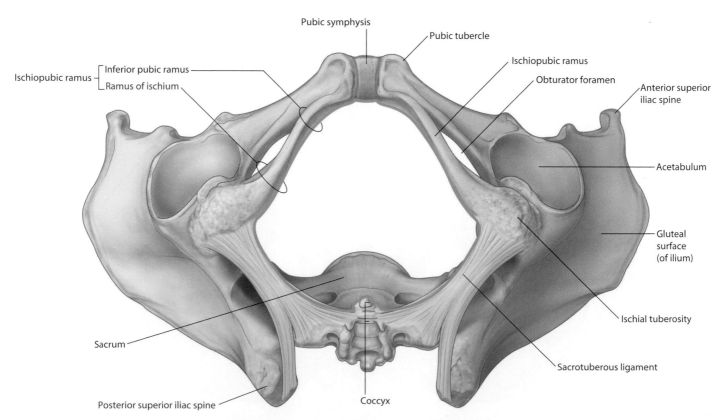

Pubic symphysis

Pubic tubercle

Ischiopubic ramus

Inferior pubic ramus

Ischiopubic ramus

Ramus of ischium

Obturator foramen

Anterior superior iliac spine

Acetabulum

Gluteal surface (of ilium)

Ischial tuberosity

Sacrotuberous ligament

Sacrum

Posterior superior iliac spine

Coccyx

Pelvic outlet (shown in green; anteroinferior view)

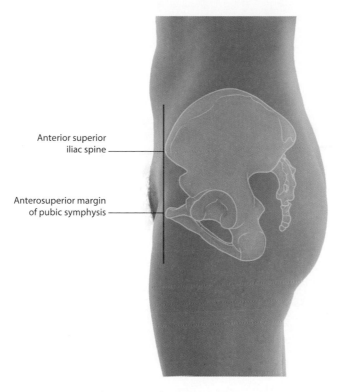

Anterior superior iliac spine

Anterosuperior margin of pubic symphysis

Pelvic orientation in anatomical position (lateral view)

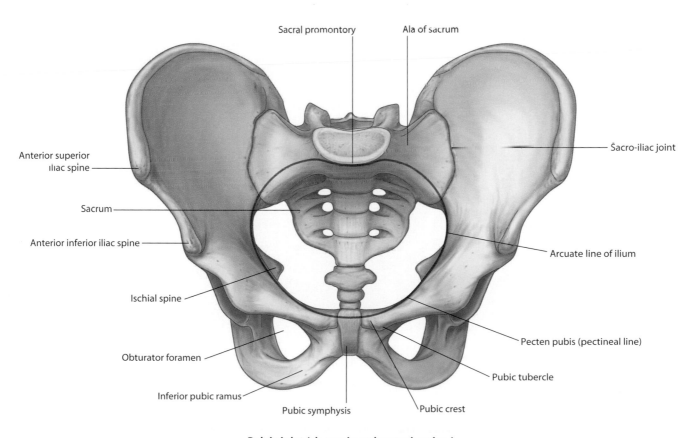

Sacral promontory

Ala of sacrum

Anterior superior iliac spine

Sacro-iliac joint

Sacrum

Anterior inferior iliac spine

Arcuate line of ilium

Ischial spine

Obturator foramen

Pecten pubis (pectineal line)

Inferior pubic ramus

Pubic tubercle

Pubic symphysis

Pubic crest

Pelvic inlet (shown in red; anterior view)

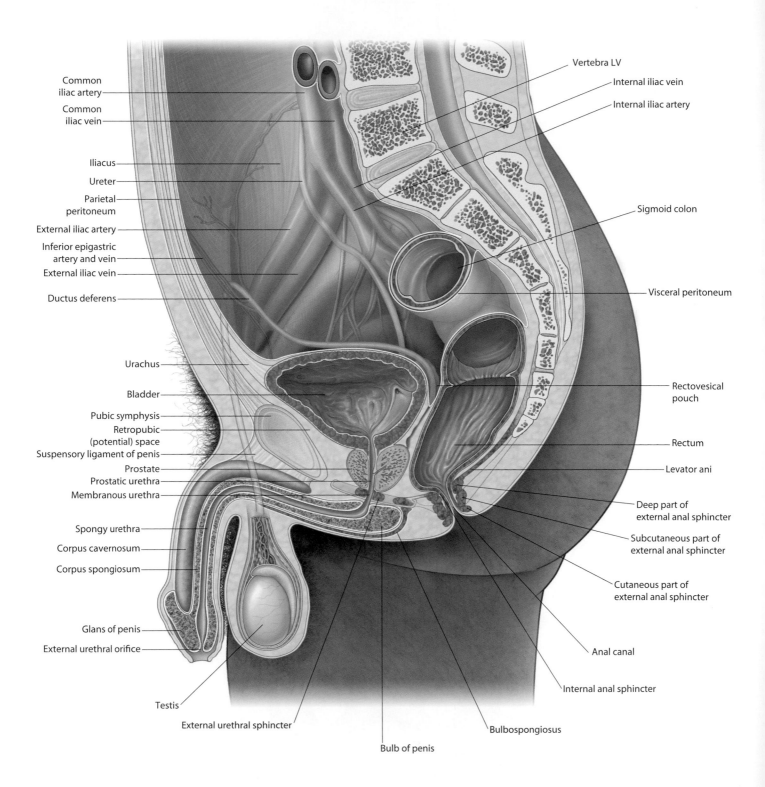

Common iliac artery

Common iliac vein

Iliacus

Ureter

Parietal peritoneum

External iliac artery

Inferior epigastric artery and vein

External iliac vein

Ductus deferens

Urachus

Bladder

Pubic symphysis

Retropubic (potential) space

Suspensory ligament of penis

Prostate

Prostatic urethra

Membranous urethra

Spongy urethra

Corpus cavernosum

Corpus spongiosum

Glans of penis

External urethral orifice

Testis

External urethral sphincter

Bulb of penis

Bulbospongiosus

Vertebra LV

Internal iliac vein

Internal iliac artery

Sigmoid colon

Visceral peritoneum

Rectovesical pouch

Rectum

Levator ani

Deep part of external anal sphincter

Subcutaneous part of external anal sphincter

Cutaneous part of external anal sphincter

Anal canal

Internal anal sphincter

Pelvic viscera and perineum in men *in situ* (sagittal section)

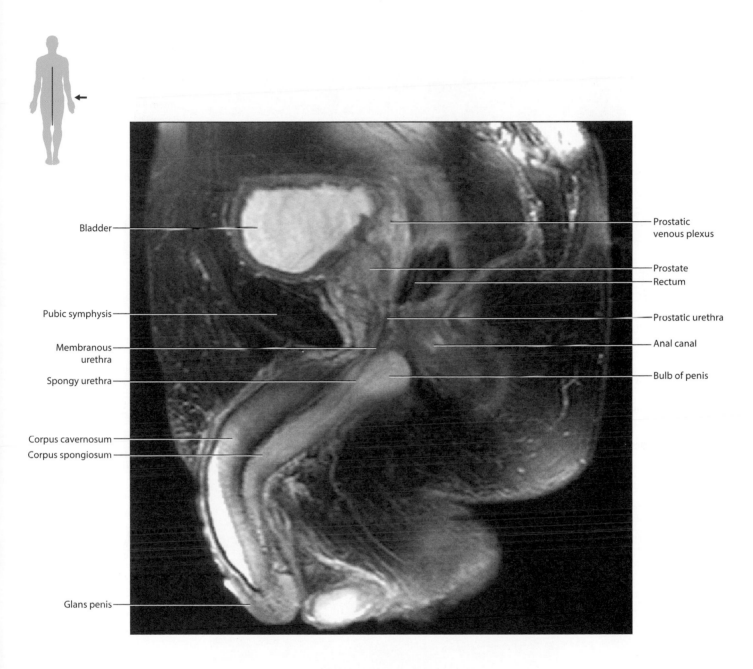

Bladder

Pubic symphysis

Membranous urethra

Spongy urethra

Corpus cavernosum

Corpus spongiosum

Glans penis

Prostatic venous plexus

Prostate

Rectum

Prostatic urethra

Anal canal

Bulb of penis

Pelvic viscera in men.
T2-weighted MR image in sagittal plane

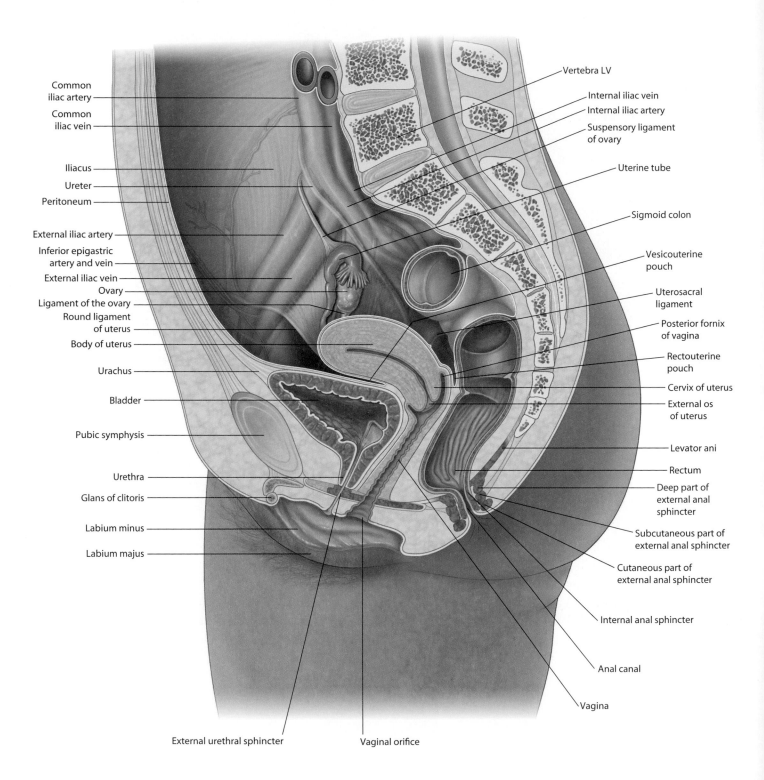

Common iliac artery

Common iliac vein

Iliacus

Ureter

Peritoneum

External iliac artery

Inferior epigastric artery and vein

External iliac vein

Ovary

Ligament of the ovary

Round ligament of uterus

Body of uterus

Urachus

Bladder

Pubic symphysis

Urethra

Glans of clitoris

Labium minus

Labium majus

External urethral sphincter

Vaginal orifice

Vertebra LV

Internal iliac vein

Internal iliac artery

Suspensory ligament of ovary

Uterine tube

Sigmoid colon

Vesicouterine pouch

Uterosacral ligament

Posterior fornix of vagina

Rectouterine pouch

Cervix of uterus

External os of uterus

Levator ani

Rectum

Deep part of external anal sphincter

Subcutaneous part of external anal sphincter

Cutaneous part of external anal sphincter

Internal anal sphincter

Anal canal

Vagina

Pelvic viscera and perineum in women *in situ* (sagittal section)

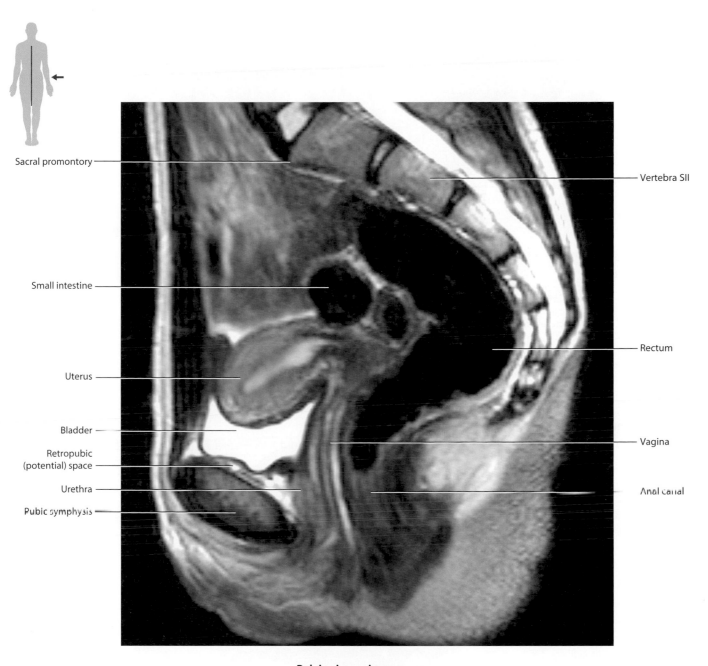

Sacral promontory

Small intestine

Uterus

Bladder

Retropubic
(potential) space

Urethra

Pubic symphysis

Vertebra SII

Rectum

Vagina

Anal canal

Pelvic viscera in women.
T2-weighted MR image in sagittal plane

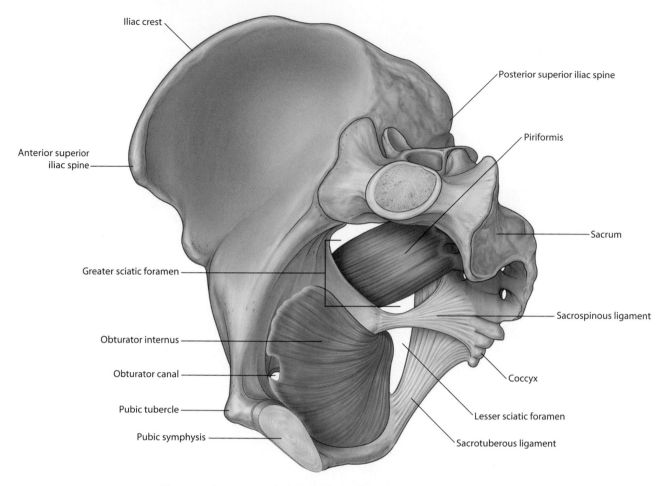

Iliac crest

Posterior superior iliac spine

Anterior superior iliac spine

Piriformis

Sacrum

Greater sciatic foramen

Obturator internus

Obturator canal

Pubic tubercle

Pubic symphysis

Sacrospinous ligament

Coccyx

Lesser sciatic foramen

Sacrotuberous ligament

Obturator internus and piriformis muscles (oblique medial view)

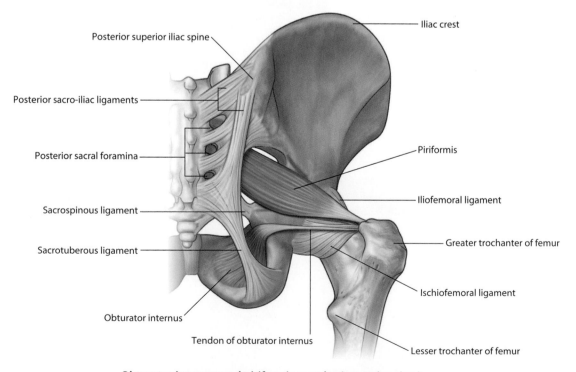

Posterior superior iliac spine

Iliac crest

Posterior sacro-iliac ligaments

Posterior sacral foramina

Sacrospinous ligament

Sacrotuberous ligament

Obturator internus

Tendon of obturator internus

Piriformis

Iliofemoral ligament

Greater trochanter of femur

Ischiofemoral ligament

Lesser trochanter of femur

Obturator internus and piriformis muscles (posterior view)

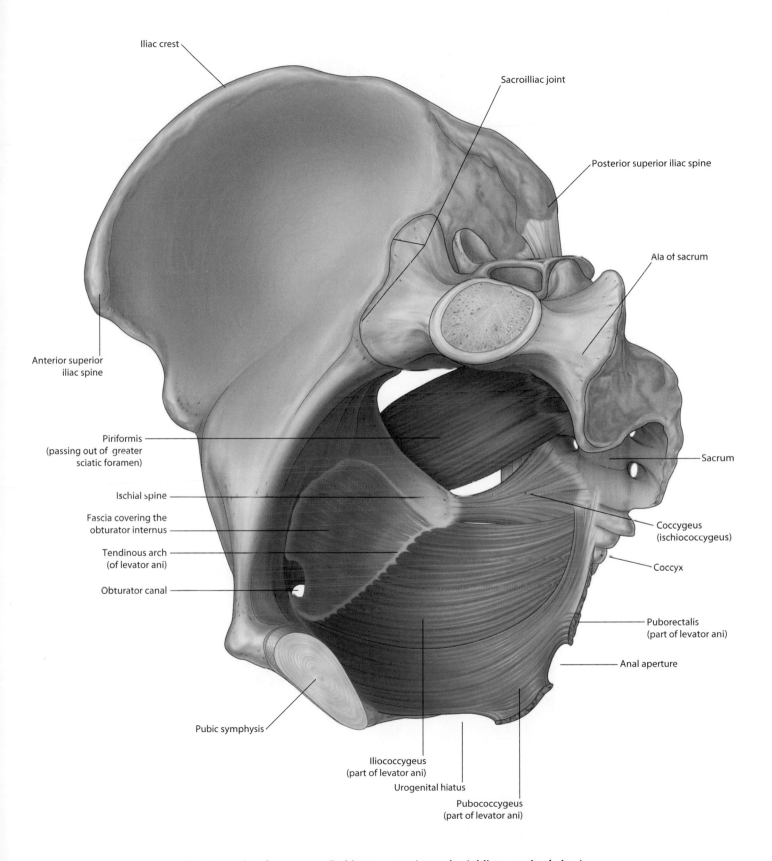

Iliac crest

Sacroilliac joint

Posterior superior iliac spine

Ala of sacrum

Anterior superior
iliac spine

Piriformis
(passing out of greater
sciatic foramen)

Ischial spine

Fascia covering the
obturator internus

Tendinous arch
(of levator ani)

Obturator canal

Pubic symphysis

Sacrum

Coccygeus
(ischiococcygeus)

Coccyx

Puborectalis
(part of levator ani)

Anal aperture

Iliococcygeus
(part of levator ani)

Urogenital hiatus

Pubococcygeus
(part of levator ani)

Levator ani and coccygeus (ischiococcygeus) muscles (oblique sagittal view)

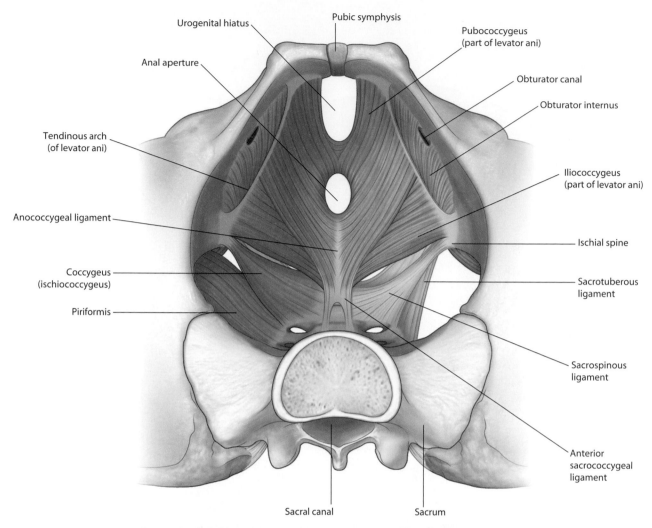

Urogenital hiatus

Pubic symphysis

Pubococcygeus
(part of levator ani)

Anal aperture

Obturator canal

Obturator internus

Tendinous arch
(of levator ani)

Iliococcygeus
(part of levator ani)

Anococcygeal ligament

Ischial spine

Coccygeus
(ischiococcygeus)

Sacrotuberous
ligament

Piriformis

Sacrospinous
ligament

Anterior
sacrococcygeal
ligament

Sacral canal

Sacrum

Levator ani and coccygeus (ischiococcygeus) muscles (anterosuperior view)

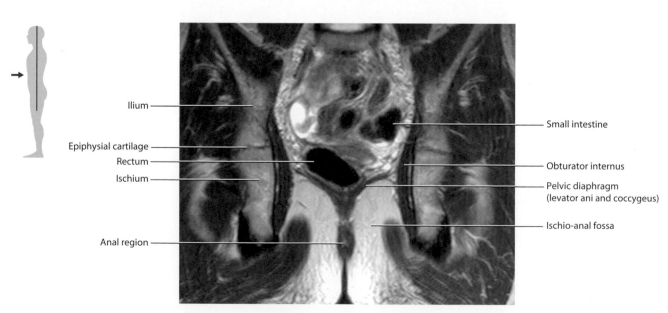

Ilium

Small intestine

Epiphysial cartilage

Rectum

Obturator internus

Ischium

Pelvic diaphragm
(levator ani and coccygeus)

Ischio-anal fossa

Anal region

**Pelvic diaphragm in relation to other structures in
the pelvic cavity and perineum.**
T2-weighted MR image in coronal plane

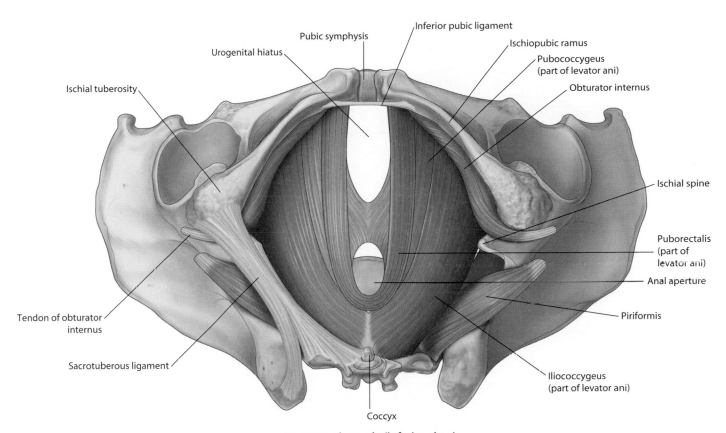

Levator ani muscle (inferior view)

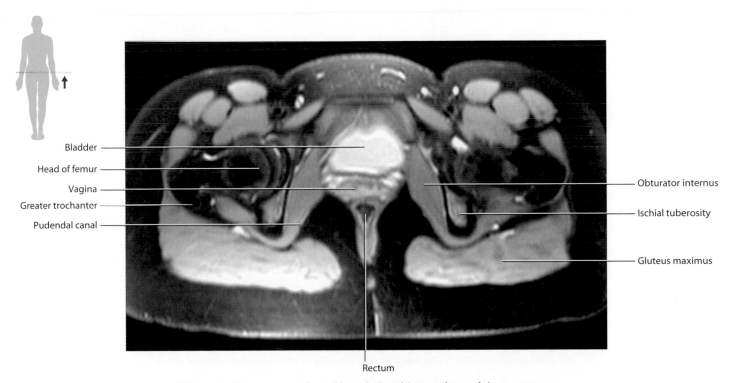

Obturator internus muscle and its relationship to other pelvic structures.
T2-weighted MR image in axial plane

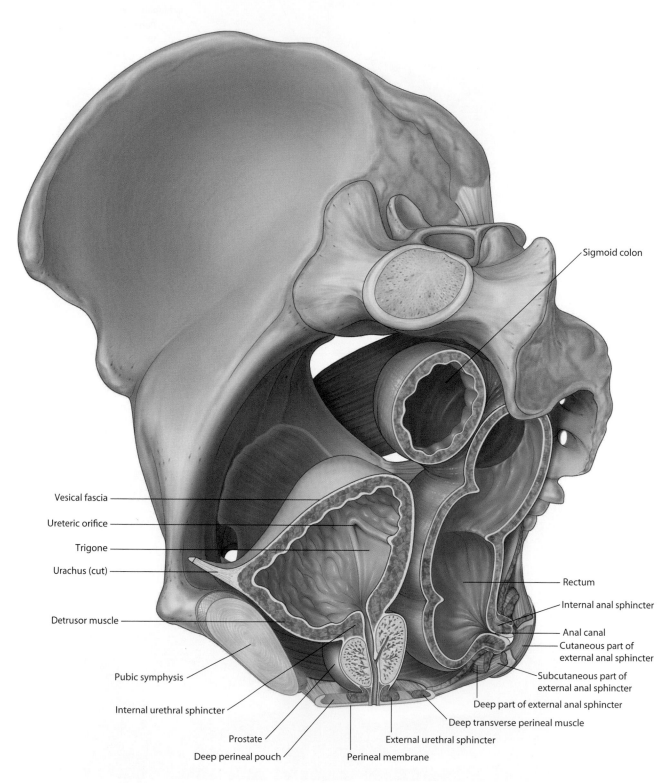

Sigmoid colon

Vesical fascia

Ureteric orifice

Trigone

Urachus (cut)

Detrusor muscle

Pubic symphysis

Internal urethral sphincter

Prostate

Deep perineal pouch

Perineal membrane

External urethral sphincter

Deep transverse perineal muscle

Deep part of external anal sphincter

Subcutaneous part of external anal sphincter

Cutaneous part of external anal sphincter

Anal canal

Internal anal sphincter

Rectum

Bladder, prostate, and rectum within pelvic cavity in men (oblique sagittal view)

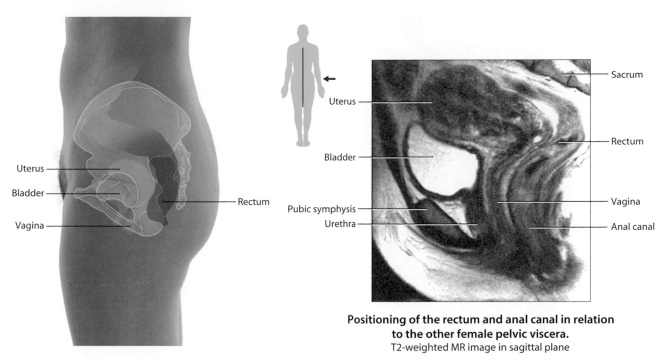

Surface projection of the rectum in women

Positioning of the rectum and anal canal in relation to the other female pelvic viscera.
T2-weighted MR image in sagittal plane

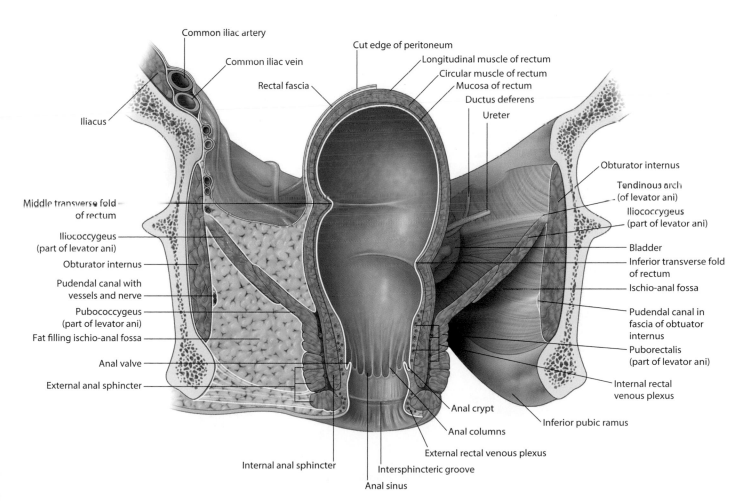

Coronal section through rectum and anal canal (posterior view)

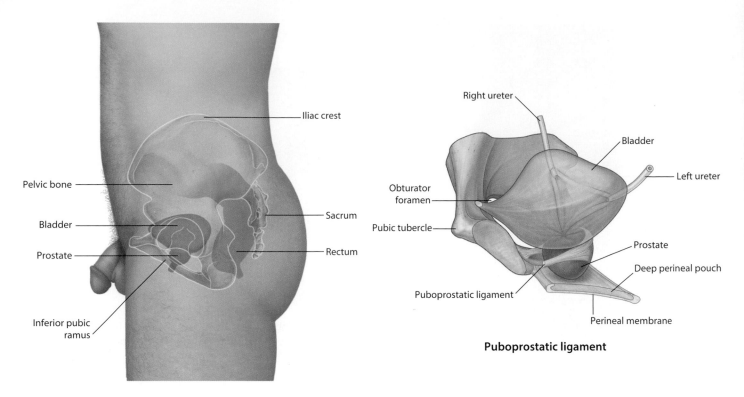

Surface projection of the bladder in men (lateral view)

Iliac crest

Pelvic bone

Bladder

Prostate

Sacrum

Rectum

Inferior pubic ramus

Right ureter

Obturator foramen

Pubic tubercle

Puboprostatic ligament

Bladder

Left ureter

Prostate

Deep perineal pouch

Perineal membrane

Puboprostatic ligament

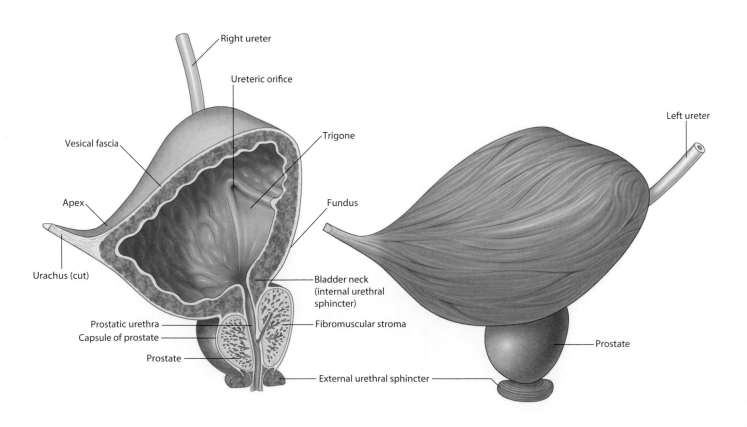

Right ureter

Ureteric orifice

Vesical fascia

Trigone

Apex

Fundus

Urachus (cut)

Left ureter

Bladder neck (internal urethral sphincter)

Prostatic urethra

Fibromuscular stroma

Capsule of prostate

Prostate

Prostate

External urethral sphincter

Urinary bladder in men

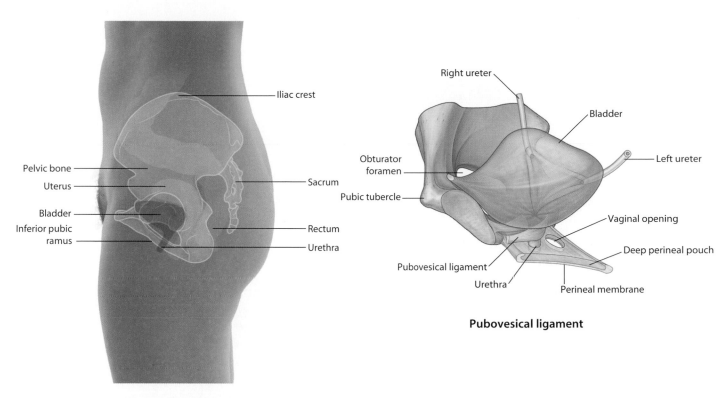

Surface projection of the bladder in women (lateral view)

Pubovesical ligament

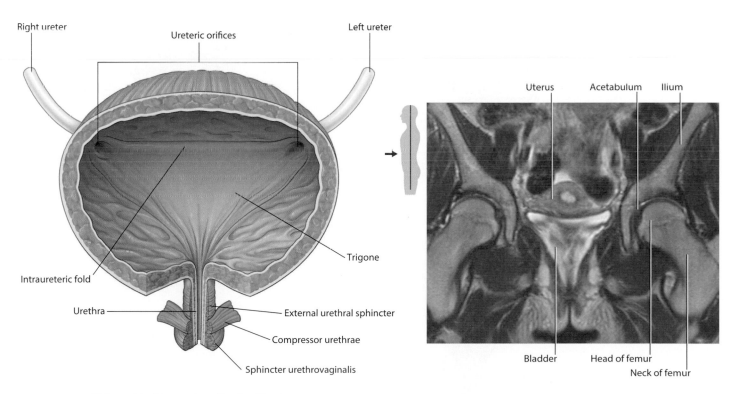

**Urinary bladder and urethral sphincter
muscles in women (anterior view of posterior wall)**

**Appearance and positioning of the bladder in relation
to other structures in the female pelvic cavity.**
T2-weighted MR image in coronal plane

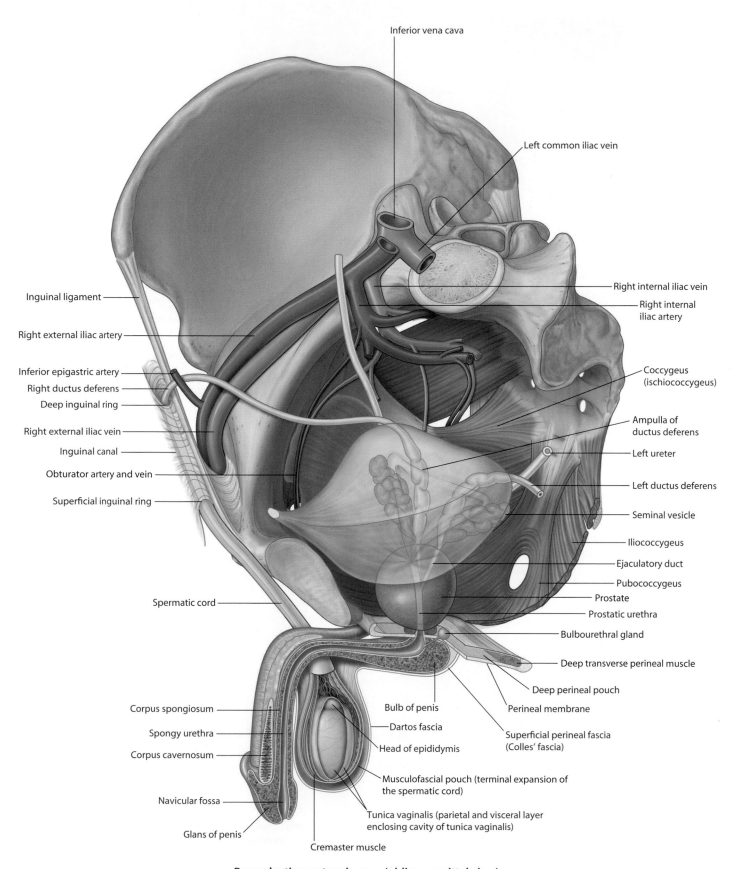

Inferior vena cava

Left common iliac vein

Right internal iliac vein

Right internal iliac artery

Inguinal ligament

Right external iliac artery

Inferior epigastric artery

Right ductus deferens

Deep inguinal ring

Right external iliac vein

Inguinal canal

Obturator artery and vein

Superficial inguinal ring

Coccygeus (ischiococcygeus)

Ampulla of ductus deferens

Left ureter

Left ductus deferens

Seminal vesicle

Iliococcygeus

Ejaculatory duct

Pubococcygeus

Prostate

Prostatic urethra

Bulbourethral gland

Deep transverse perineal muscle

Deep perineal pouch

Perineal membrane

Superficial perineal fascia (Colles' fascia)

Spermatic cord

Corpus spongiosum

Spongy urethra

Corpus cavernosum

Navicular fossa

Glans of penis

Bulb of penis

Dartos fascia

Head of epididymis

Musculofascial pouch (terminal expansion of the spermatic cord)

Tunica vaginalis (parietal and visceral layer enclosing cavity of tunica vaginalis)

Cremaster muscle

Reproductive system in men (oblique sagittal view)

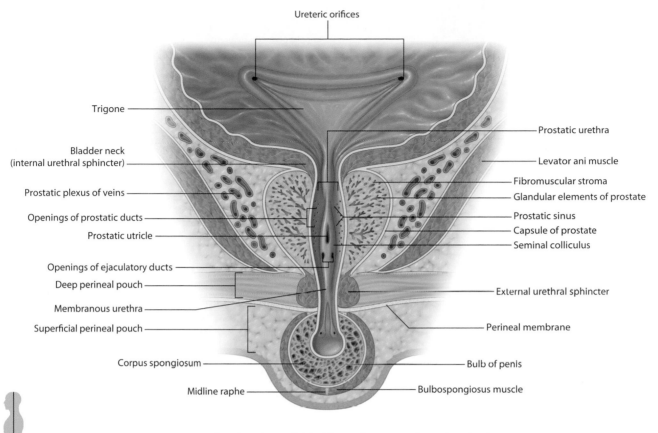

Ureteric orifices

Trigone

Bladder neck
(internal urethral sphincter)

Prostatic plexus of veins

Openings of prostatic ducts

Prostatic utricle

Openings of ejaculatory ducts

Deep perineal pouch

Membranous urethra

Superficial perineal pouch

Corpus spongiosum

Midline raphe

Prostatic urethra

Levator ani muscle

Fibromuscular stroma

Glandular elements of prostate

Prostatic sinus

Capsule of prostate

Seminal colliculus

External urethral sphincter

Perineal membrane

Bulb of penis

Bulbospongiosus muscle

Coronal secion through bladder and prostate (anterior view)

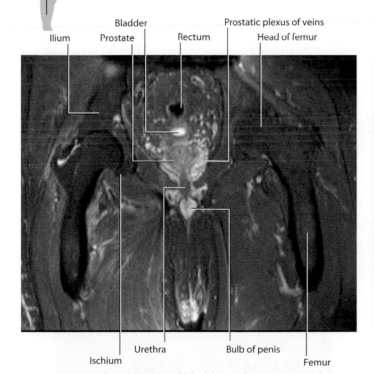

Ilium
Prostate
Bladder
Rectum
Prostatic plexus of veins
Head of femur

Ischium
Urethra
Bulb of penis
Femur

Appearance and positioning of bladder and prostate in relation to other structures in the male pelvis and perineum.
T2-weighted MR image in coronal plane

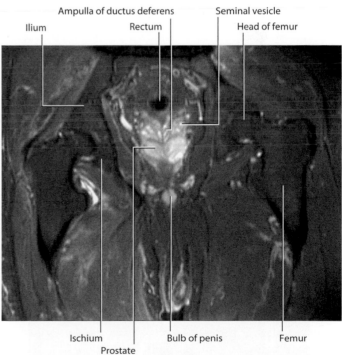

Ilium
Ampulla of ductus deferens
Rectum
Seminal vesicle
Head of femur

Ischium
Prostate
Bulb of penis
Femur

Appearance and positioning of ductus deferens, and seminal vesicles in relation to other structures in the male pelvis and perineum.
T2-weighted MR image in coronal plane

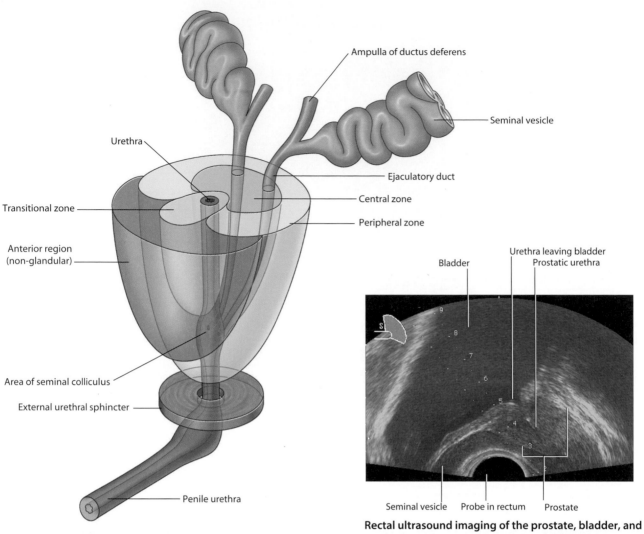

Ampulla of ductus deferens

Seminal vesicle

Urethra

Ejaculatory duct

Central zone

Transitional zone

Peripheral zone

Anterior region
(non-glandular)

Area of seminal colliculus

External urethral sphincter

Penile urethra

**Zonal anatomy of the prostate gland.
Most carcinomas originate in the peripheral zone.
Benign prostatic hypertrophy (BPH)
affects mainly the transitional zone**

Bladder

Urethra leaving bladder
Prostatic urethra

Seminal vesicle   Probe in rectum   Prostate

**Rectal ultrasound imaging of the prostate, bladder, and
seminal vesicle. Sagittal view also showing the urethra**

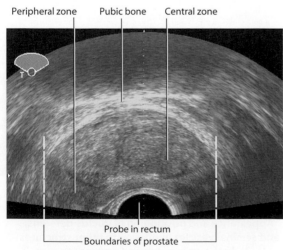

Peripheral zone   Pubic bone   Central zone

Probe in rectum
Boundaries of prostate

**Rectal ultrasound imaging of the prostate.
Axial view showing the central and peripheral zones**

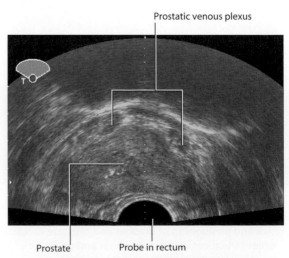

Prostatic venous plexus

Prostate   Probe in rectum

**Rectal ultrasound imaging of the prostate.
Axial view showing the surrounding plexus of veins**

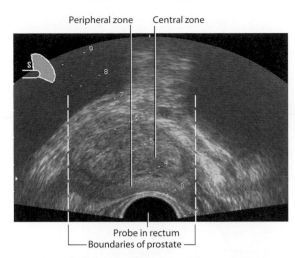

Rectal ultrasound imaging of the prostate.
Sagittal view showing the central and peripheral zones

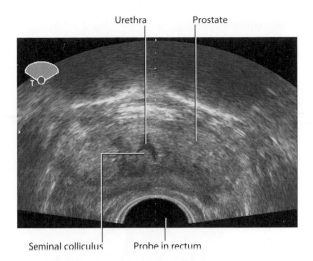

Rectal ultrasound imaging of the prostate.
Axial view showing the urethra and seminal colliculus

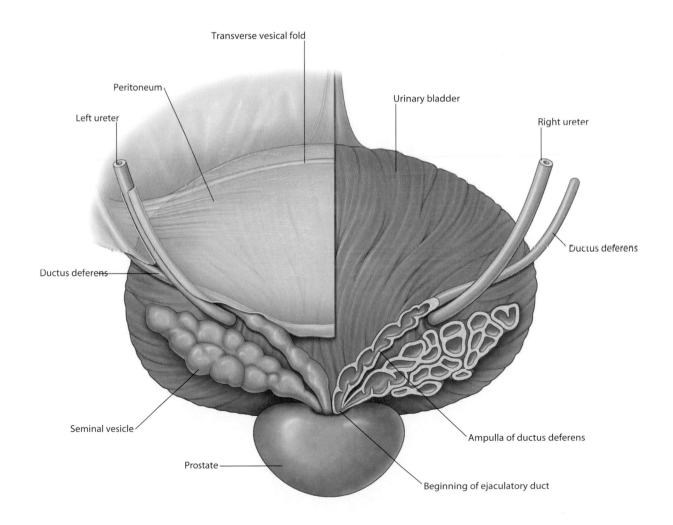

Bladder and prostate (posterior view)

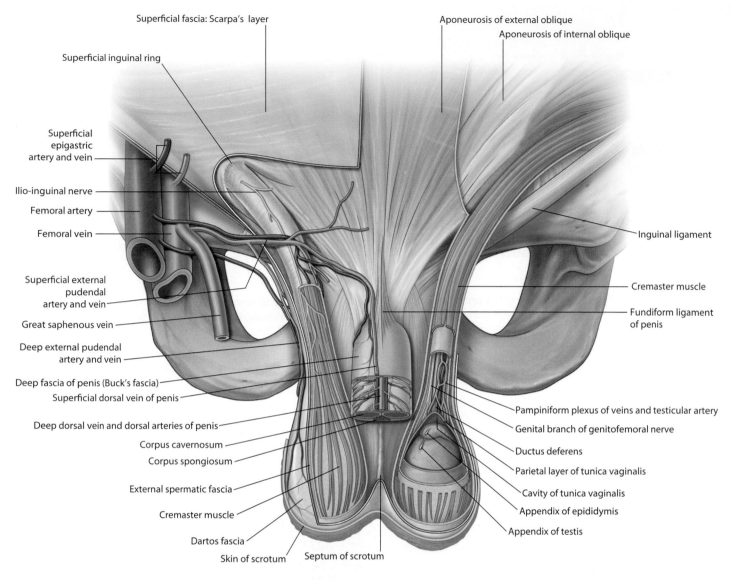

Superficial fascia: Scarpa's layer

Superficial inguinal ring

Superficial epigastric artery and vein

Ilio-inguinal nerve

Femoral artery

Femoral vein

Superficial external pudendal artery and vein

Great saphenous vein

Deep external pudendal artery and vein

Deep fascia of penis (Buck's fascia)

Superficial dorsal vein of penis

Deep dorsal vein and dorsal arteries of penis

Corpus cavernosum

Corpus spongiosum

External spermatic fascia

Cremaster muscle

Dartos fascia

Skin of scrotum

Septum of scrotum

Aponeurosis of external oblique

Aponeurosis of internal oblique

Inguinal ligament

Cremaster muscle

Fundiform ligament of penis

Pampiniform plexus of veins and testicular artery

Genital branch of genitofemoral nerve

Ductus deferens

Parietal layer of tunica vaginalis

Cavity of tunica vaginalis

Appendix of epididymis

Appendix of testis

Contents of the scrotum (anterior view)

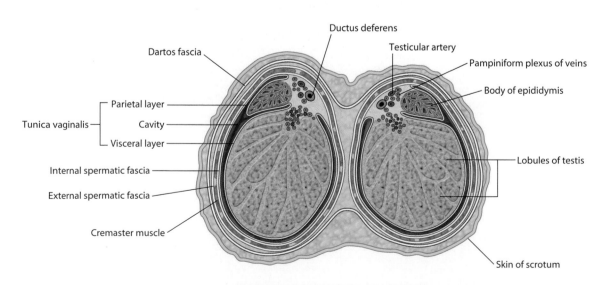

Ductus deferens

Dartos fascia

Testicular artery

Pampiniform plexus of veins

Body of epididymis

Parietal layer

Tunica vaginalis — Cavity

Visceral layer

Internal spermatic fascia

External spermatic fascia

Cremaster muscle

Lobules of testis

Skin of scrotum

Transverse section through the scrotum and testes

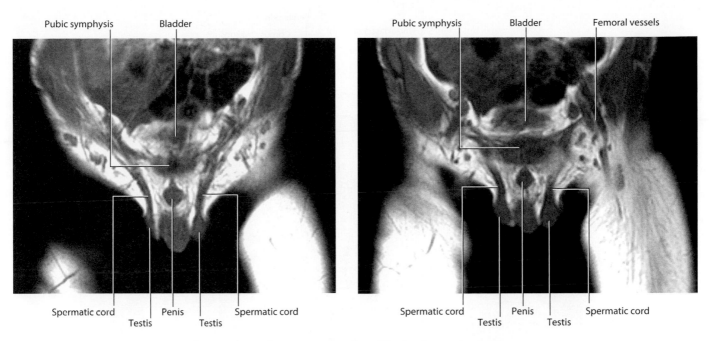

Spermatic cord appearance and positioning in a young male.
T1-weighted MR images in coronal plane

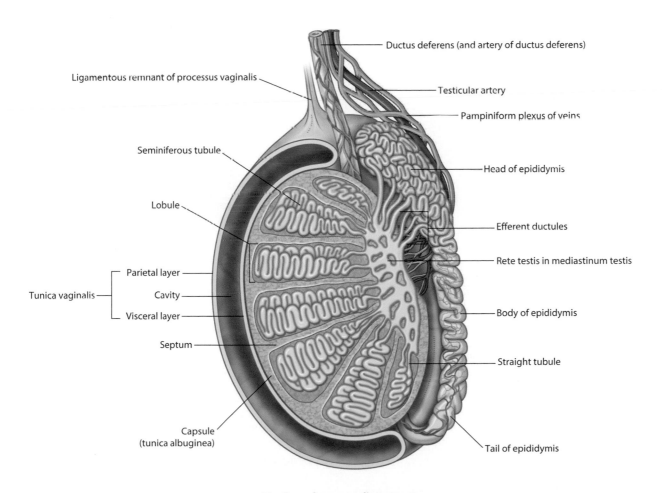

Testis and surrounding structures

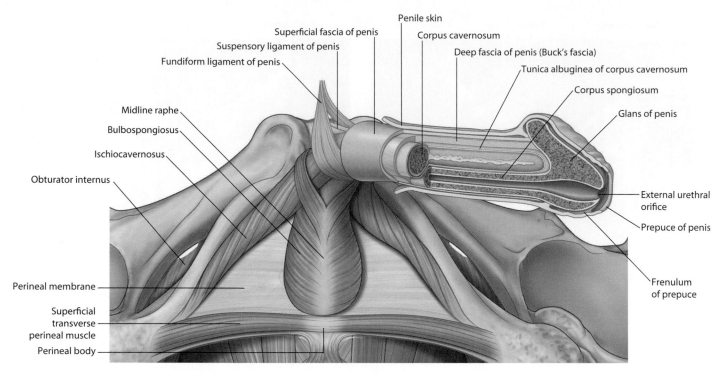

Superficial fascia of penis

Suspensory ligament of penis

Fundiform ligament of penis

Penile skin

Corpus cavernosum

Deep fascia of penis (Buck's fascia)

Tunica albuginea of corpus cavernosum

Corpus spongiosum

Glans of penis

Midline raphe

Bulbospongiosus

Ischiocavernosus

Obturator internus

Perineal membrane

Superficial transverse perineal muscle

Perineal body

External urethral orifice

Prepuce of penis

Frenulum of prepuce

Structure of the penis

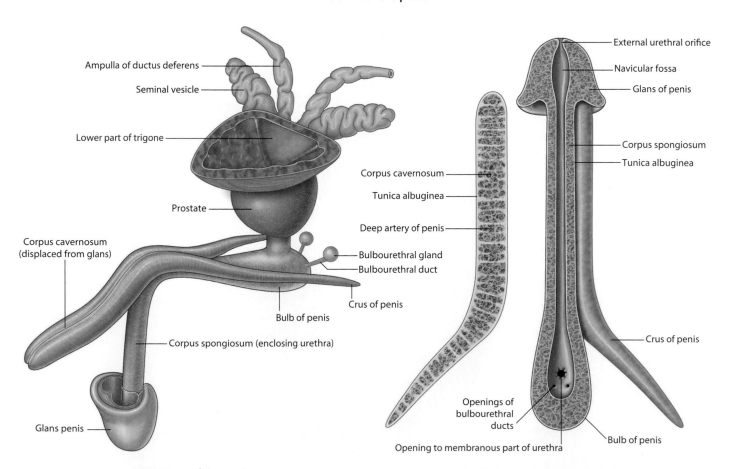

Ampulla of ductus deferens

Seminal vesicle

Lower part of trigone

Corpus cavernosum (displaced from glans)

Prostate

Bulb of penis

Corpus spongiosum (enclosing urethra)

Glans penis

Corpus cavernosum

Tunica albuginea

Deep artery of penis

Bulbourethral gland

Bulbourethral duct

Crus of penis

External urethral orifice

Navicular fossa

Glans of penis

Corpus spongiosum

Tunica albuginea

Crus of penis

Openings of bulbourethral ducts

Opening to membranous part of urethra

Bulb of penis

Structure of the penis

Roof of spongy urethra (inferior view)

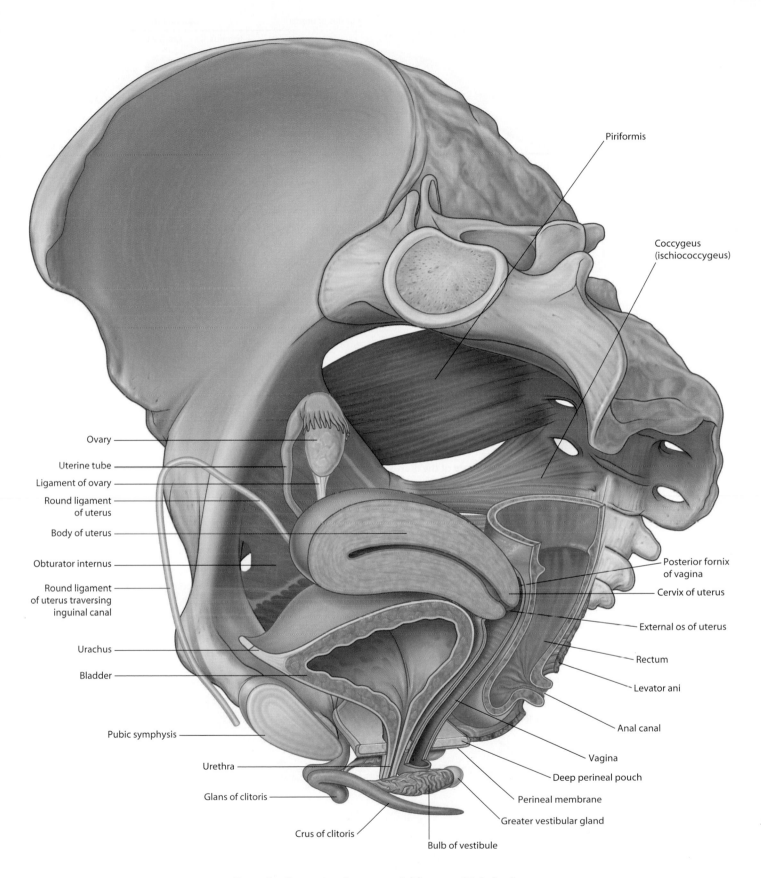

Piriformis

Coccygeus
(ischiococcygeus)

Ovary

Uterine tube

Ligament of ovary

Round ligament
of uterus

Body of uterus

Obturator internus

Round ligament
of uterus traversing
inguinal canal

Urachus

Bladder

Pubic symphysis

Urethra

Glans of clitoris

Crus of clitoris

Bulb of vestibule

Posterior fornix
of vagina

Cervix of uterus

External os of uterus

Rectum

Levator ani

Anal canal

Vagina

Deep perineal pouch

Perineal membrane

Greater vestibular gland

Reproductive system in women (oblique sagittal view)

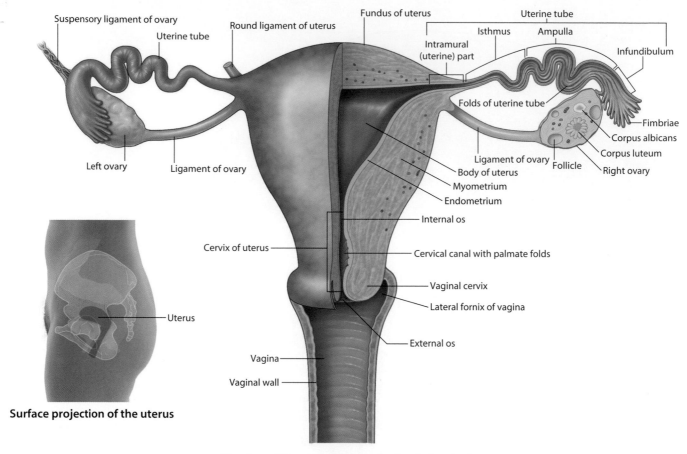

Suspensory ligament of ovary
Uterine tube
Round ligament of uterus
Fundus of uterus
Uterine tube
Isthmus
Ampulla
Intramural (uterine) part
Infundibulum
Folds of uterine tube
Fimbriae
Corpus albicans
Corpus luteum
Ligament of ovary
Follicle
Right ovary
Left ovary
Ligament of ovary
Body of uterus
Myometrium
Endometrium
Internal os
Cervix of uterus
Cervical canal with palmate folds
Vaginal cervix
Lateral fornix of vagina
External os
Vagina
Vaginal wall

Uterus

Surface projection of the uterus

Structure of the uterus and ovaries (posterior view)

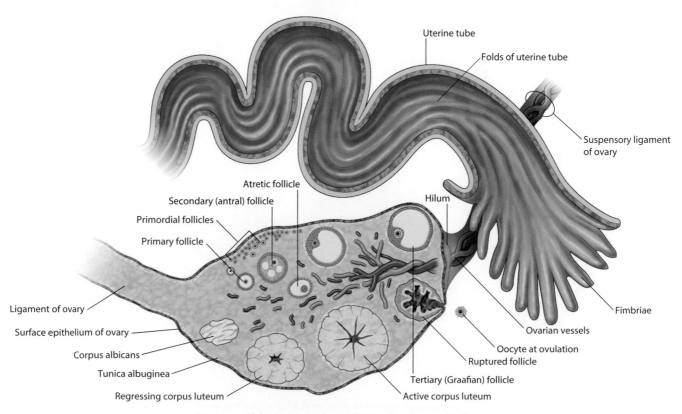

Uterine tube
Folds of uterine tube
Suspensory ligament of ovary
Atretic follicle
Secondary (antral) follicle
Primordial follicles
Primary follicle
Hilum
Ligament of ovary
Surface epithelium of ovary
Corpus albicans
Tunica albuginea
Regressing corpus luteum
Ovarian vessels
Oocyte at ovulation
Ruptured follicle
Tertiary (Graafian) follicle
Active corpus luteum
Fimbriae

Structure of the uterine tube and ovary (posterior view)

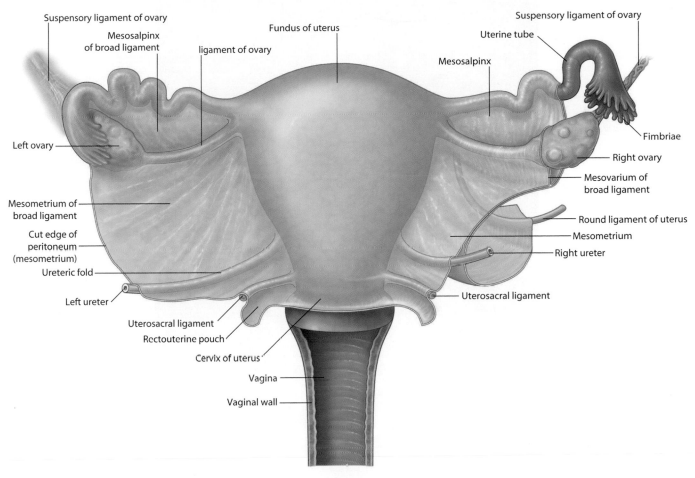

Suspensory ligament of ovary

Mesosalpinx of broad ligament

ligament of ovary

Fundus of uterus

Suspensory ligament of ovary

Uterine tube

Mesosalpinx

Fimbriae

Left ovary

Right ovary

Mesovarium of broad ligament

Mesometrium of broad ligament

Round ligament of uterus

Mesometrium

Cut edge of peritoneum (mesometrium)

Right ureter

Ureteric fold

Left ureter

Uterosacral ligament

Uterosacral ligament

Rectouterine pouch

Cervix of uterus

Vagina

Vaginal wall

Uterus and broad ligament (posterior view)

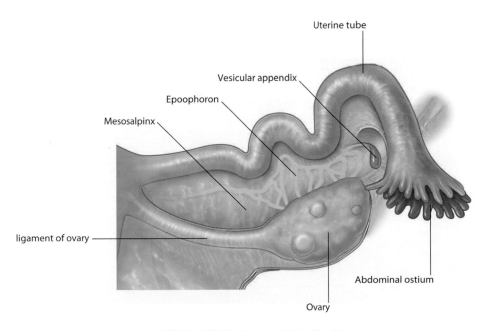

Uterine tube

Vesicular appendix

Epoophoron

Mesosalpinx

ligament of ovary

Abdominal ostium

Ovary

Uterine tube and ovary (posterior view)

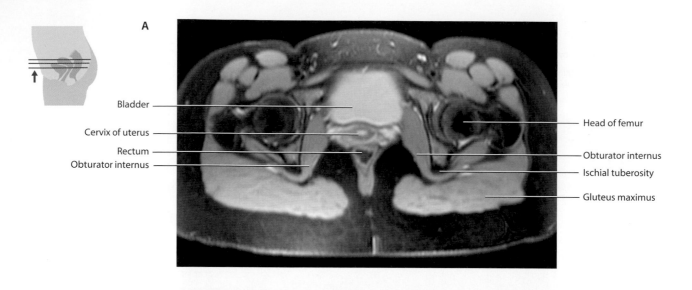

A

Bladder

Cervix of uterus

Rectum

Obturator internus

Head of femur

Obturator internus

Ischial tuberosity

Gluteus maximus

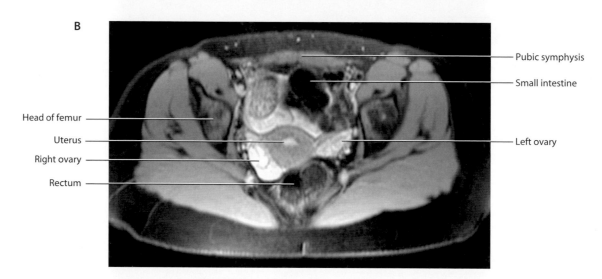

B

Head of femur

Uterus

Right ovary

Rectum

Pubic symphysis

Small intestine

Left ovary

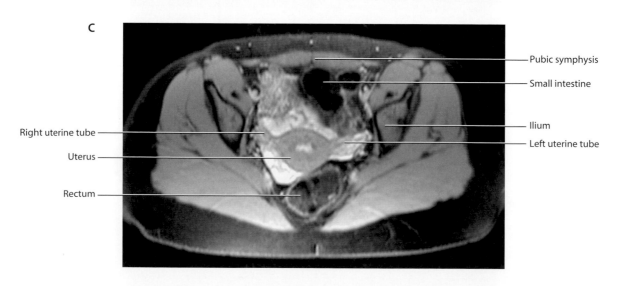

C

Right uterine tube

Uterus

Rectum

Pubic symphysis

Small intestine

Ilium

Left uterine tube

Appearance of cervix of uterus, uterus, ovaries, and uterine tubes in relation to other pelvic structures.
T2-weighted MR images in axial plane

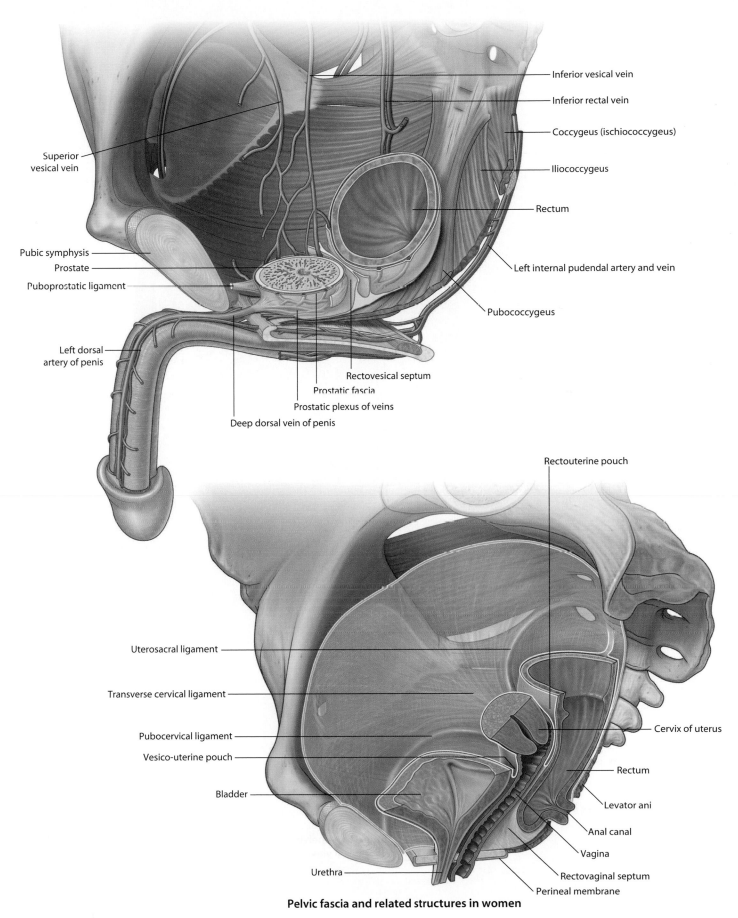

Inferior vesical vein

Inferior rectal vein

Coccygeus (ischiococcygeus)

Iliococcygeus

Rectum

Left internal pudendal artery and vein

Pubococcygeus

Superior vesical vein

Pubic symphysis

Prostate

Puboprostatic ligament

Left dorsal artery of penis

Rectovesical septum

Prostatic fascia

Prostatic plexus of veins

Deep dorsal vein of penis

Rectouterine pouch

Uterosacral ligament

Transverse cervical ligament

Pubocervical ligament

Vesico-uterine pouch

Bladder

Cervix of uterus

Rectum

Levator ani

Anal canal

Vagina

Rectovaginal septum

Urethra

Perineal membrane

Pelvic fascia and related structures in women

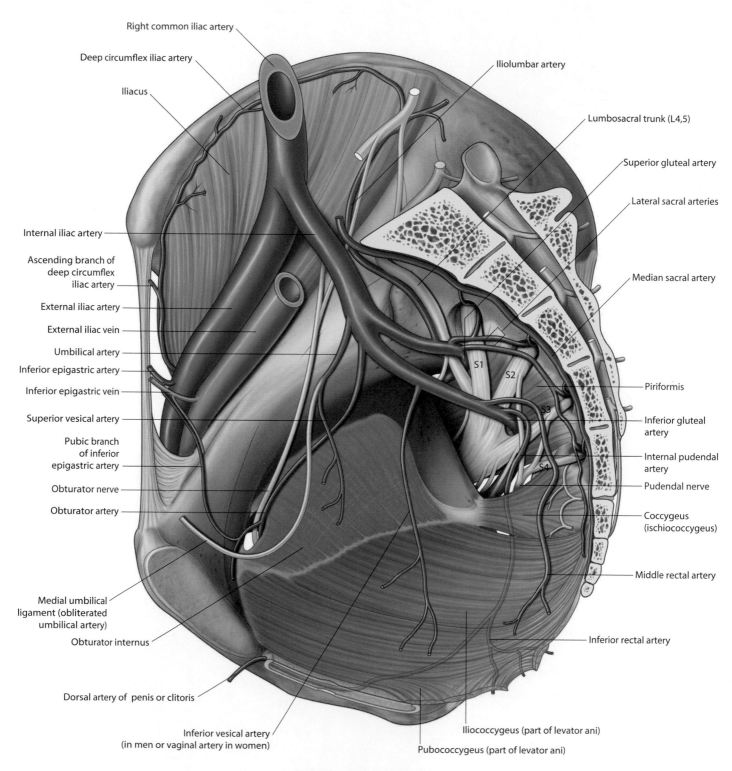

Right common iliac artery

Deep circumflex iliac artery

Iliacus

Iliolumbar artery

Lumbosacral trunk (L4,5)

Superior gluteal artery

Lateral sacral arteries

Internal iliac artery

Ascending branch of deep circumflex iliac artery

External iliac artery

External iliac vein

Umbilical artery

Inferior epigastric artery

Inferior epigastric vein

Superior vesical artery

Pubic branch of inferior epigastric artery

Obturator nerve

Obturator artery

Median sacral artery

S1

S2

S3

S4

Piriformis

Inferior gluteal artery

Internal pudendal artery

Pudendal nerve

Coccygeus (ischiococcygeus)

Middle rectal artery

Inferior rectal artery

Medial umbilical ligament (obliterated umbilical artery)

Obturator internus

Dorsal artery of penis or clitoris

Inferior vesical artery (in men or vaginal artery in women)

Pubococcygeus (part of levator ani)

Iliococcygeus (part of levator ani)

Arterial supply to the pelvis
(right side sagittal view)

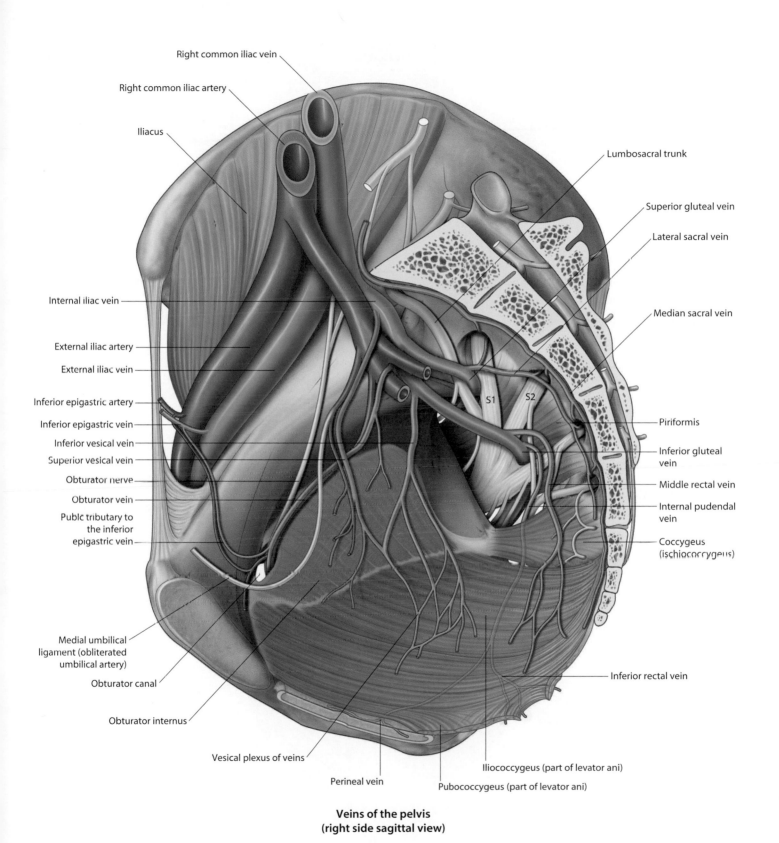

Right common iliac vein

Right common iliac artery

Iliacus

Lumbosacral trunk

Superior gluteal vein

Lateral sacral vein

Internal iliac vein

Median sacral vein

External iliac artery

External iliac vein

Inferior epigastric artery

Inferior epigastric vein

Inferior vesical vein

Superior vesical vein

Obturator nerve

Obturator vein

Pubic tributary to the inferior epigastric vein

S1

S2

Piriformis

Inferior gluteal vein

Middle rectal vein

Internal pudendal vein

Coccygeus (ischiococcygeus)

Medial umbilical ligament (obliterated umbilical artery)

Obturator canal

Obturator internus

Inferior rectal vein

Vesical plexus of veins

Perineal vein

Pubococcygeus (part of levator ani)

Iliococcygeus (part of levator ani)

**Veins of the pelvis
(right side sagittal view)**

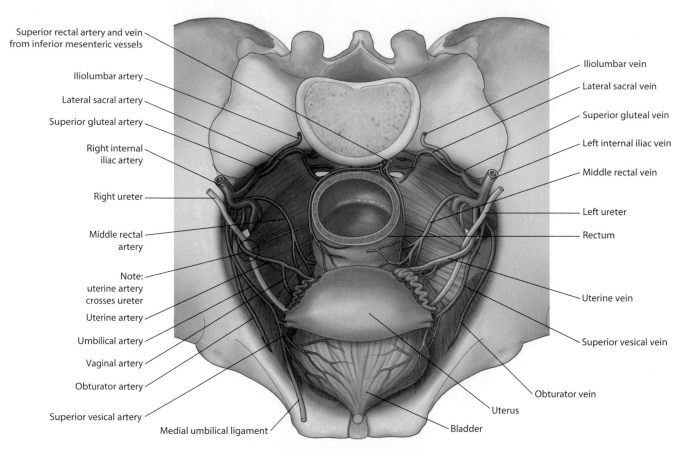

Superior rectal artery and vein from inferior mesenteric vessels

Iliolumbar artery

Lateral sacral artery

Superior gluteal artery

Right internal iliac artery

Right ureter

Middle rectal artery

Note: uterine artery crosses ureter

Uterine artery

Umbilical artery

Vaginal artery

Obturator artery

Superior vesical artery

Medial umbilical ligament

Iliolumbar vein

Lateral sacral vein

Superior gluteal vein

Left internal iliac vein

Middle rectal vein

Left ureter

Rectum

Uterine vein

Superior vesical vein

Obturator vein

Uterus

Bladder

Vasculature of the pelvic viscera in women (superior view)

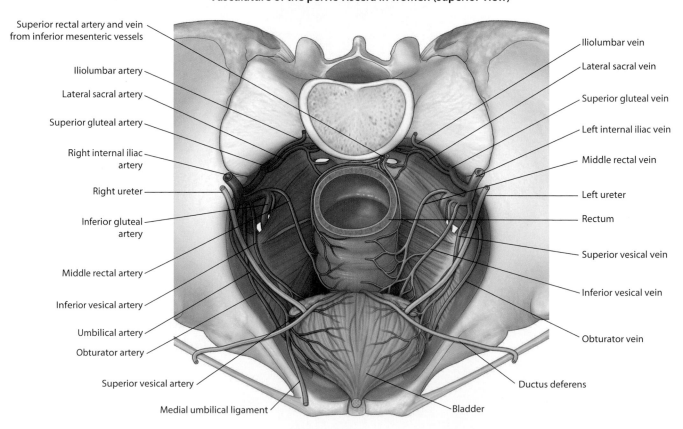

Superior rectal artery and vein from inferior mesenteric vessels

Iliolumbar artery

Lateral sacral artery

Superior gluteal artery

Right internal iliac artery

Right ureter

Inferior gluteal artery

Middle rectal artery

Inferior vesical artery

Umbilical artery

Obturator artery

Superior vesical artery

Medial umbilical ligament

Iliolumbar vein

Lateral sacral vein

Superior gluteal vein

Left internal iliac vein

Middle rectal vein

Left ureter

Rectum

Superior vesical vein

Inferior vesical vein

Obturator vein

Ductus deferens

Bladder

Vasculature of the pelvic viscera in men (superior view)

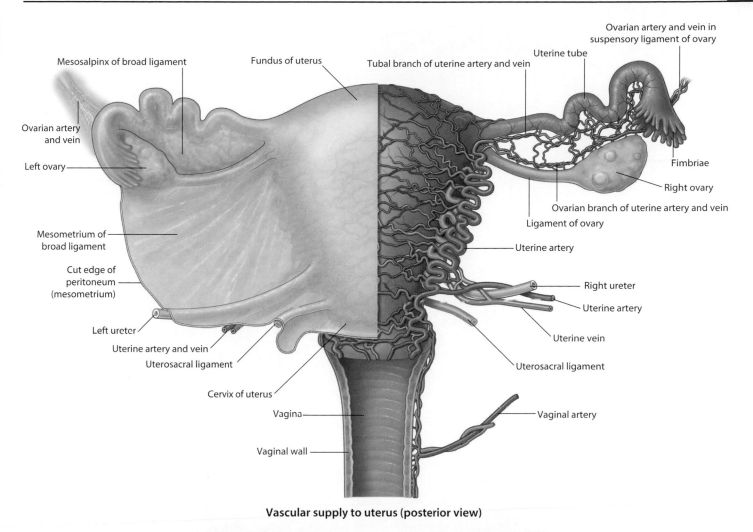

Mesosalpinx of broad ligament

Fundus of uterus

Tubal branch of uterine artery and vein

Uterine tube

Ovarian artery and vein in suspensory ligament of ovary

Ovarian artery and vein

Left ovary

Mesometrium of broad ligament

Cut edge of peritoneum (mesometrium)

Left ureter

Uterine artery and vein

Uterosacral ligament

Cervix of uterus

Vagina

Vaginal wall

Fimbriae

Right ovary

Ovarian branch of uterine artery and vein

Ligament of ovary

Uterine artery

Right ureter

Uterine artery

Uterine vein

Uterosacral ligament

Vaginal artery

Vascular supply to uterus (posterior view)

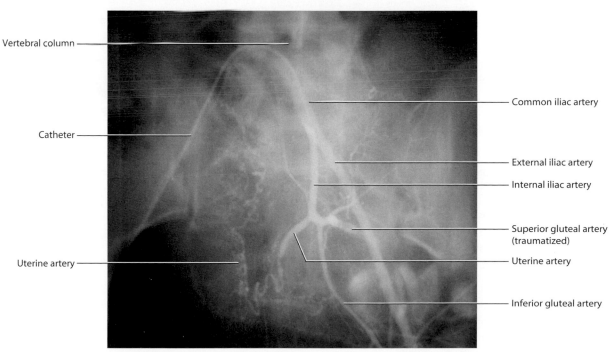

Vertebral column

Catheter

Uterine artery

Common iliac artery

External iliac artery

Internal iliac artery

Superior gluteal artery (traumatized)

Uterine artery

Inferior gluteal artery

Vascular supply to uterus.
Angiogram

251

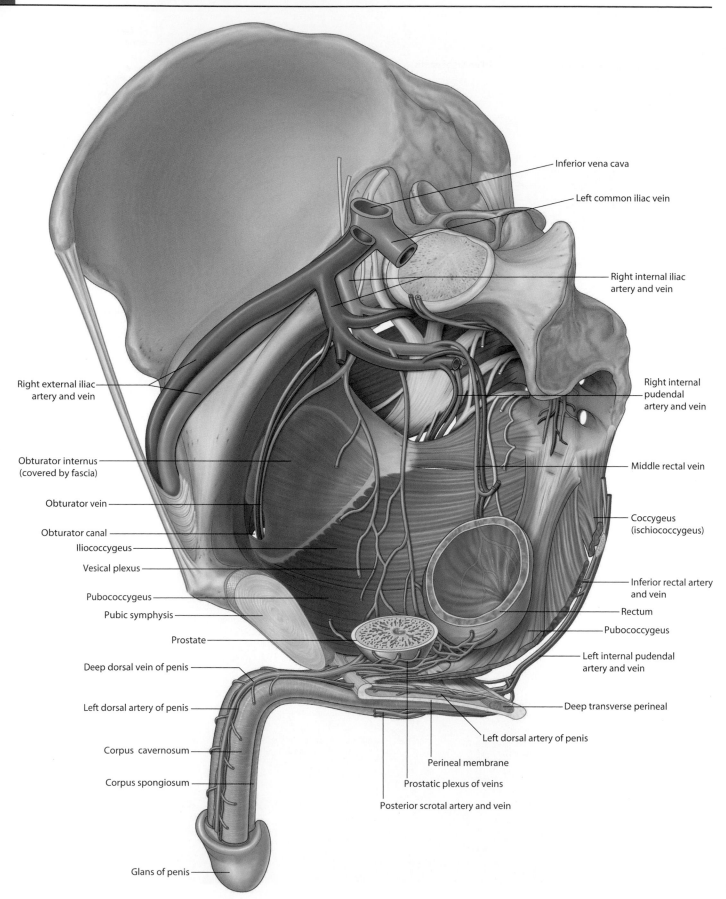

Inferior vena cava

Left common iliac vein

Right internal iliac artery and vein

Right external iliac artery and vein

Right internal pudendal artery and vein

Obturator internus (covered by fascia)

Middle rectal vein

Obturator vein

Obturator canal

Iliococcygeus

Coccygeus (ischiococcygeus)

Vesical plexus

Pubococcygeus

Inferior rectal artery and vein

Pubic symphysis

Rectum

Prostate

Pubococcygeus

Deep dorsal vein of penis

Left internal pudendal artery and vein

Left dorsal artery of penis

Deep transverse perineal

Corpus cavernosum

Left dorsal artery of penis

Corpus spongiosum

Perineal membrane

Prostatic plexus of veins

Posterior scrotal artery and vein

Glans of penis

**Venous drainage of pelvic viscera in men
(oblique sagittal view)**

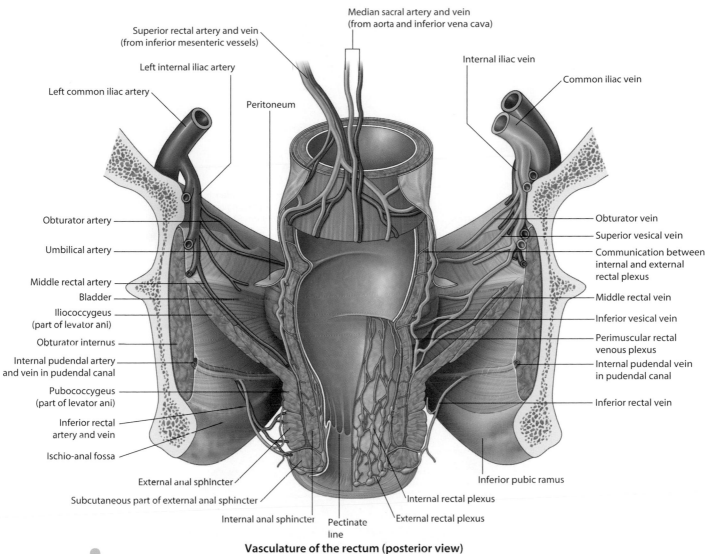

Median sacral artery and vein
(from aorta and inferior vena cava)

Superior rectal artery and vein
(from inferior mesenteric vessels)

Internal iliac vein

Left internal iliac artery

Common iliac vein

Left common iliac artery

Peritoneum

Obturator artery

Obturator vein

Umbilical artery

Superior vesical vein

Communication between
internal and external
rectal plexus

Middle rectal artery

Bladder

Middle rectal vein

Iliococcygeus
(part of levator ani)

Inferior vesical vein

Obturator internus

Perimuscular rectal
venous plexus

Internal pudendal artery
and vein in pudendal canal

Internal pudendal vein
in pudendal canal

Pubococcygeus
(part of levator ani)

Inferior rectal vein

Inferior rectal
artery and vein

Ischio-anal fossa

Inferior pubic ramus

External anal sphincter

Subcutaneous part of external anal sphincter

Internal rectal plexus

Internal anal sphincter

Pectinate
line

External rectal plexus

Vasculature of the rectum (posterior view)

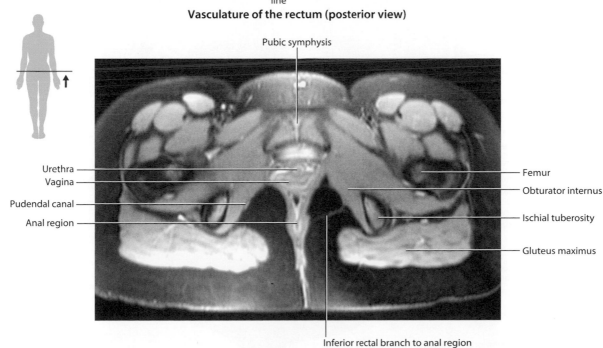

Pubic symphysis

Urethra

Femur

Vagina

Obturator internus

Pudendal canal

Ischial tuberosity

Anal region

Gluteus maximus

Inferior rectal branch to anal region

Inferior rectal neurovascular bundle crossing the ischio-anal fossa.
T2-weighted MR image in axial plane

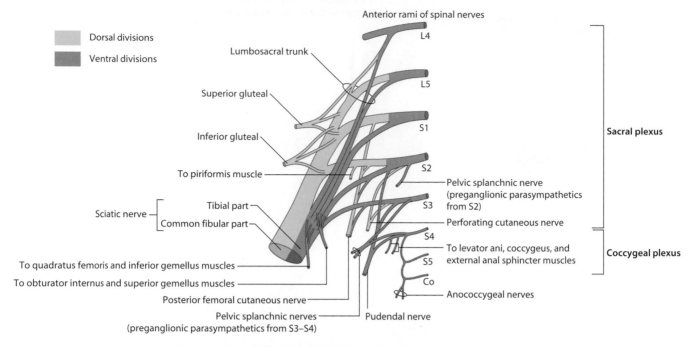

Dorsal divisions

Ventral divisions

Anterior rami of spinal nerves

L4

Lumbosacral trunk

L5

Superior gluteal

S1

Inferior gluteal

To piriformis muscle

S2

Pelvic splanchnic nerve (preganglionic parasympathetics from S2)

Sciatic nerve — Tibial part

S3

Common fibular part

Perforating cutaneous nerve

S4

To levator ani, coccygeus, and external anal sphincter muscles

S5

To quadratus femoris and inferior gemellus muscles

Co

To obturator internus and superior gemellus muscles

Anococcygeal nerves

Posterior femoral cutaneous nerve

Pelvic splanchnic nerves (preganglionic parasympathetics from S3–S4)

Pudendal nerve

Sacral plexus

Coccygeal plexus

Components and branches of the sacral and coccygeal nerve plexuses

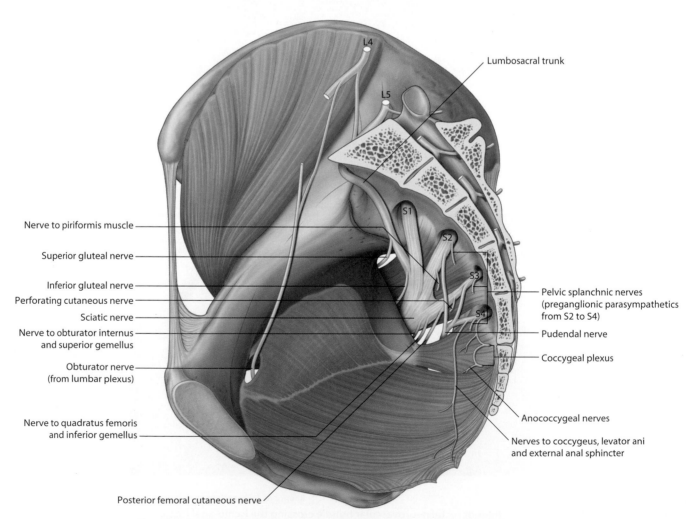

L4

Lumbosacral trunk

L5

S1

Nerve to piriformis muscle

S2

Superior gluteal nerve

S3

Inferior gluteal nerve

Perforating cutaneous nerve

Pelvic splanchnic nerves (preganglionic parasympathetics from S2 to S4)

Sciatic nerve

S4

Nerve to obturator internus and superior gemellus

Pudendal nerve

Obturator nerve (from lumbar plexus)

Coccygeal plexus

Anococcygeal nerves

Nerve to quadratus femoris and inferior gemellus

Nerves to coccygeus, levator ani and external anal sphincter

Posterior femoral cutaneous nerve

Sacral and coccygeal nerve plexuses within the pelvic cavity (sagittal view)

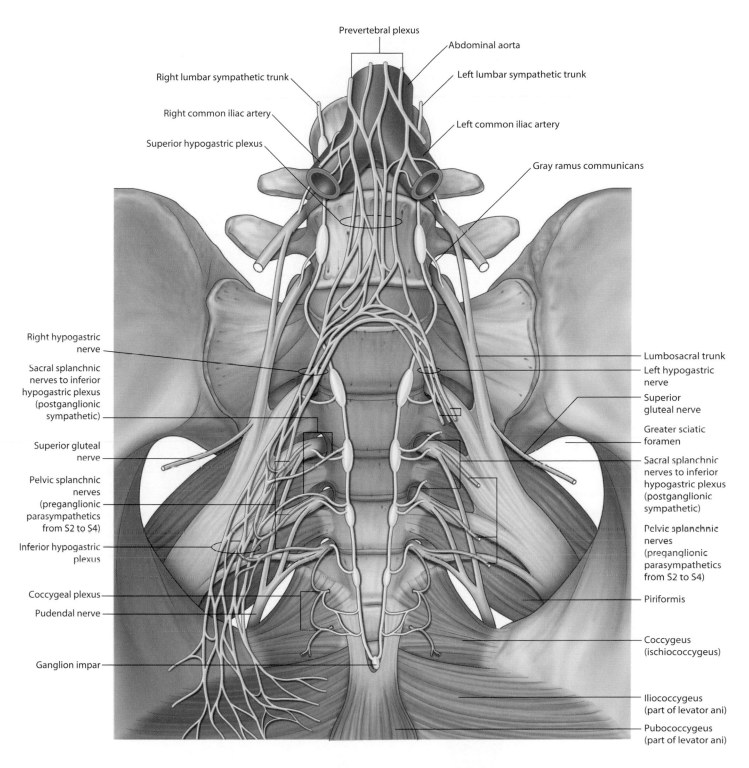

Prevertebral plexus

Abdominal aorta

Right lumbar sympathetic trunk

Left lumbar sympathetic trunk

Right common iliac artery

Left common iliac artery

Superior hypogastric plexus

Gray ramus communicans

Right hypogastric nerve

Lumbosacral trunk

Sacral splanchnic nerves to inferior hypogastric plexus (postganglionic sympathetic)

Left hypogastric nerve

Superior gluteal nerve

Greater sciatic foramen

Superior gluteal nerve

Sacral splanchnic nerves to inferior hypogastric plexus (postganglionic sympathetic)

Pelvic splanchnic nerves (preganglionic parasympathetics from S2 to S4)

Inferior hypogastric plexus

Pelvic splanchnic nerves (preganglionic parasympathetics from S2 to S4)

Coccygeal plexus

Piriformis

Pudendal nerve

Coccygeus (ischiococcygeus)

Ganglion impar

Iliococcygeus (part of levator ani)

Pubococcygeus (part of levator ani)

Pelvic extensions of the prevertebral nerve plexus (anterior view)

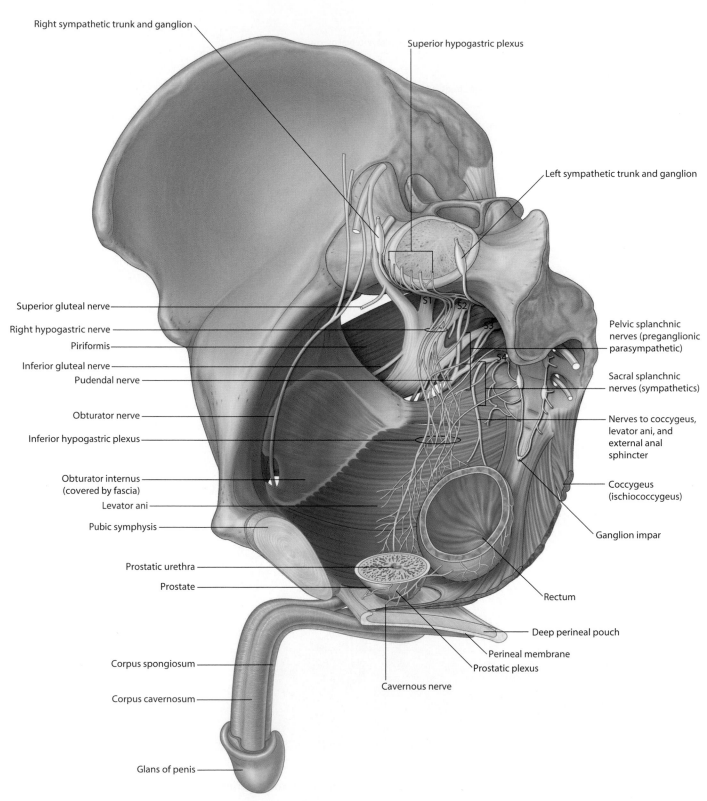

Right sympathetic trunk and ganglion

Superior hypogastric plexus

Left sympathetic trunk and ganglion

Superior gluteal nerve

Right hypogastric nerve

Piriformis

Inferior gluteal nerve

Pudendal nerve

Obturator nerve

Inferior hypogastric plexus

Obturator internus
(covered by fascia)

Levator ani

Pubic symphysis

Prostatic urethra

Prostate

Corpus spongiosum

Corpus cavernosum

Glans of penis

S1

S2

S3

S4

Pelvic splanchnic
nerves (preganglionic
parasympathetic)

Sacral splanchnic
nerves (sympathetics)

Nerves to coccygeus,
levator ani, and
external anal
sphincter

Coccygeus
(ischiococcygeus)

Ganglion impar

Rectum

Deep perineal pouch

Perineal membrane

Prostatic plexus

Cavernous nerve

**Hypogastric nerve plexuses
(oblique sagittal view)**

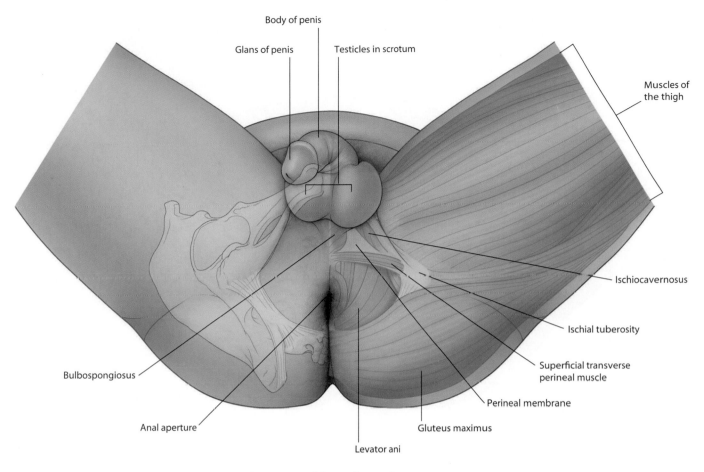

Structures of the perineum in men

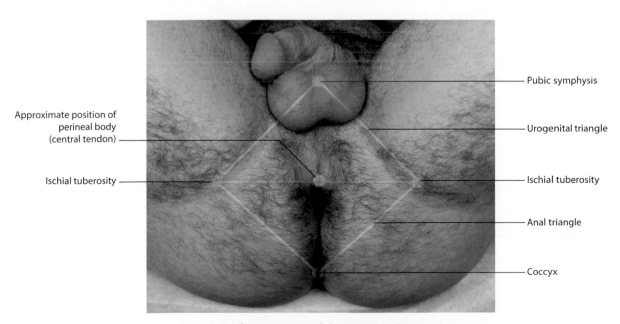

Surface anatomy of the perineum in men

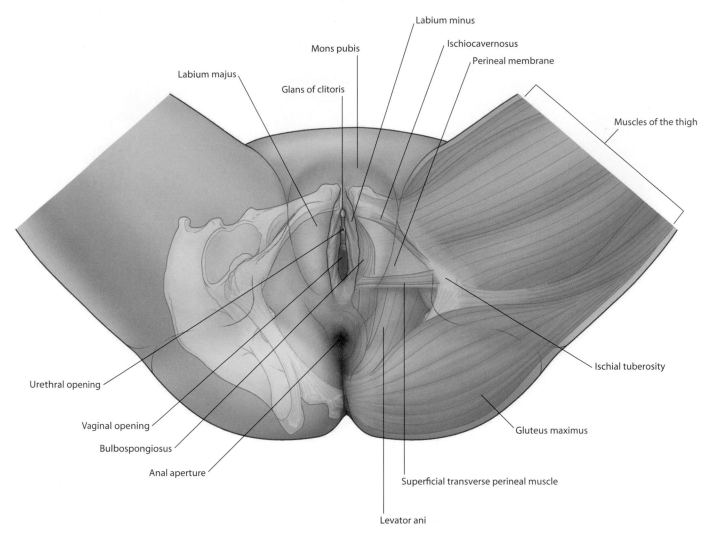

Labium minus

Mons pubis

Labium majus

Ischiocavernosus

Perineal membrane

Glans of clitoris

Muscles of the thigh

Ischial tuberosity

Urethral opening

Gluteus maximus

Vaginal opening

Bulbospongiosus

Anal aperture

Superficial transverse perineal muscle

Levator ani

Structures of the perineum in women

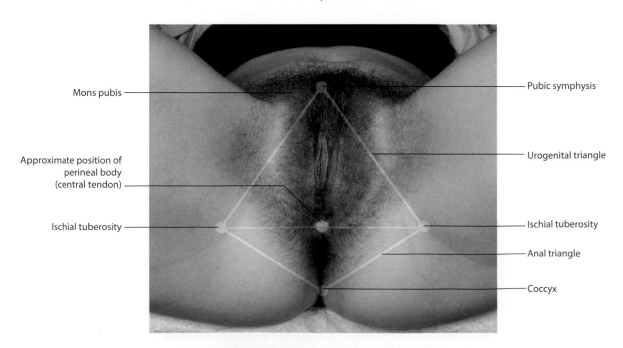

Mons pubis

Pubic symphysis

Approximate position of perineal body (central tendon)

Urogenital triangle

Ischial tuberosity

Ischial tuberosity

Anal triangle

Coccyx

Surface anatomy of the perineum in women

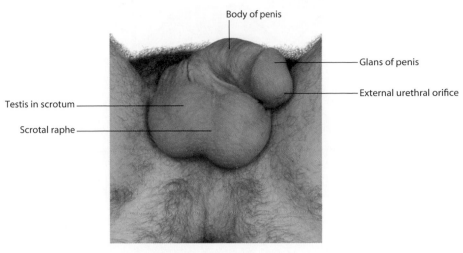

Body of penis

Glans of penis

External urethral orifice

Testis in scrotum

Scrotal raphe

Superficial features of the perineum in men

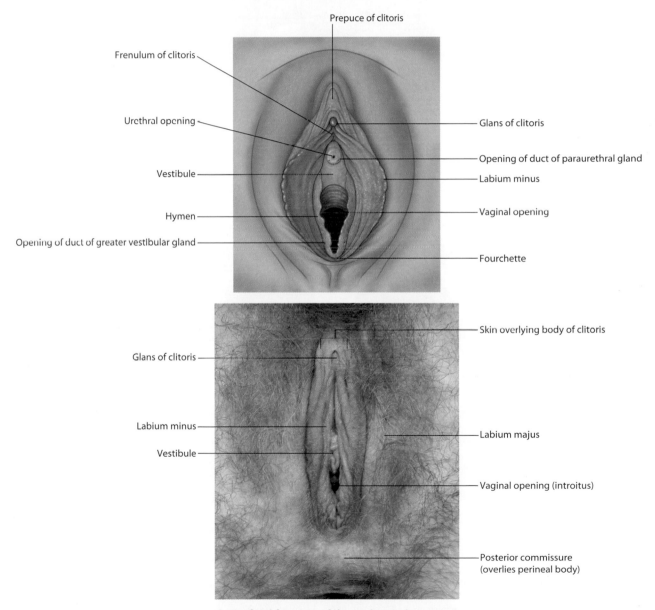

Prepuce of clitoris

Frenulum of clitoris

Urethral opening

Glans of clitoris

Opening of duct of paraurethral gland

Vestibule

Labium minus

Hymen

Vaginal opening

Opening of duct of greater vestibular gland

Fourchette

Skin overlying body of clitoris

Glans of clitoris

Labium minus

Labium majus

Vestibule

Vaginal opening (introitus)

Posterior commissure
(overlies perineal body)

Superficial features of the perineum in women

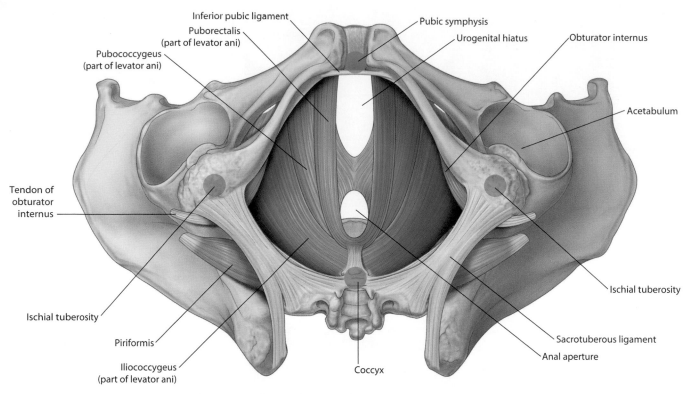

Inferior pubic ligament

Puborectalis (part of levator ani)

Pubococcygeus (part of levator ani)

Pubic symphysis

Urogenital hiatus

Obturator internus

Acetabulum

Tendon of obturator internus

Ischial tuberosity

Ischial tuberosity

Piriformis

Sacrotuberous ligament

Anal aperture

Iliococcygeus (part of levator ani)

Coccyx

Borders and ceiling of the perineum in men

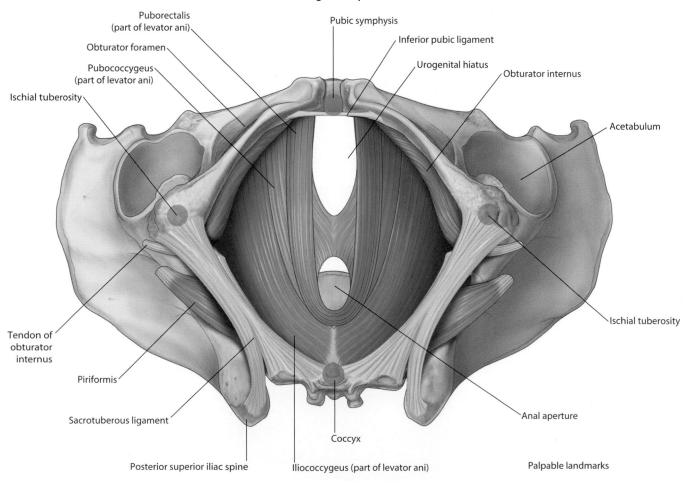

Puborectalis (part of levator ani)

Obturator foramen

Pubococcygeus (part of levator ani)

Ischial tuberosity

Pubic symphysis

Inferior pubic ligament

Urogenital hiatus

Obturator internus

Acetabulum

Ischial tuberosity

Tendon of obturator internus

Piriformis

Anal aperture

Sacrotuberous ligament

Posterior superior iliac spine

Coccyx

Iliococcygeus (part of levator ani)

Palpable landmarks

Borders and ceiling of the perineum in women

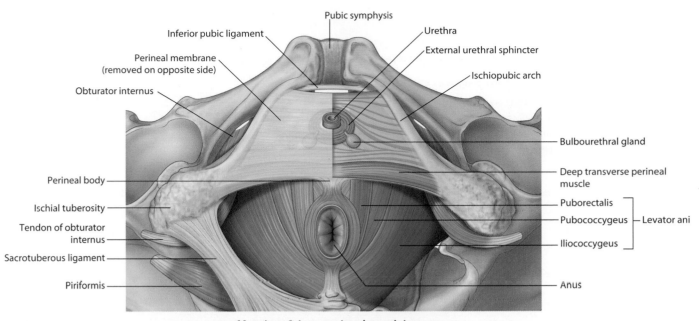

Muscles of deep perineal pouch in men
(perineal membrane removed on left side to expose deep perineal pouch)

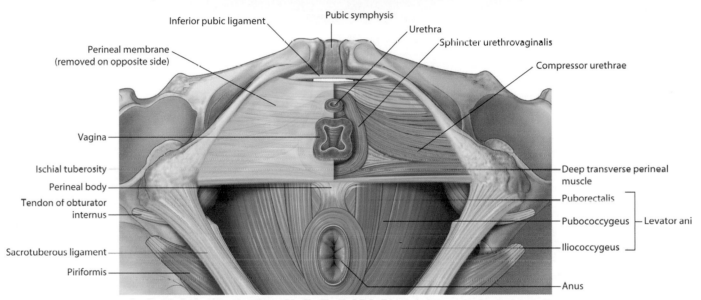

Muscles of deep perineal pouch in women
(perineal membrane removed on left side to expose deep perineal pouch)

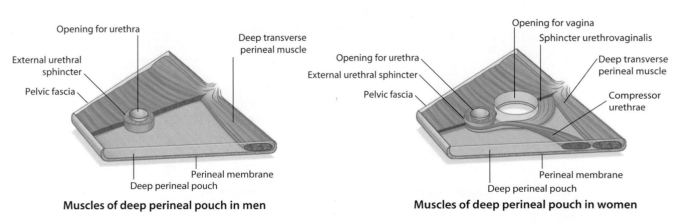

Muscles of deep perineal pouch in men   **Muscles of deep perineal pouch in women**

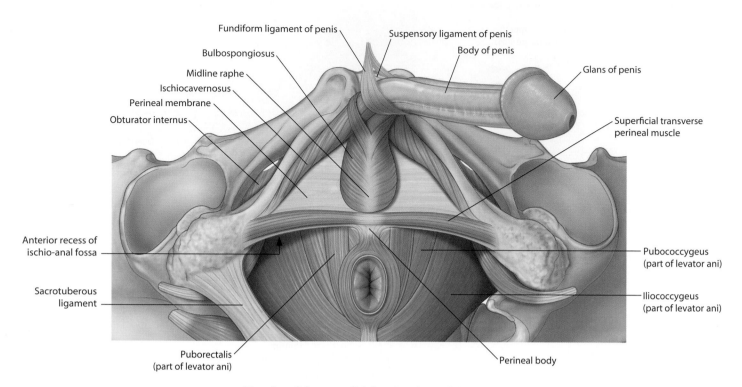

Fundiform ligament of penis

Suspensory ligament of penis

Body of penis

Bulbospongiosus

Glans of penis

Midline raphe

Ischiocavernosus

Perineal membrane

Obturator internus

Superficial transverse perineal muscle

Anterior recess of ischio-anal fossa

Pubococcygeus (part of levator ani)

Sacrotuberous ligament

Iliococcygeus (part of levator ani)

Puborectalis (part of levator ani)

Perineal body

Muscles of the superficial perineal pouch in men

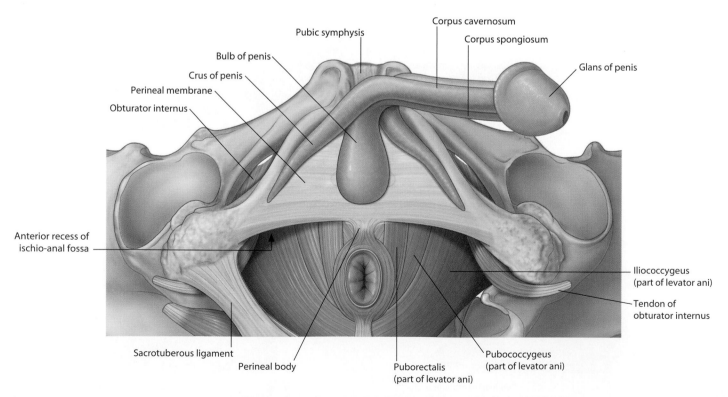

Pubic symphysis

Corpus cavernosum

Corpus spongiosum

Bulb of penis

Glans of penis

Crus of penis

Perineal membrane

Obturator internus

Anterior recess of ischio-anal fossa

Iliococcygeus (part of levator ani)

Tendon of obturator internus

Sacrotuberous ligament

Perineal body

Puborectalis (part of levator ani)

Pubococcygeus (part of levator ani)

Erectile tissues of the superficial perineal pouch in men

262

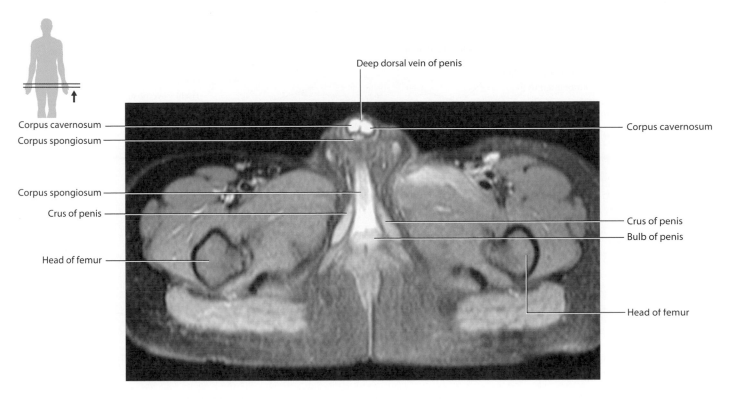

Corpus cavernosum

Corpus spongiosum

Corpus spongiosum

Crus of penis

Head of femur

Deep dorsal vein of penis

Corpus cavernosum

Crus of penis

Bulb of penis

Head of femur

Erectile tissues in relation to other structures in the male perineum.
T2-weighted MR image in axial plane

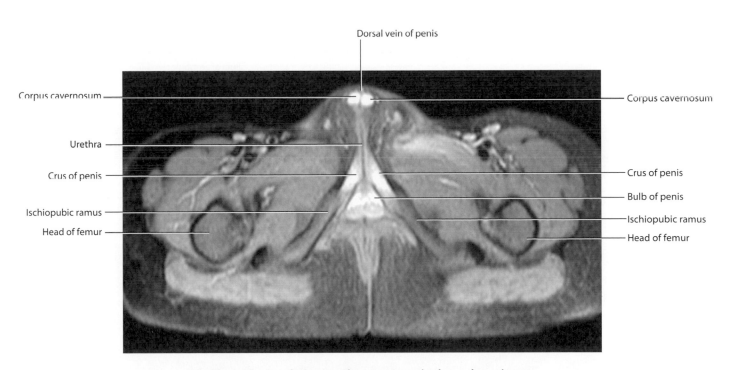

Corpus cavernosum

Urethra

Crus of penis

Ischiopubic ramus

Head of femur

Dorsal vein of penis

Corpus cavernosum

Crus of penis

Bulb of penis

Ischiopubic ramus

Head of femur

Erectile tissues in relation to other structures in the male perineum.
T2-weighted MR image in axial plane

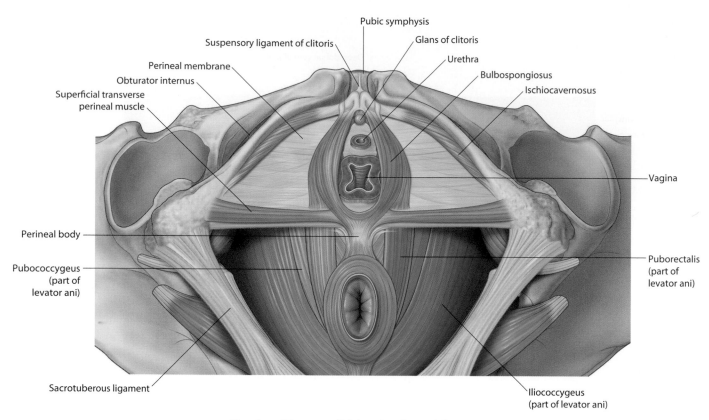

Pubic symphysis
Suspensory ligament of clitoris
Glans of clitoris
Urethra
Perineal membrane
Bulbospongiosus
Obturator internus
Ischiocavernosus
Superficial transverse perineal muscle
Vagina
Perineal body
Puborectalis (part of levator ani)
Pubococcygeus (part of levator ani)
Sacrotuberous ligament
Iliococcygeus (part of levator ani)

Muscles of the superficial perineal pouch in women

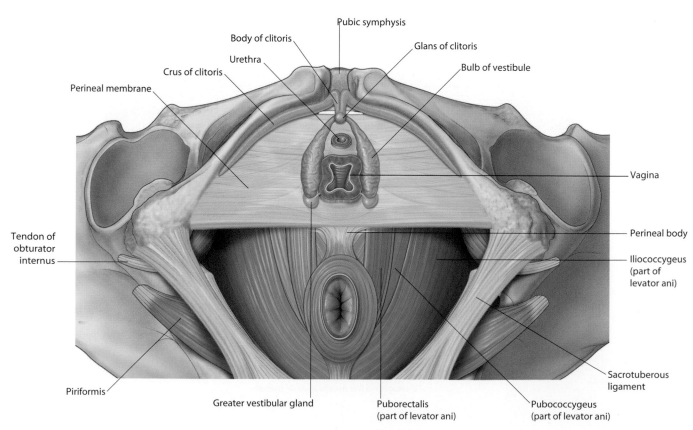

Pubic symphysis
Body of clitoris
Glans of clitoris
Urethra
Crus of clitoris
Bulb of vestibule
Perineal membrane
Vagina
Tendon of obturator internus
Perineal body
Iliococcygeus (part of levator ani)
Piriformis
Sacrotuberous ligament
Greater vestibular gland
Puborectalis (part of levator ani)
Pubococcygeus (part of levator ani)

Erectile tissues of the superficial perineal pouch in women

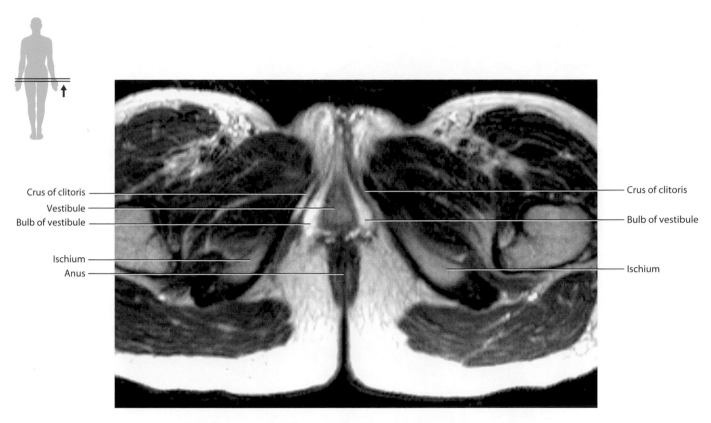

Crus of clitoris

Vestibule

Bulb of vestibule

Ischium

Anus

Crus of clitoris

Bulb of vestibule

Ischium

Erectile tissues in relation to other structures in the female perineum.
T2-weighted MR image in axial plane

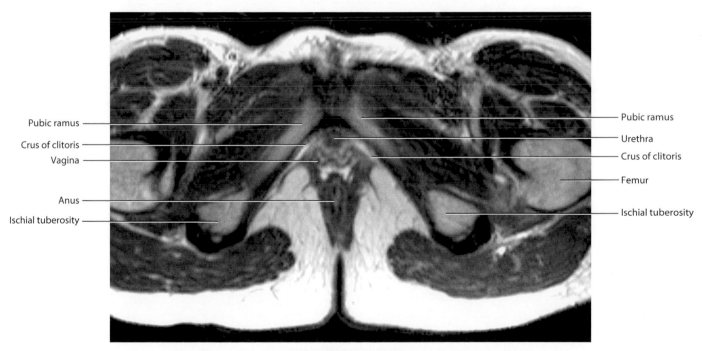

Pubic ramus

Crus of clitoris

Vagina

Anus

Ischial tuberosity

Pubic ramus

Urethra

Crus of clitoris

Femur

Ischial tuberosity

Erectile tissues in relation to other structures in the female perineum.
T2-weighted MR image in axial plane

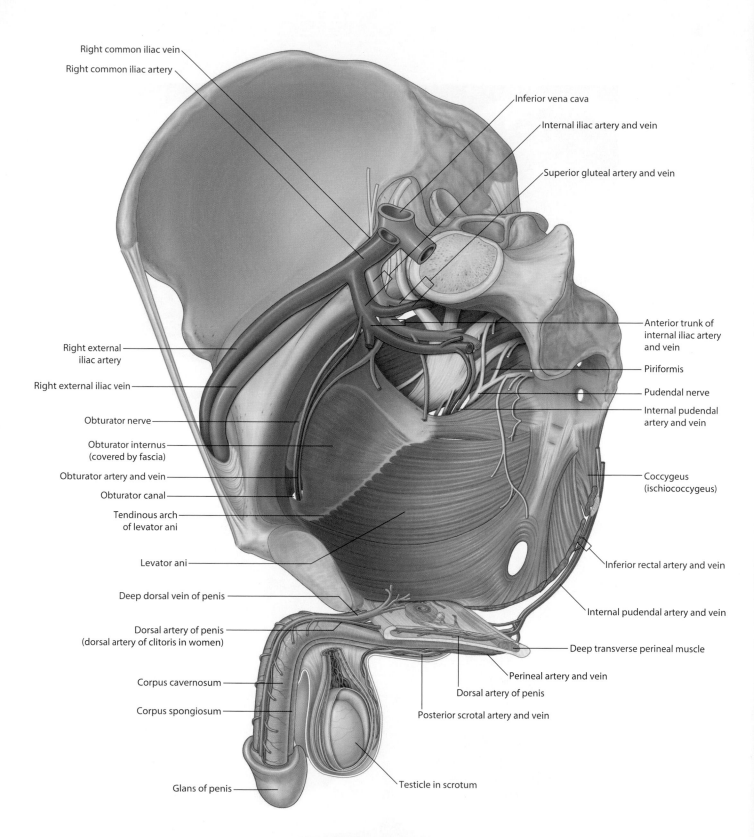

Right common iliac vein

Right common iliac artery

Inferior vena cava

Internal iliac artery and vein

Superior gluteal artery and vein

Anterior trunk of internal iliac artery and vein

Piriformis

Right external iliac artery

Pudendal nerve

Internal pudendal artery and vein

Right external iliac vein

Obturator nerve

Obturator internus (covered by fascia)

Obturator artery and vein

Obturator canal

Coccygeus (ischiococcygeus)

Tendinous arch of levator ani

Levator ani

Inferior rectal artery and vein

Deep dorsal vein of penis

Internal pudendal artery and vein

Dorsal artery of penis (dorsal artery of clitoris in women)

Deep transverse perineal muscle

Perineal artery and vein

Corpus cavernosum

Dorsal artery of penis

Corpus spongiosum

Posterior scrotal artery and vein

Testicle in scrotum

Glans of penis

Course of internal pudendal artery and vein in men (oblique sagittal view)

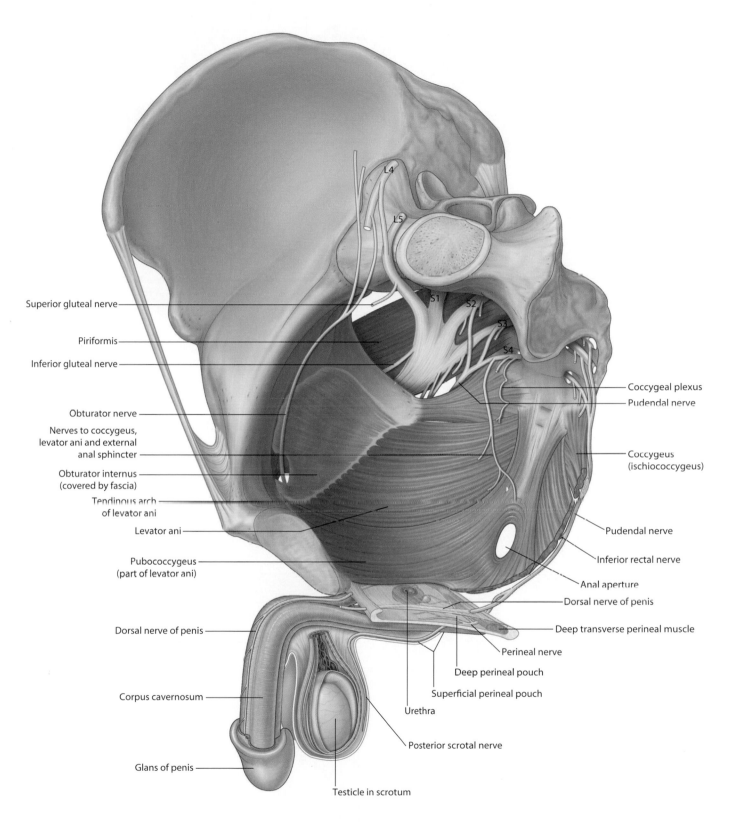

Superior gluteal nerve

Piriformis

Inferior gluteal nerve

Obturator nerve

Nerves to coccygeus, levator ani and external anal sphincter

Obturator internus (covered by fascia)

Tendinous arch of levator ani

Levator ani

Pubococcygeus (part of levator ani)

Dorsal nerve of penis

Corpus cavernosum

Glans of penis

L4

L5

S1

S2

S3

S4

Coccygeal plexus

Pudendal nerve

Coccygeus (ischiococcygeus)

Pudendal nerve

Inferior rectal nerve

Anal aperture

Dorsal nerve of penis

Deep transverse perineal muscle

Perineal nerve

Deep perineal pouch

Superficial perineal pouch

Urethra

Posterior scrotal nerve

Testicle in scrotum

**Course of pudendal nerve in men
(oblique sagittal view)**

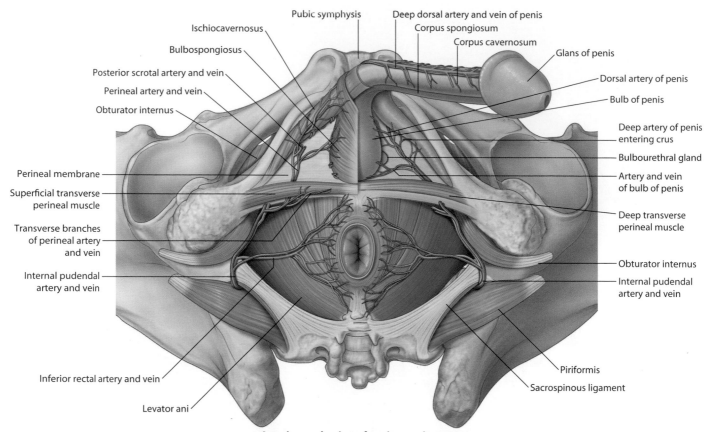

Pubic symphysis

Ischiocavernosus

Bulbospongiosus

Posterior scrotal artery and vein

Perineal artery and vein

Obturator internus

Perineal membrane

Superficial transverse perineal muscle

Transverse branches of perineal artery and vein

Internal pudendal artery and vein

Inferior rectal artery and vein

Levator ani

Deep dorsal artery and vein of penis

Corpus spongiosum

Corpus cavernosum

Glans of penis

Dorsal artery of penis

Bulb of penis

Deep artery of penis entering crus

Bulbourethral gland

Artery and vein of bulb of penis

Deep transverse perineal muscle

Obturator internus

Internal pudendal artery and vein

Piriformis

Sacrospinous ligament

Arteries and veins of perineum in men
(perineal membrane removed on left side to expose deep perineal pouch, inferior view)

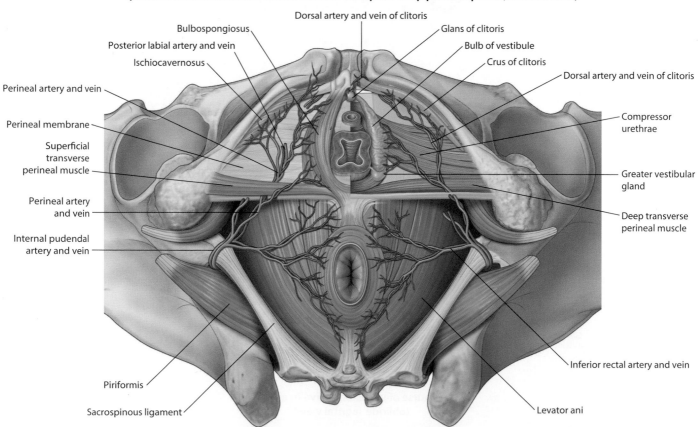

Dorsal artery and vein of clitoris

Bulbospongiosus

Posterior labial artery and vein

Ischiocavernosus

Perineal artery and vein

Perineal membrane

Superficial transverse perineal muscle

Perineal artery and vein

Internal pudendal artery and vein

Piriformis

Sacrospinous ligament

Glans of clitoris

Bulb of vestibule

Crus of clitoris

Dorsal artery and vein of clitoris

Compressor urethrae

Greater vestibular gland

Deep transverse perineal muscle

Inferior rectal artery and vein

Levator ani

Arteries and veins of perineum in women
(perineal membrane removed on left side to expose deep perineal pouch, inferior view)

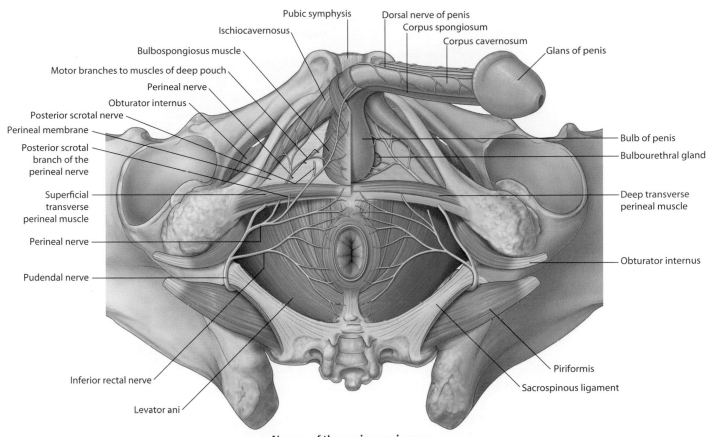

Nerves of the perineum in men
(perineal membrane removed on left side to expose deep perineal pouch, inferior view)

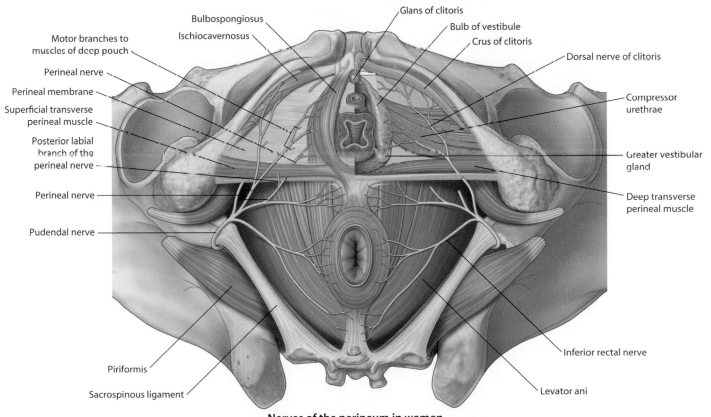

Nerves of the perineum in women
(perineal membrane removed on left side to expose deep perineal pouch, inferior view)

269

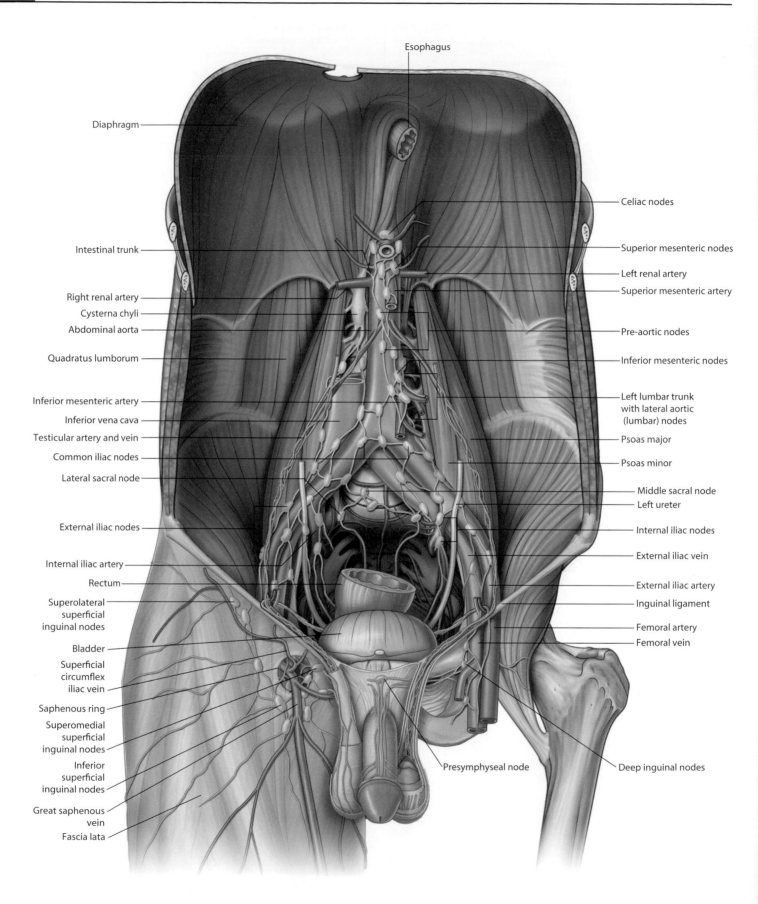

Esophagus

Diaphragm

Celiac nodes

Intestinal trunk

Superior mesenteric nodes

Left renal artery

Superior mesenteric artery

Right renal artery

Cysterna chyli

Abdominal aorta

Pre-aortic nodes

Inferior mesenteric nodes

Quadratus lumborum

Inferior mesenteric artery

Left lumbar trunk
with lateral aortic
(lumbar) nodes

Inferior vena cava

Psoas major

Testicular artery and vein

Psoas minor

Common iliac nodes

Lateral sacral node

Middle sacral node

Left ureter

Internal iliac nodes

External iliac nodes

External iliac vein

Internal iliac artery

External iliac artery

Rectum

Inguinal ligament

Superolateral
superficial
inguinal nodes

Femoral artery

Femoral vein

Bladder

Superficial
circumflex
iliac vein

Saphenous ring

Superomedial
superficial
inguinal nodes

Inferior
superficial
inguinal nodes

Presymphyseal node

Deep inguinal nodes

Great saphenous
vein

Fascia lata

Lymphatics of pelvis and perineum in men

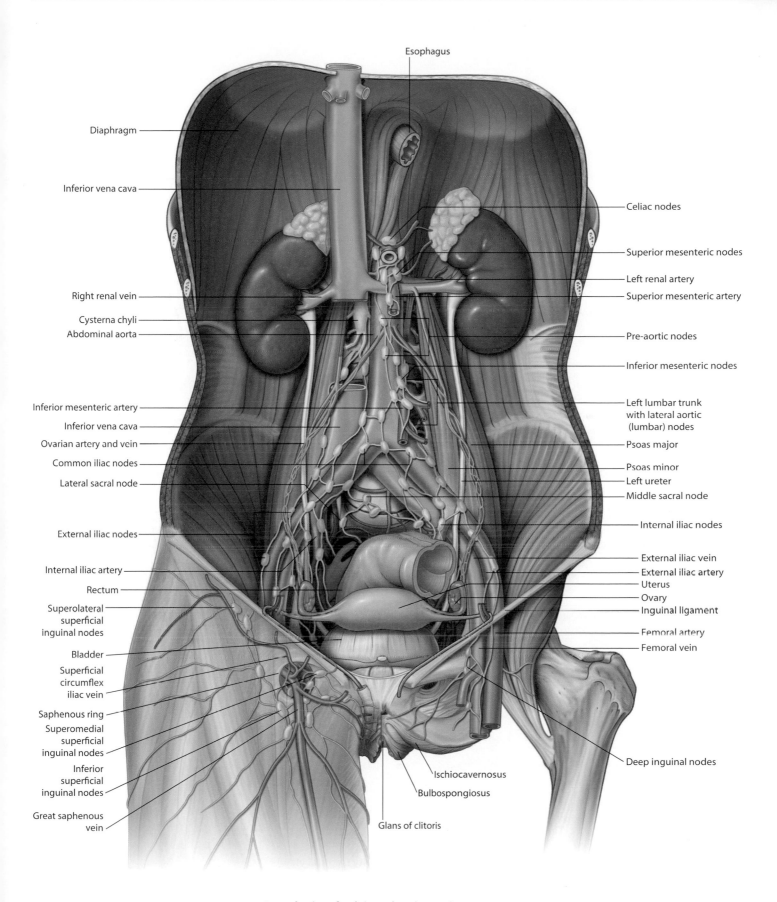

Esophagus

Diaphragm

Inferior vena cava

Celiac nodes

Superior mesenteric nodes

Left renal artery

Superior mesenteric artery

Right renal vein

Cysterna chyli

Abdominal aorta

Pre-aortic nodes

Inferior mesenteric nodes

Inferior mesenteric artery

Inferior vena cava

Ovarian artery and vein

Common iliac nodes

Lateral sacral node

Left lumbar trunk
with lateral aortic
(lumbar) nodes

Psoas major

Psoas minor

Left ureter

Middle sacral node

Internal iliac nodes

External iliac nodes

Internal iliac artery

Rectum

Superolateral
superficial
inguinal nodes

External iliac vein

External iliac artery

Uterus

Ovary

Inguinal ligament

Femoral artery

Femoral vein

Bladder

Superficial
circumflex
iliac vein

Saphenous ring

Superomedial
superficial
inguinal nodes

Inferior
superficial
inguinal nodes

Great saphenous
vein

Deep inguinal nodes

Ischiocavernosus

Bulbospongiosus

Glans of clitoris

Lymphatics of pelvis and perineum in women

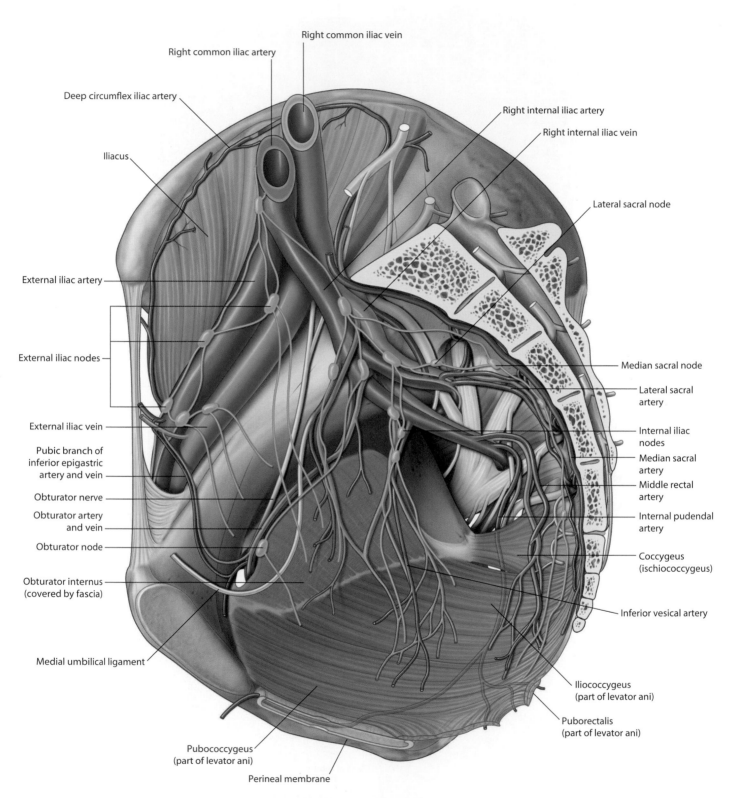

Right common iliac vein

Right common iliac artery

Deep circumflex iliac artery

Iliacus

Right internal iliac artery

Right internal iliac vein

Lateral sacral node

External iliac artery

External iliac nodes

Median sacral node

Lateral sacral artery

External iliac vein

Internal iliac nodes

Pubic branch of inferior epigastric artery and vein

Median sacral artery

Obturator nerve

Middle rectal artery

Obturator artery and vein

Internal pudendal artery

Obturator node

Coccygeus (ischiococcygeus)

Obturator internus (covered by fascia)

Inferior vesical artery

Medial umbilical ligament

Iliococcygeus (part of levator ani)

Puborectalis (part of levator ani)

Pubococcygeus (part of levator ani)

Perineal membrane

Lymphatics of pelvic cavity (sagittal view)

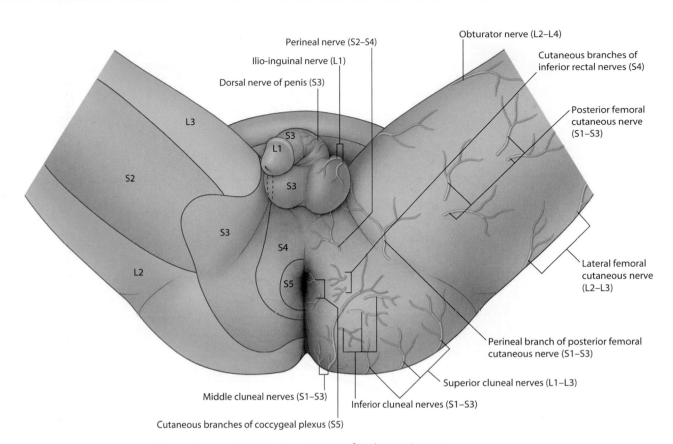

Perineal nerve (S2–S4)

Ilio-inguinal nerve (L1)

Dorsal nerve of penis (S3)

Obturator nerve (L2–L4)

Cutaneous branches of inferior rectal nerves (S4)

Posterior femoral cutaneous nerve (S1–S3)

Lateral femoral cutaneous nerve (L2–L3)

Perineal branch of posterior femoral cutaneous nerve (S1–S3)

Superior cluneal nerves (L1–L3)

Inferior cluneal nerves (S1–S3)

Middle cluneal nerves (S1–S3)

Cutaneous branches of coccygeal plexus (S5)

Dermatomes and cutaneous nerves of perineum in men

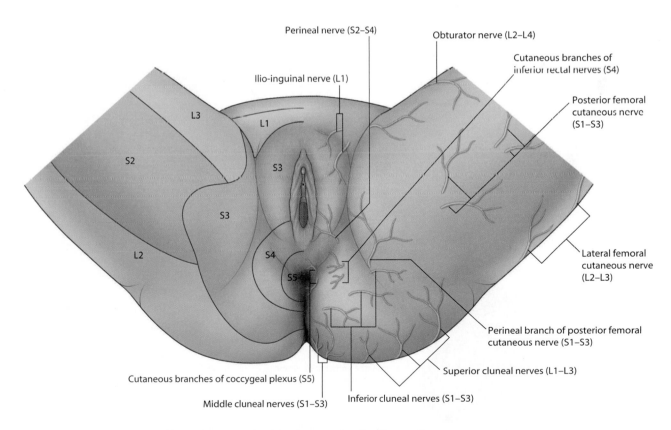

Perineal nerve (S2–S4)

Ilio-inguinal nerve (L1)

Obturator nerve (L2–L4)

Cutaneous branches of inferior rectal nerves (S4)

Posterior femoral cutaneous nerve (S1–S3)

Lateral femoral cutaneous nerve (L2–L3)

Perineal branch of posterior femoral cutaneous nerve (S1–S3)

Superior cluneal nerves (L1–L3)

Inferior cluneal nerves (S1–S3)

Cutaneous branches of coccygeal plexus (S5)

Middle cluneal nerves (S1–S3)

Dermatomes and cutaneous nerves of perineum in women

273

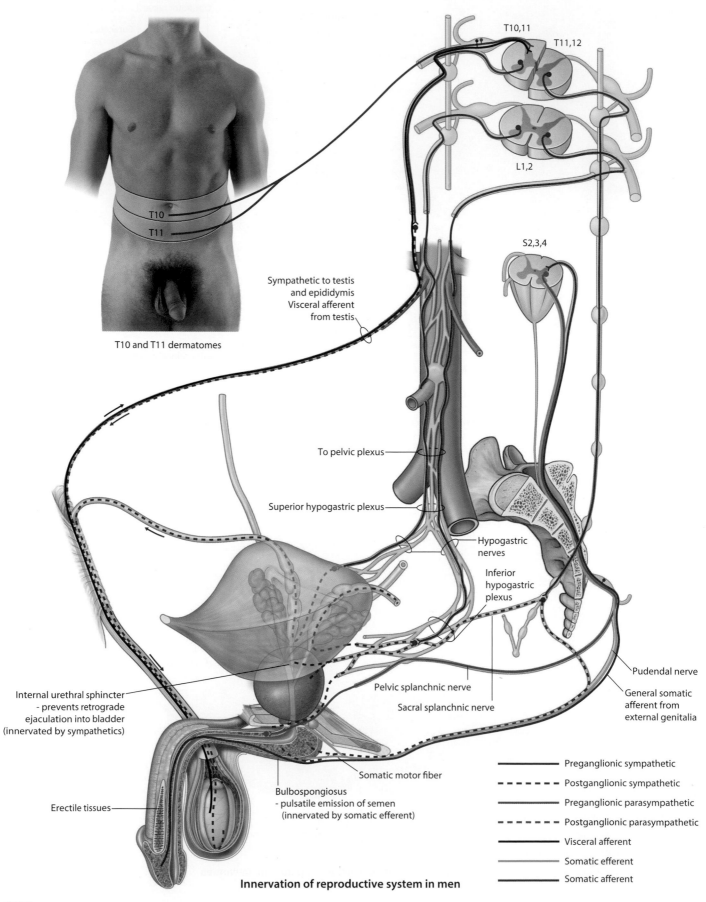

T10,11

T11,12

L1,2

S2,3,4

T10

T11

T10 and T11 dermatomes

Sympathetic to testis
and epididymis
Visceral afferent
from testis

To pelvic plexus

Superior hypogastric plexus

Hypogastric
nerves

Inferior
hypogastric
plexus

Pudendal nerve

General somatic
afferent from
external genitalia

Internal urethral sphincter
- prevents retrograde
ejaculation into bladder
(innervated by sympathetics)

Pelvic splanchnic nerve

Sacral splanchnic nerve

Somatic motor fiber

Erectile tissues

Bulbospongiosus
- pulsatile emission of semen
(innervated by somatic efferent)

Innervation of reproductive system in men

————	Preganglionic sympathetic
– – – –	Postganglionic sympathetic
————	Preganglionic parasympathetic
– – – –	Postganglionic parasympathetic
————	Visceral afferent
————	Somatic efferent
————	Somatic afferent

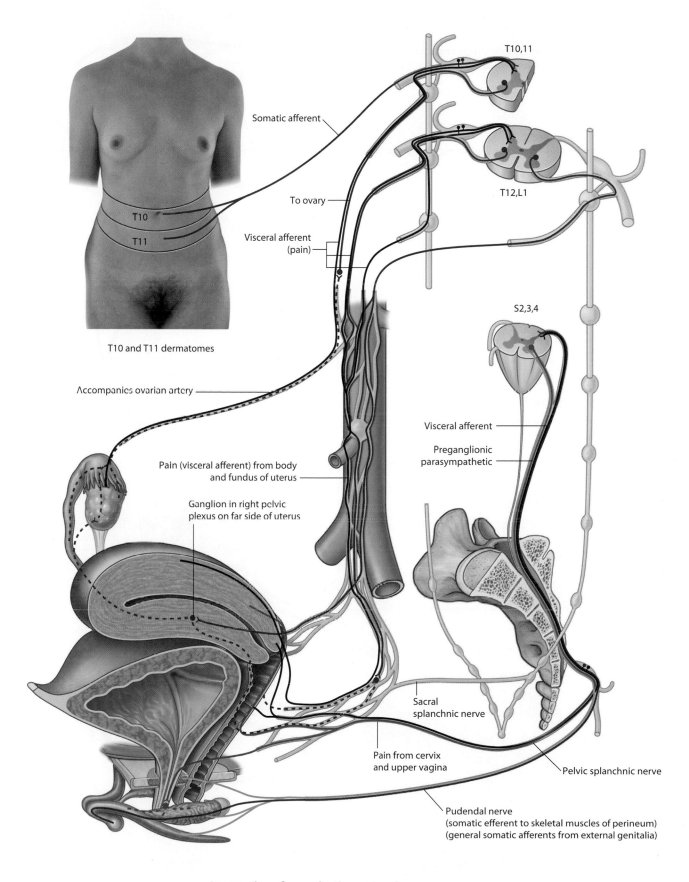

Somatic afferent

To ovary

Visceral afferent
(pain)

T10

T11

T10 and T11 dermatomes

Accompanies ovarian artery

Pain (visceral afferent) from body
and fundus of uterus

Ganglion in right pelvic
plexus on far side of uterus

T10,11

T12,L1

S2,3,4

Visceral afferent

Preganglionic
parasympathetic

Sacral
splanchnic nerve

Pain from cervix
and upper vagina

Pelvic splanchnic nerve

Pudendal nerve
(somatic efferent to skeletal muscles of perineum)
(general somatic afferents from external genitalia)

Innervation of reproductive system in women

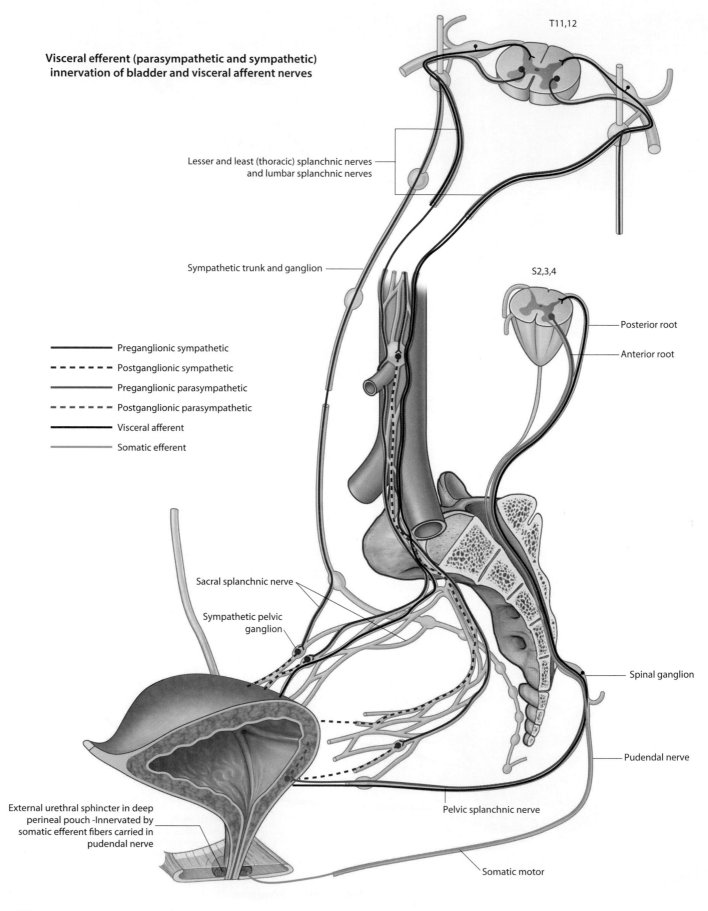

Visceral efferent (parasympathetic and sympathetic) innervation of bladder and visceral afferent nerves

T11,12

Lesser and least (thoracic) splanchnic nerves and lumbar splanchnic nerves

Sympathetic trunk and ganglion

S2,3,4

Posterior root

Anterior root

Preganglionic sympathetic

Postganglionic sympathetic

Preganglionic parasympathetic

Postganglionic parasympathetic

Visceral afferent

Somatic efferent

Sacral splanchnic nerve

Sympathetic pelvic ganglion

Spinal ganglion

Pudendal nerve

External urethral sphincter in deep perineal pouch -Innervated by somatic efferent fibers carried in pudendal nerve

Pelvic splanchnic nerve

Somatic motor

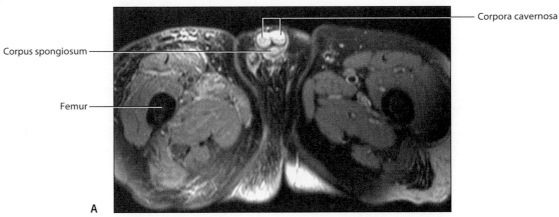

Corpus spongiosum —

Corpora cavernosa

Femur —

A

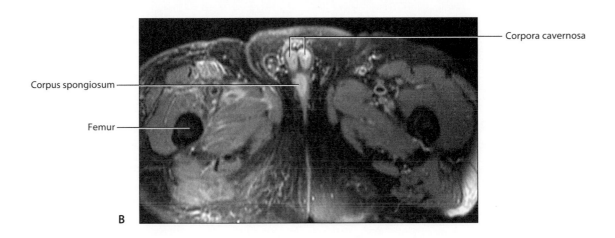

Corpus spongiosum —

Corpora cavernosa

Femur —

B

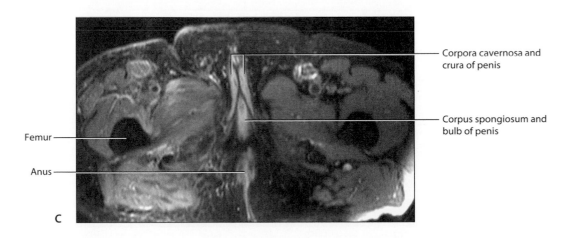

Corpora cavernosa and crura of penis

Corpus spongiosum and bulb of penis

Femur —

Anus —

C

A through C – Series of axial images that pass through the pelvic cavity and perineum from inferior to superior showing the various structures and their relationships with each other.
T2-weighted MR images in axial plane

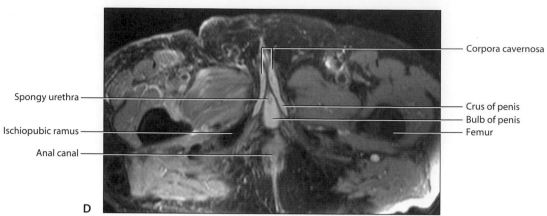

Corpora cavernosa

Spongy urethra

Crus of penis
Bulb of penis

Ischiopubic ramus

Femur

Anal canal

D

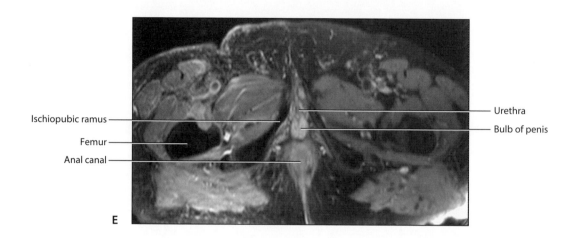

Ischiopubic ramus

Urethra

Bulb of penis

Femur

Anal canal

E

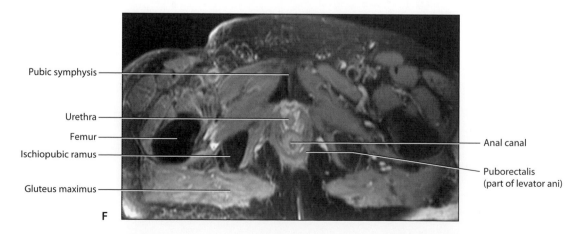

Pubic symphysis

Urethra

Femur

Ischiopubic ramus

Anal canal

Puborectalis
(part of levator ani)

Gluteus maximus

F

D through J – Series of axial images that pass through the pelvic cavity and perineum from inferior to superior showing the various structures and their relationships with each other.
T2-weighted MR images in axial plane

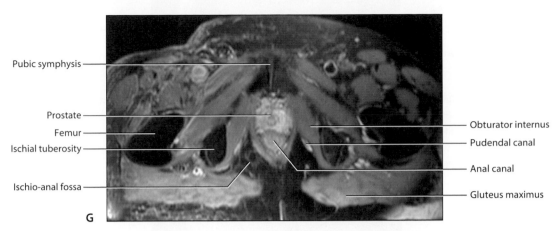

Pubic symphysis

Prostate

Femur

Ischial tuberosity

Ischio-anal fossa

Obturator internus

Pudendal canal

Anal canal

Gluteus maximus

G

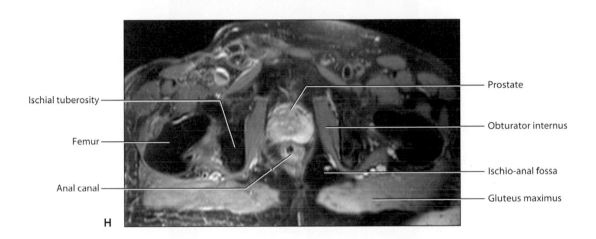

Ischial tuberosity

Femur

Anal canal

Prostate

Obturator internus

Ischio-anal fossa

Gluteus maximus

H

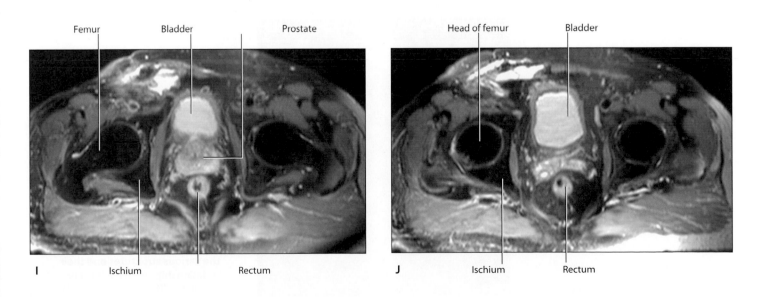

Femur   Bladder   Prostate

Head of femur   Bladder

I   Ischium   Rectum

J   Ischium   Rectum

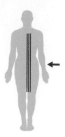

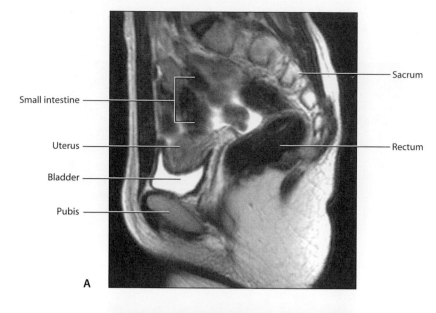

Small intestine

Uterus

Bladder

Pubis

Sacrum

Rectum

A

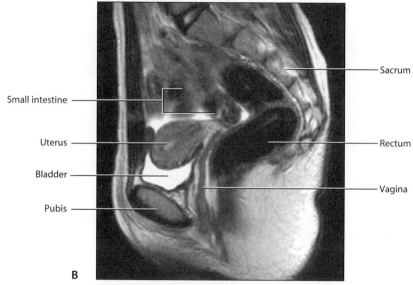

Small intestine

Uterus

Bladder

Pubis

Sacrum

Rectum

Vagina

B

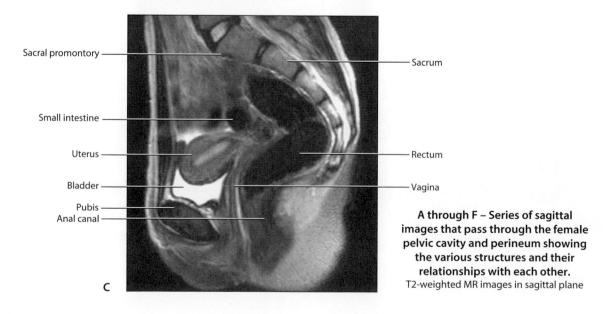

Sacral promontory

Small intestine

Uterus

Bladder

Pubis

Anal canal

Sacrum

Rectum

Vagina

A through F – Series of sagittal images that pass through the female pelvic cavity and perineum showing the various structures and their relationships with each other.
T2-weighted MR images in sagittal plane

C

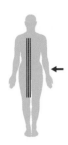

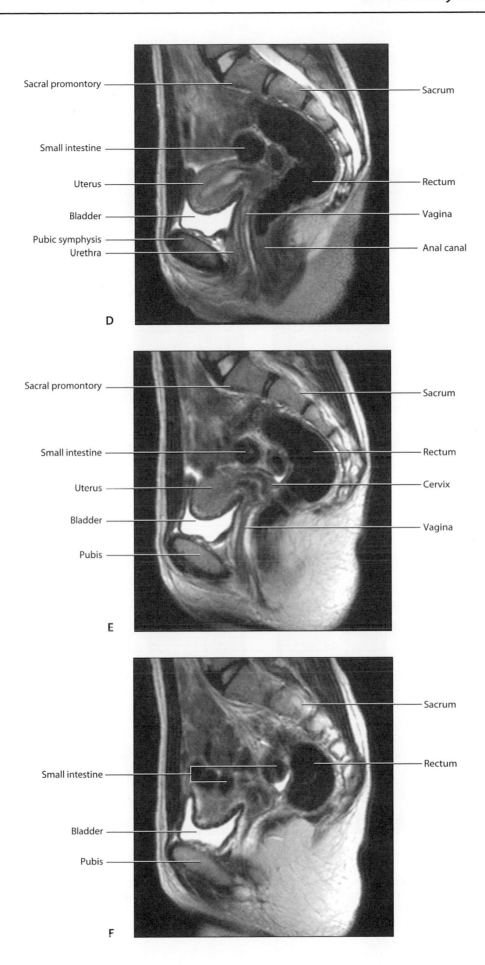

Sacral promontory — Sacrum

Small intestine

Uterus — Rectum

Bladder — Vagina

Pubic symphysis — Anal canal
Urethra

D

Sacral promontory — Sacrum

Small intestine — Rectum

Uterus — Cervix

Bladder

Pubis — Vagina

E

— Sacrum

Small intestine — Rectum

Bladder

Pubis

F

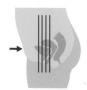

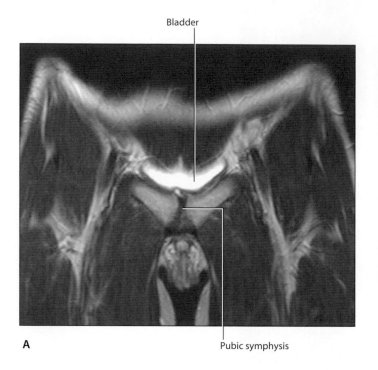

Bladder

Pubic symphysis

A

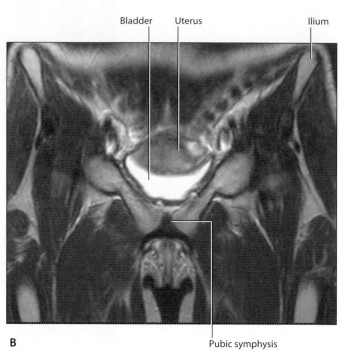

Bladder Uterus Ilium

Pubic symphysis

B

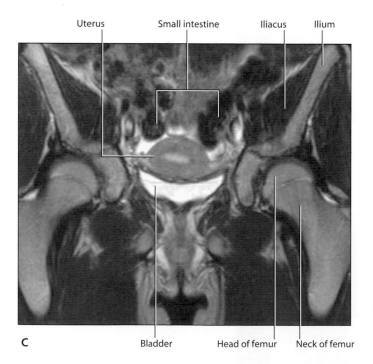

Uterus Small intestine Iliacus Ilium

Bladder Head of femur Neck of femur

C

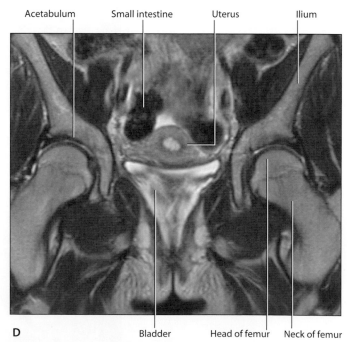

Acetabulum Small intestine Uterus Ilium

Bladder Head of femur Neck of femur

D

A through G – Series of coronal images that pass through the pelvic cavity and perineum from anterior to posterior showing the various structures and their relationships with each other.
T2-weighted MR images in coronal plane

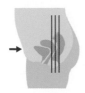

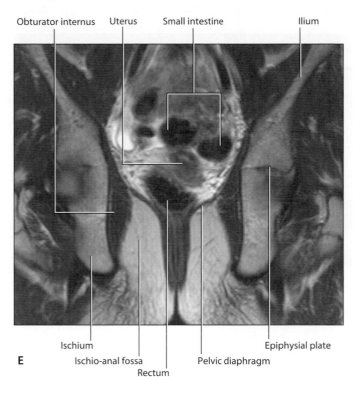

Obturator internus   Uterus   Small intestine   Ilium

Ischium

Ischio-anal fossa   Pelvic diaphragm

Rectum

Epiphysial plate

E

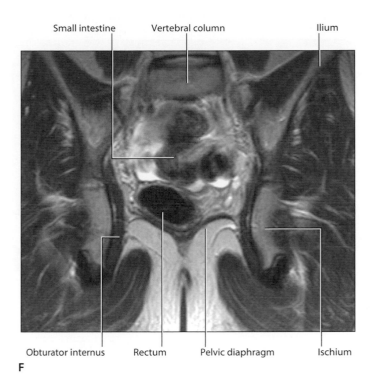

Small intestine   Vertebral column   Ilium

Obturator internus   Rectum   Pelvic diaphragm   Ischium

F

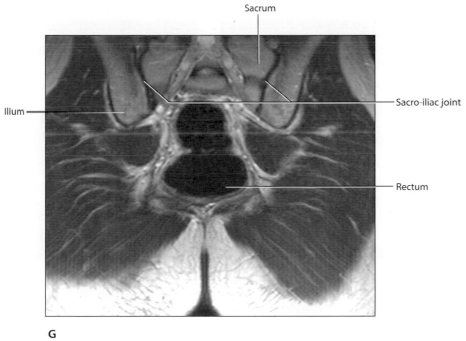

Sacrum

Ilium

Sacro-iliac joint

Rectum

G

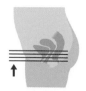

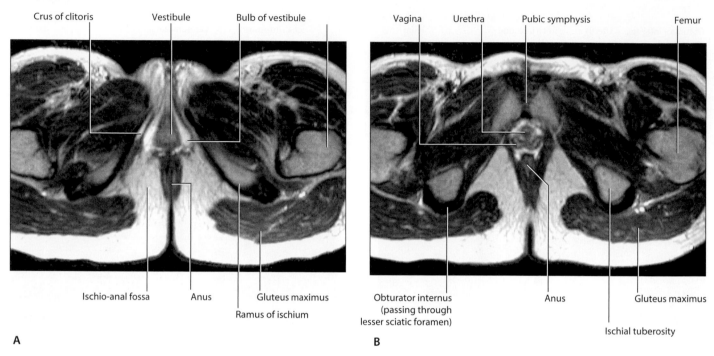

A

Crus of clitoris • Vestibule • Bulb of vestibule

Ischio-anal fossa • Anus • Gluteus maximus • Ramus of ischium

B

Vagina • Urethra • Pubic symphysis • Femur

Obturator internus (passing through lesser sciatic foramen) • Anus • Gluteus maximus • Ischial tuberosity

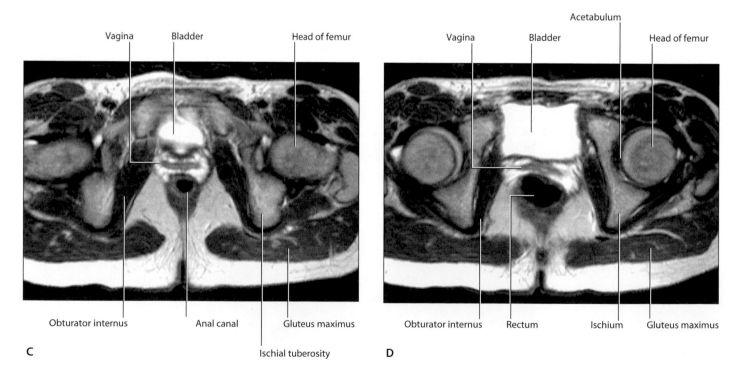

C

Vagina • Bladder • Head of femur

Obturator internus • Anal canal • Gluteus maximus • Ischial tuberosity

D

Acetabulum • Vagina • Bladder • Head of femur

Obturator internus • Rectum • Ischium • Gluteus maximus

A through H – Series of axial images that pass through the pelvic cavity and perineum from inferior to superior showing the various structures and their relationships with each other.
T2-weighted MR images in axial plane

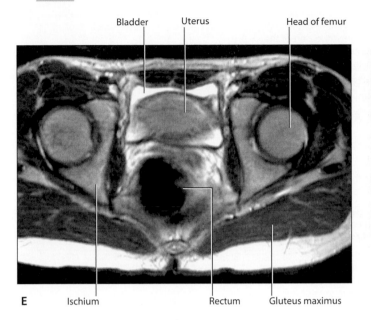

Bladder   Uterus   Head of femur

E   Ischium   Rectum   Gluteus maximus

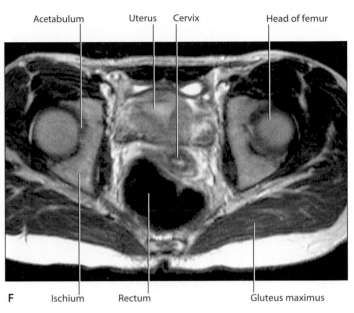

Acetabulum   Uterus   Cervix   Head of femur

F   Ischium   Rectum   Gluteus maximus

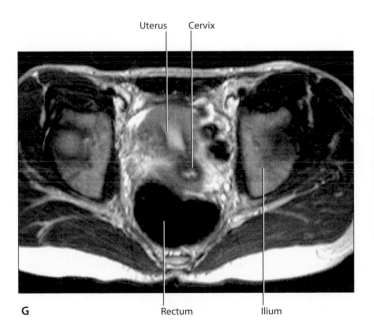

Uterus   Cervix

G   Rectum   Ilium

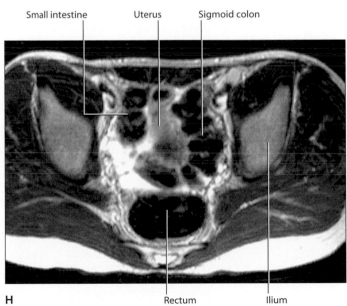

Small intestine   Uterus   Sigmoid colon

H   Rectum   Ilium

Branches of the sacral plexus
(spinal segments in parentheses do not consistently participate)

Branch		Spinal segments	Motor function	Sensory (cutaneous) function
Tibial part	1	L4 to S3	All muscles in the posterior or hamstring compartment of the thigh (including the hamstring part of the adductor magnus) except for the short head of the biceps All muscles in the posterior compartment of the leg All muscles in the sole of the foot	Skin on posterolateral and lateral surfaces of foot and sole of foot
Common fibular part	2	L4 to S2	Short head of biceps in the posterior compartment of the thigh All muscles in the anterior and lateral compartments of the leg Extensor digitorum brevis in the foot (also contributes to the supply of the first dorsal interosseous muscle)	Skin on the anterolateral surface of the leg and dorsal surface of the foot
Pudendal	3	S2 to S4	Skeletal muscles in the perineum including the external urethral and anal sphincters and levator ani (overlaps in supply of the levator ani and external sphincter with branches directly from ventral division of S4)	Most skin of the perineum. Penis and clitoris
Superior gluteal	4	L4 to S1	Gluteus medius, gluteus minimus, and tensor fasciae latae	
Inferior gluteal	5	L5 to S2	Gluteus maximus	
Nerve to obturator internus and superior gemellus	6	L5 to S2	Obturator internus and superior gemellus	
Nerve to quadratus femoris and inferior gemellus	7	L4 to S1	Quadratus femoris and inferior gemellus	
Posterior femoral cutaneous (posterior cutaneous nerve of thigh)	8	S1, S3		Skin on the posterior aspect of the thigh
Perforating cutaneous	9	S2, S3		Skin over gluteal fold (overlaps with posterior femoral cutaneous)
Nerve to piriformis	10	(L5), S1, S2	Piriformis muscle	
Nerves to levator ani, coccygeus, and external anal sphincter	11	S4	Levator ani, coccygeus, and external anal sphincter. (Overlaps with pudendal nerve)	Small patch of skin between anus and coccyx

Branch		Spinal segments	Motor function	Sensory (cutaneous) function
Pelvic splanchnic nerves	12	S2, S3 (4)	Visceral motor (preganglionic parasympathetic) to pelvic part of prevertebral plexus Stimulate erection, modulate mobility in gastrointestinal system distal to the left colic flexure, inhibitory to internal urethral sphincter	Visceral afferents from pelvic viscera and distal parts of colon. Pain from cervix and possibly from bladder and proximal urethra

Branches of the coccygeal plexus

Anococcygeal nerves	13	S4 to Co	Perianal skin	

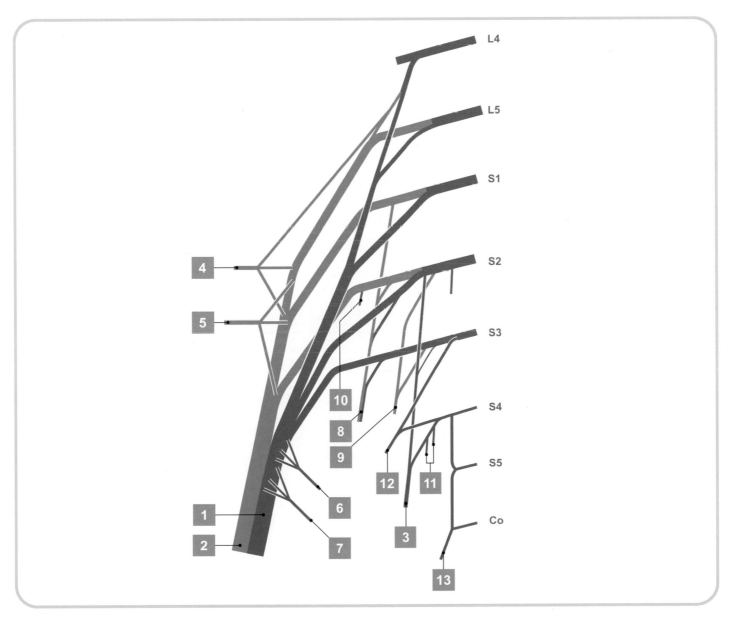

Muscles of the pelvic walls

Muscle		Origin	Insertion	Innervation	Function
Obturator internus	1	Anterolateral wall of true pelvis (deep surface of obturator membrane and surrounding bone)	Medial surface of greater trochanter of femur	Nerve to obturator internus **L5, SI**	Lateral rotation of the extended hip joint; abduction of flexed hip
Piriformis	2	Anterior surface of sacrum between anterior sacral foramina	Medial side of superior border of greater trochanter of femur	Branches from L5, **SI**, and **S2**	Lateral rotation of the extended hip joint; abduction of flexed hip

Muscles of the pelvic diaphragm

Muscle		Origin	Insertion	Innervation	Function
Levator ani	3	In a line around the pelvic wall beginning on the posterior aspect of the pubic bone and extending across the obturator internus muscle as a tendinous arch (thickening of the obturator internus fascia) to the ischial spine	The anterior part is attached to the superior surface of the perineal membrane; the posterior part meets its partner on the other side at the perineal body, around the anal canal, and along the anococcygeal ligament	Branches direct from the anterior ramus of S4, and by the inferior rectal branch of the pudendal nerve (S2 to S4)	Contributes to the formation of the pelvic floor, which supports the pelvic viscera; maintains an angle between the rectum and anal canal. Reinforces the external anal sphincter and, in women, functions as a vaginal sphincter
Coccygeus	4	Ischial spine and pelvic surface of the sacrospinous ligament	Lateral margin of coccyx and related border of sacrum	Branches from the anterior rami of S3 and S4	Contributes to the formation of the pelvic floor, which supports the pelvic viscera; pulls coccyx forward after defecation

Muscles within the deep perineal pouch

Muscle		Origin	Insertion	Innervation	Function
External urethral sphincter	5	From the inferior ramus of the pubis on each side and adjacent walls of the deep perineal pouch	Surrounds membranous part of urethra	Perineal branches of the pudendal nerve (S2 to S4)	Compresses the membranous urethra; relaxes during micturition
Deep transverse perineal	6	Medial aspect of ischial ramus	Perineal body	Perineal branches of the pudendal nerve (S2 to S4)	Stabilizes the position of the perineal body
Compressor urethrae (in women only)	7	Ischiopubic ramus on each side	Blends with partner on other side anterior to the urethra	Perineal branches of the pudendal nerve (S2 to S4)	Functions as an accessory sphincter of the urethra
Sphincter urethrovaginalis (in women only)	8	Perineal body	Passes forward lateral to the vagina to blend with partner on other side anterior to the urethra	Perineal branches of the pudendal nerve (S2 to S4)	Functions as an accessory sphincter of the urethra (also may facilitate closing the vagina)

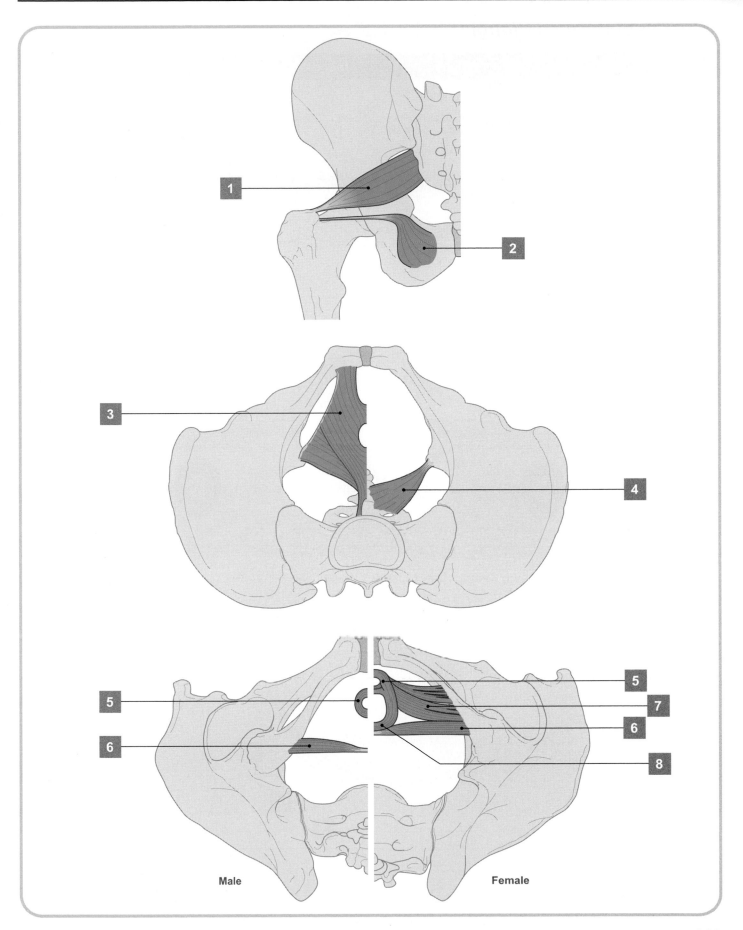

Male

Female

Muscles of the anal triangle

Muscle		Origin	Insertion	Innervation	Function
EXTERNAL ANAL SPHINCTER					
Deep part	1	Surrounds superior aspect of anal canal		Pudendal nerve (S2 and S3) and branches directly from S4	Closes anal canal
Superficial part	2	Surrounds lower part of anal canal	Anchored to perineal body and anococcygeal body		
Subcutaneous part	3	Surrounds anal aperture			

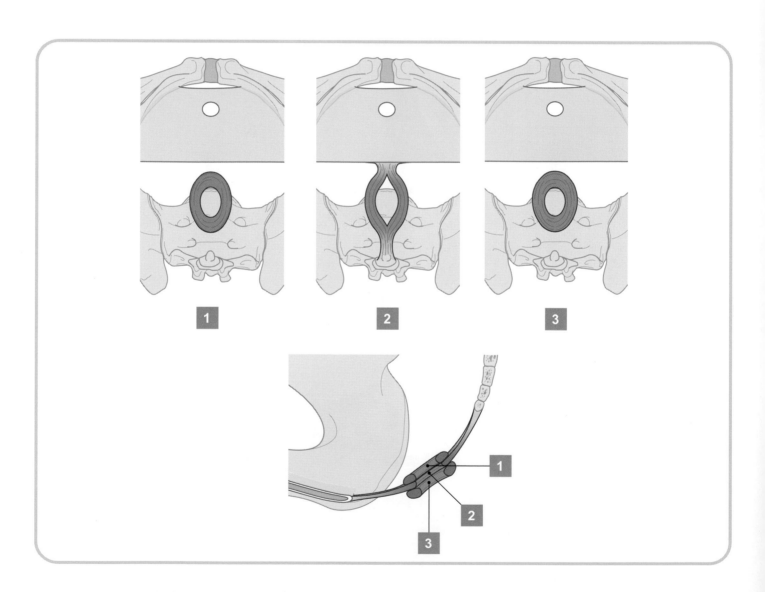

Muscles of the superficial perineal pouch

Muscle		Origin	Insertion	Innervation	Function
Ischiocavernosus	1	Ischial tuberosity and ramus	Crus of penis and clitoris	Pudendal nerve (S2 to S4)	Move blood from crura into the body of the erect penis and clitoris
Bulbospongiosus	2	In women: perineal body In men: perineal body, midline raphe	In women: bulb of vestibule, perineal membrane, body of clitoris, and corpus cavernosum In men: bulbospongiosus, perineal membrane, corpus cavernosum	Pudendal nerve (S2 to S4)	Move blood from attached parts of the clitoris and penis into the glans In men: removal of residual urine from urethra after urination; pulsatile emission of semen during ejaculation
Superficial transverse perineal	3	Ischial tuberosity and ramus	Perineal body	Pudendal nerve (S2 to S4)	Stabilize the perineal body

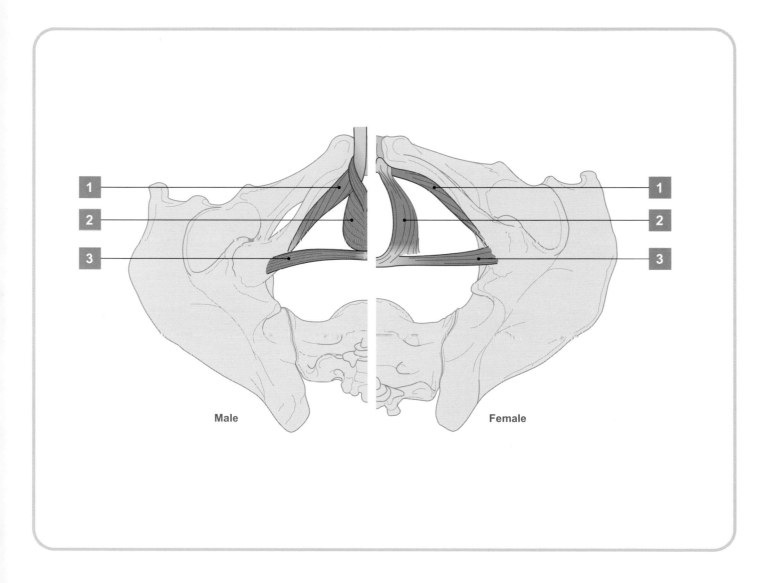

Male Female

6

LOWER LIMB

CONTENTS

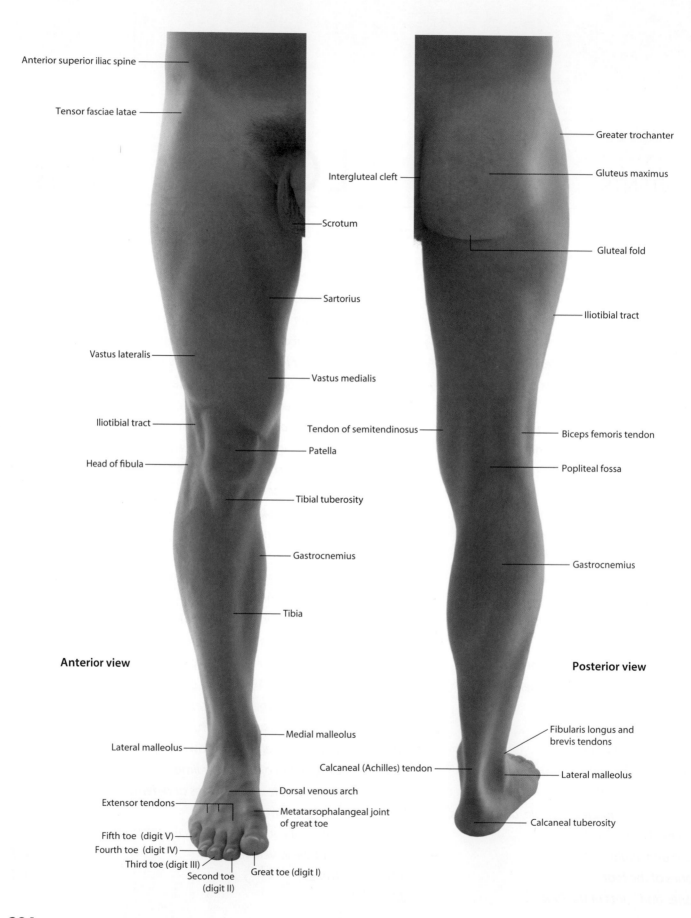

Anterior superior iliac spine

Tensor fasciae latae

Greater trochanter

Intergluteal cleft

Gluteus maximus

Scrotum

Gluteal fold

Sartorius

Iliotibial tract

Vastus lateralis

Vastus medialis

Iliotibial tract

Tendon of semitendinosus

Biceps femoris tendon

Patella

Head of fibula

Popliteal fossa

Tibial tuberosity

Gastrocnemius

Gastrocnemius

Tibia

Anterior view

Posterior view

Medial malleolus

Lateral malleolus

Fibularis longus and
brevis tendons

Calcaneal (Achilles) tendon

Lateral malleolus

Dorsal venous arch

Extensor tendons

Metatarsophalangeal joint
of great toe

Fifth toe (digit V)

Fourth toe (digit IV)

Calcaneal tuberosity

Third toe (digit III)

Second toe
(digit II)

Great toe (digit I)

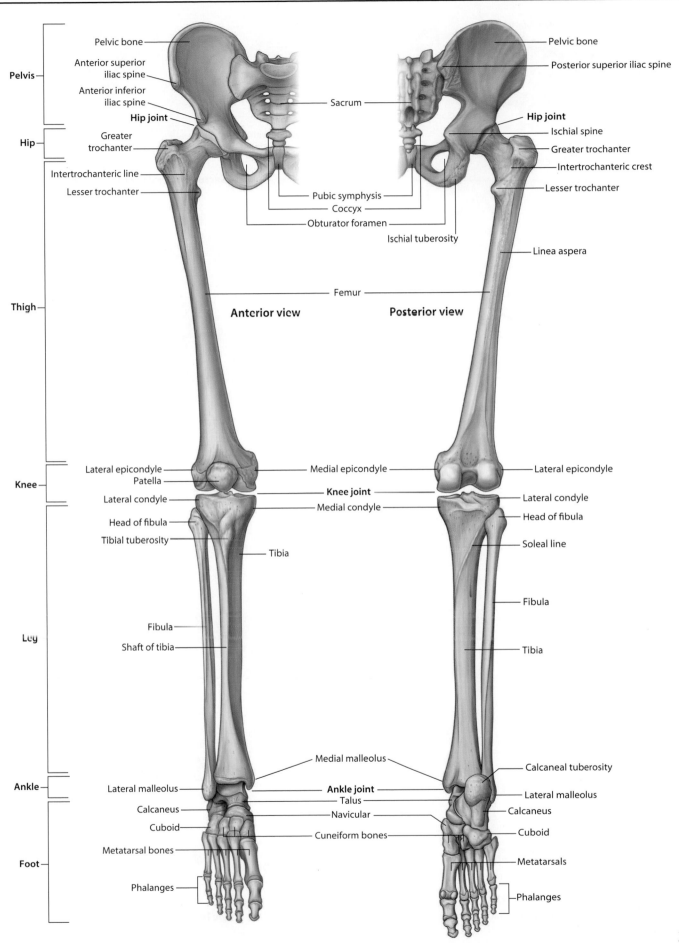

Pelvis

Pelvic bone

Anterior superior iliac spine

Anterior inferior iliac spine

Hip joint

Sacrum

Pelvic bone

Posterior superior iliac spine

Hip

Greater trochanter

Intertrochanteric line

Lesser trochanter

Hip joint

Ischial spine

Greater trochanter

Intertrochanteric crest

Lesser trochanter

Pubic symphysis

Coccyx

Obturator foramen

Ischial tuberosity

Linea aspera

Thigh

Femur

Anterior view

Posterior view

Knee

Lateral epicondyle

Patella

Lateral condyle

Head of fibula

Tibial tuberosity

Medial epicondyle

Knee joint

Medial condyle

Lateral epicondyle

Lateral condyle

Head of fibula

Soleal line

Tibia

Leg

Fibula

Shaft of tibia

Fibula

Tibia

Medial malleolus

Calcaneal tuberosity

Ankle

Lateral malleolus

Ankle joint

Talus

Lateral malleolus

Calcaneus

Cuboid

Navicular

Calcaneus

Foot

Metatarsal bones

Cuneiform bones

Cuboid

Metatarsals

Phalanges

Phalanges

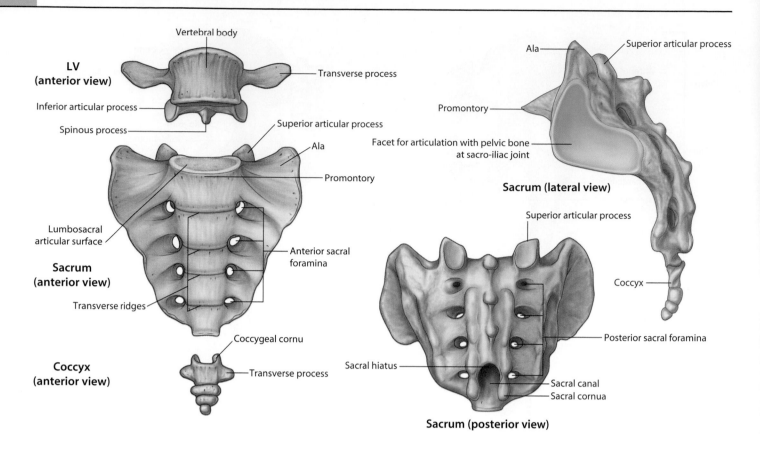

LV
(anterior view)

Vertebral body

Transverse process

Inferior articular process

Spinous process

Superior articular process

Ala

Promontory

Lumbosacral
articular surface

Sacrum
(anterior view)

Transverse ridges

Anterior sacral
foramina

Coccygeal cornu

Coccyx
(anterior view)

Transverse process

Ala

Superior articular process

Promontory

Facet for articulation with pelvic bone
at sacro-iliac joint

Sacrum (lateral view)

Superior articular process

Coccyx

Sacral hiatus

Posterior sacral foramina

Sacral canal
Sacral cornua

Sacrum (posterior view)

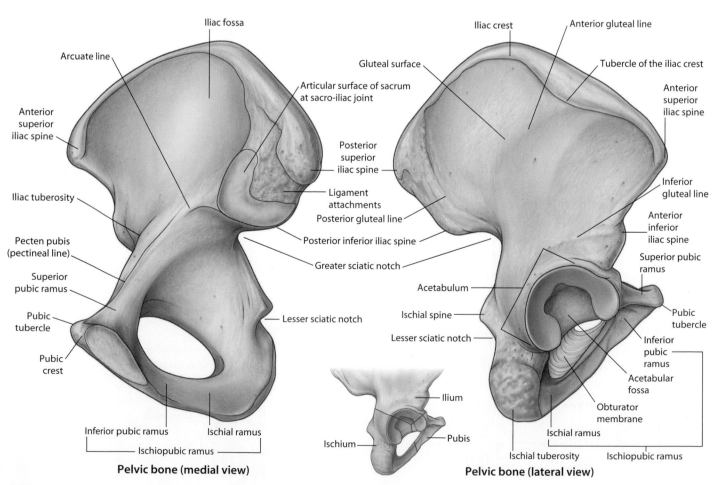

Iliac fossa

Arcuate line

Anterior
superior
iliac spine

Iliac tuberosity

Pecten pubis
(pectineal line)

Superior
pubic ramus

Pubic
tubercle

Pubic
crest

Inferior pubic ramus   Ischial ramus

Ischiopubic ramus

Pelvic bone (medial view)

Gluteal surface

Articular surface of sacrum
at sacro-iliac joint

Posterior
superior
iliac spine

Ligament
attachments

Posterior gluteal line

Posterior inferior iliac spine

Greater sciatic notch

Lesser sciatic notch

Iliac crest

Anterior gluteal line

Tubercle of the iliac crest

Anterior
superior
iliac spine

Inferior
gluteal line

Anterior
inferior
iliac spine

Superior pubic
ramus

Pubic
tubercle

Inferior
pubic
ramus

Acetabular
fossa

Obturator
membrane

Acetabulum

Ischial spine

Lesser sciatic notch

Ilium

Ischium

Pubis

Ischial ramus

Ischial tuberosity   Ischiopubic ramus

Pelvic bone (lateral view)

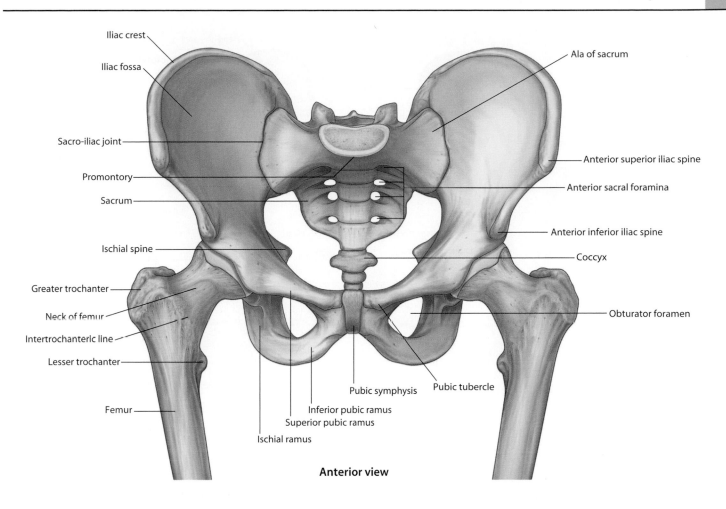

Iliac crest
Iliac fossa
Sacro-iliac joint
Promontory
Sacrum
Ischial spine
Greater trochanter
Neck of femur
Intertrochanteric line
Lesser trochanter
Femur

Ala of sacrum
Anterior superior iliac spine
Anterior sacral foramina
Anterior inferior iliac spine
Coccyx
Obturator foramen

Ischial ramus
Superior pubic ramus
Inferior pubic ramus
Pubic symphysis
Pubic tubercle

Anterior view

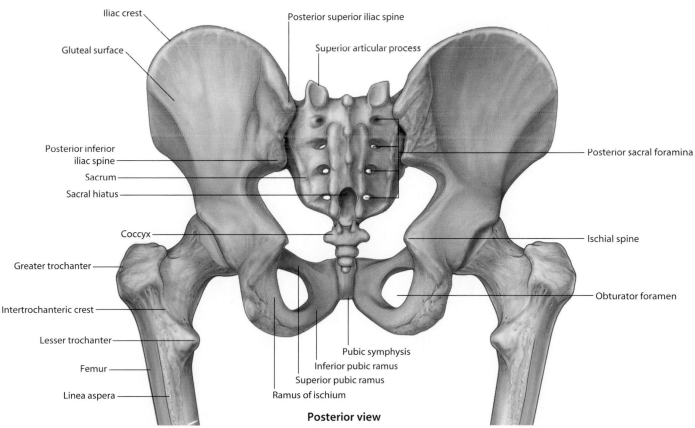

Iliac crest
Gluteal surface
Posterior inferior iliac spine
Sacrum
Sacral hiatus
Coccyx
Greater trochanter
Intertrochanteric crest
Lesser trochanter
Femur
Linea aspera

Posterior superior iliac spine
Superior articular process
Posterior sacral foramina
Ischial spine
Obturator foramen

Ramus of ischium
Superior pubic ramus
Inferior pubic ramus
Pubic symphysis

Posterior view

297

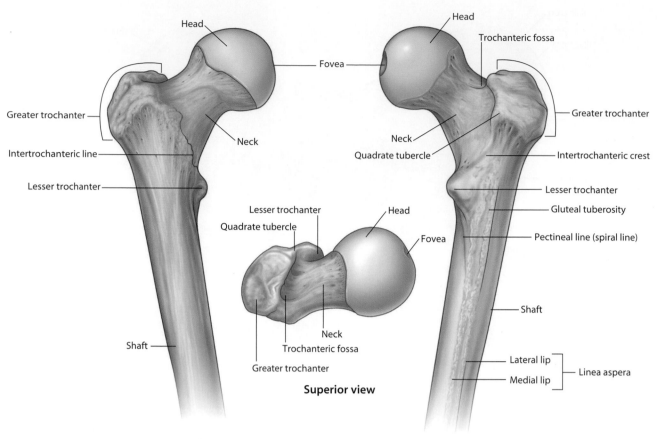

Head

Fovea

Neck

Greater trochanter

Intertrochanteric line

Lesser trochanter

Shaft

Head

Trochanteric fossa

Greater trochanter

Neck

Quadrate tubercle

Intertrochanteric crest

Lesser trochanter

Gluteal tuberosity

Pectineal line (spiral line)

Shaft

Lateral lip

Medial lip

Linea aspera

Lesser trochanter

Quadrate tubercle

Head

Fovea

Neck

Trochanteric fossa

Greater trochanter

Superior view

Anterior view

Posterior view

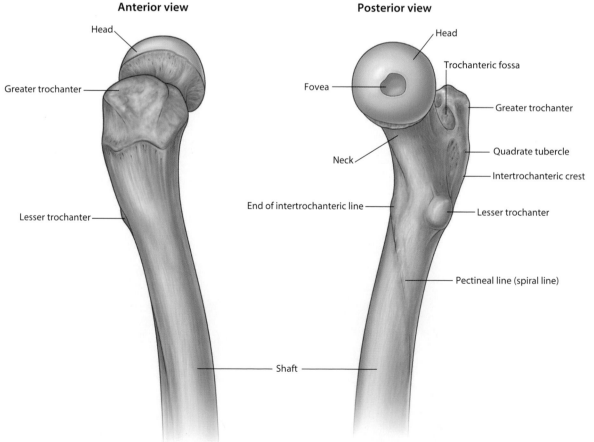

Head

Greater trochanter

Lesser trochanter

Shaft

Head

Fovea

Neck

Trochanteric fossa

Greater trochanter

Quadrate tubercle

Intertrochanteric crest

End of intertrochanteric line

Lesser trochanter

Pectineal line (spiral line)

Shaft

Lateral view

Medial view

298

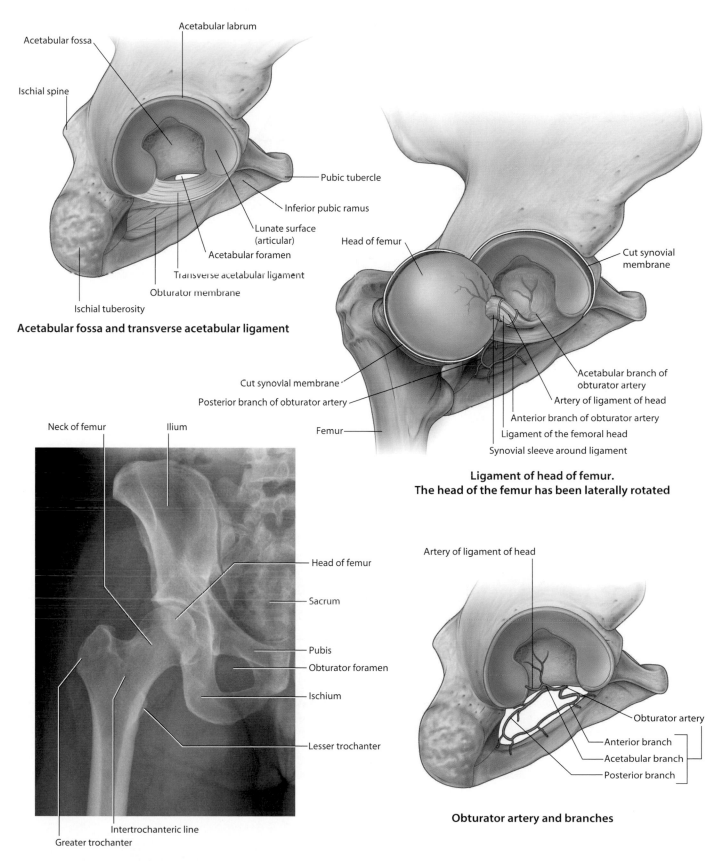

Acetabular fossa and transverse acetabular ligament

Acetabular fossa
Ischial spine
Acetabular labrum
Pubic tubercle
Inferior pubic ramus
Lunate surface (articular)
Acetabular foramen
Transverse acetabular ligament
Obturator membrane
Ischial tuberosity

Ligament of head of femur.
The head of the femur has been laterally rotated

Head of femur
Cut synovial membrane
Cut synovial membrane
Posterior branch of obturator artery
Femur
Acetabular branch of obturator artery
Artery of ligament of head
Anterior branch of obturator artery
Ligament of the femoral head
Synovial sleeve around ligament

Normal hip joint.
Radiograph, AP view

Neck of femur
Ilium
Head of femur
Sacrum
Pubis
Obturator foramen
Ischium
Lesser trochanter
Intertrochanteric line
Greater trochanter

Obturator artery and branches

Artery of ligament of head
Obturator artery
Anterior branch
Acetabular branch
Posterior branch

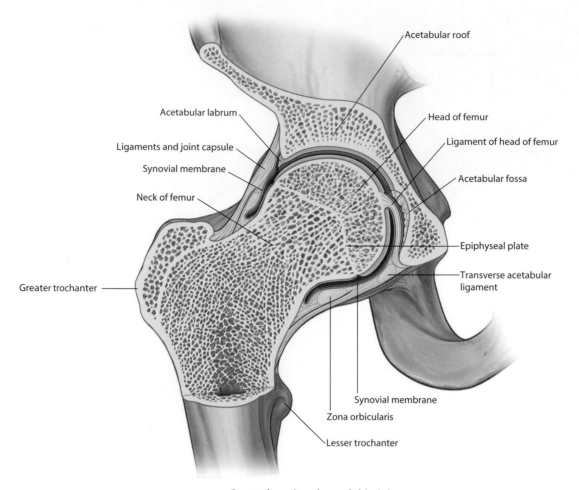

Acetabular roof

Acetabular labrum

Ligaments and joint capsule

Synovial membrane

Neck of femur

Greater trochanter

Head of femur

Ligament of head of femur

Acetabular fossa

Epiphyseal plate

Transverse acetabular ligament

Synovial membrane

Zona orbicularis

Lesser trochanter

Coronal section through hip joint

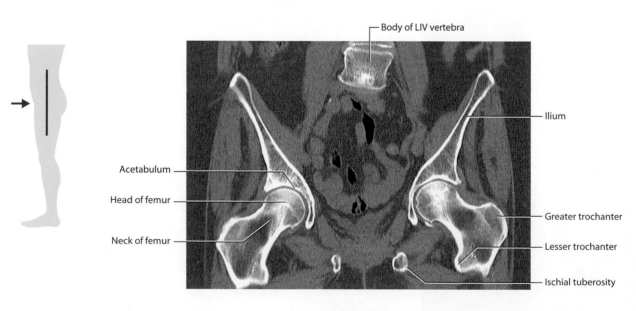

Body of LIV vertebra

Ilium

Acetabulum

Head of femur

Neck of femur

Greater trochanter

Lesser trochanter

Ischial tuberosity

Hip joints.
CT image in coronal plane

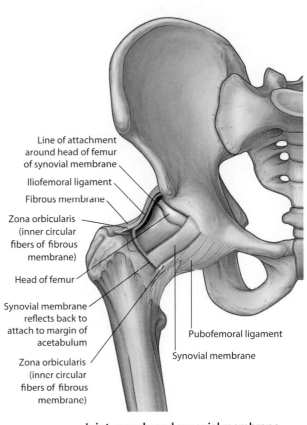

Line of attachment around head of femur of synovial membrane

Iliofemoral ligament

Fibrous membrane

Zona orbicularis (inner circular fibers of fibrous membrane)

Head of femur

Synovial membrane reflects back to attach to margin of acetabulum

Zona orbicularis (inner circular fibers of fibrous membrane)

Pubofemoral ligament

Synovial membrane

Joint capsule and synovial membrane

Iliofemoral ligament

Ischial spine

Greater trochanter

Intertrochanteric crest

Lesser trochanter

Ischial tuberosity

Ischiofemoral ligament

Femur

Ischiofemoral ligament (posterior view)

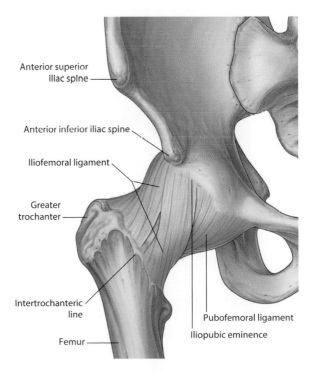

Anterior superior iliac spine

Anterior inferior iliac spine

Iliofemoral ligament

Greater trochanter

Intertrochanteric line

Femur

Pubofemoral ligament

Iliopubic eminence

Iliofemoral and pubofemoral ligaments (anterior view)

Internal iliac artery

Superior gluteal artery

External iliac artery

Obturator artery

Inferior gluteal artery

Abdominal aorta

Deep circumflex iliac artery

Superficial circumflex iliac artery

Superficial epigastric artery

Ascending branch of lateral circumflex femoral artery

Transverse branch of lateral circumflex femoral artery

Medial circumflex femoral artery

Descending branch of lateral circumflex femoral artery

First perforating artery

Deep artery of thigh

Femoral artery

Deep external pudendal artery

Posterior branch of obturator artery and acetabular branch

Superficial external pudendal artery

Arterial supply of the hip joint

301

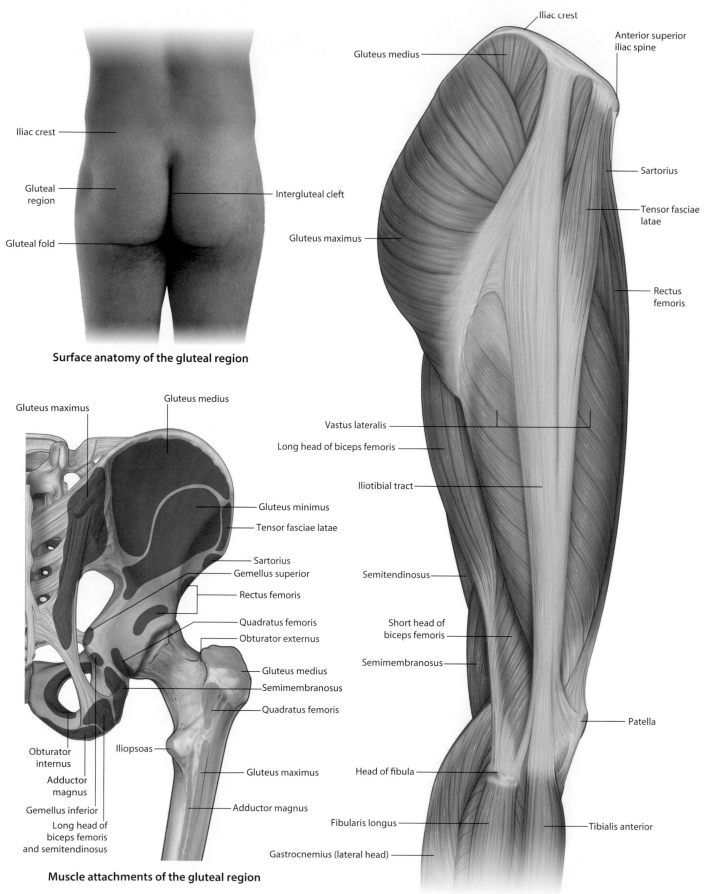

Surface anatomy of the gluteal region

Iliac crest

Gluteal region

Gluteal fold

Intergluteal cleft

Gluteus maximus

Gluteus medius

Gluteus minimus

Tensor fasciae latae

Sartorius

Gemellus superior

Rectus femoris

Quadratus femoris

Obturator externus

Gluteus medius

Semimembranosus

Quadratus femoris

Gluteus maximus

Adductor magnus

Iliopsoas

Obturator internus

Adductor magnus

Gemellus inferior

Long head of biceps femoris and semitendinosus

Muscle attachments of the gluteal region

Iliac crest

Gluteus medius

Anterior superior iliac spine

Sartorius

Tensor fasciae latae

Rectus femoris

Vastus lateralis

Long head of biceps femoris

Iliotibial tract

Semitendinosus

Short head of biceps femoris

Semimembranosus

Patella

Head of fibula

Fibularis longus

Tibialis anterior

Gastrocnemius (lateral head)

Muscles of the hip and thigh (lateral view)

302

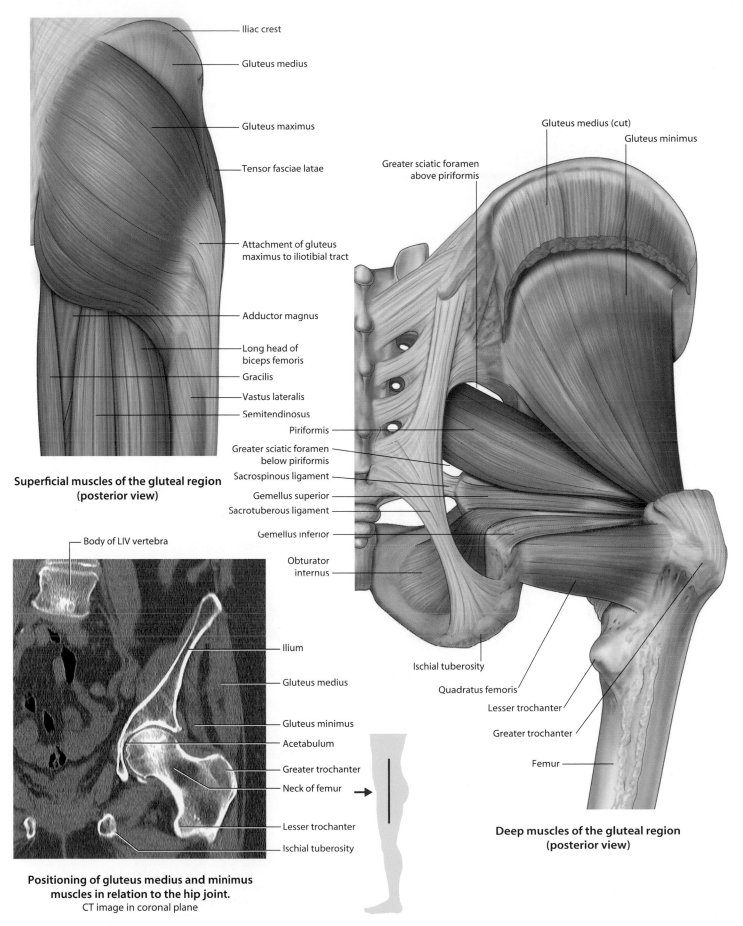

Iliac crest

Gluteus medius

Gluteus maximus

Tensor fasciae latae

Attachment of gluteus maximus to iliotibial tract

Adductor magnus

Long head of biceps femoris

Gracilis

Vastus lateralis

Semitendinosus

Superficial muscles of the gluteal region (posterior view)

Gluteus medius (cut)

Gluteus minimus

Greater sciatic foramen above piriformis

Piriformis

Greater sciatic foramen below piriformis

Sacrospinous ligament

Gemellus superior

Sacrotuberous ligament

Gemellus inferior

Obturator internus

Ischial tuberosity

Quadratus femoris

Lesser trochanter

Greater trochanter

Femur

Deep muscles of the gluteal region (posterior view)

Body of LIV vertebra

Ilium

Gluteus medius

Gluteus minimus

Acetabulum

Greater trochanter

Neck of femur

Lesser trochanter

Ischial tuberosity

Positioning of gluteus medius and minimus muscles in relation to the hip joint.
CT image in coronal plane

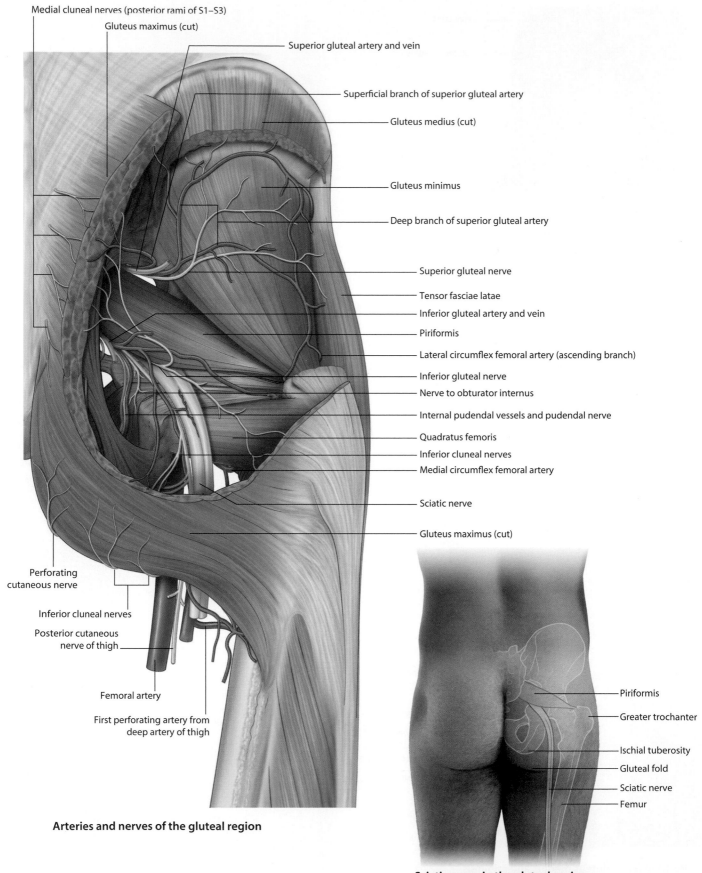

Medial cluneal nerves (posterior rami of S1–S3)

Gluteus maximus (cut)

Superior gluteal artery and vein

Superficial branch of superior gluteal artery

Gluteus medius (cut)

Gluteus minimus

Deep branch of superior gluteal artery

Superior gluteal nerve

Tensor fasciae latae

Inferior gluteal artery and vein

Piriformis

Lateral circumflex femoral artery (ascending branch)

Inferior gluteal nerve

Nerve to obturator internus

Internal pudendal vessels and pudendal nerve

Quadratus femoris

Inferior cluneal nerves

Medial circumflex femoral artery

Sciatic nerve

Gluteus maximus (cut)

Perforating cutaneous nerve

Inferior cluneal nerves

Posterior cutaneous nerve of thigh

Femoral artery

First perforating artery from deep artery of thigh

Arteries and nerves of the gluteal region

Piriformis

Greater trochanter

Ischial tuberosity

Gluteal fold

Sciatic nerve

Femur

Sciatic nerve in the gluteal region as it relates to the surface (posterior view)

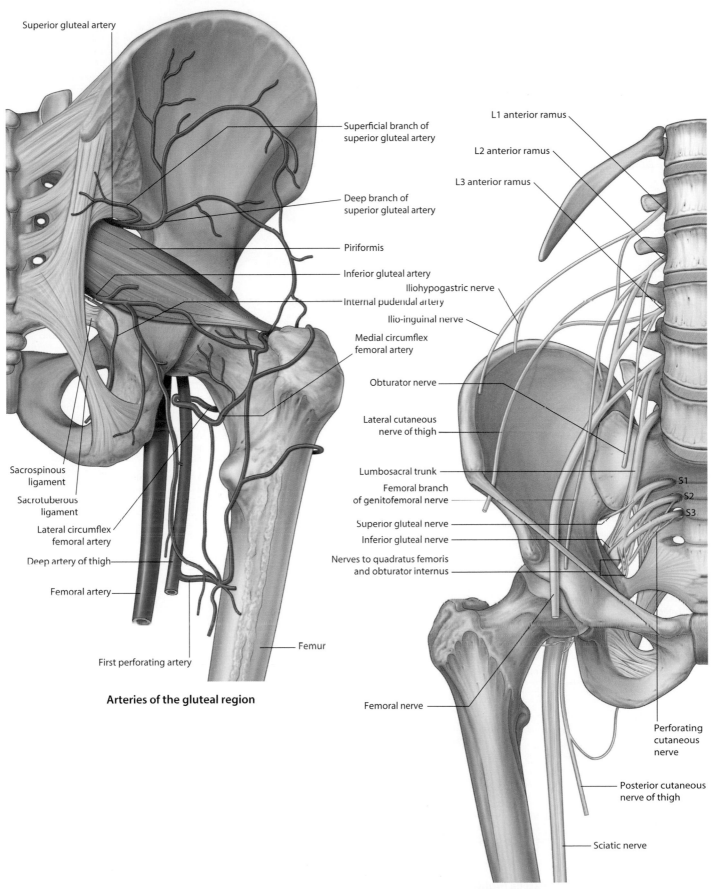

Superior gluteal artery

Superficial branch of
superior gluteal artery

Deep branch of
superior gluteal artery

Piriformis

Inferior gluteal artery

Internal pudendal artery

Medial circumflex
femoral artery

Sacrospinous
ligament

Sacrotuberous
ligament

Lateral circumflex
femoral artery

Deep artery of thigh

Femoral artery

First perforating artery

Femur

Arteries of the gluteal region

L1 anterior ramus

L2 anterior ramus

L3 anterior ramus

Iliohypogastric nerve

Ilio-inguinal nerve

Obturator nerve

Lateral cutaneous
nerve of thigh

Lumbosacral trunk

Femoral branch
of genitofemoral nerve

Superior gluteal nerve

Inferior gluteal nerve

Nerves to quadratus femoris
and obturator internus

Femoral nerve

S1

S2

S3

Perforating
cutaneous
nerve

Posterior cutaneous
nerve of thigh

Sciatic nerve

Branches of the lumbosacral plexus related to lower limb

305

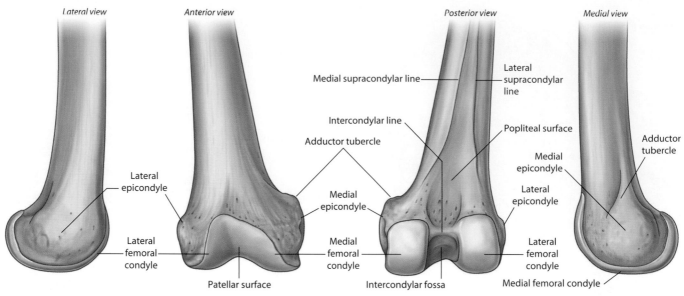

Lateral view

Anterior view

Posterior view

Medial view

Medial supracondylar line

Lateral supracondylar line

Intercondylar line

Popliteal surface

Adductor tubercle

Lateral epicondyle

Adductor tubercle

Medial epicondyle

Lateral femoral condyle

Lateral epicondyle

Medial epicondyle

Lateral femoral condyle

Medial femoral condyle

Lateral femoral condyle

Patellar surface

Medial femoral condyle

Intercondylar fossa

Medial femoral condyle

Distal end of (right) femur

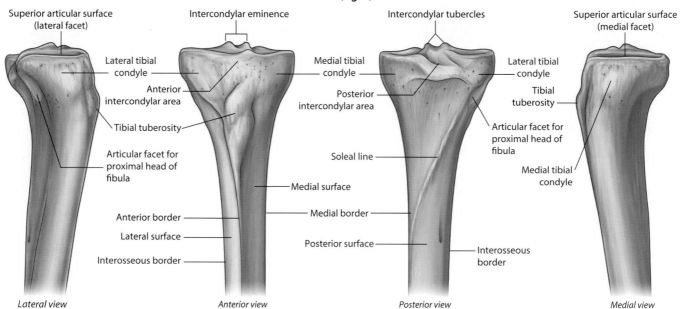

Superior articular surface (lateral facet)

Intercondylar eminence

Intercondylar tubercles

Superior articular surface (medial facet)

Lateral tibial condyle

Medial tibial condyle

Lateral tibial condyle

Anterior intercondylar area

Posterior intercondylar area

Tibial tuberosity

Tibial tuberosity

Articular facet for proximal head of fibula

Articular facet for proximal head of fibula

Soleal line

Medial tibial condyle

Medial surface

Anterior border

Medial border

Lateral surface

Posterior surface

Interosseous border

Interosseous border

Lateral view

Anterior view

Posterior view

Medial view

Proximal end of (right) tibia

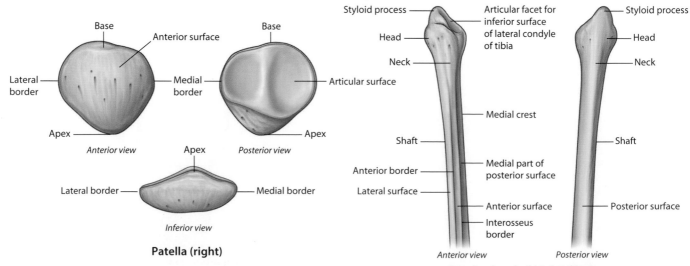

Base

Anterior surface

Base

Styloid process

Articular facet for inferior surface of lateral condyle of tibia

Styloid process

Lateral border

Medial border

Medial border

Head

Head

Apex

Articular surface

Neck

Neck

Apex

Anterior view

Posterior view

Apex

Medial crest

Lateral border

Medial border

Shaft

Shaft

Inferior view

Anterior border

Medial part of posterior surface

Patella (right)

Lateral surface

Anterior surface

Posterior surface

Interosseus border

Anterior view

Posterior view

Proximal end of (right) fibula

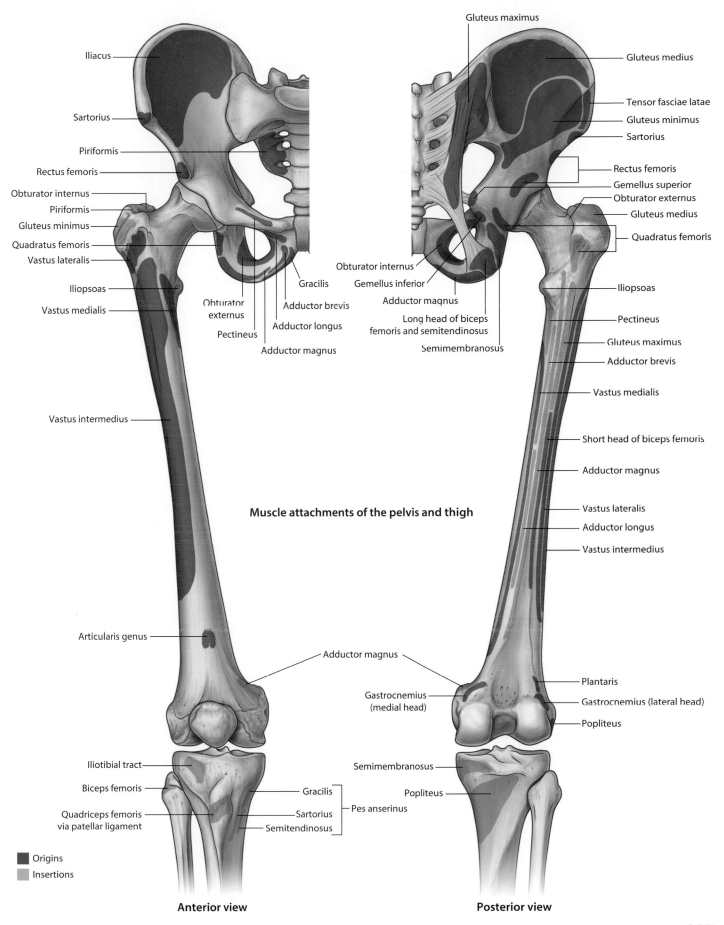

Iliacus

Sartorius

Piriformis

Rectus femoris

Obturator internus
Piriformis
Gluteus minimus
Quadratus femoris
Vastus lateralis

Iliopsoas

Vastus medialis

Obturator externus

Pectineus

Gracilis

Adductor brevis

Adductor longus

Adductor magnus

Vastus intermedius

Gluteus maximus

Gluteus medius

Tensor fasciae latae
Gluteus minimus
Sartorius

Rectus femoris
Gemellus superior
Obturator externus
Gluteus medius

Quadratus femoris

Obturator internus
Gemellus inferior
Adductor magnus

Long head of biceps
femoris and semitendinosus

Semimembranosus

Iliopsoas

Pectineus

Gluteus maximus

Adductor brevis

Vastus medialis

Short head of biceps femoris

Adductor magnus

Vastus lateralis
Adductor longus
Vastus intermedius

Muscle attachments of the pelvis and thigh

Articularis genus

Adductor magnus

Iliotibial tract

Biceps femoris

Quadriceps femoris
via patellar ligament

Gracilis

Sartorius

Semitendinosus

Pes anserinus

Gastrocnemius
(medial head)

Semimembranosus

Popliteus

Plantaris

Gastrocnemius (lateral head)

Popliteus

■ Origins
■ Insertions

Anterior view

Posterior view

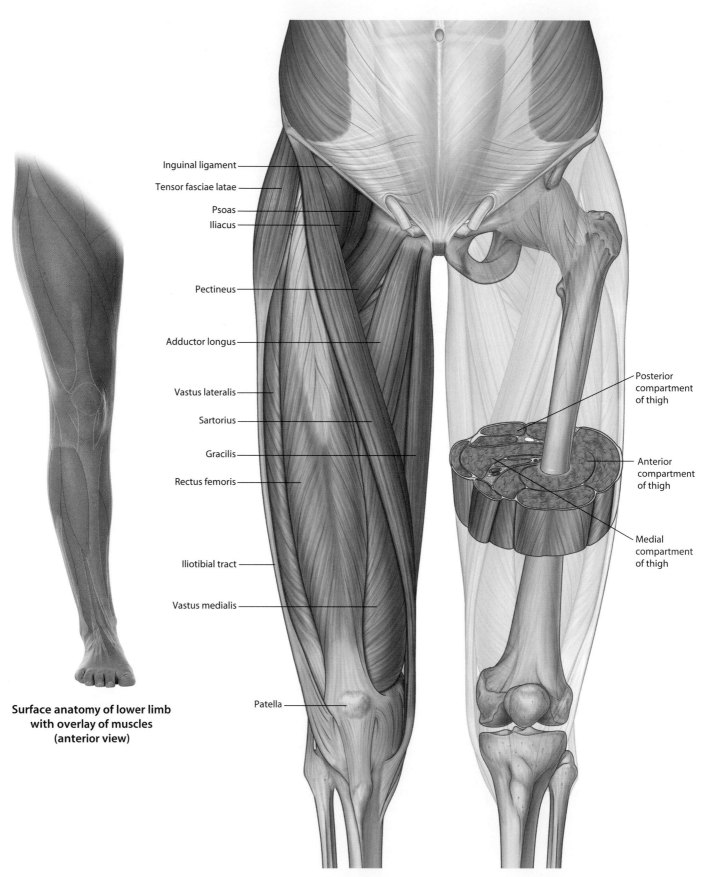

Inguinal ligament

Tensor fasciae latae

Psoas

Iliacus

Pectineus

Adductor longus

Vastus lateralis

Sartorius

Gracilis

Rectus femoris

Iliotibial tract

Vastus medialis

Patella

Posterior compartment of thigh

Anterior compartment of thigh

Medial compartment of thigh

Surface anatomy of lower limb with overlay of muscles (anterior view)

Superficial muscles of the thigh (anterior view)

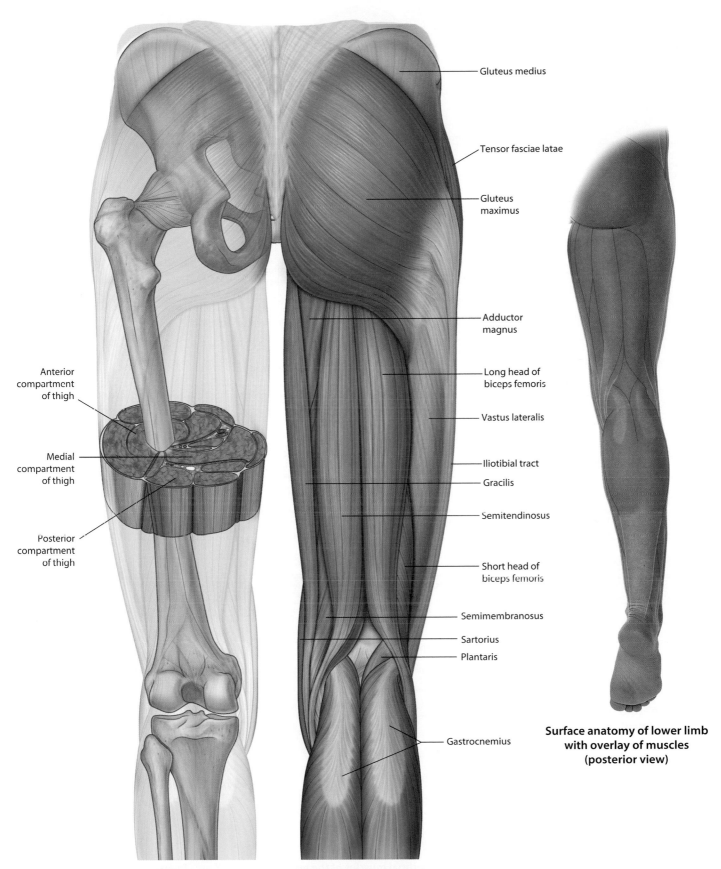

Gluteus medius

Tensor fasciae latae

Gluteus maximus

Adductor magnus

Long head of biceps femoris

Vastus lateralis

Iliotibial tract

Gracilis

Semitendinosus

Short head of biceps femoris

Semimembranosus

Sartorius

Plantaris

Gastrocnemius

Anterior compartment of thigh

Medial compartment of thigh

Posterior compartment of thigh

Superficial muscles of the thigh (posterior view)

Surface anatomy of lower limb with overlay of muscles (posterior view)

309

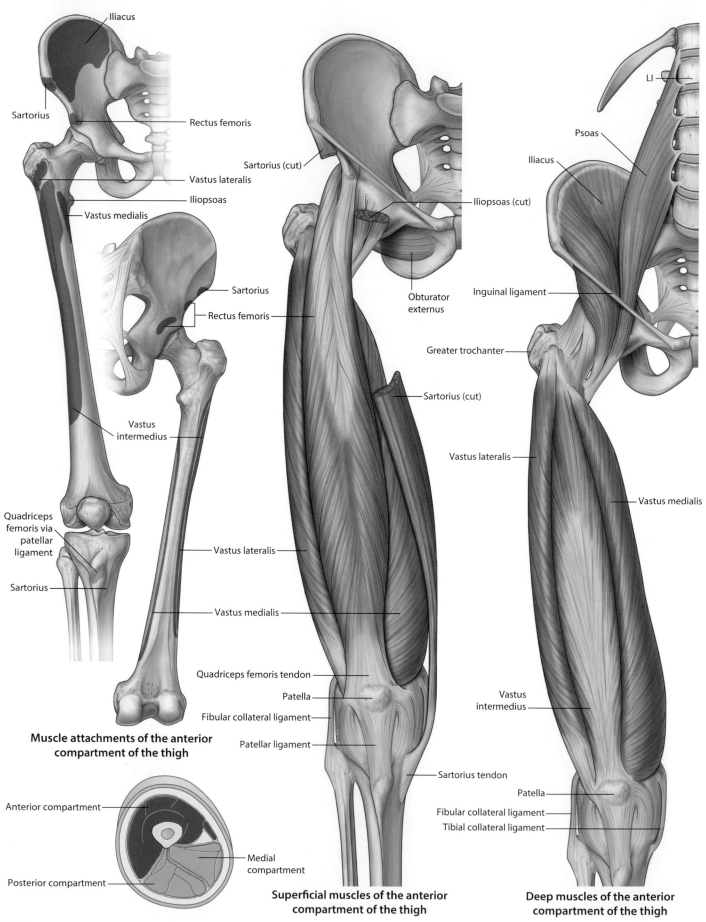

Iliacus

Sartorius

Rectus femoris

Vastus lateralis

Iliopsoas

Vastus medialis

Sartorius

Rectus femoris

Vastus intermedius

Quadriceps femoris via patellar ligament

Sartorius

Muscle attachments of the anterior compartment of the thigh

Anterior compartment

Posterior compartment

Medial compartment

Sartorius (cut)

Iliopsoas (cut)

Obturator externus

Sartorius (cut)

Vastus lateralis

Vastus medialis

Quadriceps femoris tendon

Patella

Fibular collateral ligament

Patellar ligament

Sartorius tendon

Superficial muscles of the anterior compartment of the thigh

LI

Psoas

Iliacus

Inguinal ligament

Greater trochanter

Vastus lateralis

Vastus medialis

Vastus intermedius

Patella

Fibular collateral ligament

Tibial collateral ligament

Deep muscles of the anterior compartment of the thigh

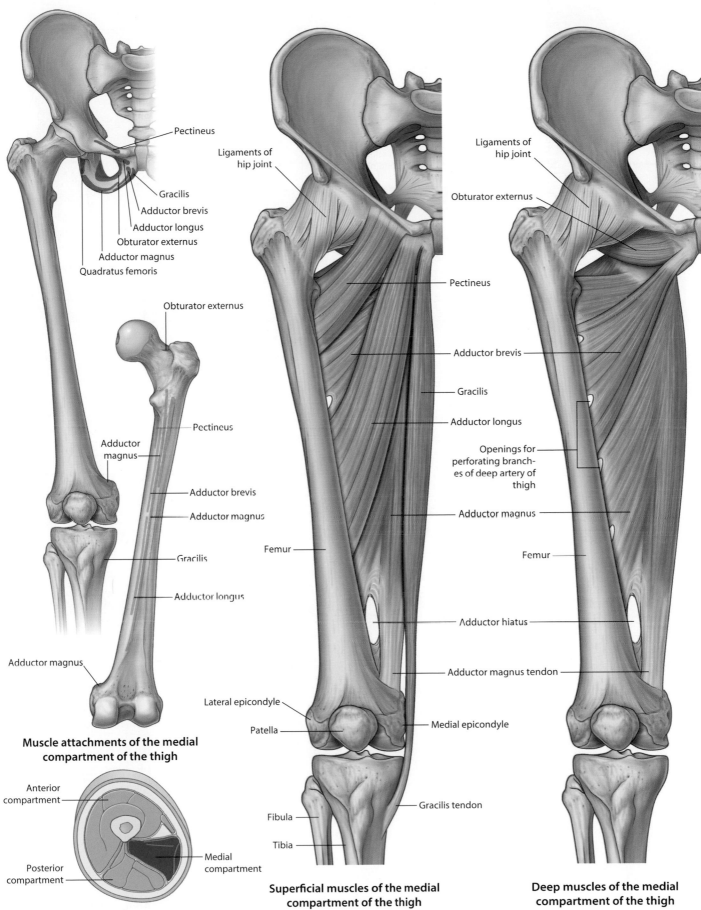

Pectineus

Ligaments of
hip joint

Gracilis

Adductor brevis

Adductor longus

Obturator externus

Adductor magnus

Quadratus femoris

Obturator externus

Pectineus

Adductor
magnus

Adductor brevis

Adductor magnus

Gracilis

Adductor longus

Adductor magnus

**Muscle attachments of the medial
compartment of the thigh**

Anterior
compartment

Posterior
compartment

Medial
compartment

Ligaments of
hip joint

Obturator externus

Pectineus

Adductor brevis

Gracilis

Adductor longus

Openings for
perforating branch-
es of deep artery of
thigh

Adductor magnus

Femur

Adductor hiatus

Adductor magnus tendon

Lateral epicondyle

Patella

Medial epicondyle

Femur

Gracilis tendon

Fibula

Tibia

**Superficial muscles of the medial
compartment of the thigh**

**Deep muscles of the medial
compartment of the thigh**

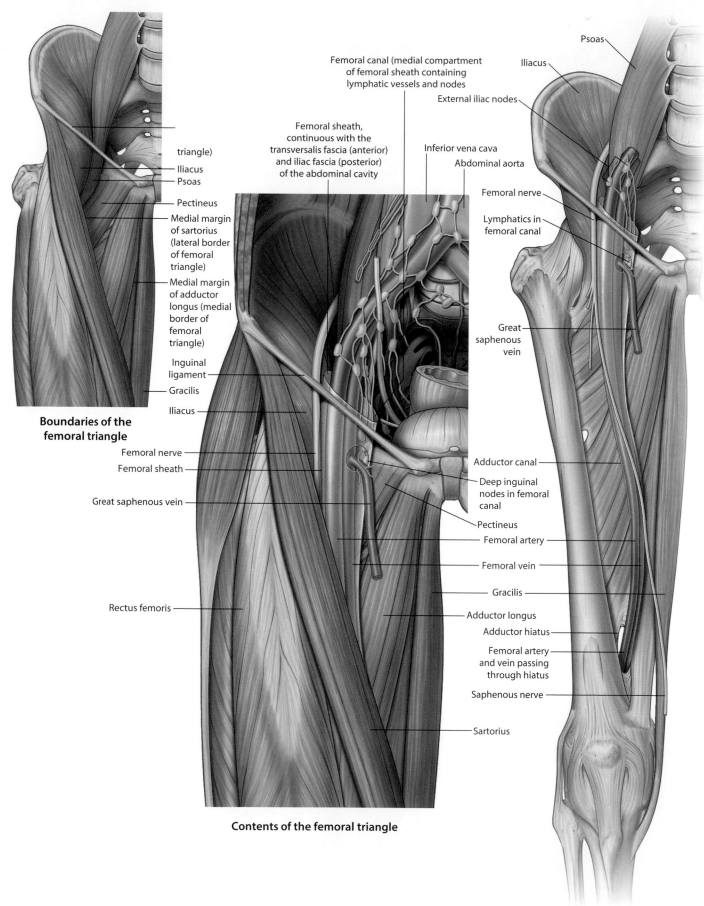

triangle)

Iliacus

Psoas

Pectineus

Medial margin
of sartorius
(lateral border
of femoral
triangle)

Medial margin
of adductor
longus (medial
border of
femoral
triangle)

Inguinal
ligament

Gracilis

Iliacus

**Boundaries of the
femoral triangle**

Femoral nerve

Femoral sheath

Great saphenous vein

Rectus femoris

Femoral canal (medial compartment
of femoral sheath containing
lymphatic vessels and nodes

Femoral sheath,
continuous with the
transversalis fascia (anterior)
and iliac fascia (posterior)
of the abdominal cavity

Inferior vena cava

Abdominal aorta

Contents of the femoral triangle

Psoas

Iliacus

External iliac nodes

Femoral nerve

Lymphatics in
femoral canal

Great
saphenous
vein

Adductor canal

Deep inguinal
nodes in femoral
canal

Pectineus

Femoral artery

Femoral vein

Gracilis

Adductor longus

Adductor hiatus

Femoral artery
and vein passing
through hiatus

Saphenous nerve

Sartorius

Adductor canal

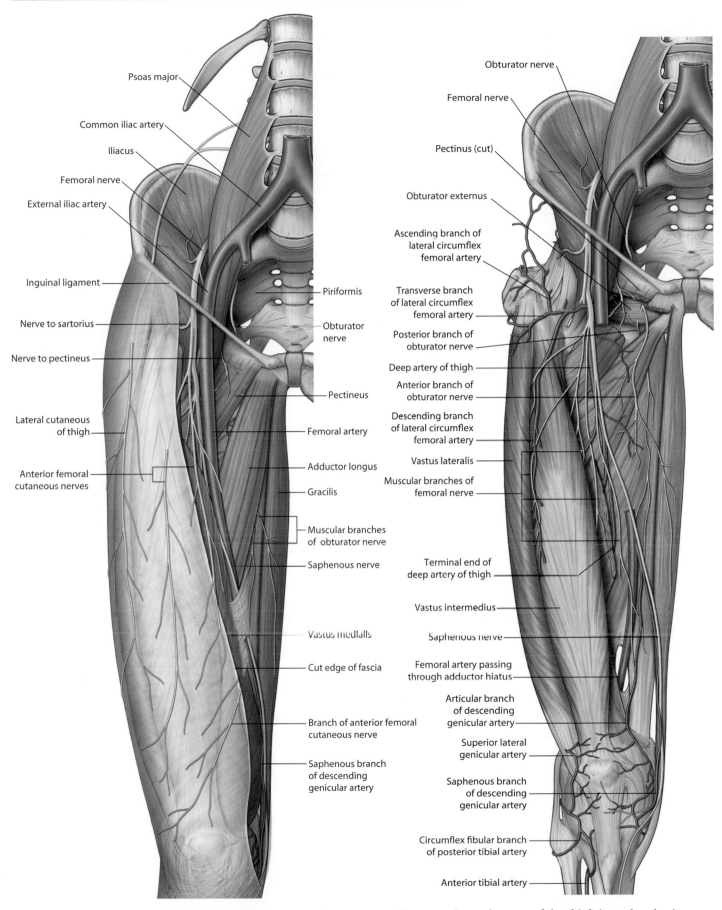

Psoas major

Common iliac artery

Iliacus

Femoral nerve

External iliac artery

Inguinal ligament

Nerve to sartorius

Nerve to pectineus

Lateral cutaneous of thigh

Anterior femoral cutaneous nerves

Piriformis

Obturator nerve

Pectineus

Femoral artery

Adductor longus

Gracilis

Muscular branches of obturator nerve

Saphenous nerve

Vastus medialis

Cut edge of fascia

Branch of anterior femoral cutaneous nerve

Saphenous branch of descending genicular artery

Obturator nerve

Femoral nerve

Pectinus (cut)

Obturator externus

Ascending branch of lateral circumflex femoral artery

Transverse branch of lateral circumflex femoral artery

Posterior branch of obturator nerve

Deep artery of thigh

Anterior branch of obturator nerve

Descending branch of lateral circumflex femoral artery

Vastus lateralis

Muscular branches of femoral nerve

Terminal end of deep artery of thigh

Vastus intermedius

Saphenous nerve

Femoral artery passing through adductor hiatus

Articular branch of descending genicular artery

Superior lateral genicular artery

Saphenous branch of descending genicular artery

Circumflex fibular branch of posterior tibial artery

Anterior tibial artery

Superficial arteries and nerves of the thigh (anterior view)

Deep arteries and nerves of the thigh (anterior view)

313

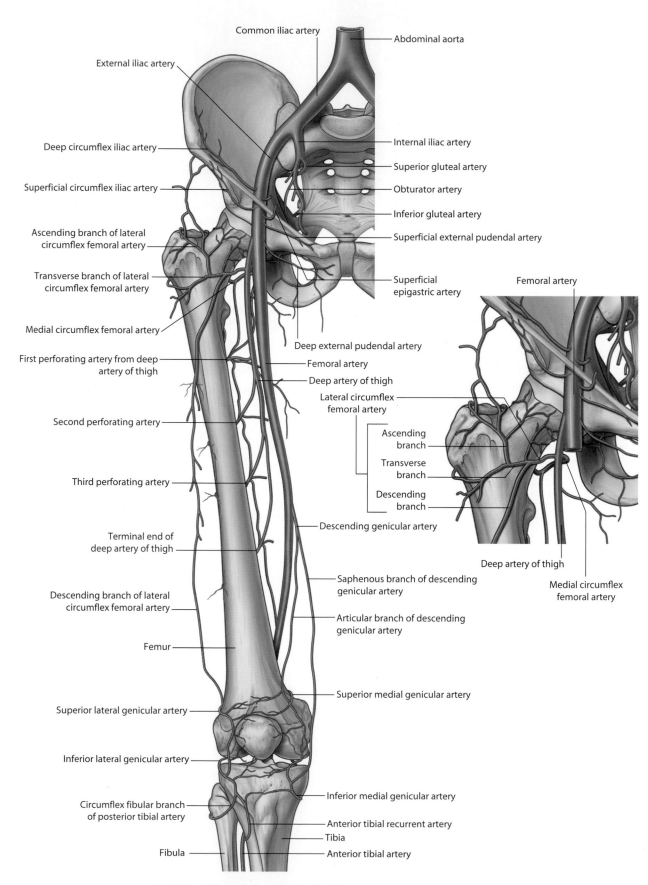

Common iliac artery

Abdominal aorta

External iliac artery

Deep circumflex iliac artery

Internal iliac artery

Superior gluteal artery

Superficial circumflex iliac artery

Obturator artery

Inferior gluteal artery

Ascending branch of lateral circumflex femoral artery

Superficial external pudendal artery

Transverse branch of lateral circumflex femoral artery

Superficial epigastric artery

Medial circumflex femoral artery

Femoral artery

First perforating artery from deep artery of thigh

Deep external pudendal artery

Femoral artery

Second perforating artery

Deep artery of thigh

Lateral circumflex femoral artery

Ascending branch

Transverse branch

Third perforating artery

Descending branch

Terminal end of deep artery of thigh

Descending genicular artery

Deep artery of thigh

Descending branch of lateral circumflex femoral artery

Saphenous branch of descending genicular artery

Medial circumflex femoral artery

Femur

Articular branch of descending genicular artery

Superior medial genicular artery

Superior lateral genicular artery

Inferior lateral genicular artery

Inferior medial genicular artery

Circumflex fibular branch of posterior tibial artery

Anterior tibial recurrent artery

Tibia

Fibula

Anterior tibial artery

Arteries of the thigh (anterior view)

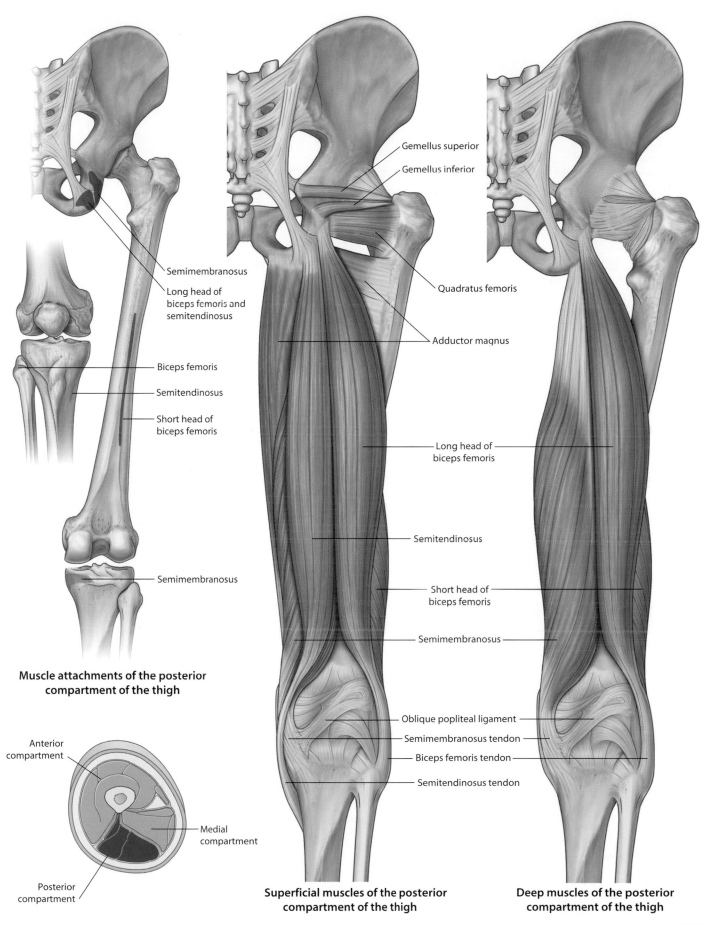

Semimembranosus

Long head of
biceps femoris and
semitendinosus

Biceps femoris

Semitendinosus

Short head of
biceps femoris

Semimembranosus

**Muscle attachments of the posterior
compartment of the thigh**

Anterior
compartment

Medial
compartment

Posterior
compartment

Gemellus superior

Gemellus inferior

Quadratus femoris

Adductor magnus

Long head of
biceps femoris

Semitendinosus

Short head of
biceps femoris

Semimembranosus

Oblique popliteal ligament

Semimembranosus tendon

Biceps femoris tendon

Semitendinosus tendon

**Superficial muscles of the posterior
compartment of the thigh**

**Deep muscles of the posterior
compartment of the thigh**

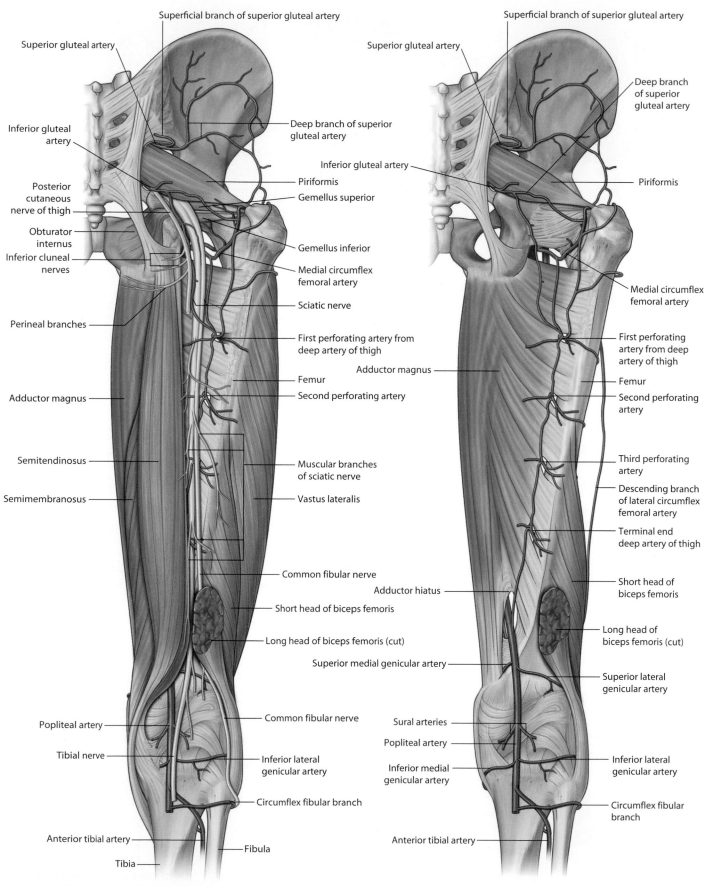

Superficial branch of superior gluteal artery

Superior gluteal artery

Inferior gluteal artery

Posterior cutaneous nerve of thigh

Obturator internus

Inferior cluneal nerves

Perineal branches

Adductor magnus

Semitendinosus

Semimembranosus

Popliteal artery

Tibial nerve

Anterior tibial artery

Tibia

Deep branch of superior gluteal artery

Piriformis

Gemellus superior

Gemellus inferior

Medial circumflex femoral artery

Sciatic nerve

First perforating artery from deep artery of thigh

Femur

Second perforating artery

Muscular branches of sciatic nerve

Vastus lateralis

Common fibular nerve

Short head of biceps femoris

Long head of biceps femoris (cut)

Superior medial genicular artery

Common fibular nerve

Inferior lateral genicular artery

Circumflex fibular branch

Fibula

Arteries and nerves of the thigh (posterior view)

Superficial branch of superior gluteal artery

Superior gluteal artery

Inferior gluteal artery

Deep branch of superior gluteal artery

Piriformis

Medial circumflex femoral artery

First perforating artery from deep artery of thigh

Femur

Second perforating artery

Third perforating artery

Descending branch of lateral circumflex femoral artery

Terminal end deep artery of thigh

Short head of biceps femoris

Adductor hiatus

Adductor magnus

Long head of biceps femoris (cut)

Superior lateral genicular artery

Sural arteries

Popliteal artery

Inferior medial genicular artery

Inferior lateral genicular artery

Circumflex fibular branch

Anterior tibial artery

Deep arteries of the thigh (posterior view)

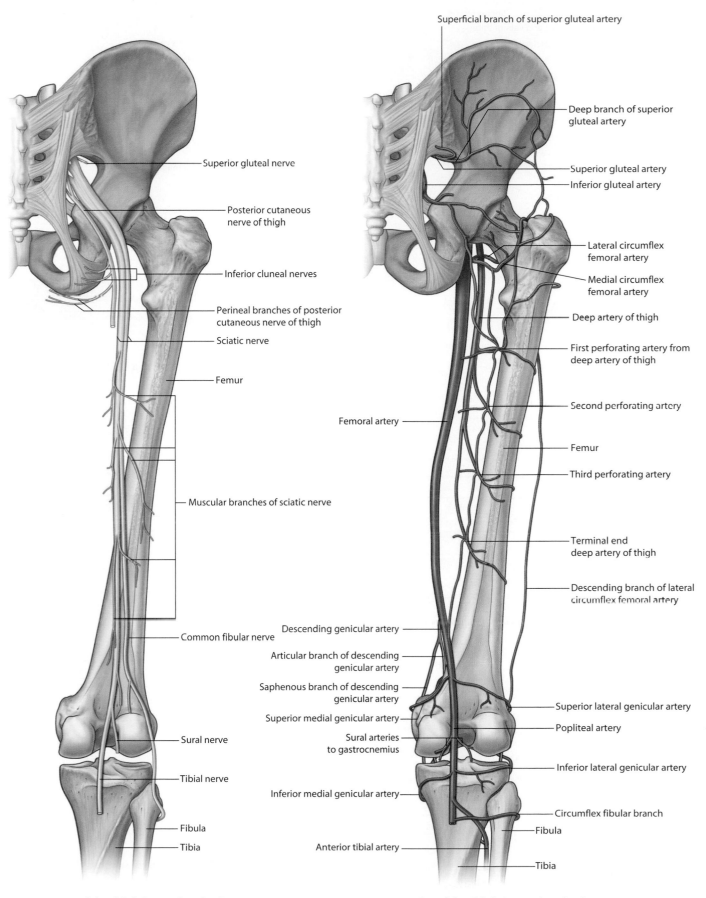

Superficial branch of superior gluteal artery

Deep branch of superior gluteal artery

Superior gluteal nerve

Posterior cutaneous nerve of thigh

Superior gluteal artery

Inferior gluteal artery

Lateral circumflex femoral artery

Inferior cluneal nerves

Medial circumflex femoral artery

Perineal branches of posterior cutaneous nerve of thigh

Deep artery of thigh

Sciatic nerve

First perforating artery from deep artery of thigh

Femur

Second perforating artery

Femoral artery

Femur

Third perforating artery

Muscular branches of sciatic nerve

Terminal end deep artery of thigh

Descending branch of lateral circumflex femoral artery

Common fibular nerve

Descending genicular artery

Articular branch of descending genicular artery

Saphenous branch of descending genicular artery

Superior medial genicular artery

Superior lateral genicular artery

Popliteal artery

Sural nerve

Sural arteries to gastrocnemius

Tibial nerve

Inferior lateral genicular artery

Inferior medial genicular artery

Circumflex fibular branch

Fibula

Fibula

Tibia

Anterior tibial artery

Tibia

Nerves of the thigh (posterior view)

Arteries of the thigh (posterior view)

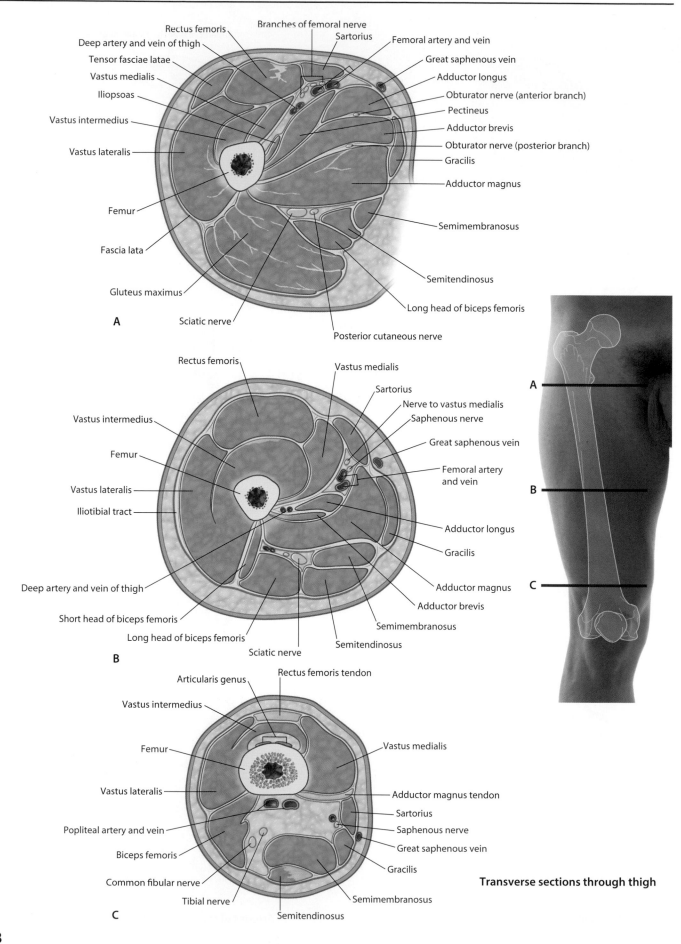

A

Rectus femoris
Deep artery and vein of thigh
Tensor fasciae latae
Vastus medialis
Iliopsoas
Vastus intermedius
Vastus lateralis
Femur
Fascia lata
Gluteus maximus
Sciatic nerve

Branches of femoral nerve
Sartorius
Femoral artery and vein
Great saphenous vein
Adductor longus
Obturator nerve (anterior branch)
Pectineus
Adductor brevis
Obturator nerve (posterior branch)
Gracilis
Adductor magnus
Semimembranosus
Semitendinosus
Long head of biceps femoris
Posterior cutaneous nerve

B

Rectus femoris
Vastus intermedius
Femur
Vastus lateralis
Iliotibial tract
Deep artery and vein of thigh
Short head of biceps femoris
Long head of biceps femoris
Sciatic nerve

Vastus medialis
Sartorius
Nerve to vastus medialis
Saphenous nerve
Great saphenous vein
Femoral artery and vein
Adductor longus
Gracilis
Adductor magnus
Adductor brevis
Semimembranosus
Semitendinosus

C

Articularis genus
Vastus intermedius
Femur
Vastus lateralis
Popliteal artery and vein
Biceps femoris
Common fibular nerve
Tibial nerve
Semitendinosus

Rectus femoris tendon
Vastus medialis
Adductor magnus tendon
Sartorius
Saphenous nerve
Great saphenous vein
Gracilis
Semimembranosus

A
B
C

Transverse sections through thigh

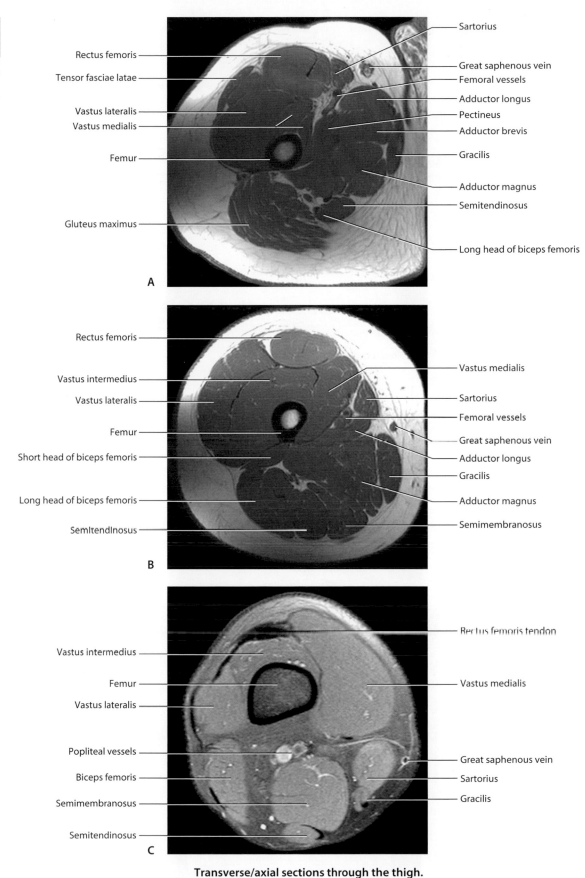

Rectus femoris
Tensor fasciae latae
Vastus lateralis
Vastus medialis
Femur
Gluteus maximus

Sartorius
Great saphenous vein
Femoral vessels
Adductor longus
Pectineus
Adductor brevis
Gracilis
Adductor magnus
Semitendinosus
Long head of biceps femoris

A

Rectus femoris
Vastus intermedius
Vastus lateralis
Femur
Short head of biceps femoris
Long head of biceps femoris
Semltendlnosus

Vastus medialis
Sartorius
Femoral vessels
Great saphenous vein
Adductor longus
Gracilis
Adductor magnus
Semimembranosus

B

Vastus intermedius
Femur
Vastus lateralis
Popliteal vessels
Biceps femoris
Semimembranosus
Semitendinosus

Rectus femoris tendon
Vastus medialis
Great saphenous vein
Sartorius
Gracilis

C

Transverse/axial sections through the thigh.
A. Proximal/upper thigh. T1-weighted MR image in axial plane
B. Middle thigh. T1-weighted MR image in axial plane
C. Distal/lower thigh. T2-weighted MR image in axial plane

319

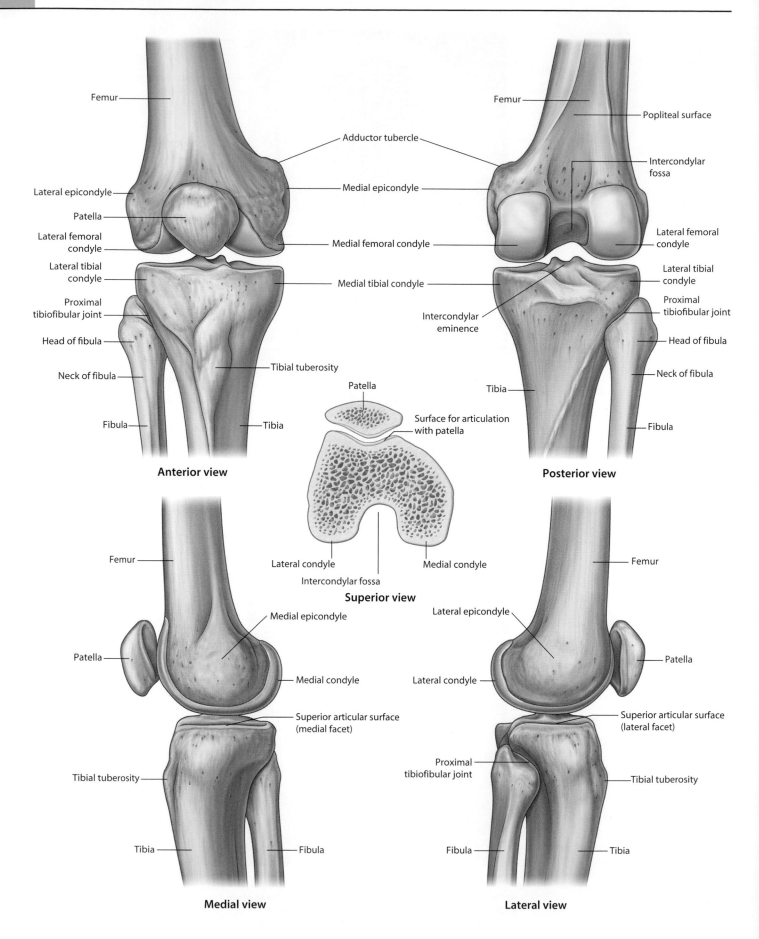

Femur

Adductor tubercle

Medial epicondyle

Lateral epicondyle

Patella

Lateral femoral condyle

Medial femoral condyle

Lateral tibial condyle

Medial tibial condyle

Proximal tibiofibular joint

Head of fibula

Neck of fibula

Tibial tuberosity

Fibula

Tibia

Anterior view

Femur

Popliteal surface

Intercondylar fossa

Lateral femoral condyle

Lateral tibial condyle

Intercondylar eminence

Proximal tibiofibular joint

Head of fibula

Tibia

Neck of fibula

Fibula

Posterior view

Patella

Surface for articulation with patella

Lateral condyle

Medial condyle

Intercondylar fossa

Superior view

Femur

Medial epicondyle

Patella

Medial condyle

Superior articular surface (medial facet)

Tibial tuberosity

Tibia

Fibula

Medial view

Femur

Lateral epicondyle

Lateral condyle

Patella

Superior articular surface (lateral facet)

Proximal tibiofibular joint

Tibial tuberosity

Fibula

Tibia

Lateral view

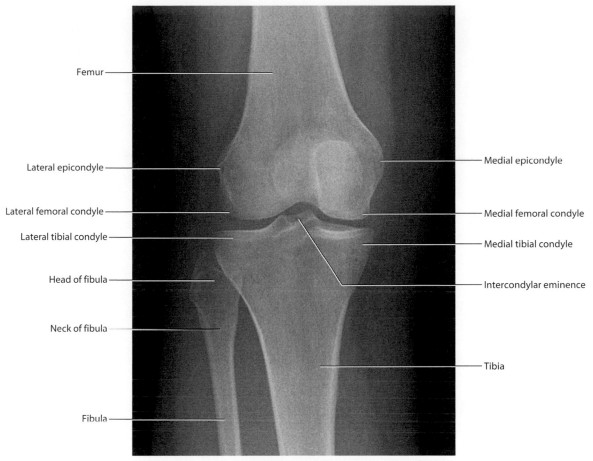

Femur

Lateral epicondyle

Lateral femoral condyle

Lateral tibial condyle

Head of fibula

Neck of fibula

Fibula

Medial epicondyle

Medial femoral condyle

Medial tibial condyle

Intercondylar eminence

Tibia

Normal knee joint.
Radiograph, AP view

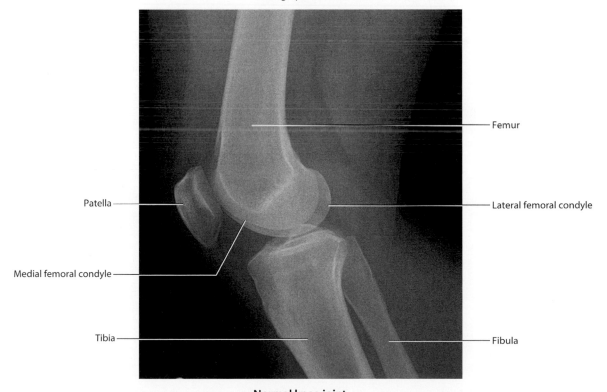

Patella

Medial femoral condyle

Tibia

Femur

Lateral femoral condyle

Fibula

Normal knee joint.
Radiograph, lateral view

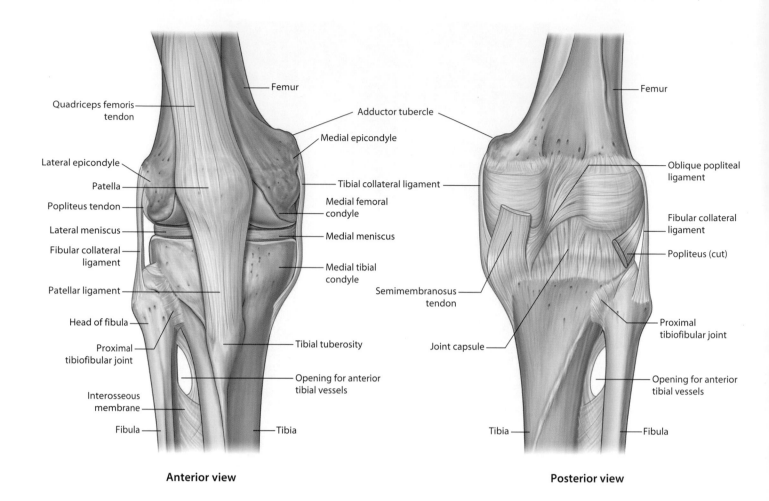

Quadriceps femoris tendon

Lateral epicondyle

Patella

Popliteus tendon

Lateral meniscus

Fibular collateral ligament

Patellar ligament

Head of fibula

Proximal tibiofibular joint

Interosseous membrane

Fibula

Femur

Adductor tubercle

Medial epicondyle

Tibial collateral ligament

Medial femoral condyle

Medial meniscus

Medial tibial condyle

Tibial tuberosity

Opening for anterior tibial vessels

Tibia

Anterior view

Femur

Adductor tubercle

Medial epicondyle

Oblique popliteal ligament

Tibial collateral ligament

Fibular collateral ligament

Popliteus (cut)

Semimembranosus tendon

Joint capsule

Proximal tibiofibular joint

Opening for anterior tibial vessels

Tibia

Fibula

Posterior view

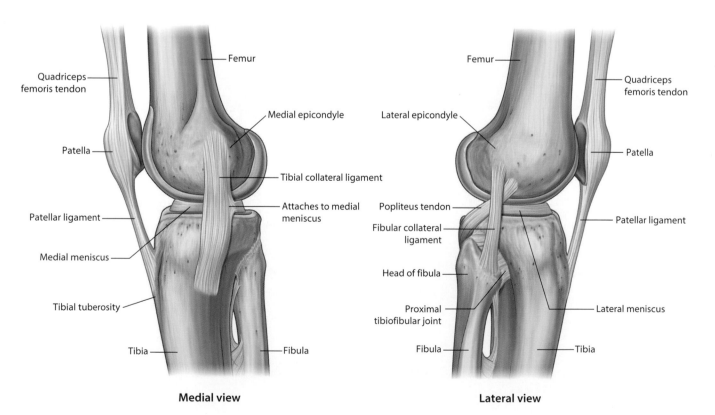

Quadriceps femoris tendon

Patella

Patellar ligament

Medial meniscus

Tibial tuberosity

Tibia

Femur

Medial epicondyle

Tibial collateral ligament

Attaches to medial meniscus

Fibula

Medial view

Femur

Lateral epicondyle

Popliteus tendon

Fibular collateral ligament

Head of fibula

Proximal tibiofibular joint

Fibula

Quadriceps femoris tendon

Patella

Patellar ligament

Lateral meniscus

Tibia

Lateral view

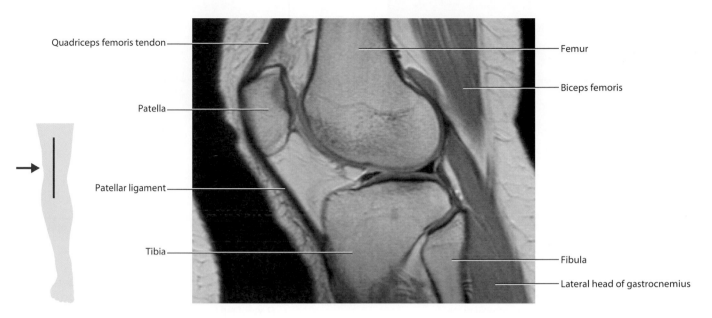

Quadriceps femoris tendon

Patella

Patellar ligament

Tibia

Femur

Biceps femoris

Fibula

Lateral head of gastrocnemius

Normal knee joint.
T2-weighted MR image in sagittal plane

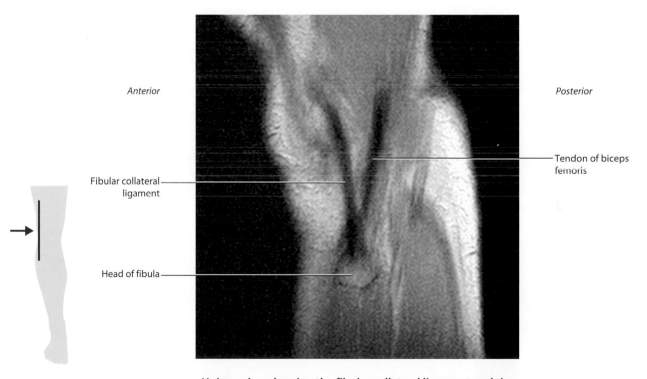

Anterior

Posterior

Fibular collateral ligament

Head of fibula

Tendon of biceps femoris

**Unique view showing the fibular collateral ligament and the
tendon of the biceps femoris muscle attaching to the head of the fibula.**
T2-weighted MR image in sagittal plane

323

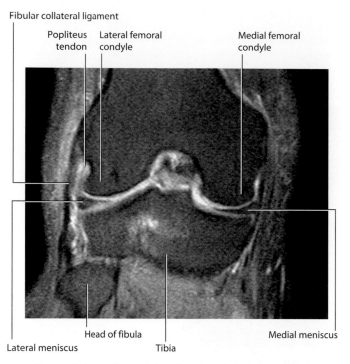

Fibular collateral ligament

Popliteus tendon

Lateral femoral condyle

Medial femoral condyle

Lateral meniscus

Head of fibula

Tibia

Medial meniscus

Coronal view of knee joint showing the fibular collateral ligament and its relationship to surrounding structures.
T2-weighted MR image in coronal plane

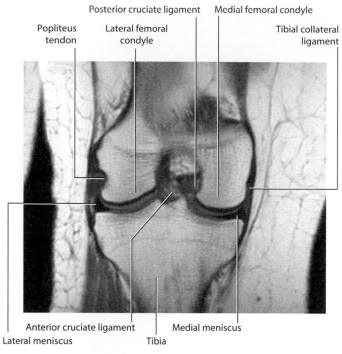

Popliteus tendon

Posterior cruciate ligament

Lateral femoral condyle

Medial femoral condyle

Tibial collateral ligament

Lateral meniscus

Anterior cruciate ligament

Medial meniscus

Tibia

Anterior view of knee joint showing the relationship between the tibial collateral ligament and the medial meniscus.
T1-weighted MR image in coronal plane

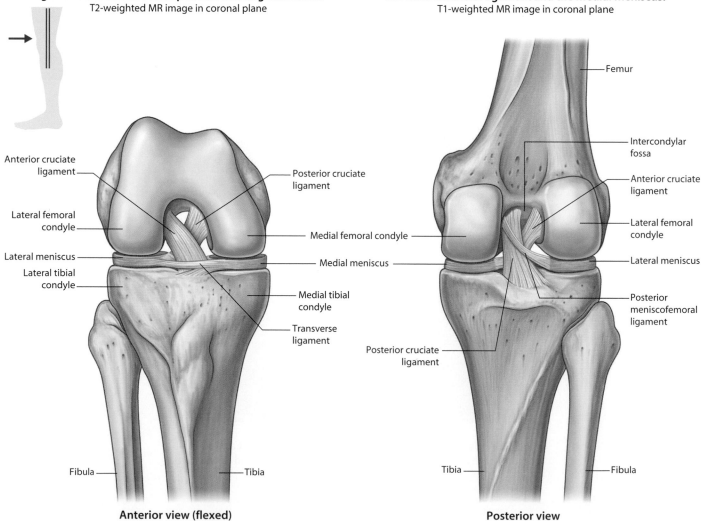

Anterior cruciate ligament

Posterior cruciate ligament

Lateral femoral condyle

Lateral meniscus

Medial femoral condyle

Lateral tibial condyle

Medial meniscus

Medial tibial condyle

Transverse ligament

Fibula

Tibia

Anterior view (flexed)

Femur

Intercondylar fossa

Anterior cruciate ligament

Lateral femoral condyle

Lateral meniscus

Posterior meniscofemoral ligament

Posterior cruciate ligament

Tibia

Fibula

Posterior view

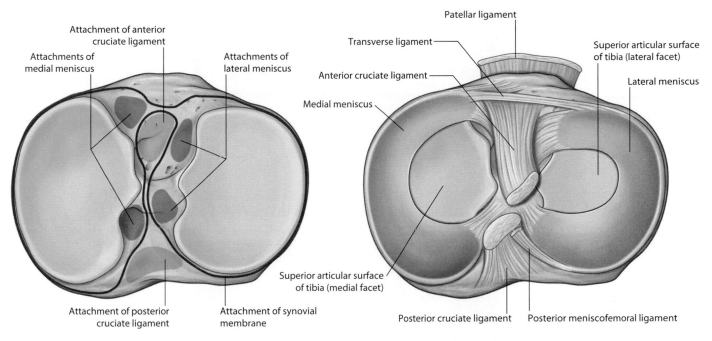

Attachments of menisci, cruciate ligaments, and synovial membrane of the right tibia.
(superior view)

Menisci of the right knee joint.
(superior view)

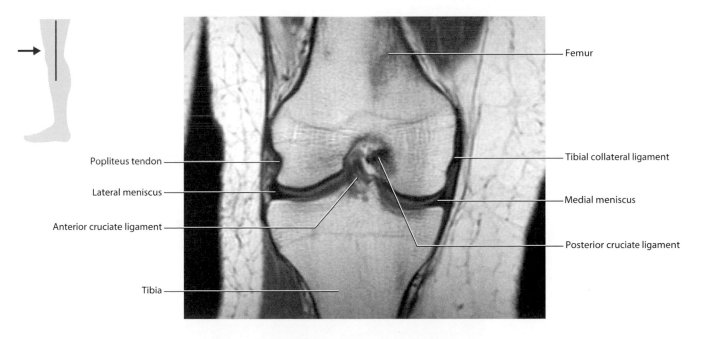

Anterior view of knee joint showing the anterior and posterior cruciate ligaments.
T2-weighted MR image in coronal plane

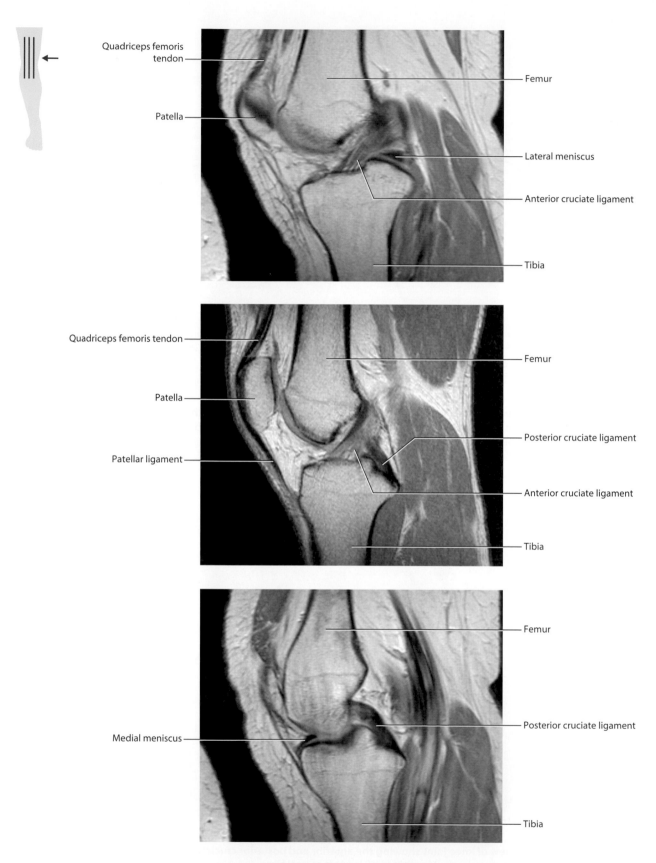

Quadriceps femoris tendon

Patella

Femur

Lateral meniscus

Anterior cruciate ligament

Tibia

Quadriceps femoris tendon

Patella

Patellar ligament

Femur

Posterior cruciate ligament

Anterior cruciate ligament

Tibia

Medial meniscus

Femur

Posterior cruciate ligament

Tibia

A series of images moving from lateral to medial showing the relationship between anterior and posterior cruciate ligaments.
T2-weighted MR images in sagittal plane

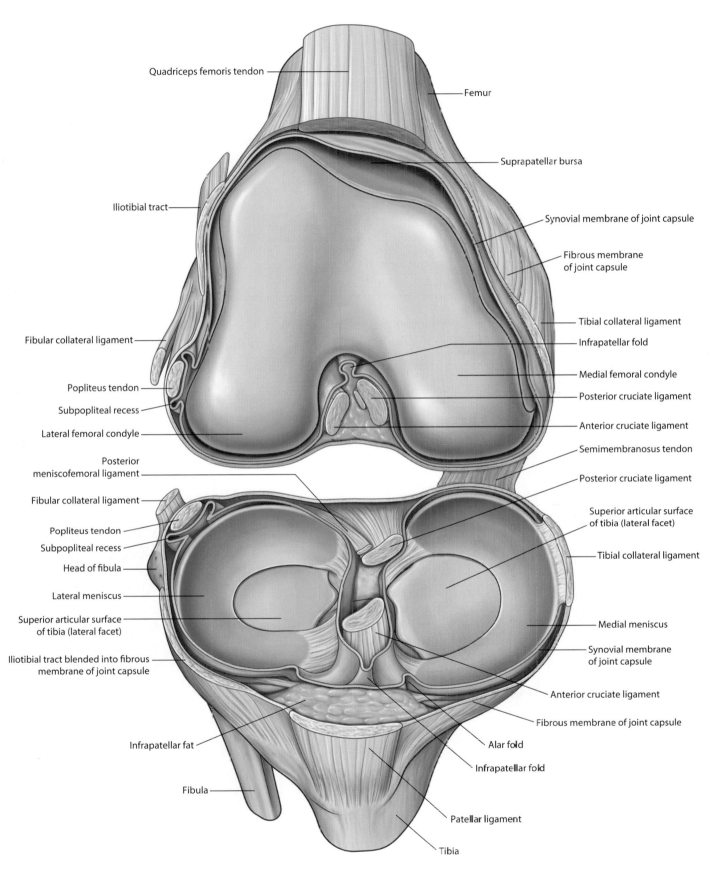

Quadriceps femoris tendon

Femur

Suprapatellar bursa

Iliotibial tract

Synovial membrane of joint capsule

Fibrous membrane of joint capsule

Tibial collateral ligament

Infrapatellar fold

Fibular collateral ligament

Medial femoral condyle

Popliteus tendon

Posterior cruciate ligament

Subpopliteal recess

Anterior cruciate ligament

Lateral femoral condyle

Semimembranosus tendon

Posterior meniscofemoral ligament

Posterior cruciate ligament

Fibular collateral ligament

Superior articular surface of tibia (lateral facet)

Popliteus tendon

Subpopliteal recess

Tibial collateral ligament

Head of fibula

Lateral meniscus

Medial meniscus

Superior articular surface of tibia (lateral facet)

Synovial membrane of joint capsule

Iliotibial tract blended into fibrous membrane of joint capsule

Anterior cruciate ligament

Fibrous membrane of joint capsule

Infrapatellar fat

Alar fold

Infrapatellar fold

Fibula

Patellar ligament

Tibia

Knee joint with patella removed (anterosuperior view)

327

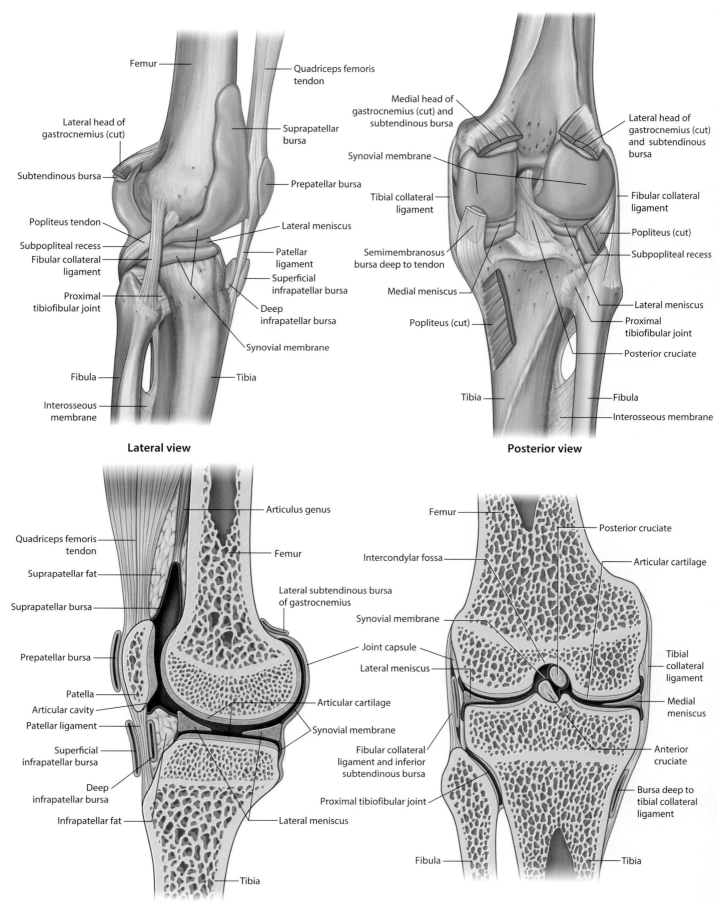

Femur

Quadriceps femoris tendon

Lateral head of gastrocnemius (cut)

Suprapatellar bursa

Subtendinous bursa

Prepatellar bursa

Popliteus tendon

Lateral meniscus

Subpopliteal recess

Fibular collateral ligament

Patellar ligament

Proximal tibiofibular joint

Superficial infrapatellar bursa

Deep infrapatellar bursa

Synovial membrane

Fibula

Tibia

Interosseous membrane

Lateral view

Medial head of gastrocnemius (cut) and subtendinous bursa

Synovial membrane

Lateral head of gastrocnemius (cut) and subtendinous bursa

Tibial collateral ligament

Fibular collateral ligament

Semimembranosus bursa deep to tendon

Popliteus (cut)

Subpopliteal recess

Medial meniscus

Lateral meniscus

Popliteus (cut)

Proximal tibiofibular joint

Posterior cruciate

Tibia

Fibula

Interosseous membrane

Posterior view

Articulus genus

Quadriceps femoris tendon

Suprapatellar fat

Femur

Suprapatellar bursa

Lateral subtendinous bursa of gastrocnemius

Prepatellar bursa

Patella

Articular cavity

Articular cartilage

Patellar ligament

Synovial membrane

Superficial infrapatellar bursa

Deep infrapatellar bursa

Infrapatellar fat

Lateral meniscus

Tibia

Paramedian section through knee joint

Femur

Posterior cruciate

Intercondylar fossa

Articular cartilage

Synovial membrane

Joint capsule

Tibial collateral ligament

Lateral meniscus

Medial meniscus

Fibular collateral ligament and inferior subtendinous bursa

Anterior cruciate

Proximal tibiofibular joint

Bursa deep to tibial collateral ligament

Fibula

Tibia

Coronal section through knee joint (anterior view)

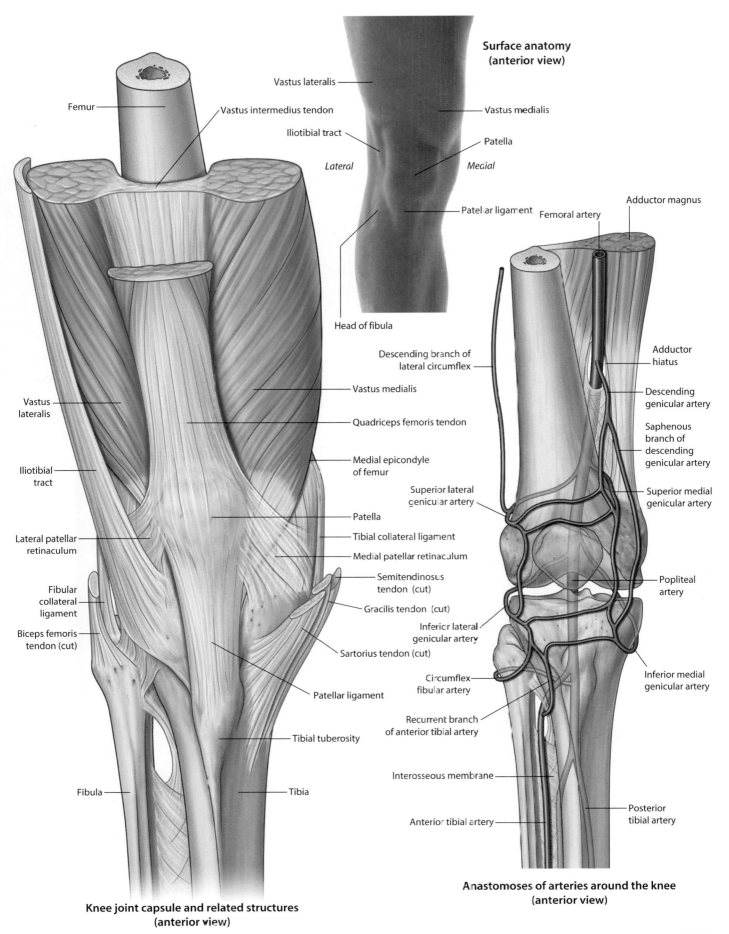

**Surface anatomy
(anterior view)**

Vastus lateralis

Iliotibial tract

Lateral

Vastus medialis

Patella

Medial

Patellar ligament

Head of fibula

Femur

Vastus intermedius tendon

Vastus lateralis

Iliotibial tract

Lateral patellar retinaculum

Fibular collateral ligament

Biceps femoris tendon (cut)

Fibula

Vastus medialis

Quadriceps femoris tendon

Medial epicondyle of femur

Patella

Tibial collateral ligament

Medial patellar retinaculum

Semitendinosus tendon (cut)

Gracilis tendon (cut)

Sartorius tendon (cut)

Patellar ligament

Tibial tuberosity

Tibia

**Knee joint capsule and related structures
(anterior view)**

Femoral artery

Adductor magnus

Descending branch of lateral circumflex

Adductor hiatus

Descending genicular artery

Saphenous branch of descending genicular artery

Superior medial genicular artery

Superior lateral genicular artery

Popliteal artery

Inferior lateral genicular artery

Inferior medial genicular artery

Circumflex fibular artery

Recurrent branch of anterior tibial artery

Interosseous membrane

Anterior tibial artery

Posterior tibial artery

**Anastomoses of arteries around the knee
(anterior view)**

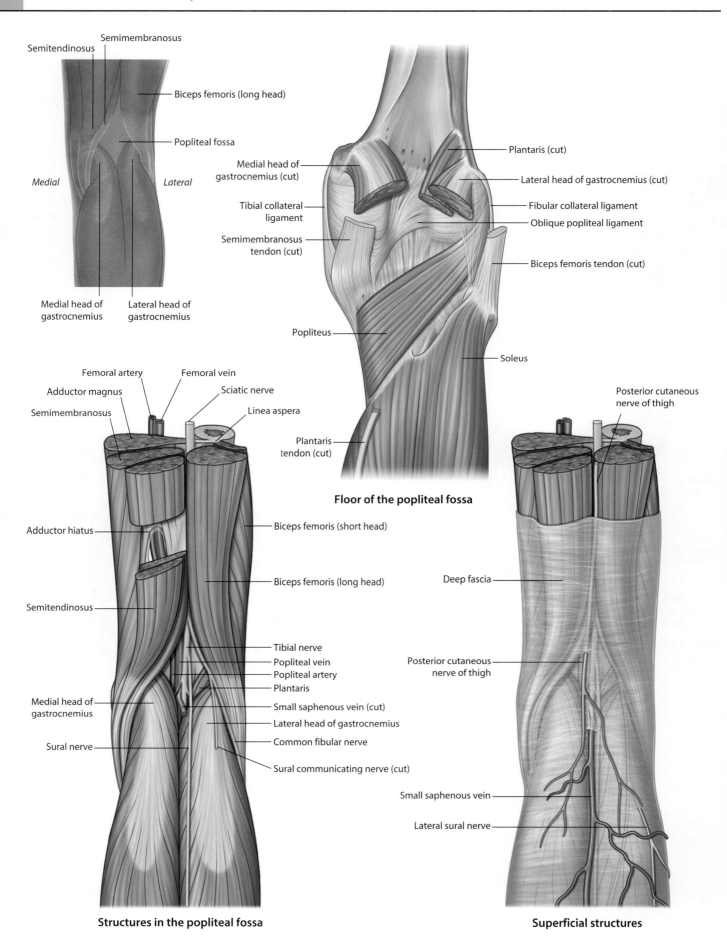

Semitendinosus

Semimembranosus

Biceps femoris (long head)

Popliteal fossa

Medial

Lateral

Medial head of
gastrocnemius

Lateral head of
gastrocnemius

Medial head of
gastrocnemius (cut)

Tibial collateral
ligament

Semimembranosus
tendon (cut)

Plantaris (cut)

Lateral head of gastrocnemius (cut)

Fibular collateral ligament

Oblique popliteal ligament

Biceps femoris tendon (cut)

Popliteus

Soleus

Plantaris
tendon (cut)

Floor of the popliteal fossa

Femoral artery

Femoral vein

Adductor magnus

Sciatic nerve

Semimembranosus

Linea aspera

Posterior cutaneous
nerve of thigh

Adductor hiatus

Biceps femoris (short head)

Biceps femoris (long head)

Semitendinosus

Deep fascia

Tibial nerve

Popliteal vein

Popliteal artery

Plantaris

Medial head of
gastrocnemius

Small saphenous vein (cut)

Lateral head of gastrocnemius

Common fibular nerve

Sural nerve

Sural communicating nerve (cut)

Posterior cutaneous
nerve of thigh

Small saphenous vein

Lateral sural nerve

Structures in the popliteal fossa

Superficial structures

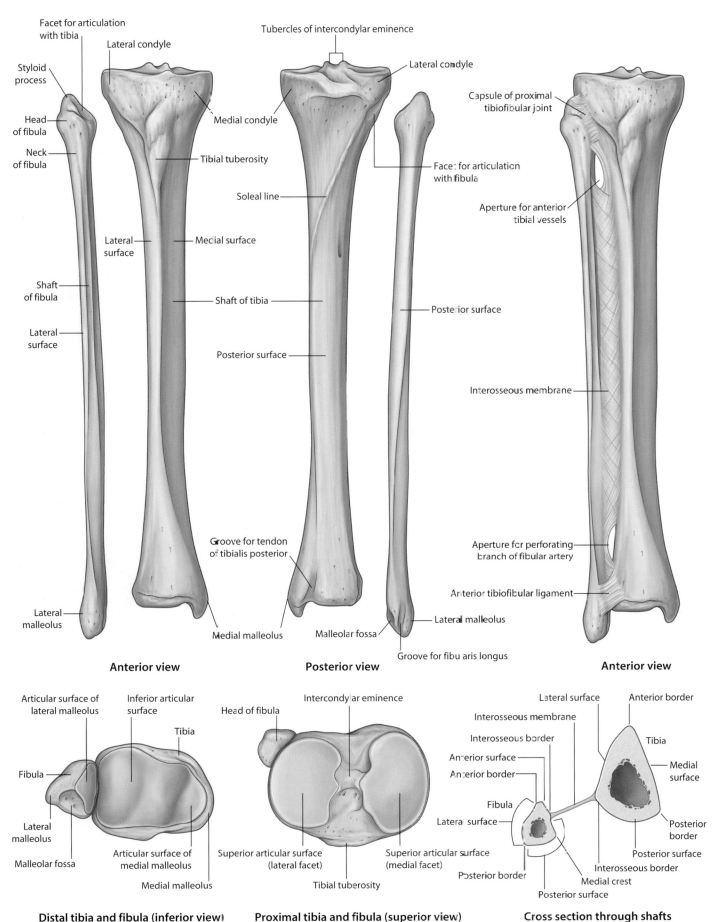

Facet for articulation with tibia

Styloid process

Head of fibula

Neck of fibula

Lateral condyle

Medial condyle

Tibial tuberosity

Lateral surface

Medial surface

Shaft of fibula

Lateral surface

Shaft of tibia

Posterior surface

Lateral malleolus

Groove for tendon of tibialis posterior

Medial malleolus

Anterior view

Tubercles of intercondylar eminence

Lateral condyle

Facet for articulation with fibula

Soleal line

Posterior surface

Malleolar fossa

Lateral malleolus

Groove for fibularis longus

Posterior view

Capsule of proximal tibiofibular joint

Aperture for anterior tibial vessels

Interosseous membrane

Aperture for perforating branch of fibular artery

Anterior tibiofibular ligament

Lateral malleolus

Anterior view

Articular surface of lateral malleolus

Inferior articular surface

Tibia

Fibula

Lateral malleolus

Malleolar fossa

Articular surface of medial malleolus

Medial malleolus

Distal tibia and fibula (inferior view)

Intercondylar eminence

Head of fibula

Superior articular surface (lateral facet)

Tibial tuberosity

Superior articular surface (medial facet)

Proximal tibia and fibula (superior view)

Lateral surface

Interosseous membrane

Interosseous border

Anterior surface

Anterior border

Fibula

Lateral surface

Posterior border

Posterior surface

Anterior border

Tibia

Medial surface

Posterior border

Posterior surface

Interosseous border

Medial crest

Cross section through shafts

331

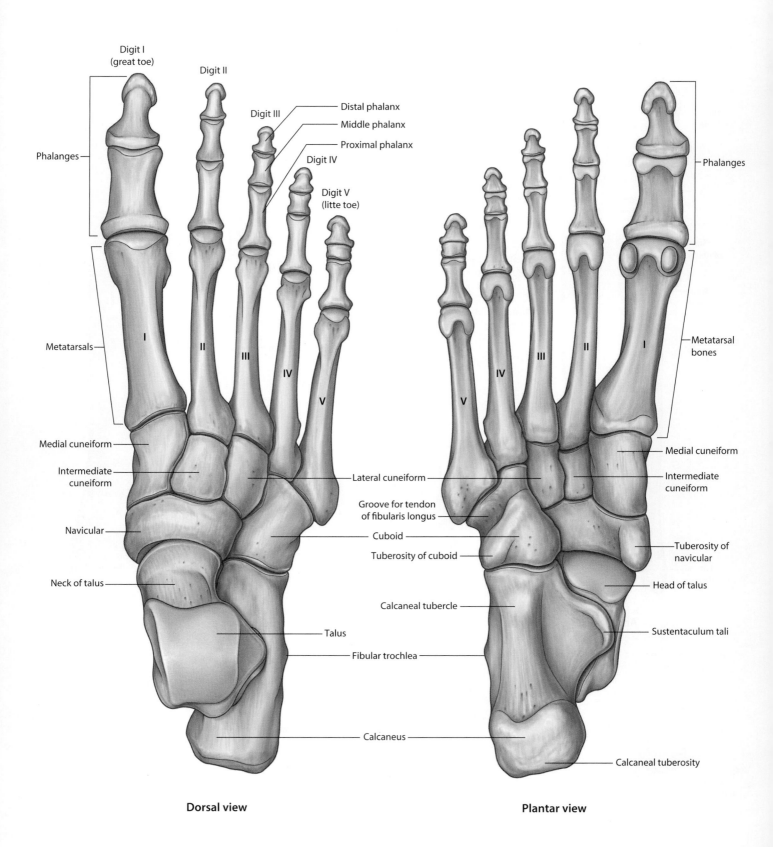

Digit I
(great toe)

Digit II

Digit III

Distal phalanx

Middle phalanx

Proximal phalanx

Digit IV

Phalanges

Digit V
(litte toe)

Phalanges

Metatarsals

Metatarsal
bones

Medial cuneiform

Medial cuneiform

Intermediate
cuneiform

Lateral cuneiform

Intermediate
cuneiform

Groove for tendon
of fibularis longus

Navicular

Cuboid

Neck of talus

Tuberosity of cuboid

Tuberosity of
navicular

Head of talus

Talus

Calcaneal tubercle

Sustentaculum tali

Fibular trochlea

Calcaneus

Calcaneal tuberosity

Dorsal view

Plantar view

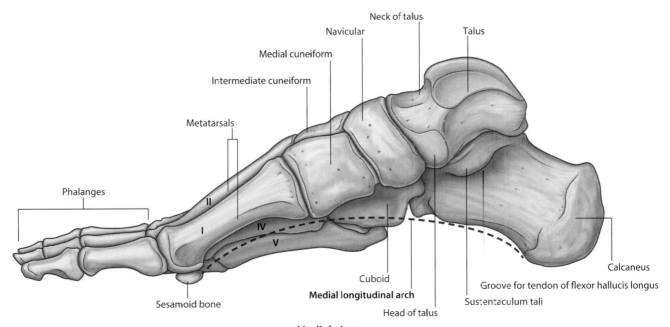

Neck of talus
Navicular
Talus
Medial cuneiform
Intermediate cuneiform
Metatarsals
Phalanges
II
I
IV
V
Sesamoid bone
Cuboid
Medial longitudinal arch
Head of talus
Groove for tendon of flexor hallucis longus
Sustentaculum tali
Calcaneus

Medial view

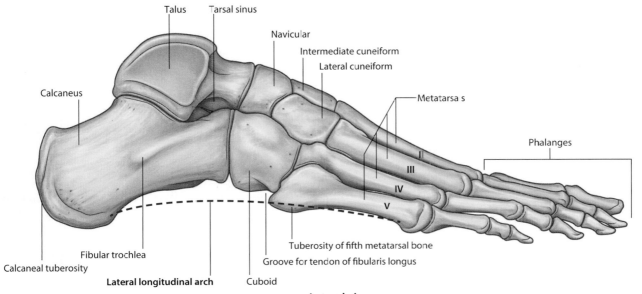

Talus
Tarsal sinus
Navicular
Intermediate cuneiform
Lateral cuneiform
Metatarsals
Phalanges
Calcaneus
I
III
IV
V
Fibular trochlea
Calcaneal tuberosity
Lateral longitudinal arch
Cuboid
Tuberosity of fifth metatarsal bone
Groove for tendon of fibularis longus

Lateral view

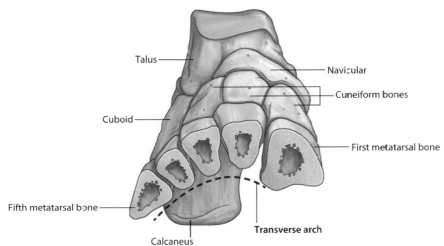

Talus
Navicular
Cuneiform bones
Cuboid
First metatarsal bone
Fifth metatarsal bone
Calcaneus
Transverse arch

Cross section through the foot bones

333

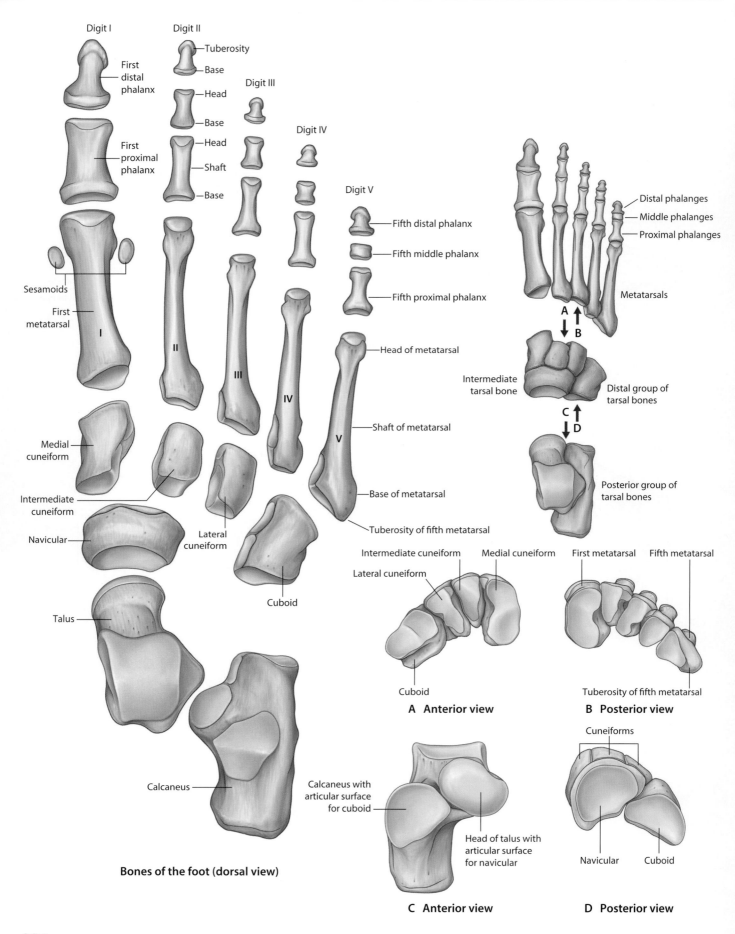

Digit I

First distal phalanx

First proximal phalanx

Sesamoids

First metatarsal

I

Medial cuneiform

Intermediate cuneiform

Navicular

Talus

Calcaneus

Digit II

Tuberosity

Base

Head

Base

Head

Shaft

Base

II

Digit III

Head

Shaft

Base

III

Lateral cuneiform

Digit IV

IV

Cuboid

Digit V

Fifth distal phalanx

Fifth middle phalanx

Fifth proximal phalanx

Head of metatarsal

V

Shaft of metatarsal

Base of metatarsal

Tuberosity of fifth metatarsal

Distal phalanges

Middle phalanges

Proximal phalanges

Metatarsals

A

B

Intermediate tarsal bone

Distal group of tarsal bones

C

D

Posterior group of tarsal bones

Bones of the foot (dorsal view)

Intermediate cuneiform

Lateral cuneiform

Medial cuneiform

First metatarsal

Fifth metatarsal

Cuboid

A Anterior view

Tuberosity of fifth metatarsal

B Posterior view

Calcaneus with articular surface for cuboid

Head of talus with articular surface for navicular

C Anterior view

Cuneiforms

Navicular

Cuboid

D Posterior view

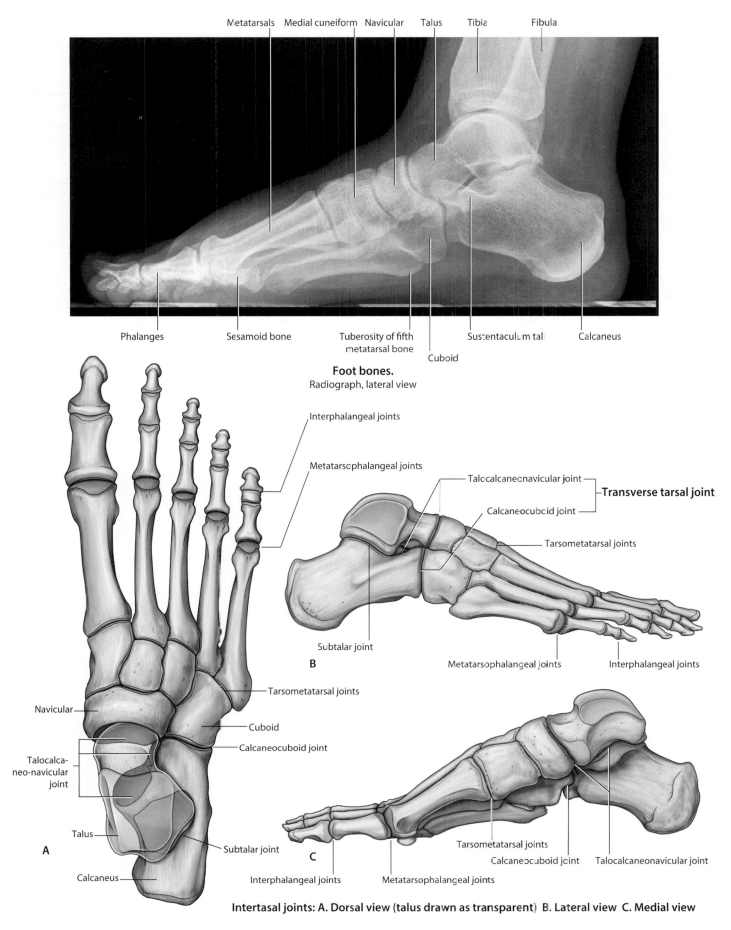

Metatarsals Medial cuneiform Navicular Talus Tibia Fibula

Phalanges Sesamoid bone Tuberosity of fifth metatarsal bone Cuboid Sustentaculum tali Calcaneus

Foot bones.
Radiograph, lateral view

Interphalangeal joints

Metatarsophalangeal joints

Talocalcaneonavicular joint
Calcaneocuboid joint **Transverse tarsal joint**
Tarsometatarsal joints

Subtalar joint

B

Metatarsophalangeal joints Interphalangeal joints

Tarsometatarsal joints

Navicular

Cuboid

Calcaneocuboid joint

Talocalca-neo-navicular joint

Talus

Subtalar joint

A

Calcaneus

C

Tarsometatarsal joints

Calcaneocuboid joint Talocalcaneonavicular joint

Interphalangeal joints Metatarsophalangeal joints

Intertasal joints: A. Dorsal view (talus drawn as transparent) B. Lateral view C. Medial view

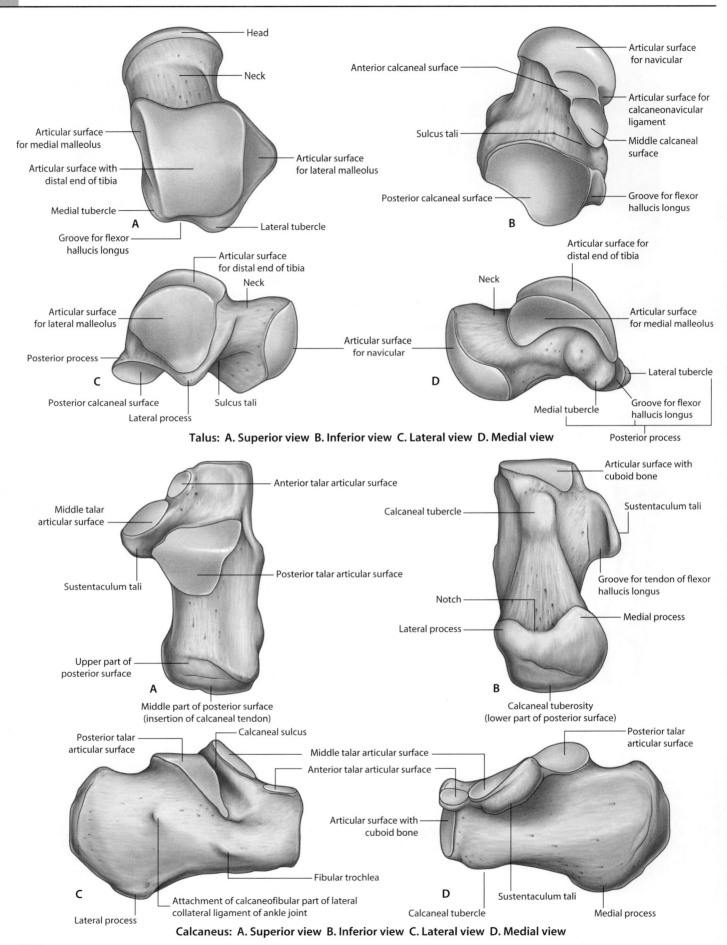

Head

Neck

Articular surface
for medial malleolus

Articular surface with
distal end of tibia

Medial tubercle

Groove for flexor
hallucis longus

Articular surface
for lateral malleolus

Lateral tubercle

A

Anterior calcaneal surface

Sulcus tali

Posterior calcaneal surface

Articular surface
for navicular

Articular surface for
calcaneonavicular
ligament

Middle calcaneal
surface

Groove for flexor
hallucis longus

B

Articular surface
for distal end of tibia

Neck

Articular surface
for lateral malleolus

Posterior process

C

Posterior calcaneal surface

Lateral process

Sulcus tali

Articular surface
for navicular

Articular surface for
distal end of tibia

Neck

Articular surface
for medial malleolus

Lateral tubercle

Medial tubercle

Groove for flexor
hallucis longus

Posterior process

D

Talus: A. Superior view B. Inferior view C. Lateral view D. Medial view

Middle talar
articular surface

Sustentaculum tali

Upper part of
posterior surface

Anterior talar articular surface

Posterior talar articular surface

Middle part of posterior surface
(insertion of calcaneal tendon)

A

Articular surface with
cuboid bone

Calcaneal tubercle

Sustentaculum tali

Notch

Lateral process

Groove for tendon of flexor
hallucis longus

Medial process

Calcaneal tuberosity
(lower part of posterior surface)

B

Posterior talar
articular surface

Calcaneal sulcus

Middle talar articular surface

Anterior talar articular surface

Articular surface with
cuboid bone

Fibular trochlea

Attachment of calcaneofibular part of lateral
collateral ligament of ankle joint

Lateral process

C

Posterior talar
articular surface

Sustentaculum tali

Calcaneal tubercle

Medial process

D

Calcaneus: A. Superior view B. Inferior view C. Lateral view D. Medial view

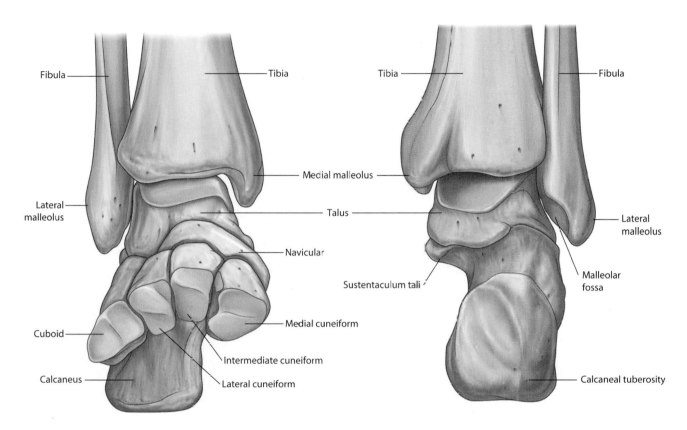

Anterior view
(metatarsals and phalanges removed)

Posterior view

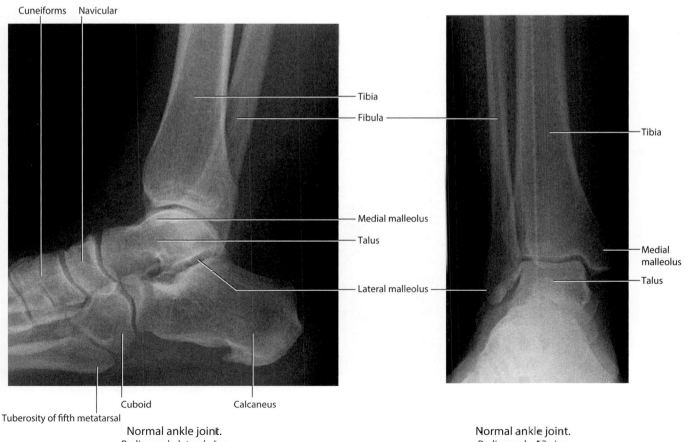

Normal ankle joint.
Radiograph, lateral view

Normal ankle joint.
Radiograph, AP view

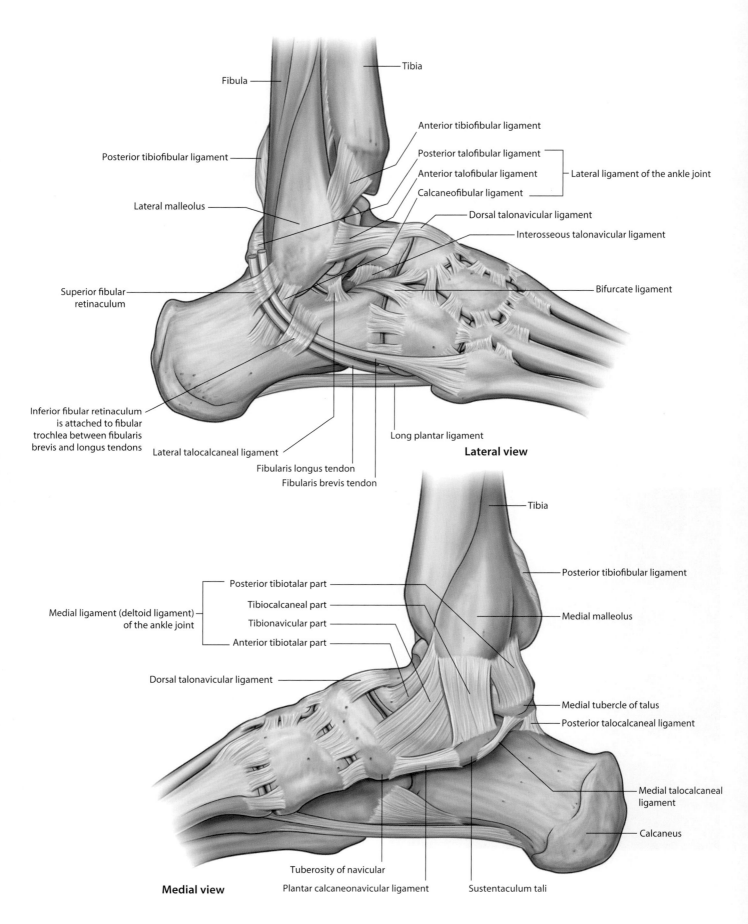

Fibula

Tibia

Anterior tibiofibular ligament

Posterior tibiofibular ligament

Posterior talofibular ligament

Anterior talofibular ligament

Lateral ligament of the ankle joint

Calcaneofibular ligament

Lateral malleolus

Dorsal talonavicular ligament

Interosseous talonavicular ligament

Superior fibular retinaculum

Bifurcate ligament

Inferior fibular retinaculum is attached to fibular trochlea between fibularis brevis and longus tendons

Lateral talocalcaneal ligament

Long plantar ligament

Lateral view

Fibularis longus tendon

Fibularis brevis tendon

Tibia

Posterior tibiofibular ligament

Posterior tibiotalar part

Tibiocalcaneal part

Tibionavicular part

Anterior tibiotalar part

Medial ligament (deltoid ligament) of the ankle joint

Medial malleolus

Dorsal talonavicular ligament

Medial tubercle of talus

Posterior talocalcaneal ligament

Medial talocalcaneal ligament

Calcaneus

Tuberosity of navicular

Medial view

Plantar calcaneonavicular ligament

Sustentaculum tali

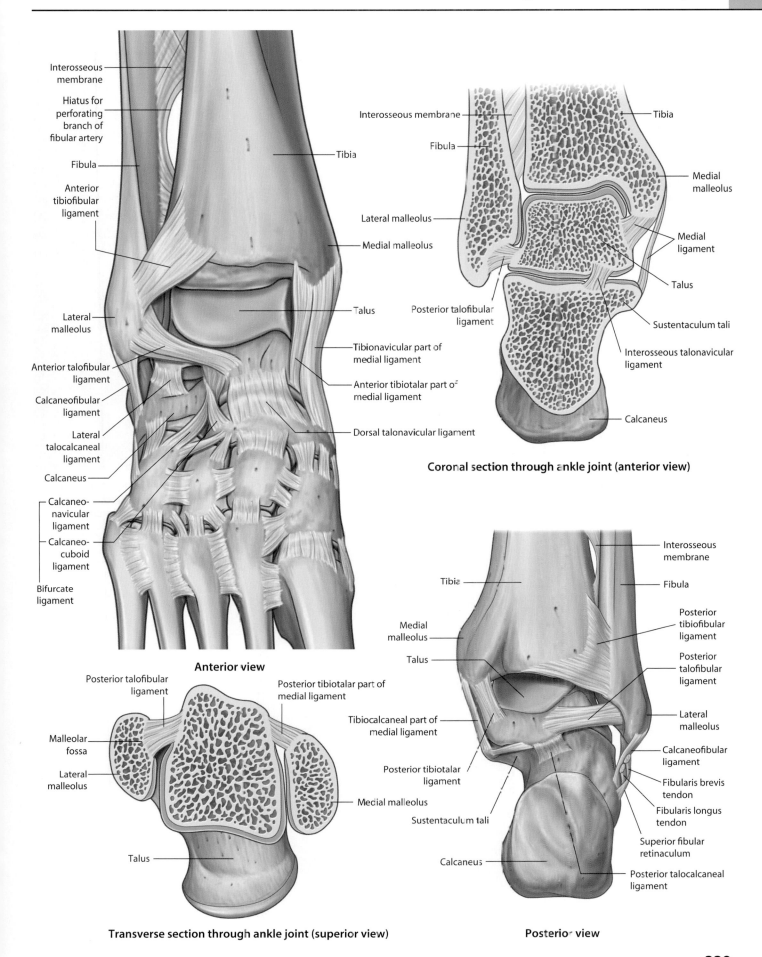

Interosseous membrane

Hiatus for perforating branch of fibular artery

Fibula

Anterior tibiofibular ligament

Lateral malleolus

Anterior talofibular ligament

Calcaneofibular ligament

Lateral talocalcaneal ligament

Calcaneus

Calcaneo-navicular ligament

Calcaneo-cuboid ligament

Bifurcate ligament

Tibia

Talus

Tibionavicular part of medial ligament

Anterior tibiotalar part of medial ligament

Dorsal talonavicular ligament

Anterior view

Interosseous membrane

Fibula

Lateral malleolus

Posterior talofibular ligament

Tibia

Medial malleolus

Medial ligament

Talus

Sustentaculum tali

Interosseous talonavicular ligament

Calcaneus

Coronal section through ankle joint (anterior view)

Posterior talofibular ligament

Malleolar fossa

Lateral malleolus

Talus

Posterior tibiotalar part of medial ligament

Medial malleolus

Transverse section through ankle joint (superior view)

Tibia

Medial malleolus

Talus

Tibiocalcaneal part of medial ligament

Posterior tibiotalar ligament

Sustentaculum tali

Calcaneus

Interosseous membrane

Fibula

Posterior tibiofibular ligament

Posterior talofibular ligament

Lateral malleolus

Calcaneofibular ligament

Fibularis brevis tendon

Fibularis longus tendon

Superior fibular retinaculum

Posterior talocalcaneal ligament

Posterior view

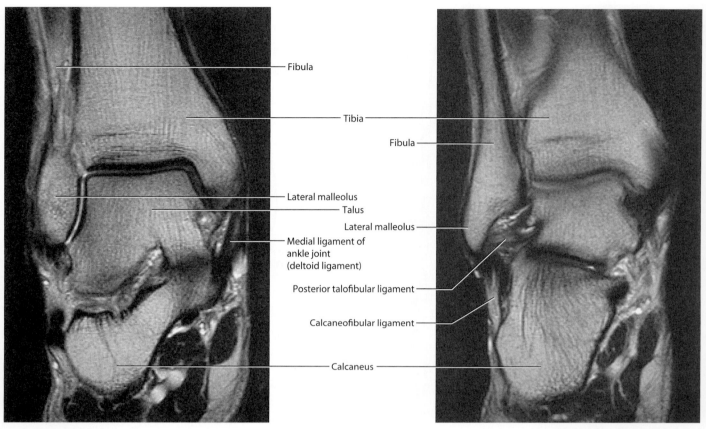

Coronal view of the ankle joint showing the medial ligament of the ankle joint (deltoid ligament).
T2-weighted MR image in coronal plane

Fibula

Tibia

Fibula

Lateral malleolus

Talus

Lateral malleolus

Medial ligament of ankle joint (deltoid ligament)

Posterior talofibular ligament

Calcaneofibular ligament

Calcaneus

Coronal view of the ankle joint showing the posterior talofibular and calcaneofibular ligaments.
T2-weighted MR image in coronal plane

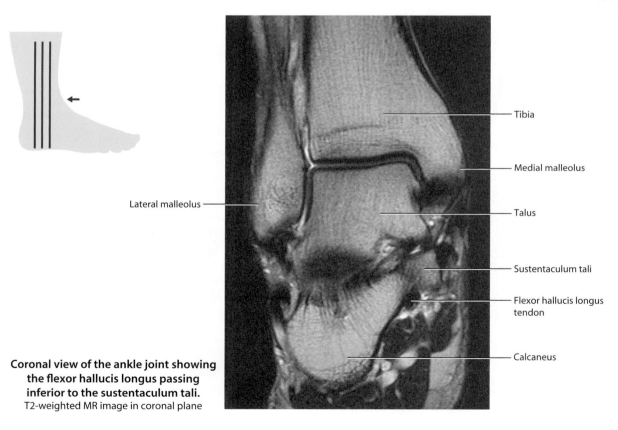

Coronal view of the ankle joint showing the flexor hallucis longus passing inferior to the sustentaculum tali.
T2-weighted MR image in coronal plane

Lateral malleolus

Tibia

Medial malleolus

Talus

Sustentaculum tali

Flexor hallucis longus tendon

Calcaneus

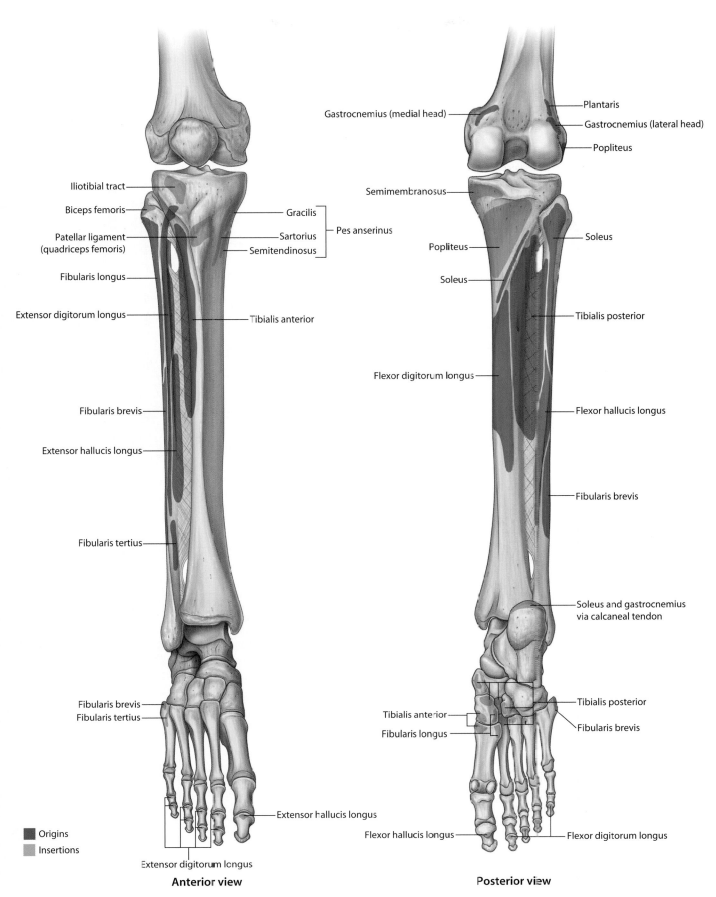

Gastrocnemius (medial head)

Plantaris

Gastrocnemius (lateral head)

Popliteus

Iliotibial tract

Biceps femoris

Gracilis

Patellar ligament
(quadriceps femoris)

Sartorius

Pes anserinus

Semitendinosus

Semimembranosus

Fibularis longus

Soleus

Extensor digitorum longus

Popliteus

Tibialis anterior

Soleus

Fibularis brevis

Tibialis posterior

Extensor hallucis longus

Flexor digitorum longus

Flexor hallucis longus

Fibularis tertius

Fibularis brevis

Soleus and gastrocnemius
via calcaneal tendon

Fibularis brevis

Fibularis tertius

Tibialis posterior

Tibialis anterior

Fibularis brevis

Fibularis longus

Extensor hallucis longus

Origins

Insertions

Flexor hallucis longus

Flexor digitorum longus

Extensor digitorum longus

Anterior view

Posterior view

341

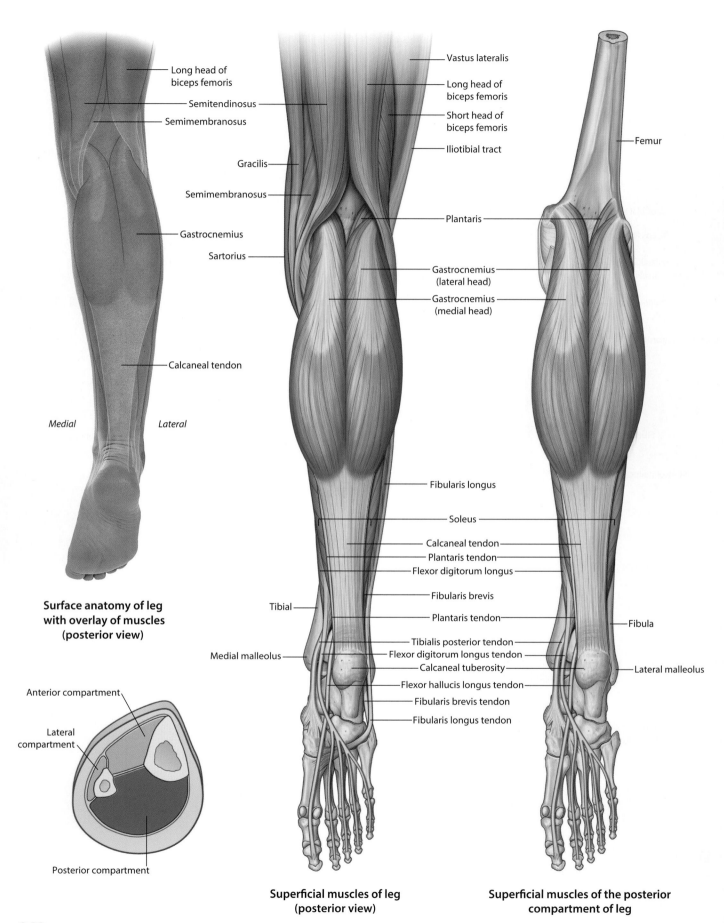

Long head of
biceps femoris

Semitendinosus

Semimembranosus

Gracilis

Semimembranosus

Gastrocnemius

Sartorius

Calcaneal tendon

Medial　　*Lateral*

**Surface anatomy of leg
with overlay of muscles
(posterior view)**

Anterior compartment

Lateral
compartment

Posterior compartment

Vastus lateralis

Long head of
biceps femoris

Short head of
biceps femoris

Iliotibial tract

Femur

Plantaris

Gastrocnemius
(lateral head)

Gastrocnemius
(medial head)

Fibularis longus

Soleus

Calcaneal tendon

Plantaris tendon

Flexor digitorum longus

Fibularis brevis

Tibial

Plantaris tendon

Fibula

Tibialis posterior tendon

Medial malleolus

Flexor digitorum longus tendon

Calcaneal tuberosity

Lateral malleolus

Flexor hallucis longus tendon

Fibularis brevis tendon

Fibularis longus tendon

**Superficial muscles of leg
(posterior view)**

**Superficial muscles of the posterior
compartment of leg**

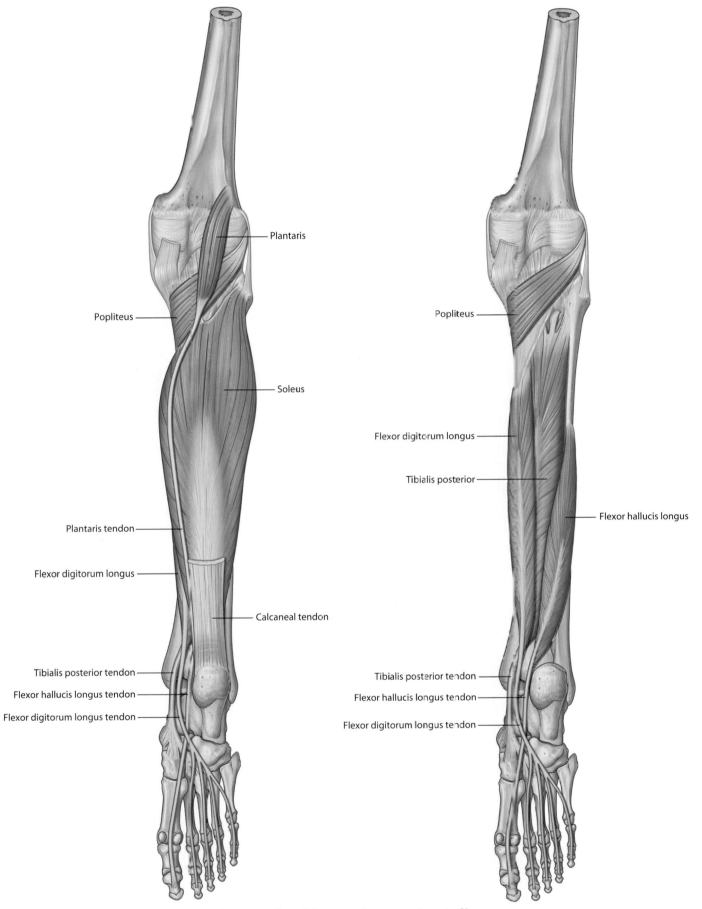

Plantaris

Popliteus

Soleus

Plantaris tendon

Flexor digitorum longus

Calcaneal tendon

Tibialis posterior tendon

Flexor hallucis longus tendon

Flexor digitorum longus tendon

Popliteus

Flexor digitorum longus

Tibialis posterior

Flexor hallucis longus

Tibialis posterior tendon

Flexor hallucis longus tendon

Flexor digitorum longus tendon

Deep muscles of the posterior compartment of leg

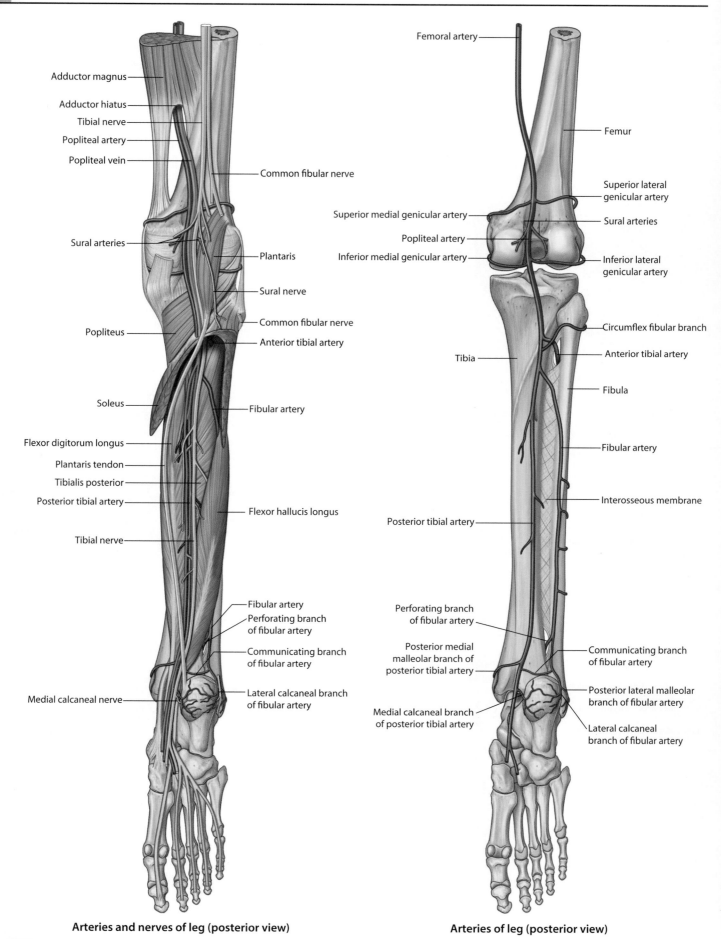

Adductor magnus

Adductor hiatus

Tibial nerve

Popliteal artery

Popliteal vein

Common fibular nerve

Sural arteries

Plantaris

Sural nerve

Common fibular nerve

Anterior tibial artery

Popliteus

Soleus

Fibular artery

Flexor digitorum longus

Plantaris tendon

Tibialis posterior

Posterior tibial artery

Flexor hallucis longus

Tibial nerve

Fibular artery

Perforating branch of fibular artery

Communicating branch of fibular artery

Medial calcaneal nerve

Lateral calcaneal branch of fibular artery

Femoral artery

Femur

Superior lateral genicular artery

Superior medial genicular artery

Sural arteries

Popliteal artery

Inferior medial genicular artery

Inferior lateral genicular artery

Circumflex fibular branch

Tibia

Anterior tibial artery

Fibula

Fibular artery

Interosseous membrane

Posterior tibial artery

Perforating branch of fibular artery

Communicating branch of fibular artery

Posterior medial malleolar branch of posterior tibial artery

Posterior lateral malleolar branch of fibular artery

Medial calcaneal branch of posterior tibial artery

Lateral calcaneal branch of fibular artery

Arteries and nerves of leg (posterior view)

Arteries of leg (posterior view)

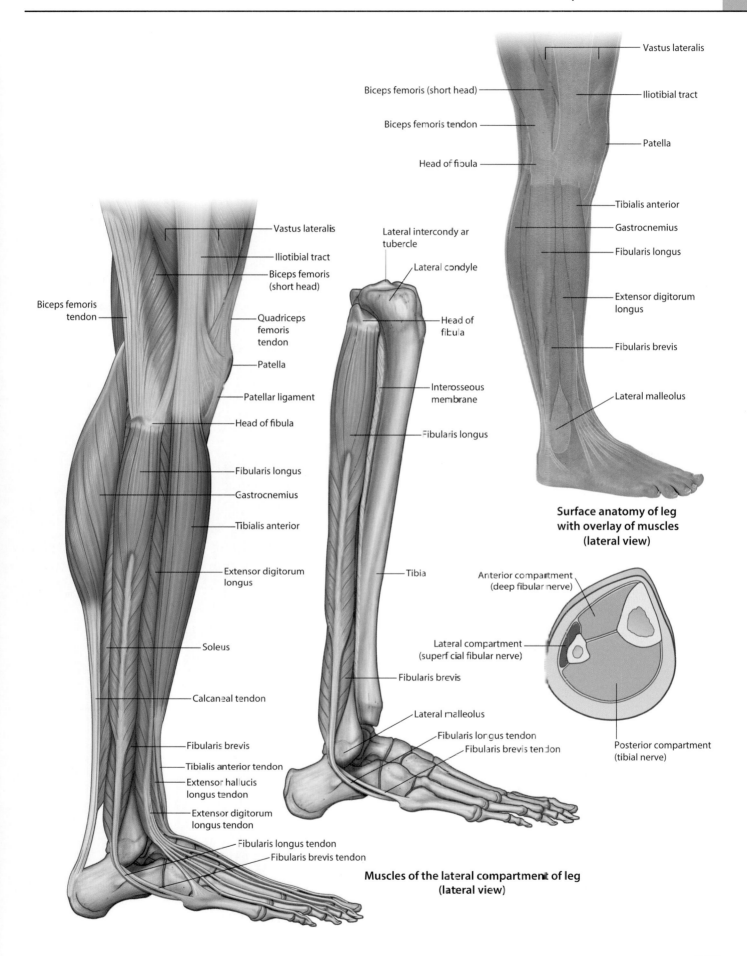

Vastus lateralis

Biceps femoris (short head)

Biceps femoris tendon

Head of fibula

Vastus lateralis

Iliotibial tract

Patella

Tibialis anterior

Gastrocnemius

Fibularis longus

Extensor digitorum longus

Fibularis brevis

Lateral malleolus

**Surface anatomy of leg
with overlay of muscles
(lateral view)**

Biceps femoris tendon

Vastus lateralis

Iliotibial tract

Biceps femoris (short head)

Quadriceps femoris tendon

Patella

Patellar ligament

Head of fibula

Fibularis longus

Gastrocnemius

Tibialis anterior

Extensor digitorum longus

Soleus

Calcaneal tendon

Fibularis brevis

Tibialis anterior tendon

Extensor hallucis longus tendon

Extensor digitorum longus tendon

Fibularis longus tendon

Fibularis brevis tendon

Lateral intercondylar tubercle

Lateral condyle

Head of fibula

Interosseous membrane

Fibularis longus

Tibia

Fibularis brevis

Lateral malleolus

Fibularis longus tendon

Fibularis brevis tendon

Anterior compartment
(deep fibular nerve)

Lateral compartment
(superficial fibular nerve)

Posterior compartment
(tibial nerve)

**Muscles of the lateral compartment of leg
(lateral view)**

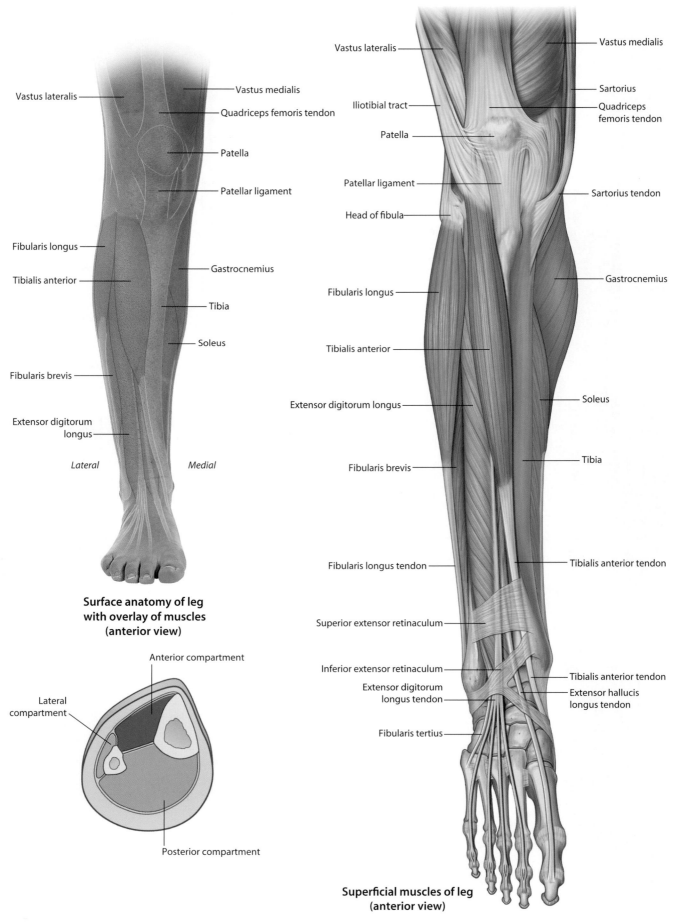

Vastus lateralis

Vastus medialis

Quadriceps femoris tendon

Patella

Patellar ligament

Fibularis longus

Tibialis anterior

Gastrocnemius

Tibia

Soleus

Fibularis brevis

Extensor digitorum longus

Lateral

Medial

**Surface anatomy of leg
with overlay of muscles
(anterior view)**

Anterior compartment

Lateral compartment

Posterior compartment

Vastus lateralis

Vastus medialis

Iliotibial tract

Sartorius

Patella

Quadriceps femoris tendon

Patellar ligament

Head of fibula

Sartorius tendon

Fibularis longus

Tibialis anterior

Gastrocnemius

Extensor digitorum longus

Soleus

Fibularis brevis

Tibia

Fibularis longus tendon

Tibialis anterior tendon

Superior extensor retinaculum

Inferior extensor retinaculum

Tibialis anterior tendon

Extensor digitorum longus tendon

Extensor hallucis longus tendon

Fibularis tertius

**Superficial muscles of leg
(anterior view)**

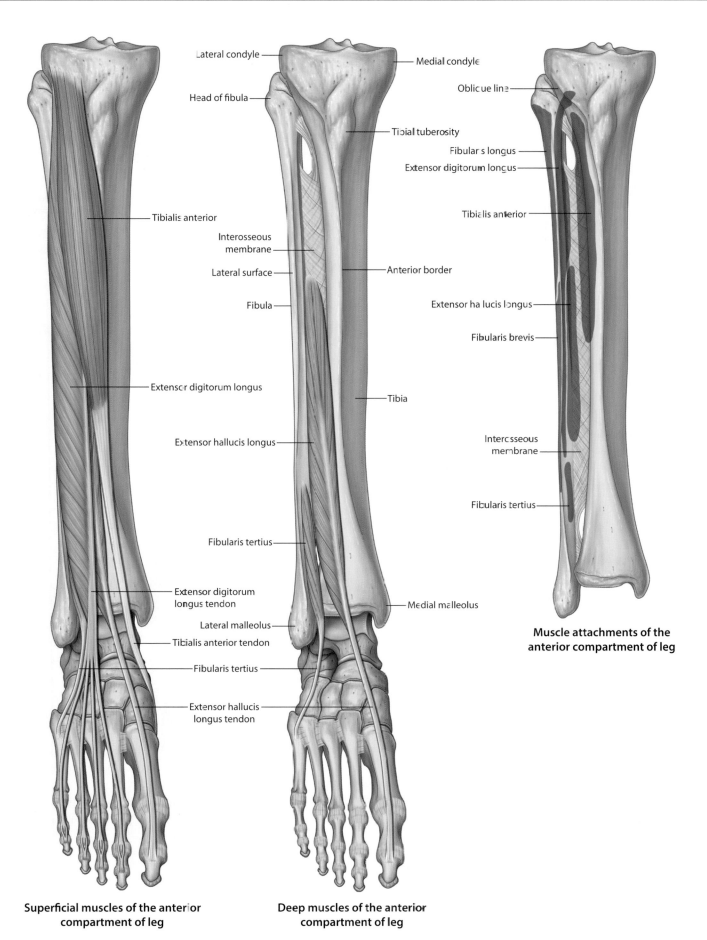

Lateral condyle

Medial condyle

Head of fibula

Oblique line

Tibial tuberosity

Fibularis longus

Extensor digitorum longus

Tibialis anterior

Tibialis anterior

Interosseous membrane

Lateral surface

Anterior border

Fibula

Extensor hallucis longus

Extensor digitorum longus

Fibularis brevis

Tibia

Extensor hallucis longus

Fibularis tertius

Interosseous membrane

Extensor digitorum longus tendon

Fibularis tertius

Medial malleolus

Lateral malleolus

Tibialis anterior tendon

Fibularis tertius

Extensor hallucis longus tendon

Muscle attachments of the anterior compartment of leg

Superficial muscles of the anterior compartment of leg

Deep muscles of the anterior compartment of leg

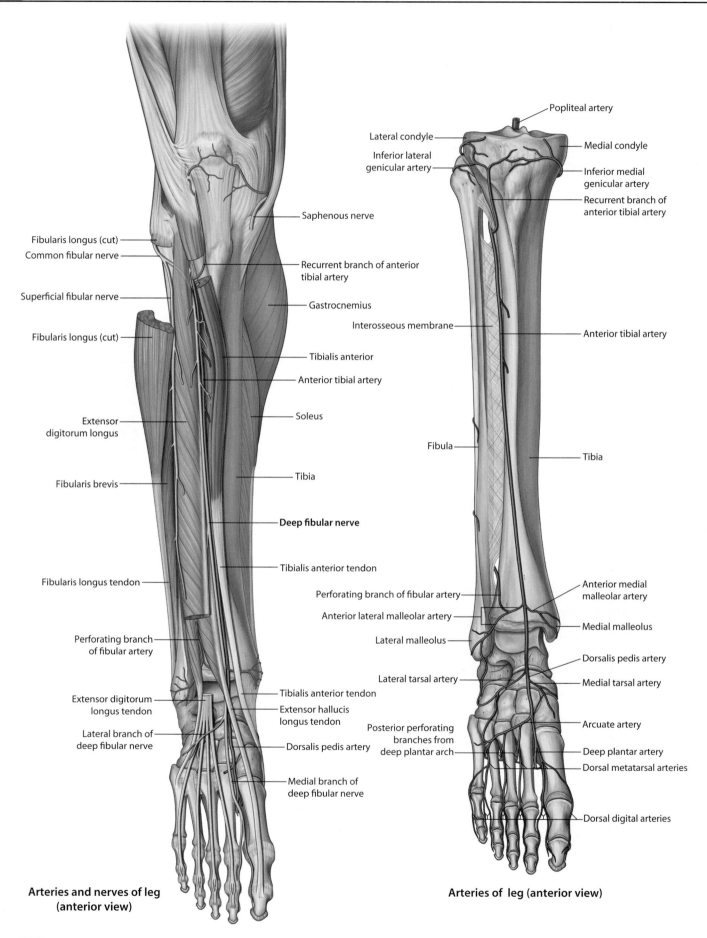

Popliteal artery

Lateral condyle

Inferior lateral
genicular artery

Medial condyle

Inferior medial
genicular artery

Recurrent branch of
anterior tibial artery

Saphenous nerve

Fibularis longus (cut)

Common fibular nerve

Recurrent branch of anterior
tibial artery

Superficial fibular nerve

Gastrocnemius

Interosseous membrane

Anterior tibial artery

Fibularis longus (cut)

Tibialis anterior

Anterior tibial artery

Extensor
digitorum longus

Soleus

Fibula

Tibia

Fibularis brevis

Tibia

Deep fibular nerve

Fibularis longus tendon

Tibialis anterior tendon

Perforating branch of fibular artery

Anterior medial
malleolar artery

Anterior lateral malleolar artery

Medial malleolus

Perforating branch
of fibular artery

Lateral malleolus

Dorsalis pedis artery

Lateral tarsal artery

Medial tarsal artery

Extensor digitorum
longus tendon

Tibialis anterior tendon

Extensor hallucis
longus tendon

Posterior perforating
branches from
deep plantar arch

Arcuate artery

Lateral branch of
deep fibular nerve

Dorsalis pedis artery

Deep plantar artery

Dorsal metatarsal arteries

Medial branch of
deep fibular nerve

Dorsal digital arteries

**Arteries and nerves of leg
(anterior view)**

Arteries of leg (anterior view)

348

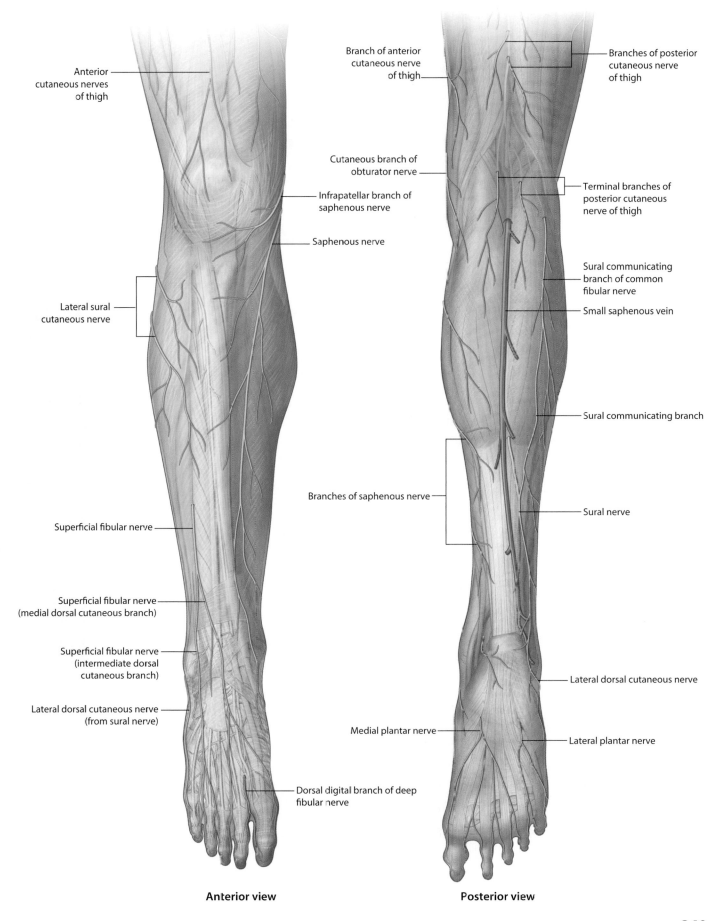

Anterior
cutaneous nerves
of thigh

Lateral sural
cutaneous nerve

Superficial fibular nerve

Superficial fibular nerve
(medial dorsal cutaneous branch)

Superficial fibular nerve
(intermediate dorsal
cutaneous branch)

Lateral dorsal cutaneous nerve
(from sural nerve)

Branch of anterior
cutaneous nerve
of thigh

Cutaneous branch of
obturator nerve

Infrapatellar branch of
saphenous nerve

Saphenous nerve

Branches of saphenous nerve

Medial plantar nerve

Dorsal digital branch of deep
fibular nerve

Branches of posterior
cutaneous nerve
of thigh

Terminal branches of
posterior cutaneous
nerve of thigh

Sural communicating
branch of common
fibular nerve

Small saphenous vein

Sural communicating branch

Sural nerve

Lateral dorsal cutaneous nerve

Lateral plantar nerve

Anterior view

Posterior view

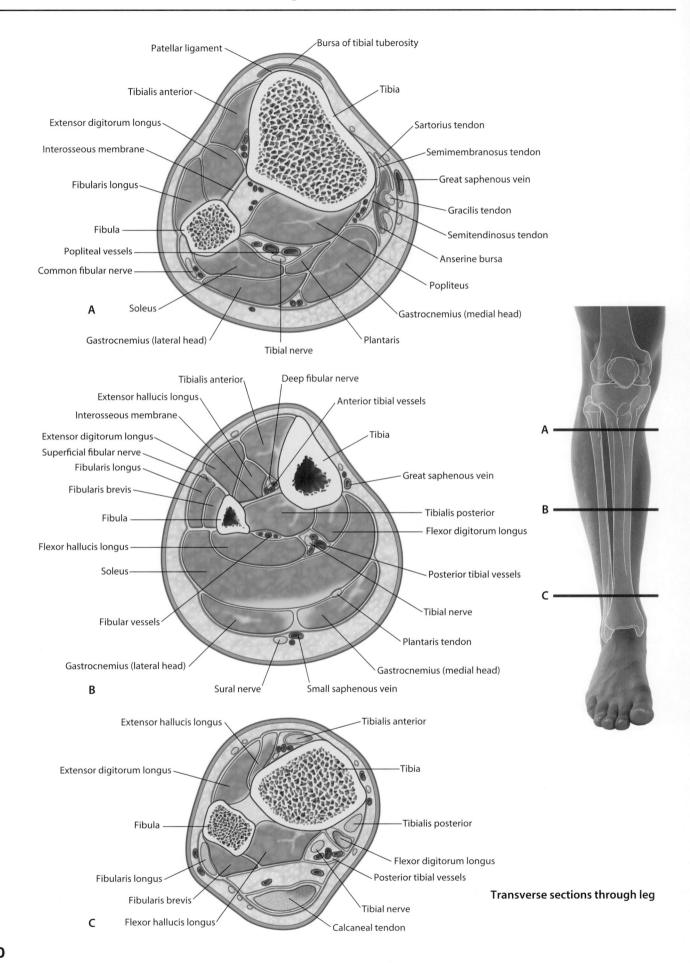

A

Patellar ligament
Bursa of tibial tuberosity
Tibialis anterior
Tibia
Extensor digitorum longus
Sartorius tendon
Interosseous membrane
Semimembranosus tendon
Fibularis longus
Great saphenous vein
Fibula
Gracilis tendon
Popliteal vessels
Semitendinosus tendon
Common fibular nerve
Anserine bursa
Soleus
Popliteus
Gastrocnemius (lateral head)
Gastrocnemius (medial head)
Tibial nerve
Plantaris

B

Tibialis anterior
Deep fibular nerve
Extensor hallucis longus
Anterior tibial vessels
Interosseous membrane
Extensor digitorum longus
Tibia
Superficial fibular nerve
Fibularis longus
Great saphenous vein
Fibularis brevis
Tibialis posterior
Fibula
Flexor digitorum longus
Flexor hallucis longus
Soleus
Posterior tibial vessels
Fibular vessels
Tibial nerve
Gastrocnemius (lateral head)
Plantaris tendon
Sural nerve
Gastrocnemius (medial head)
Small saphenous vein

C

Extensor hallucis longus
Tibialis anterior
Extensor digitorum longus
Tibia
Fibula
Tibialis posterior
Fibularis longus
Flexor digitorum longus
Fibularis brevis
Posterior tibial vessels
Flexor hallucis longus
Tibial nerve
Calcaneal tendon

A
B
C

Transverse sections through leg

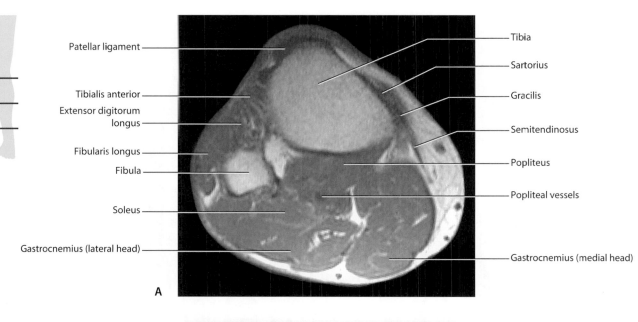

Patellar ligament

Tibialis anterior

Extensor digitorum longus

Fibularis longus

Fibula

Soleus

Gastrocnemius (lateral head)

Tibia

Sartorius

Gracilis

Semitendinosus

Popliteus

Popliteal vessels

Gastrocnemius (medial head)

A

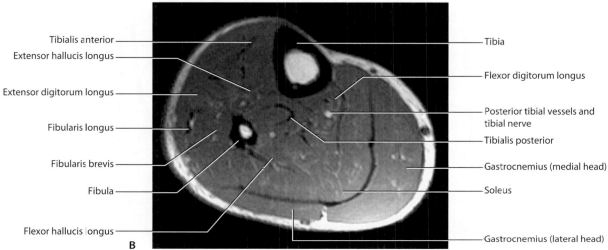

Tibialis anterior

Extensor hallucis longus

Extensor digitorum longus

Fibularis longus

Fibularis brevis

Fibula

Flexor hallucis longus

Tibia

Flexor digitorum longus

Posterior tibial vessels and tibial nerve

Tibialis posterior

Gastrocnemius (medial head)

Soleus

Gastrocnemius (lateral head)

B

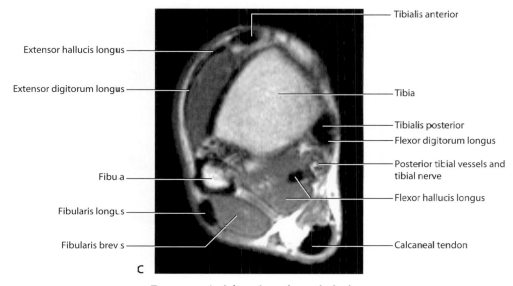

Tibialis anterior

Extensor hallucis longus

Extensor digitorum longus

Fibula

Fibularis longus

Fibularis brevis

Tibia

Tibialis posterior

Flexor digitorum longus

Posterior tibial vessels and tibial nerve

Flexor hallucis longus

Calcaneal tendon

C

Transverse/axial sections through the leg.

A. Proximal/upper leg. T1-weighted MR image in axial plane
B. Middle leg. T1-weighted MR image in axial plane
C. Distal/lower leg. T1-weighted MR image in axial plane

Muscle attachments of the foot

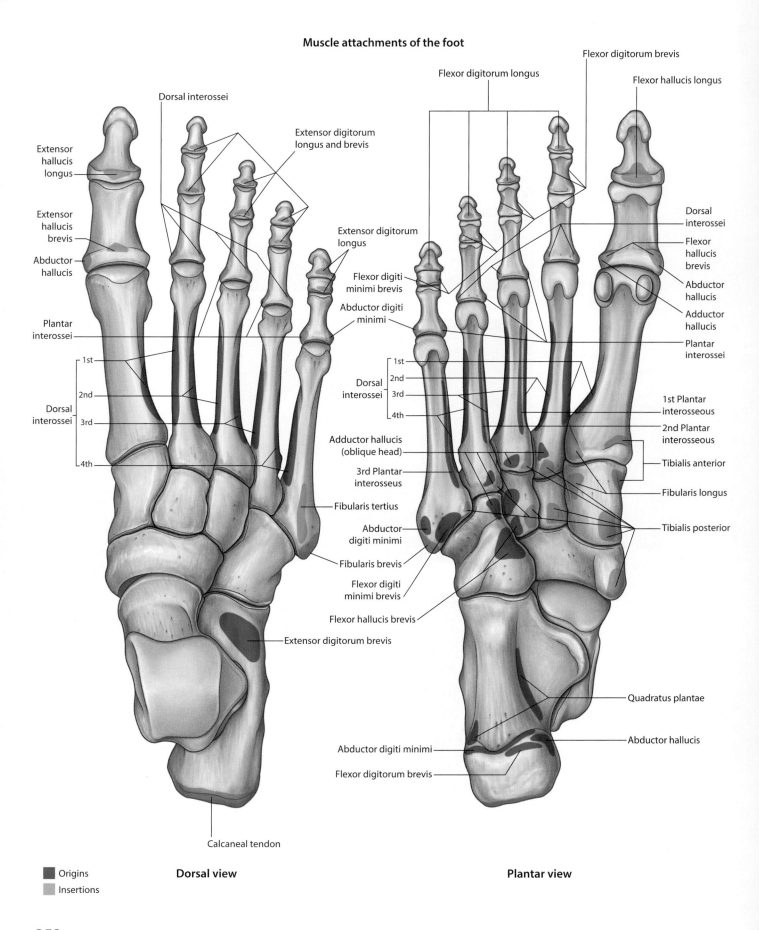

Dorsal interossei

Extensor digitorum longus and brevis

Extensor hallucis longus

Extensor hallucis brevis

Abductor hallucis

Extensor digitorum longus

Plantar interossei

Flexor digiti minimi brevis

Abductor digiti minimi

1st
2nd
3rd
4th

Dorsal interossei

Adductor hallucis (oblique head)

3rd Plantar interosseus

Fibularis tertius

Abductor digiti minimi

Fibularis brevis

Flexor digiti minimi brevis

Flexor hallucis brevis

Extensor digitorum brevis

Calcaneal tendon

Flexor digitorum longus

Flexor digitorum brevis

Flexor hallucis longus

Dorsal interossei

Flexor hallucis brevis

Abductor hallucis

Adductor hallucis

Plantar interossei

1st Plantar interosseous

2nd Plantar interosseous

Tibialis anterior

Fibularis longus

Tibialis posterior

1st
2nd
3rd
4th

Dorsal interossei

Quadratus plantae

Abductor hallucis

Abductor digiti minimi

Flexor digitorum brevis

Origins
Insertions

Dorsal view

Plantar view

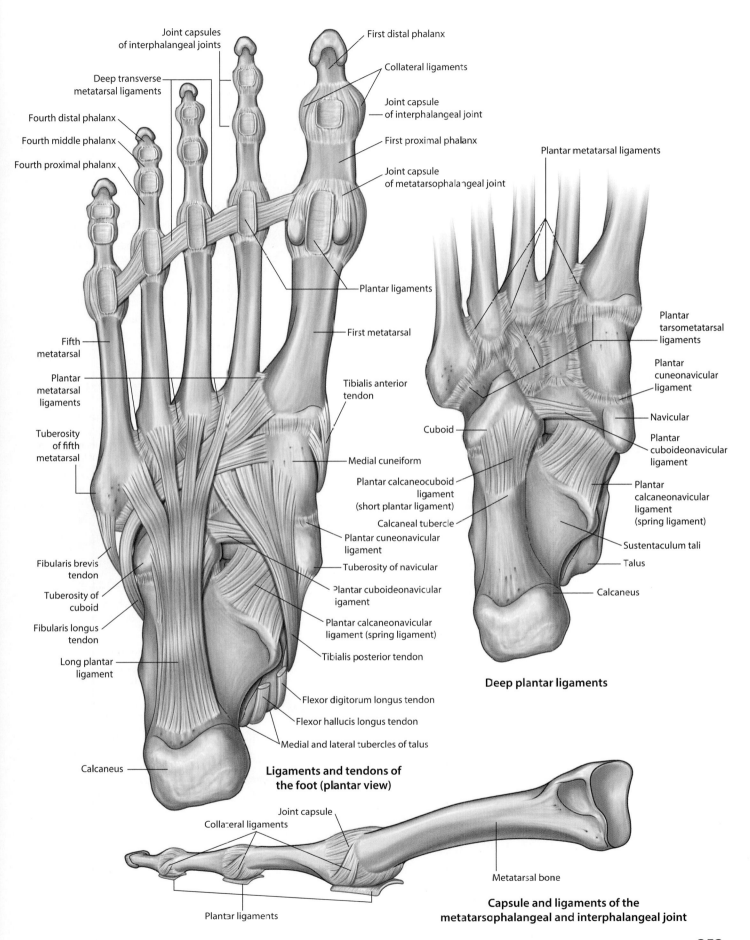

Joint capsules
of interphalangeal joints

First distal phalanx

Collateral ligaments

Deep transverse
metatarsal ligaments

Joint capsule
of interphalangeal joint

Fourth distal phalanx

First proximal phalanx

Fourth middle phalanx

Joint capsule
of metatarsophalangeal joint

Fourth proximal phalanx

Plantar metatarsal ligaments

Plantar
tarsometatarsal
ligaments

Plantar ligaments

Plantar
cuneonavicular
ligament

Fifth
metatarsal

First metatarsal

Navicular

Plantar
metatarsal
ligaments

Tibialis anterior
tendon

Cuboid

Plantar
cuboideonavicular
ligament

Tuberosity
of fifth
metatarsal

Medial cuneiform

Plantar
calcaneonavicular
ligament
(spring ligament)

Plantar calcaneocuboid
ligament
(short plantar ligament)

Fibularis brevis
tendon

Sustentaculum tali

Calcaneal tubercle

Talus

Tuberosity of
cuboid

Plantar cuneonavicular
ligament

Calcaneus

Fibularis longus
tendon

Tuberosity of navicular

Long plantar
ligament

Plantar cuboideonavicular
ligament

Deep plantar ligaments

Plantar calcaneonavicular
ligament (spring ligament)

Tibialis posterior tendon

Flexor digitorum longus tendon

Flexor hallucis longus tendon

Calcaneus

Medial and lateral tubercles of talus

**Ligaments and tendons of
the foot (plantar view)**

Joint capsule

Collateral ligaments

Metatarsal bone

Plantar ligaments

**Capsule and ligaments of the
metatarsophalangeal and interphalangeal joint**

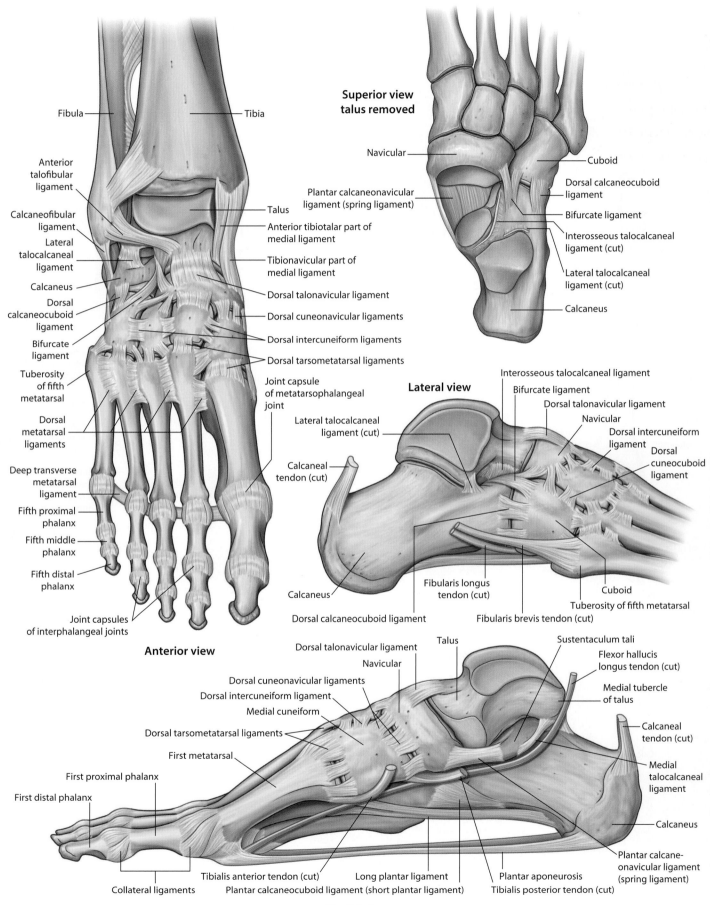

Superior view talus removed

Navicular

Plantar calcaneonavicular ligament (spring ligament)

Cuboid

Dorsal calcaneocuboid ligament

Bifurcate ligament

Interosseous talocalcaneal ligament (cut)

Lateral talocalcaneal ligament (cut)

Calcaneus

Fibula

Tibia

Anterior talofibular ligament

Calcaneofibular ligament

Lateral talocalcaneal ligament

Calcaneus

Dorsal calcaneocuboid ligament

Bifurcate ligament

Tuberosity of fifth metatarsal

Dorsal metatarsal ligaments

Deep transverse metatarsal ligament

Fifth proximal phalanx

Fifth middle phalanx

Fifth distal phalanx

Joint capsules of interphalangeal joints

Talus

Anterior tibiotalar part of medial ligament

Tibionavicular part of medial ligament

Dorsal talonavicular ligament

Dorsal cuneonavicular ligaments

Dorsal intercuneiform ligaments

Dorsal tarsometatarsal ligaments

Joint capsule of metatarsophalangeal joint

Anterior view

Lateral view

Interosseous talocalcaneal ligament

Bifurcate ligament

Dorsal talonavicular ligament

Navicular

Dorsal intercuneiform ligament

Dorsal cuneocuboid ligament

Lateral talocalcaneal ligament (cut)

Calcaneal tendon (cut)

Calcaneus

Dorsal calcaneocuboid ligament

Fibularis longus tendon (cut)

Fibularis brevis tendon (cut)

Cuboid

Tuberosity of fifth metatarsal

Dorsal talonavicular ligament

Talus

Sustentaculum tali

Flexor hallucis longus tendon (cut)

Medial tubercle of talus

Calcaneal tendon (cut)

Medial talocalcaneal ligament

Calcaneus

Plantar calcaneonavicular ligament (spring ligament)

Navicular

Dorsal cuneonavicular ligaments

Dorsal intercuneiform ligament

Medial cuneiform

Dorsal tarsometatarsal ligaments

First metatarsal

First proximal phalanx

First distal phalanx

Collateral ligaments

Tibialis anterior tendon (cut)

Plantar calcaneocuboid ligament (short plantar ligament)

Long plantar ligament

Plantar aponeurosis

Tibialis posterior tendon (cut)

Medial view

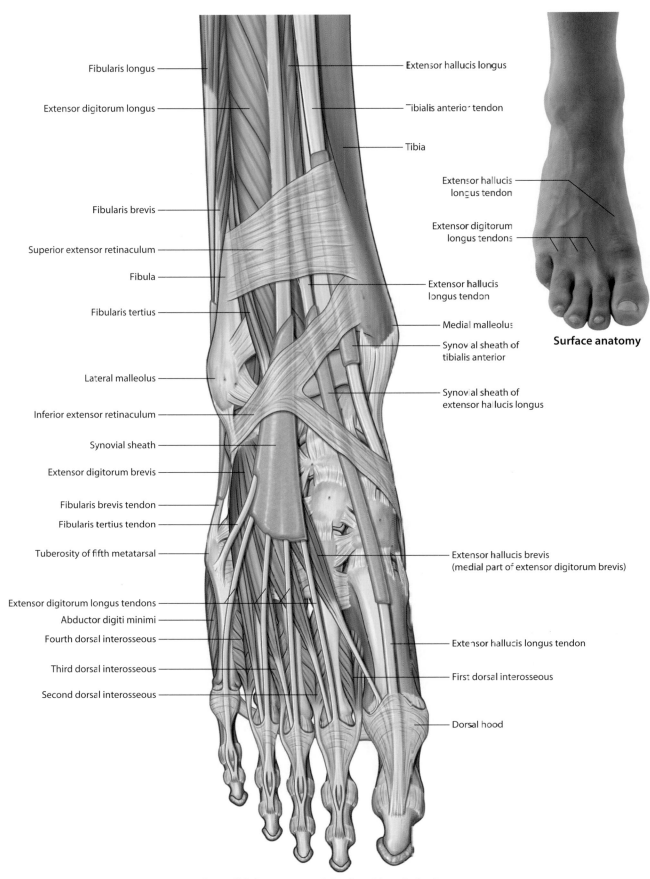

Fibularis longus

Extensor digitorum longus

Fibularis brevis

Superior extensor retinaculum

Fibula

Fibularis tertius

Lateral malleolus

Inferior extensor retinaculum

Synovial sheath

Extensor digitorum brevis

Fibularis brevis tendon

Fibularis tertius tendon

Tuberosity of fifth metatarsal

Extensor digitorum longus tendons

Abductor digiti minimi

Fourth dorsal interosseous

Third dorsal interosseous

Second dorsal interosseous

Extensor hallucis longus

Tibialis anterior tendon

Tibia

Extensor hallucis longus tendon

Extensor digitorum longus tendons

Surface anatomy

Extensor hallucis longus tendon

Medial malleolus

Synovial sheath of tibialis anterior

Synovial sheath of extensor hallucis longus

Extensor hallucis brevis (medial part of extensor digitorum brevis)

Extensor hallucis longus tendon

First dorsal interosseous

Dorsal hood

Superficial structures of the foot (dorsal view)

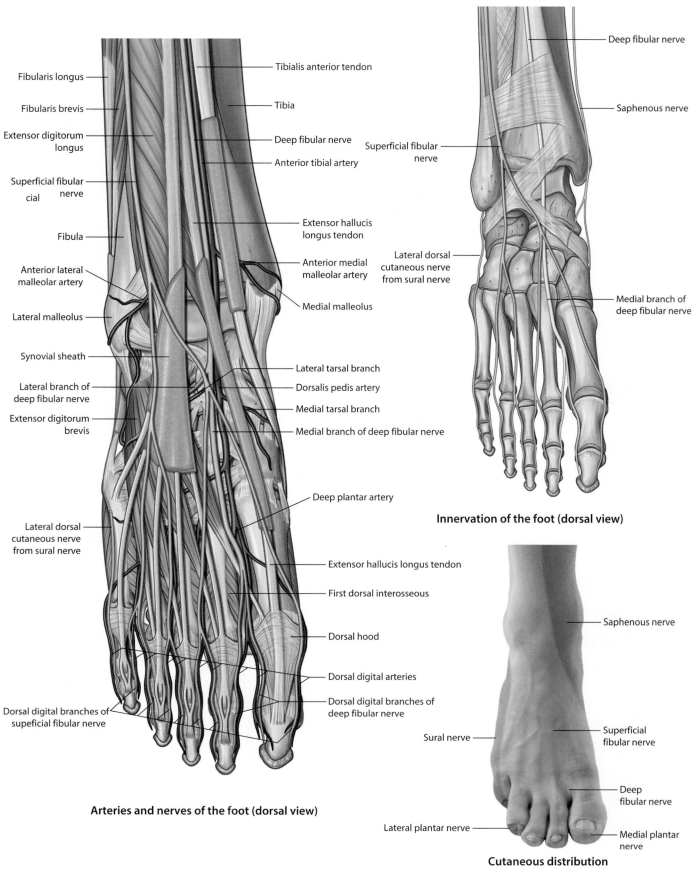

Fibularis longus

Fibularis brevis

Extensor digitorum longus

Superficial fibular cial nerve

Fibula

Anterior lateral malleolar artery

Lateral malleolus

Synovial sheath

Lateral branch of deep fibular nerve

Extensor digitorum brevis

Lateral dorsal cutaneous nerve from sural nerve

Dorsal digital branches of supeficial fibular nerve

Tibialis anterior tendon

Tibia

Deep fibular nerve

Anterior tibial artery

Extensor hallucis longus tendon

Anterior medial malleolar artery

Medial malleolus

Lateral tarsal branch

Dorsalis pedis artery

Medial tarsal branch

Medial branch of deep fibular nerve

Deep plantar artery

Extensor hallucis longus tendon

First dorsal interosseous

Dorsal hood

Dorsal digital arteries

Dorsal digital branches of deep fibular nerve

Arteries and nerves of the foot (dorsal view)

Deep fibular nerve

Saphenous nerve

Superficial fibular nerve

Lateral dorsal cutaneous nerve from sural nerve

Medial branch of deep fibular nerve

Innervation of the foot (dorsal view)

Saphenous nerve

Sural nerve

Superficial fibular nerve

Deep fibular nerve

Lateral plantar nerve

Medial plantar nerve

Cutaneous distribution

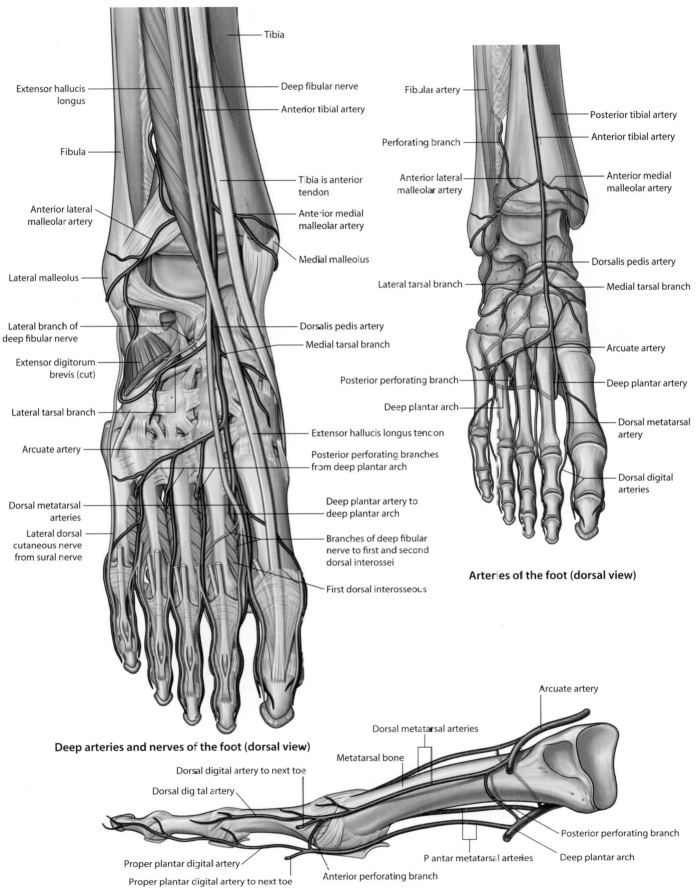

Extensor hallucis longus

Tibia

Deep fibular nerve

Anterior tibial artery

Tibia is anterior tendon

Fibula

Anterior medial malleolar artery

Anterior lateral malleolar artery

Medial malleolus

Lateral malleolus

Dorsalis pedis artery

Lateral branch of deep fibular nerve

Medial tarsal branch

Extensor digitorum brevis (cut)

Lateral tarsal branch

Arcuate artery

Extensor hallucis longus tendon

Dorsal metatarsal arteries

Posterior perforating branches from deep plantar arch

Lateral dorsal cutaneous nerve from sural nerve

Deep plantar artery to deep plantar arch

Branches of deep fibular nerve to first and second dorsal interossei

First dorsal interosseous

Deep arteries and nerves of the foot (dorsal view)

Fibular artery

Posterior tibial artery

Perforating branch

Anterior tibial artery

Anterior lateral malleolar artery

Anterior medial malleolar artery

Dorsalis pedis artery

Lateral tarsal branch

Medial tarsal branch

Arcuate artery

Posterior perforating branch

Deep plantar artery

Deep plantar arch

Dorsal metatarsal artery

Dorsal digital arteries

Arteries of the foot (dorsal view)

Arcuate artery

Dorsal metatarsal arteries

Metatarsal bone

Dorsal digital artery to next toe

Dorsal digital artery

Posterior perforating branch

Proper plantar digital artery

Plantar metatarsal arteries

Deep plantar arch

Anterior perforating branch

Proper plantar digital artery to next toe

Arteries of digit III (middle toe)

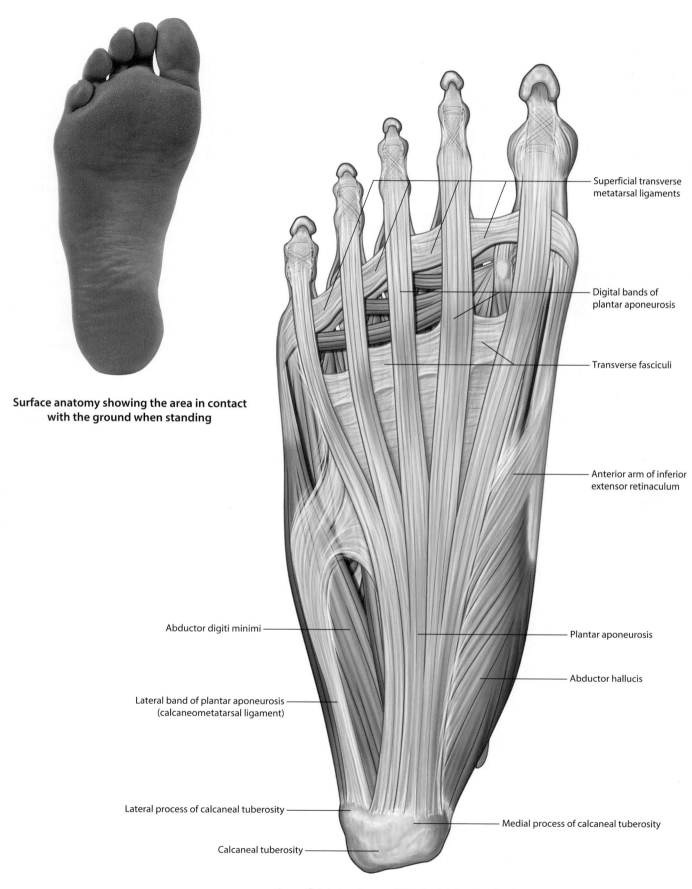

Surface anatomy showing the area in contact with the ground when standing

Superficial transverse metatarsal ligaments

Digital bands of plantar aponeurosis

Transverse fasciculi

Anterior arm of inferior extensor retinaculum

Abductor digiti minimi

Lateral band of plantar aponeurosis (calcaneometatarsal ligament)

Plantar aponeurosis

Abductor hallucis

Lateral process of calcaneal tuberosity

Medial process of calcaneal tuberosity

Calcaneal tuberosity

Superficial structures of the foot (plantar view)

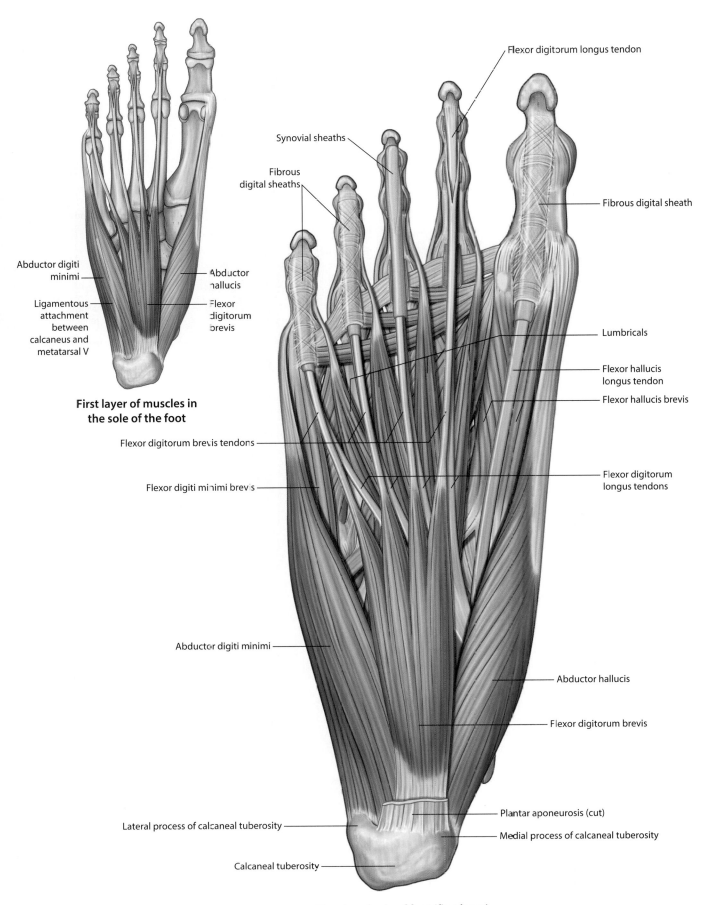

Flexor digitorum longus tendon

Synovial sheaths

Fibrous
digital sheaths

Fibrous digital sheath

Abductor digiti
minimi

Abductor
hallucis

Ligamentous
attachment
between
calcaneus and
metatarsal V

Flexor
digitorum
brevis

Lumbricals

Flexor hallucis
longus tendon

Flexor hallucis brevis

**First layer of muscles in
the sole of the foot**

Flexor digitorum longus tendons

Flexor digitorum brevis tendons

Flexor digiti minimi brevis

Abductor digiti minimi

Abductor hallucis

Flexor digitorum brevis

Plantar aponeurosis (cut)

Lateral process of calcaneal tuberosity

Medial process of calcaneal tuberosity

Calcaneal tuberosity

Muscles of sole of foot (first layer)

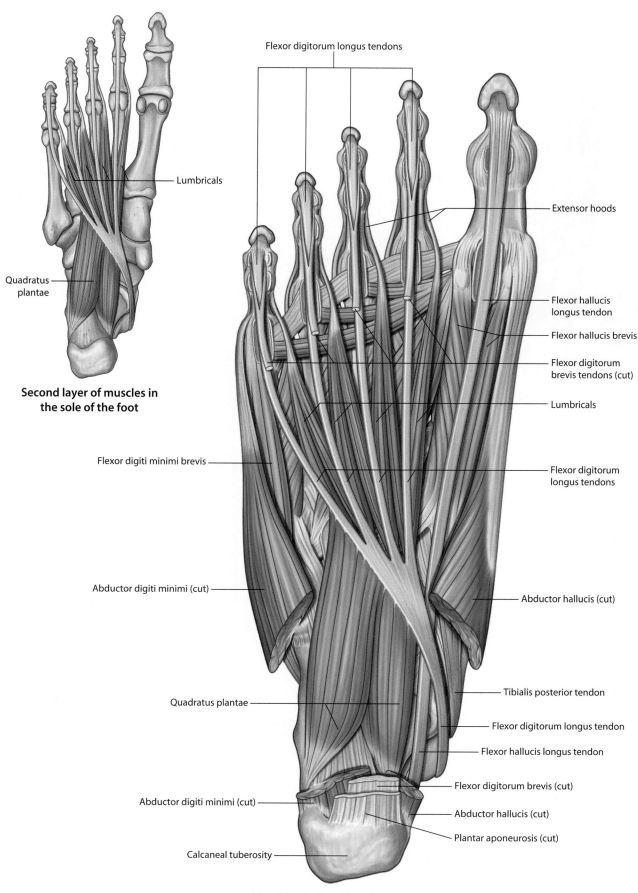

Flexor digitorum longus tendons

Lumbricals

Quadratus plantae

Second layer of muscles in the sole of the foot

Extensor hoods

Flexor hallucis longus tendon

Flexor hallucis brevis

Flexor digitorum brevis tendons (cut)

Lumbricals

Flexor digiti minimi brevis

Flexor digitorum longus tendons

Abductor digiti minimi (cut)

Abductor hallucis (cut)

Tibialis posterior tendon

Quadratus plantae

Flexor digitorum longus tendon

Flexor hallucis longus tendon

Flexor digitorum brevis (cut)

Abductor digiti minimi (cut)

Abductor hallucis (cut)

Plantar aponeurosis (cut)

Calcaneal tuberosity

Muscles of sole of foot (second layer)

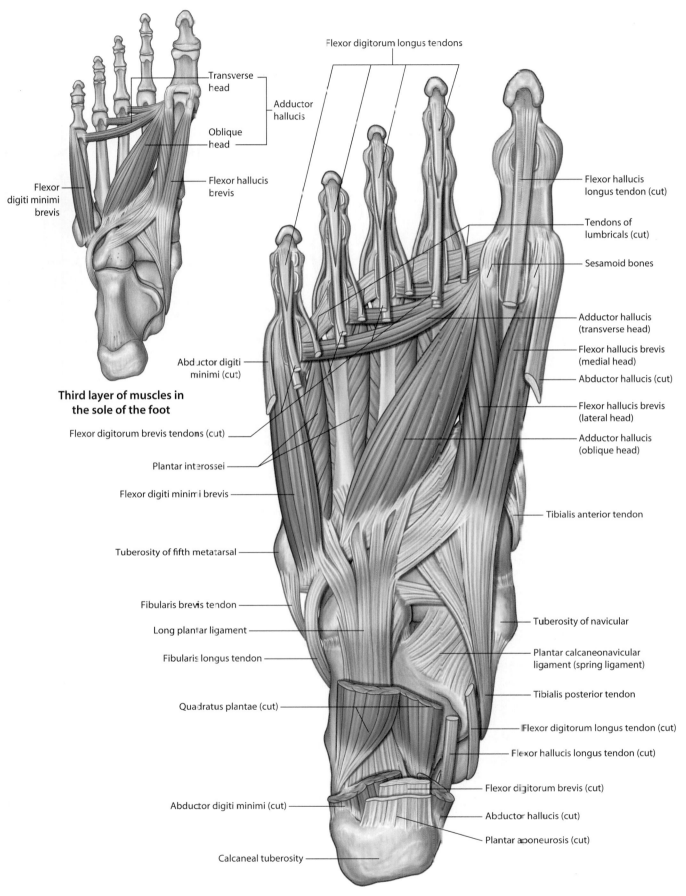

Flexor digitorum longus tendons

Transverse head

Adductor hallucis

Oblique head

Flexor hallucis brevis

Flexor digiti minimi brevis

Third layer of muscles in the sole of the foot

Flexor hallucis longus tendon (cut)

Tendons of lumbricals (cut)

Sesamoid bones

Adductor hallucis (transverse head)

Flexor hallucis brevis (medial head)

Abductor hallucis (cut)

Flexor hallucis brevis (lateral head)

Adductor hallucis (oblique head)

Abductor digiti minimi (cut)

Flexor digitorum brevis tendons (cut)

Plantar interossei

Flexor digiti minimi brevis

Tibialis anterior tendon

Tuberosity of fifth metatarsal

Fibularis brevis tendon

Long plantar ligament

Fibularis longus tendon

Tuberosity of navicular

Plantar calcaneonavicular ligament (spring ligament)

Tibialis posterior tendon

Quadratus plantae (cut)

Flexor digitorum longus tendon (cut)

Flexor hallucis longus tendon (cut)

Flexor digitorum brevis (cut)

Abductor digiti minimi (cut)

Abductor hallucis (cut)

Plantar aponeurosis (cut)

Calcaneal tuberosity

Muscles of sole of foot (third layer)

361

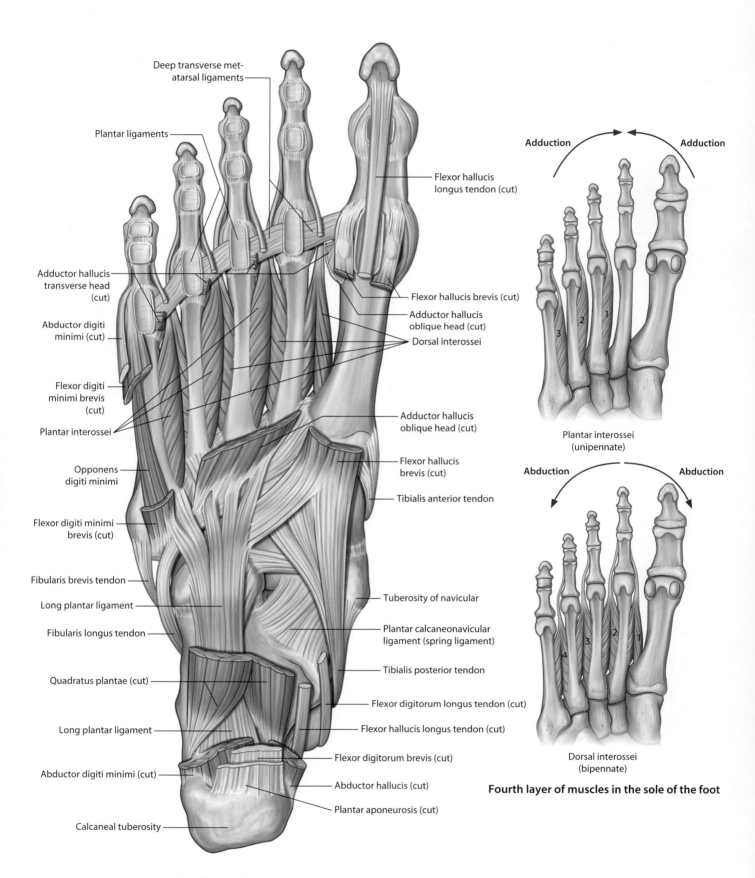

Deep transverse met-
atarsal ligaments

Plantar ligaments

Adductor hallucis
transverse head
(cut)

Abductor digiti
minimi (cut)

Flexor digiti
minimi brevis
(cut)

Plantar interossei

Opponens
digiti minimi

Flexor digiti minimi
brevis (cut)

Fibularis brevis tendon

Long plantar ligament

Fibularis longus tendon

Quadratus plantae (cut)

Long plantar ligament

Abductor digiti minimi (cut)

Calcaneal tuberosity

Flexor hallucis
longus tendon (cut)

Flexor hallucis brevis (cut)

Adductor hallucis
oblique head (cut)

Dorsal interossei

Adductor hallucis
oblique head (cut)

Flexor hallucis
brevis (cut)

Tibialis anterior tendon

Tuberosity of navicular

Plantar calcaneonavicular
ligament (spring ligament)

Tibialis posterior tendon

Flexor digitorum longus tendon (cut)

Flexor hallucis longus tendon (cut)

Flexor digitorum brevis (cut)

Abductor hallucis (cut)

Plantar aponeurosis (cut)

Muscles of sole of foot (fourth layer)

Adduction — **Adduction**

3   2   1

Plantar interossei
(unipennate)

Abduction — **Abduction**

4   3   2   1

Dorsal interossei
(bipennate)

Fourth layer of muscles in the sole of the foot

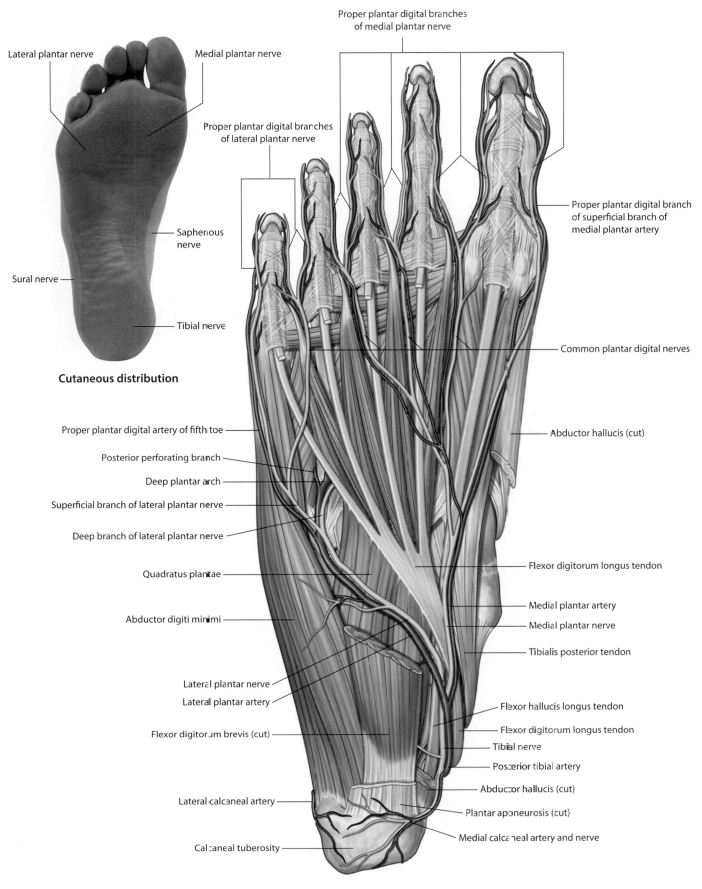

Lateral plantar nerve

Medial plantar nerve

Proper plantar digital branches
of medial plantar nerve

Proper plantar digital branches
of lateral plantar nerve

Saphenous
nerve

Sural nerve

Tibial nerve

Cutaneous distribution

Proper plantar digital branch
of superficial branch of
medial plantar artery

Common plantar digital nerves

Abductor hallucis (cut)

Proper plantar digital artery of fifth toe

Posterior perforating branch

Deep plantar arch

Superficial branch of lateral plantar nerve

Deep branch of lateral plantar nerve

Quadratus plantae

Abductor digiti minimi

Lateral plantar nerve

Lateral plantar artery

Flexor digitorum brevis (cut)

Lateral calcaneal artery

Calcaneal tuberosity

Flexor digitorum longus tendon

Medial plantar artery

Medial plantar nerve

Tibialis posterior tendon

Flexor hallucis longus tendon

Flexor digitorum longus tendon

Tibial nerve

Posterior tibial artery

Abductor hallucis (cut)

Plantar aponeurosis (cut)

Medial calcaneal artery and nerve

Arteries and nerves of sole of foot (plantar view)

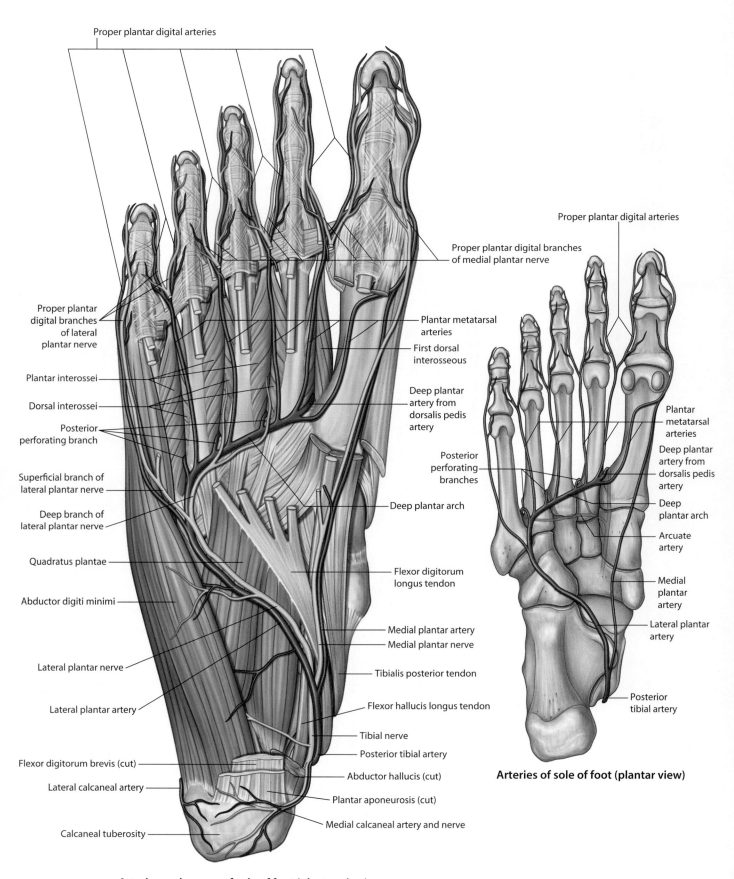

Proper plantar digital arteries

Proper plantar digital branches
of medial plantar nerve

Proper plantar
digital branches
of lateral
plantar nerve

Plantar metatarsal
arteries

First dorsal
interosseous

Plantar interossei

Dorsal interossei

Posterior
perforating branch

Deep plantar
artery from
dorsalis pedis
artery

Superficial branch of
lateral plantar nerve

Deep branch of
lateral plantar nerve

Deep plantar arch

Quadratus plantae

Flexor digitorum
longus tendon

Abductor digiti minimi

Lateral plantar nerve

Medial plantar artery

Medial plantar nerve

Tibialis posterior tendon

Lateral plantar artery

Flexor hallucis longus tendon

Tibial nerve

Posterior tibial artery

Flexor digitorum brevis (cut)

Lateral calcaneal artery

Abductor hallucis (cut)

Plantar aponeurosis (cut)

Calcaneal tuberosity

Medial calcaneal artery and nerve

Arteries and nerves of sole of foot (plantar view)

Proper plantar digital arteries

Plantar
metatarsal
arteries

Posterior
perforating
branches

Deep plantar
artery from
dorsalis pedis
artery

Deep
plantar arch

Arcuate
artery

Medial
plantar
artery

Lateral plantar
artery

Posterior
tibial artery

Arteries of sole of foot (plantar view)

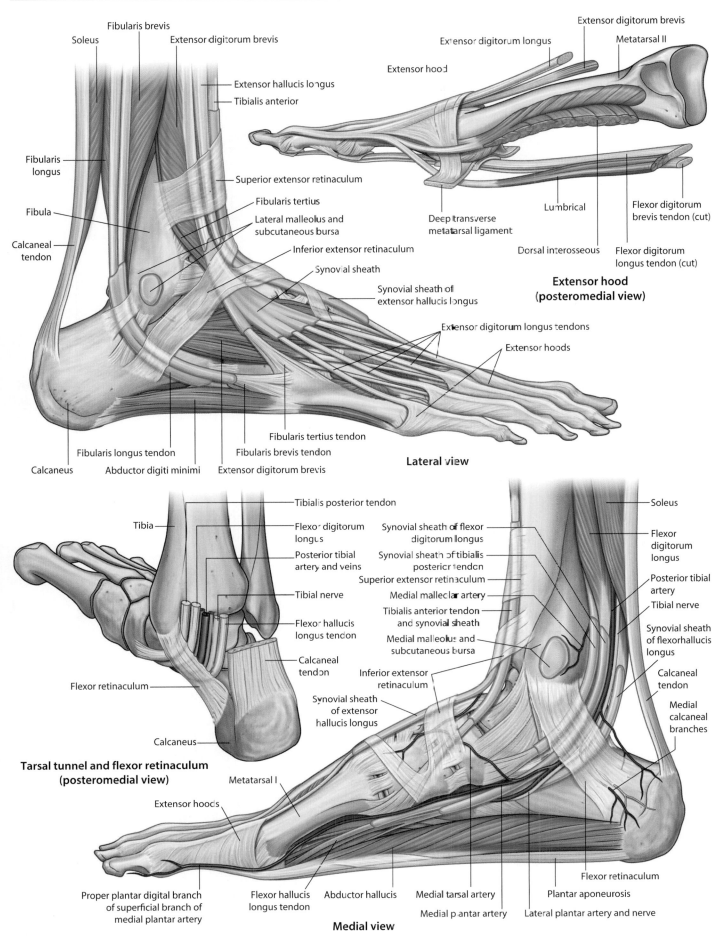

Soleus
Fibularis brevis
Extensor digitorum brevis
Extensor hallucis longus
Tibialis anterior
Fibularis longus
Fibula
Calcaneal tendon
Superior extensor retinaculum
Fibularis tertius
Lateral malleolus and subcutaneous bursa
Inferior extensor retinaculum
Synovial sheath
Synovial sheath of extensor hallucis longus
Fibularis longus tendon
Abductor digiti minimi
Extensor digitorum brevis
Fibularis brevis tendon
Fibularis tertius tendon
Calcaneus
Extensor digitorum longus tendons
Extensor hoods

Lateral view

Extensor digitorum longus
Extensor hood
Extensor digitorum brevis
Metatarsal II
Deep transverse metatarsal ligament
Lumbrical
Dorsal interosseous
Flexor digitorum brevis tendon (cut)
Flexor digitorum longus tendon (cut)

Extensor hood (posteromedial view)

Tibialis posterior tendon
Tibia
Flexor digitorum longus
Posterior tibial artery and veins
Tibial nerve
Flexor hallucis longus tendon
Calcaneal tendon
Flexor retinaculum
Calcaneus

Tarsal tunnel and flexor retinaculum (posteromedial view)

Synovial sheath of flexor digitorum longus
Synovial sheath of tibialis posterior tendon
Superior extensor retinaculum
Medial malleolar artery
Tibialis anterior tendon and synovial sheath
Medial malleolus and subcutaneous bursa
Inferior extensor retinaculum
Synovial sheath of extensor hallucis longus
Metatarsal I
Extensor hoods
Proper plantar digital branch of superficial branch of medial plantar artery
Flexor hallucis longus tendon
Abductor hallucis
Medial tarsal artery
Medial plantar artery

Soleus
Flexor digitorum longus
Posterior tibial artery
Tibial nerve
Synovial sheath of flexor hallucis longus
Calcaneal tendon
Medial calcaneal branches
Flexor retinaculum
Plantar aponeurosis
Lateral plantar artery and nerve

Medial view

365

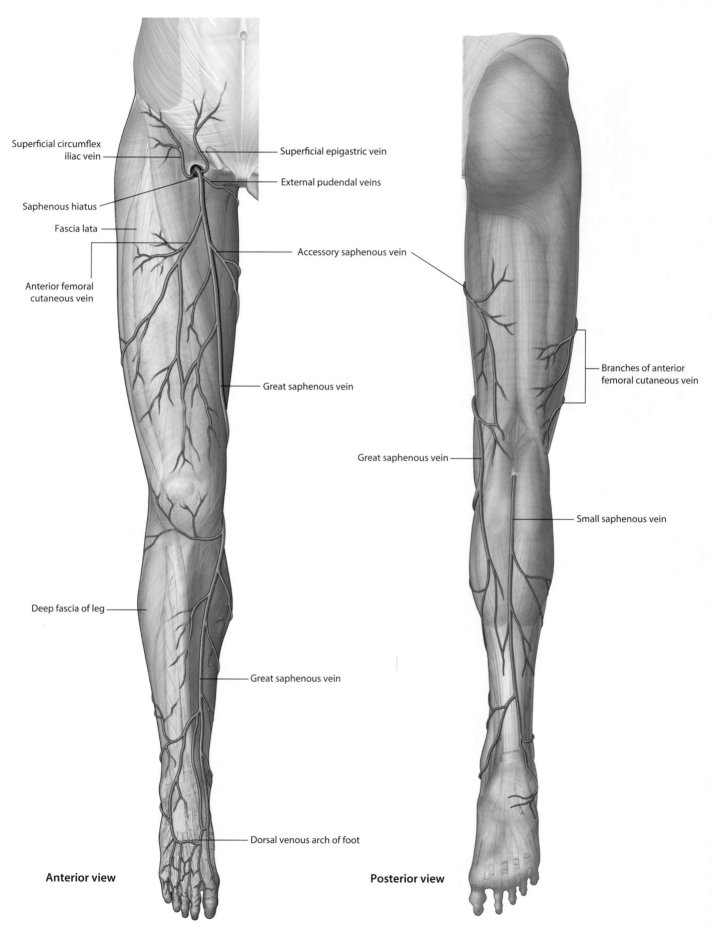

Superficial circumflex iliac vein

Saphenous hiatus

Fascia lata

Anterior femoral cutaneous vein

Deep fascia of leg

Superficial epigastric vein

External pudendal veins

Accessory saphenous vein

Great saphenous vein

Great saphenous vein

Dorsal venous arch of foot

Branches of anterior femoral cutaneous vein

Great saphenous vein

Small saphenous vein

Anterior view

Posterior view

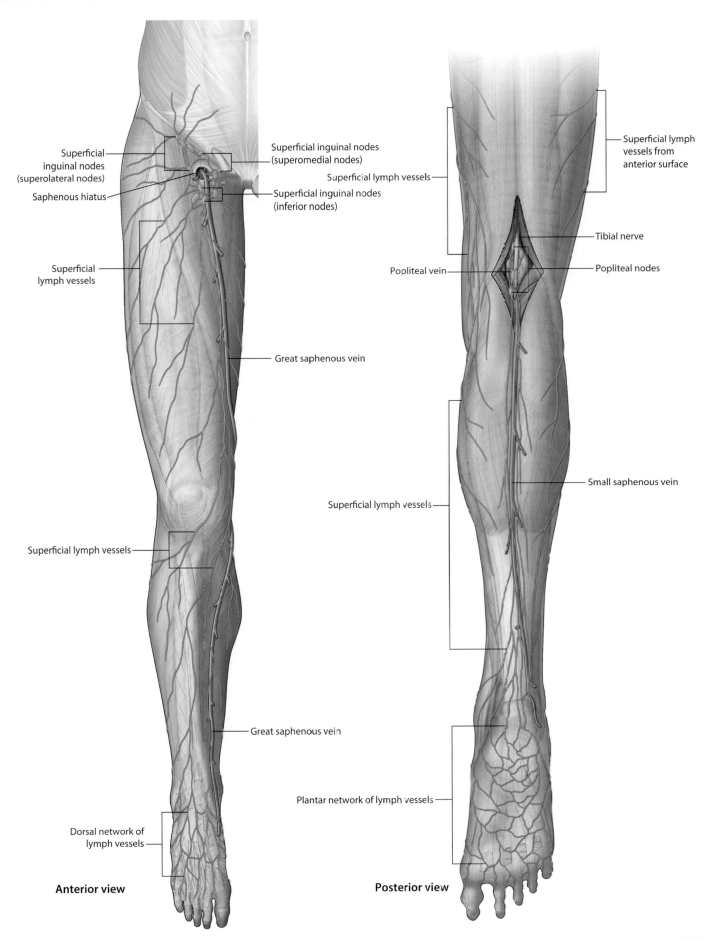

Superficial inguinal nodes (superolateral nodes)

Saphenous hiatus

Superficial lymph vessels

Superficial lymph vessels

Dorsal network of lymph vessels

Anterior view

Superficial inguinal nodes (superomedial nodes)

Superficial lymph vessels

Superficial inguinal nodes (inferior nodes)

Great saphenous vein

Great saphenous vein

Superficial lymph vessels from anterior surface

Tibial nerve

Popliteal vein

Popliteal nodes

Small saphenous vein

Superficial lymph vessels

Plantar network of lymph vessels

Posterior view

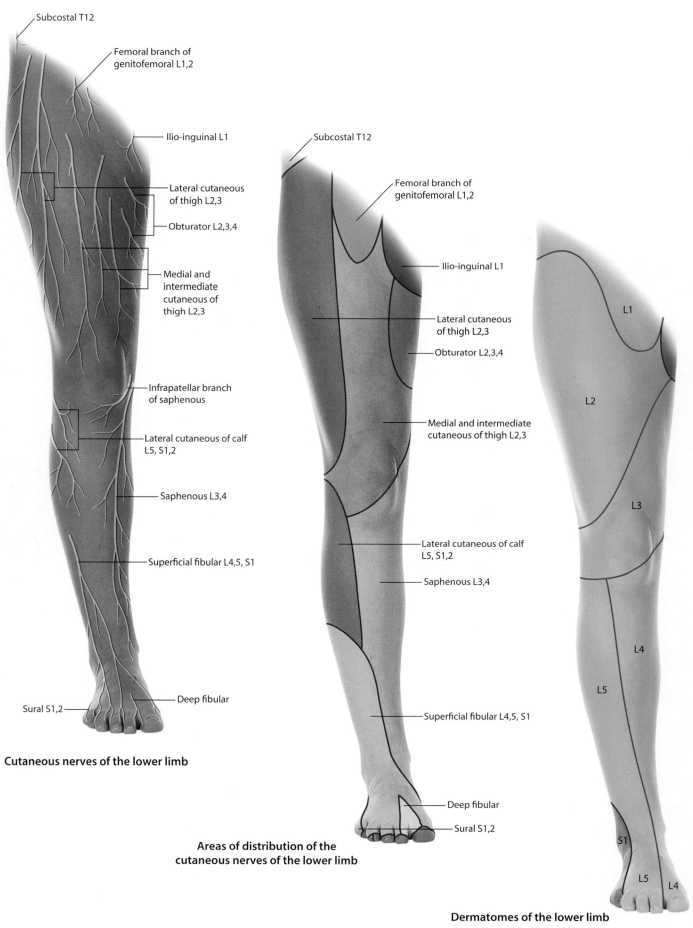

Subcostal T12

Femoral branch of
genitofemoral L1,2

Ilio-inguinal L1

Lateral cutaneous
of thigh L2,3

Obturator L2,3,4

Medial and
intermediate
cutaneous of
thigh L2,3

Infrapatellar branch
of saphenous

Lateral cutaneous of calf
L5, S1,2

Saphenous L3,4

Superficial fibular L4,5, S1

Sural S1,2

Deep fibular

Cutaneous nerves of the lower limb

Subcostal T12

Femoral branch of
genitofemoral L1,2

Ilio-inguinal L1

Lateral cutaneous
of thigh L2,3

Obturator L2,3,4

Medial and intermediate
cutaneous of thigh L2,3

Lateral cutaneous of calf
L5, S1,2

Saphenous L3,4

Superficial fibular L4,5, S1

Deep fibular

Sural S1,2

**Areas of distribution of the
cutaneous nerves of the lower limb**

L1

L2

L3

L4

L5

S1

L5

L4

Dermatomes of the lower limb

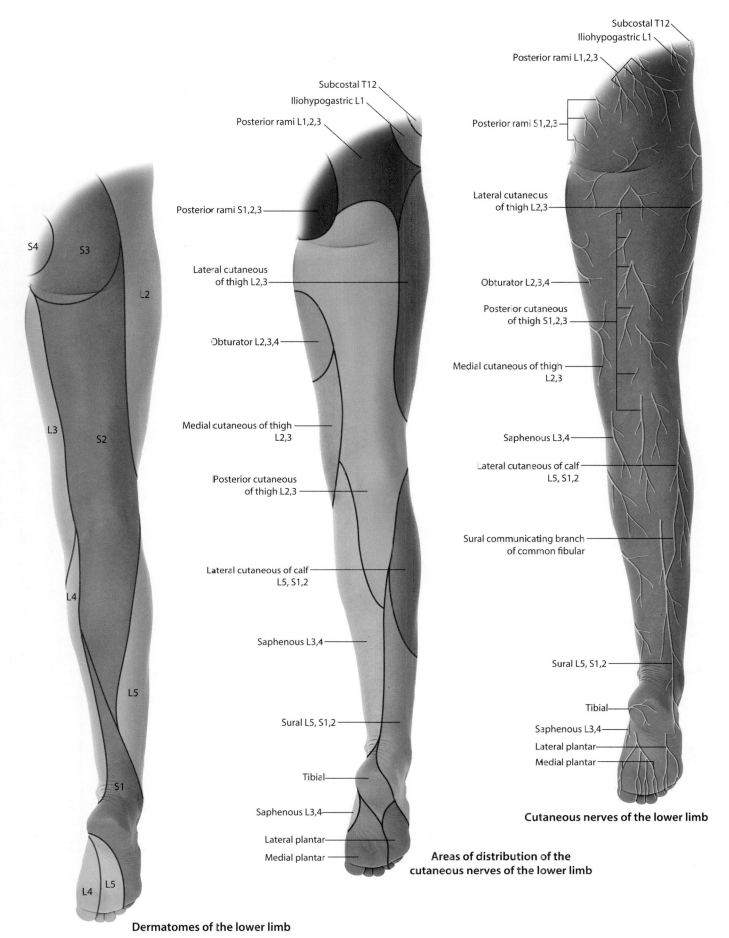

Subcostal T12
Iliohypogastric L1
Posterior rami L1,2,3

Posterior rami S1,2,3

Lateral cutaneous
of thigh L2,3

Obturator L2,3,4

Posterior cutaneous
of thigh S1,2,3

Medial cutaneous of thigh
L2,3

Saphenous L3,4

Lateral cutaneous of calf
L5, S1,2

Sural communicating branch
of common fibular

Sural L5, S1,2

Tibial

Saphenous L3,4

Lateral plantar

Medial plantar

Cutaneous nerves of the lower limb

Subcostal T12
Iliohypogastric L1
Posterior rami L1,2,3

Posterior rami S1,2,3

Lateral cutaneous
of thigh L2,3

Obturator L2,3,4

Medial cutaneous of thigh
L2,3

Posterior cutaneous
of thigh L2,3

Lateral cutaneous of calf
L5, S1,2

Saphenous L3,4

Sural L5, S1,2

Tibial

Saphenous L3,4

Lateral plantar

Medial plantar

**Areas of distribution of the
cutaneous nerves of the lower limb**

S4   S3

L2

L3   S2

L4

L5

S1

L4   L5

Dermatomes of the lower limb

Branches of the lumbosacral plexus associated with the lower limb

Branch		Spinal segments	Function: motor	Function: sensory (cutaneous)
Ilio-inguinal	1	L1	No motor function in lower limb, but innervates muscles of the abdominal wall	Skin over anteromedial part of upper thigh and adjacent skin of perineum
Genitofemoral	2	L1, L2	No motor function in lower limb, but genital branch innervates cremaster muscle in the wall of the spermatic cord in men	Femoral branch innervates skin on anterior central part of upper thigh; the genital branch innervates skin in anterior part of perineum (anterior scrotum in men, and mons pubis and anterior labia majora in women)
Femoral	3	L2 to L4	All muscles in the anterior compartment of thigh; in the abdomen, also gives rise to branches that supply iliacus and pectineus	Skin over the anterior thigh, anteromedial knee, medial side of the leg, and the medial side of the foot
Obturator	4	L2 to L4	All muscles in the medial compartment of thigh (except pectineus and the part of adductor magnus attached to the ischium); also innervates obturator externus	Skin over upper medial aspect of thigh
Sciatic	5	L4 to S3	All muscles in the posterior compartment of thigh and the part of adductor magnus attached to the ischium; all muscles in the leg and foot	Skin over lateral side of leg and foot, and over the sole and dorsal surface of foot
Superior gluteal	6	L4 to S1	Muscles of the gluteal region (gluteus medius, gluteus minimus, tensor fasciae latae)	
Inferior gluteal	7	L5 to S2	Muscle of the gluteal region (gluteus maximus)	
Lateral cutaneous nerve of thigh	8	L2, L3		Parietal peritoneum in iliac fossa; skin over anterolateral thigh
Posterior cutaneous nerve of thigh	9	S1 to S3		Skin over gluteal fold and upper medial aspect of thigh and adjacent perineum, posterior aspect of thigh and upper posterior leg
Nerve to quadratus femoris	10	L4 to S1	Muscles of gluteal region (quadratus femoris and gemellus inferior)	
Nerve to obturator internus	11	L5 to S2	Muscles of gluteal region (obturator internus and gemellus superior)	
Perforating cutaneous nerve	12	S2, S3		Skin over medial aspect of gluteal fold

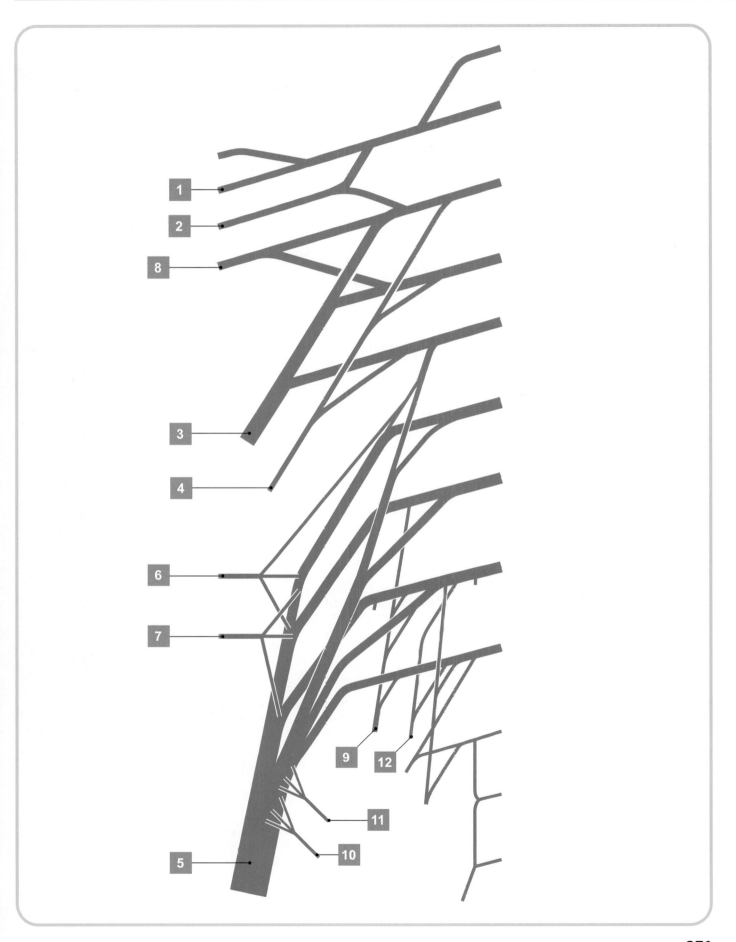

Muscles of the gluteal region

(spinal segments in bold are the major segments innervating the muscle)

Muscle		Origin	Insertion	Innervation	Function
Piriformis	1	Anterior surface of sacrum between anterior sacral foramina	Medial side of superior border of greater trochanter of femur	Branches from **L5**, **S1**, **S2**	Laterally rotates the extended femur at hip joint; abducts flexed femur at hip joint
Obturator internus	2	Anterolateral wall of true pelvis; deep surface of obturator membrane and surrounding bone	Medial side of greater trochanter of femur	Nerve to obturator internus (L5, **S1**)	Laterally rotates the extended femur at hip joint; abducts flexed femur at hip joint
Gemellus superior	3	External surface of ischial spine	Along length of superior surface of the obturator internus tendon and into the medial side of greater trochanter of femur with obturator internus tendon	Nerve to obturator internus (L5, **S1**)	Laterally rotates the extended femur at hip joint; abducts flexed femur at hip joint
Gemellus inferior	4	Upper aspect of ischial tuberosity	Along length of inferior surface of the obturator internus tendon and into the medial side of greater trochanter of femur with obturator internus tendon	Nerve to quadratus femoris (**L5**, **S1**)	Laterally rotates the extended femur at hip joint; abducts flexed femur at hip joint
Quadratus femoris	5	Lateral aspect of the ischium just anterior to the ischial tuberosity	Quadrate tubercle on the intertrochanteric crest of the proximal femur	Nerve to quadratus femoris (**L5**, **S1**)	Laterally rotates femur at hip joint
Gluteus minimus	6	External surface of ilium between inferior and anterior gluteal lines	Linear facet on the anterolateral aspect of the greater trochanter	Superior gluteal nerve (**L4**, **L5**, S1)	Abducts femur at hip joint; holds pelvis secure over stance leg and prevents pelvic drop on the opposite swing side during walking; medially rotates thigh
Gluteus medius	7	External surface of ilium between anterior and posterior gluteal lines	Elongate facet on the lateral surface of the greater trochanter	Superior gluteal nerve (**L4**, **L5**, S1)	Abducts femur at hip joint; holds pelvis secure over stance leg and prevents pelvic drop on the opposite swing side during walking; medially rotates thigh
Gluteus maximus	8	Fascia covering gluteus medius, external surface of ilium behind posterior gluteal line, fascia of erector spinae, dorsal surface of lower sacrum, lateral margin of coccyx, external surface of sacrotuberous ligament	Posterior aspect of iliotibial tract of fascia lata and gluteal tuberosity of proximal femur	Inferior gluteal nerve (**L5**, **S1**, S2)	Powerful extensor of flexed femur at hip joint; lateral stabilizer of hip joint and knee joint; laterally rotates and abducts thigh
Tensor fasciae latae	9	Lateral aspect of crest of ilium between anterior superior iliac spine and tubercle of the crest	Iliotibial tract of fascia lata	Superior gluteal nerve (**L4**, **L5**, S1)	Stabilizes the knee in extension

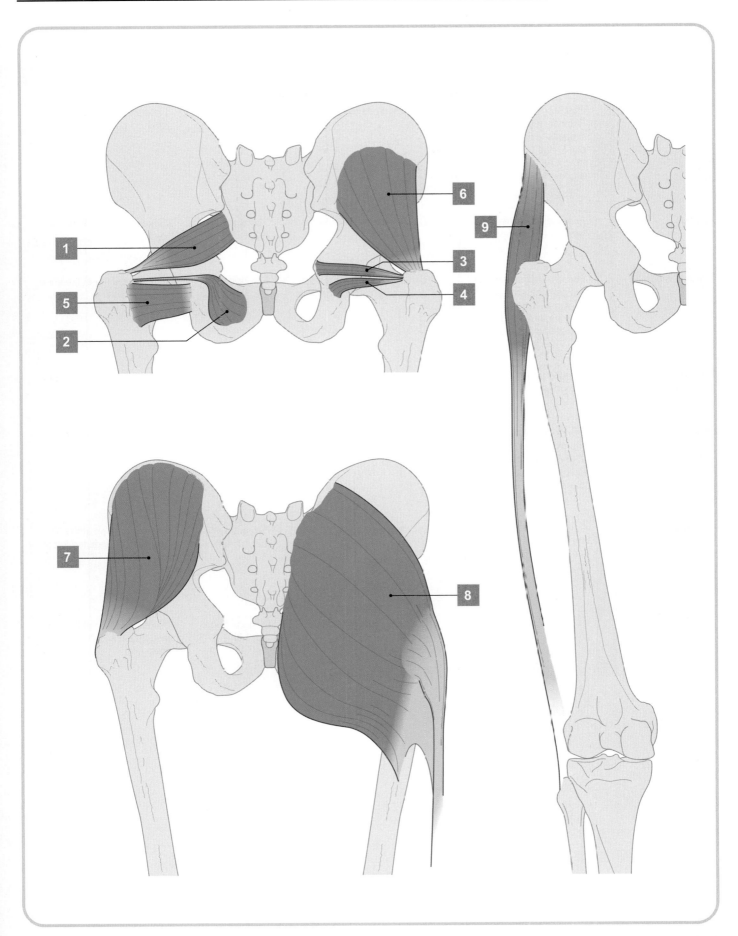

Muscles of the anterior compartment of thigh

(spinal segments in bold are the major segments innervating the muscle)

Muscle		Origin	Insertion	Innervation	Function
Psoas major	1	Posterior abdominal wall (lumbar transverse processes, intervertebral discs, and adjacent bodies from TXII to LV and tendinous arches between these points)	Lesser trochanter of femur	Anterior rami [**L1**, **L2**, L3]	Flexes the thigh at the hip joint
Iliacus	2	Posterior abdominal wall (iliac fossa)	Lesser trochanter of femur	Femoral nerve [**L2**, L3]	Flexes the thigh at the hip joint
Vastus medialis	3	Femur—medial part of intertrochanteric line, pectineal line, medial lip of the linea aspera, medial supracondylar line	Quadriceps femoris tendon and medial border of patella	Femoral nerve [L2, **L3**, **L4**]	Extends the leg at the knee joint
Vastus intermedius	4	Femur—upper two-thirds of anterior and lateral surfaces	Quadriceps femoris tendon and lateral margin of patella	Femoral nerve [L2, **L3**, **L4**]	Extends the leg at the knee joint
Vastus lateralis	5	Femur—lateral part of intertrochanteric line, margin of greater trochanter, lateral margin of gluteal tuberosity, lateral lip of the linea aspera	Quadriceps femoris tendon	Femoral nerve [L2, **L3**, **L4**]	Extends the leg at the knee joint
Rectus femoris	6	Straight head originates from the anterior inferior iliac spine; reflected head originates from the ilium just superior to the acetabulum	Quadriceps femoris tendon	Femoral nerve [L2, **L3**, **L4**]	Flexes the thigh at the hip joint and extends the leg at the knee joint
Sartorius	7	Anterior superior iliac spine	Medial surface of tibia just inferomedial to tibial tuberosity	Femoral nerve [**L2**, **L3**]	Flexes the thigh at the hip joint and flexes the leg at the knee joint

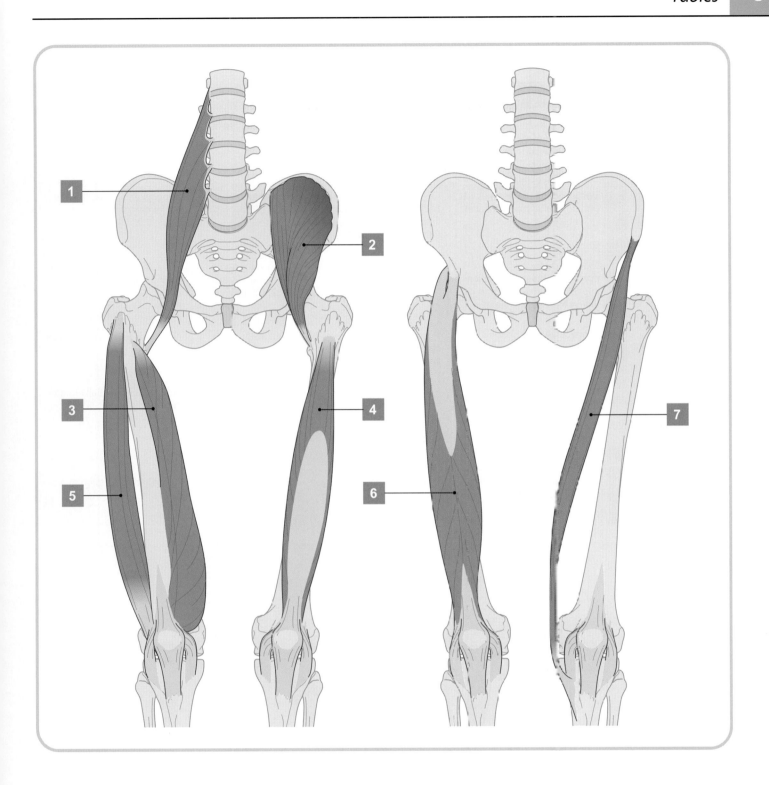

Muscles of the medial compartment of thigh
(spinal segments in bold are the major segments innervating the muscle)

Muscle		Origin	Insertion	Innervation	Function
Gracilis	1	A line on the external surfaces of the body of the pubis, the inferior pubic ramus, and the ramus of the ischium	Medial surface of proximal shaft of tibia	Obturator nerve [**L2**, L3]	Adducts thigh at hip joint and flexes leg at knee joint
Pectineus	2	Pectineal line (pecten pubis) and adjacent bone of pelvis	Oblique line extending from base of lesser trochanter to linea aspera on posterior surface of proximal femur	Femoral nerve [**L2**, L3]	Adducts and flexes thigh at hip joint
Adductor longus	3	External surface of body of pubis (triangular depression inferior to pubic crest and lateral to pubic symphysis)	Linea aspera on middle one-third of shaft of femur	Obturator nerve (anterior division) [**L2**, **L3**, L4]	Adducts and medially rotates thigh at hip joint
Adductor brevis	4	External surface of body of pubis and inferior pubic ramus	Posterior surface of proximal femur and upper one-third of linea aspera	Obturator nerve [**L2**, **L3**]	Adducts and medially rotates thigh at hip joint
Adductor magnus	5	Adductor part—ischiopubic ramus Hamstring part—ischial tuberosity	Posterior surface of proximal femur, linea aspera, medial supracondylar line Adductor tubercle and supracondylar line	Obturator nerve [**L2**, **L3**, L4] Sciatic nerve (tibial division) [**L2**, **L3**, L4]	Adducts and medially rotates thigh at hip joint
Obturator externus	6	External surface of obturator membrane and adjacent bone	Trochanteric fossa	Obturator nerve (posterior division) [L3, **L4**]	Laterally rotates thigh at hip joint

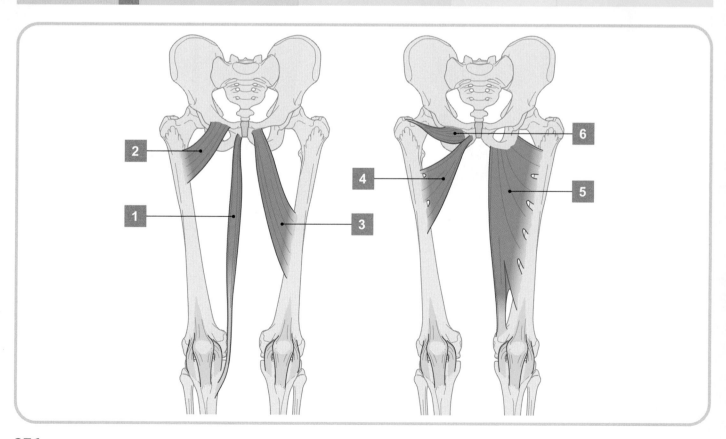

Muscles of the posterior compartment of thigh

(spinal segments in bold are the major segments innervating the muscle)

Muscle		Origin	Insertion	Innervation	Function
Biceps femoris	1	Long head—inferomedial part of the upper area of the ischial tuberosity; short head—lateral lip of linea aspera	Head of fibula	Sciatic nerve [L5, **S1**, S2]	Flexes leg at knee joint; extends and laterally rotates thigh at hip joint and laterally rotates leg at knee joint
Semitendinosus	2	Inferomedial part of the upper area of the ischial tuberosity	Medial surface of proximal tibia	Sciatic nerve [L5, **S1**, S2]	Flexes leg at knee joint and extends thigh at hip joint; medially rotates thigh at hip joint and leg at knee joint
Semimembranosus	3	Superolateral impression on the ischial tuberosity	Groove and adjacent bone on medial and posterior surface of medial tibial condyle	Sciatic nerve [L5, **S1**, S2]	Flexes leg at knee joint and extends thigh at hip joint; medially rotates thigh at hip joint and leg at knee joint

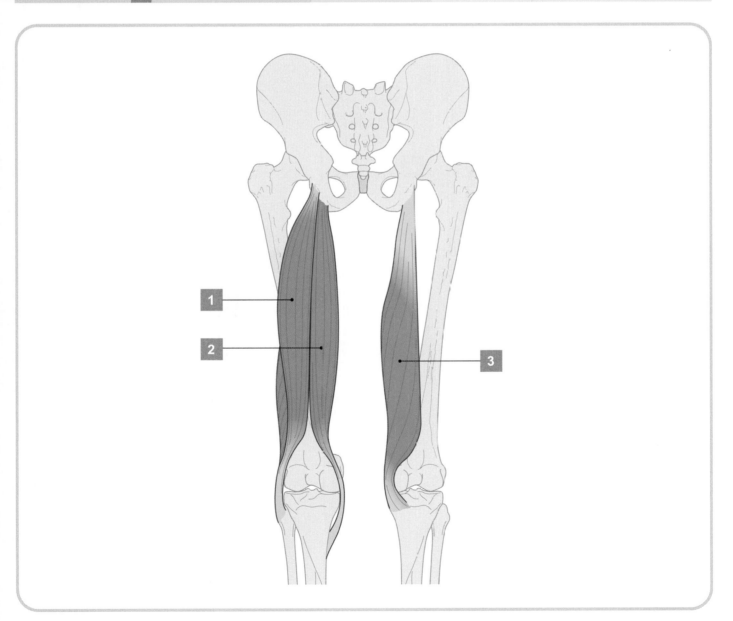

Superficial group of muscles in the posterior compartment of leg

(spinal segments in bold are the major segments innervating the muscle)

Muscle		Origin	Insertion	Innervation	Function
Gastrocnemius	1	Medial head—posterior surface of distal femur just superior to medial condyle; lateral head—upper posterolateral surface of lateral femoral condyle	Via calcaneal tendon, to posterior surface of calcaneus	Tibial nerve [**S1**, **S2**]	Plantarflexes foot and flexes knee
Plantaris	2	Inferior part of lateral supracondylar line of femur and oblique popliteal ligament of knee	Via calcaneal tendon, to posterior surface of calcaneus	Tibial nerve [**S1**, **S2**]	Plantarflexes foot and flexes knee
Soleus	3	Soleal line and medial border of tibia; posterior aspect of fibular head and adjacent surfaces of neck and proximal shaft; tendinous arch between tibial and fibular attachments	Via calcaneal tendon, to posterior surface of calcaneus	Tibial nerve [**S1**, **S2**]	Plantarflexes the foot

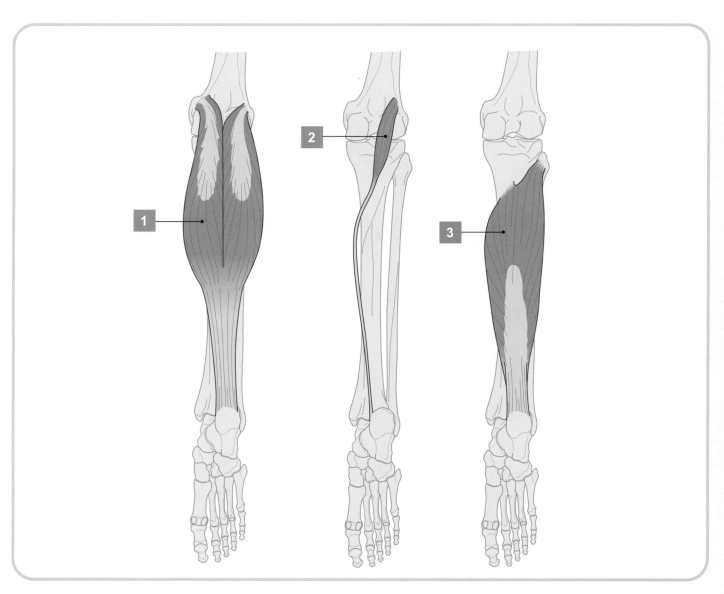

Deep group of muscles in the posterior compartment of leg

(spinal segments in bold are the major segments innervating the muscle)

Muscle		Origin	Insertion	Innervation	Function
Popliteus	1	Lateral femoral condyle	Posterior surface of proximal tibia	Tibial nerve [L4 to S1]	Stabilizes knee joint (resists lateral rotation of tibia on femur) Unlocks knee joint (laterally rotates femur on fixed tibia)
Flexor hallucis longus	2	Posterior surface of fibula and adjacent interosseous membrane	Plantar surface of distal phalanx of great toe	Tibial nerve [**S2**, S3]	Flexes great toe
Flexor digitorum longus	3	Medial side of posterior surface of the tibia	Plantar surfaces of bases of distal phalanges of the lateral four toes	Tibial nerve [**S2**, S3]	Flexes lateral four toes
Tibialis posterior	4	Posterior surfaces of interosseous membrane and adjacent regions of tibia and fibula	Mainly to tuberosity of navicular and adjacent region of medial cuneiform	Tibial nerve [L4, L5]	Inversion and plantarflexion of foot; support of medial arch of foot during walking

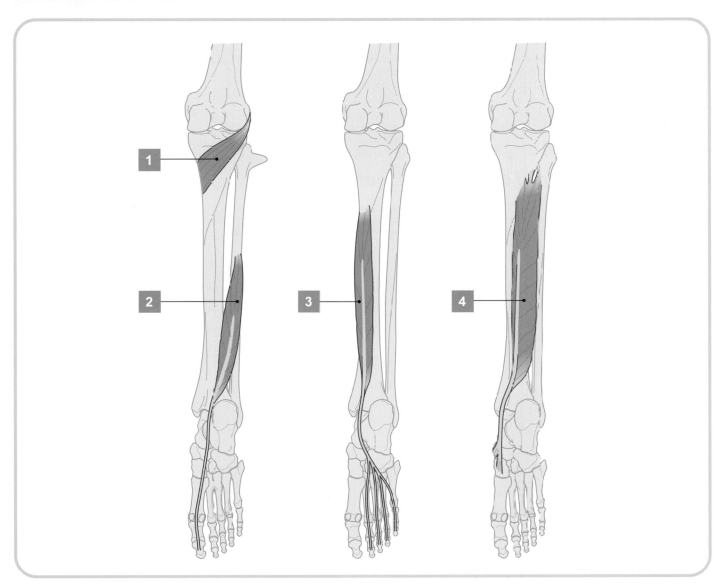

Muscles of the lateral compartment of leg

(spinal segments in bold are the major segments innervating the muscle)

Muscle		Origin	Insertion	Innervation	Function
Fibularis longus	1	Upper lateral surface of fibula, head of fibula, and occasionally the lateral tibial condyle	Undersurface of lateral sides of distal end of medial cuneiform and base of metatarsal I	Superficial fibular nerve [**L5**, **S1**, S2]	Eversion and plantarflexion of foot; supports arches of foot
Fibularis brevis	2	Lower two-thirds of lateral surface of shaft of fibula	Lateral tubercle at base of metatarsal V	Superficial fibular nerve [**L5**, **S1**, S2]	Eversion of foot

Muscles of the anterior compartment of leg

Muscle		Origin	Insertion	Innervation	Function
Tibialis anterior	3	Lateral surface of tibia and adjacent interosseous membrane	Medial and inferior surfaces of medial cuneiform and adjacent surfaces on base of metatarsal I	Deep fibular nerve [**L4**, L5]	Dorsiflexion of foot at ankle joint; inversion of foot; dynamic support of medial arch of foot
Extensor hallucis longus	4	Middle one-half of medial surface of fibula and adjacent surface of interosseous membrane	Dorsal surface of base of distal phalanx of great toe	Deep fibular nerve [**L5**, **S1**]	Extension of great toe and dorsiflexion of foot
Extensor digitorum longus	5	Proximal one-half of medial surface of fibula and related surface of lateral tibial condyle	Via dorsal digital expansions into bases of distal and middle phalanges of lateral four toes	Deep fibular nerve [**L5**, **S1**]	Extension of lateral four toes and dorsiflexion of foot
Fibularis tertius	6	Distal part of medial surface of fibula	Dorsomedial surface of base of metatarsal V	Deep fibular nerve [**L5**, **S1**]	Dorsiflexion and eversion of foot

Muscles of the dorsal aspect of the foot

Muscle		Origin	Insertion	Innervation	Function
Extensor digitorum brevis	7	Superolateral surface of the calcaneus	Lateral sides of the tendons of extensor digitorum longus of toes II to IV	Deep fibular nerve [**S1**, **S2**]	Extension of metatarsophalangeal joints of toes II to IV
Extensor hallucis brevis	8	Superolateral surface of calcaneus	Base of proximal phalanx of great toe	Deep fibular nerve [S1, S2]	Extension of metatarsophalangeal joint of great toe

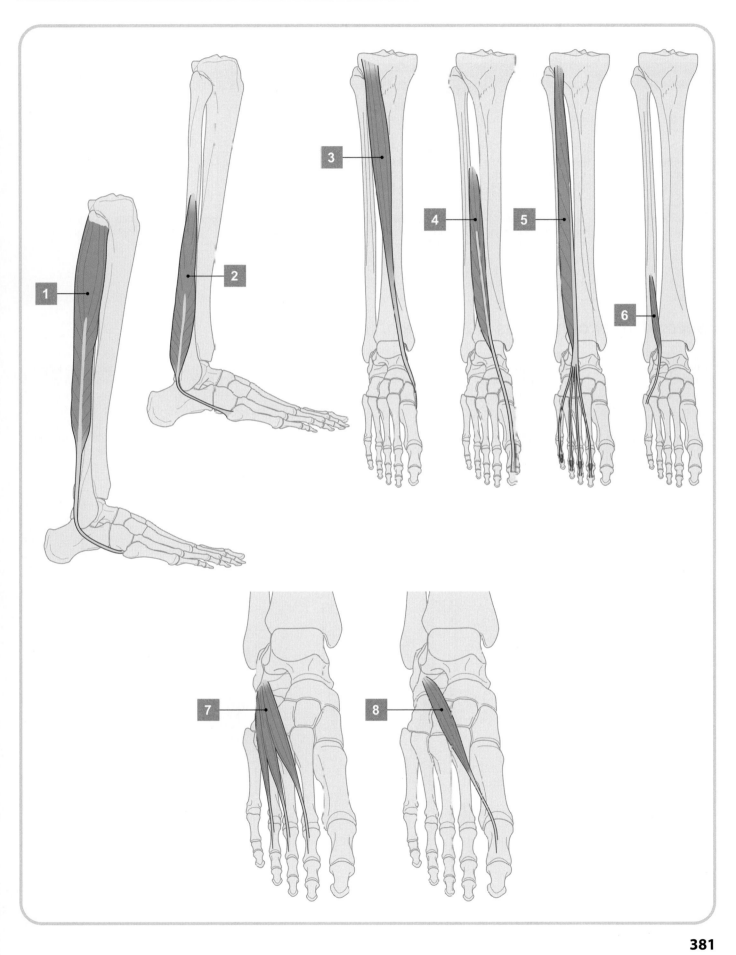

First layer of muscles in the sole of the foot

(spinal segments in bold are the major segments innervating the muscle)

Muscle		Origin	Insertion	Innervation	Function
Abductor hallucis	1	Medial process of calcaneal tuberosity	Medial side of base of proximal phalanx of great toe	Medial plantar nerve from the tibial nerve [**S1**, **S2**, S3]	Abducts and flexes great toe at metatarsophalangeal joint
Flexor digitorum brevis	2	Medial process of calcaneal tuberosity and plantar aponeurosis	Sides of plantar surface of middle phalanges of lateral four toes	Medial plantar nerve from the tibial nerve [**S1**, **S2**, S3]	Flexes lateral four toes at proximal interphalangeal joint
Abductor digiti minimi	3	Lateral and medial processes of calcaneal tuberosity, and band of connective tissue connecting calcaneus with base of metatarsal V	Lateral side of base of proximal phalanx of little toe	Lateral plantar nerve from the tibial nerve [**S1**, **S2**, S3]	Abducts little toe at the metatarsophalangeal joint

Second layer of muscles in the sole of the foot

Quadratus plantae	4	Medial surface of calcaneus and lateral process of calcaneal tuberosity	Lateral side of tendon of flexor digitorum longus in proximal sole of the foot	Lateral plantar nerve from tibial nerve [**S1**, **S2**, S3]	Assists flexor digitorum longus tendon in flexing toes II to V
Lumbricals	5	First lumbrical—medial side of tendon of flexor digitorum longus associated with toe II; second, third, and fourth lumbricals—adjacent surfaces of adjacent tendons of flexor digitorum longus	Medial free margins of extensor hoods of toes II to V	First lumbrical—medial plantar nerve from the tibial nerve; second, third, and fourth lumbricals—lateral plantar nerve from the tibial nerve [**S2**, **S3**]	Flexion of metatarsophalangeal joint and extension of interphalangeal joints

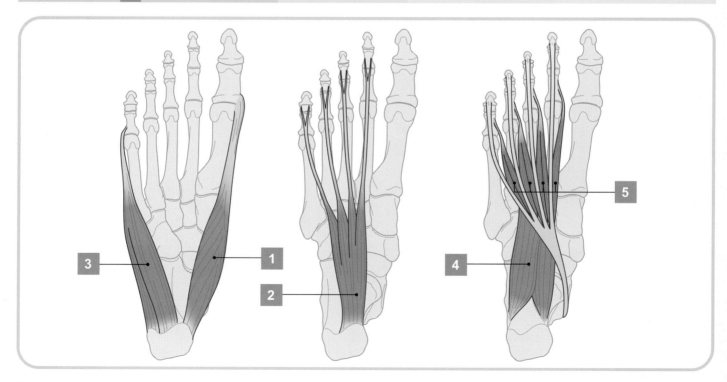

Third layer of muscles in the sole of the foot

(spinal segments in bold are the major segments innervating the muscle)

Muscle		Origin	Insertion	Innervation	Function
Flexor hallucis brevis	1	Plantar surface of cuboid and lateral cuneiform; tendon of tibialis posterior	Lateral and medial sides of base of proximal phalanx of the great toe	Medial plantar nerve from tibial nerve [**S1**, S2]	Flexes metatarsophalangeal joint of the great toe
Adductor hallucis	2	Transverse head—ligaments associated with metatarsophalangeal joints of lateral three toes; oblique head—bases of metatarsals II to IV and from sheath covering fibularis longus	Lateral side of base of proximal phalanx of great toe	Lateral plantar nerve from tibial nerve [**S2**, S3]	Adducts great toe at metatarsophalangeal joint
Flexor digiti minimi brevis	3	Base of metatarsal V and related sheath of fibularis longus tendon	Lateral side of base of proximal phalanx of little toe	Lateral plantar nerve from tibial nerve [**S2**, S3]	Flexes little toe at metatarsophalangeal joint

Fourth layer of muscles in the sole of the foot

Muscle		Origin	Insertion	Innervation	Function
Dorsal interossei	4	Sides of adjacent metatarsals	Extensor hoods and bases of proximal phalanges of toes II to IV	Lateral plantar nerve from tibial nerve; first and second dorsal interossei also innervated by deep fibular nerve [**S2**, **S3**]	Abduction of toes II to IV at metatarsophalangeal joints; resist extension of metatarsophalangeal joints and flexion of interphalangeal joints
Plantar interossei	5	Medial sides of metatarsals of toes III to V	Extensor hoods and bases of proximal phalanges of toes III to V	Lateral plantar nerve from tibial nerve [**S2**, **S3**]	Adduction of toes III to V at metatarsophalangeal joints; resist extension of the metatarsophalangeal joints and flexion of the interphalangeal joints

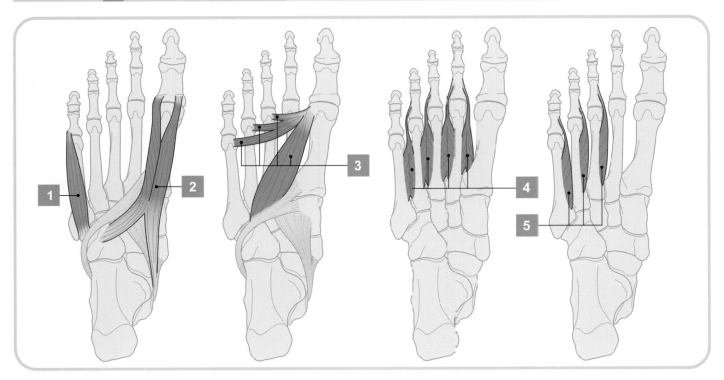

CONTENTS

UPPER LIMB

7

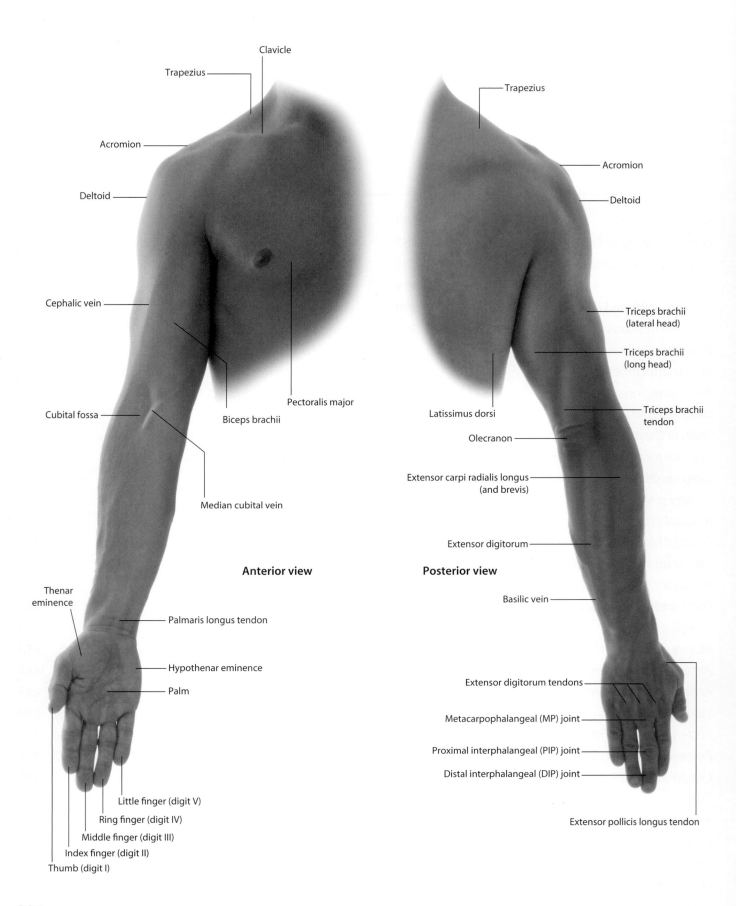

Clavicle

Trapezius

Acromion

Deltoid

Cephalic vein

Cubital fossa

Biceps brachii

Pectoralis major

Median cubital vein

Anterior view

Thenar eminence

Palmaris longus tendon

Hypothenar eminence

Palm

Little finger (digit V)

Ring finger (digit IV)

Middle finger (digit III)

Index finger (digit II)

Thumb (digit I)

Trapezius

Acromion

Deltoid

Triceps brachii (lateral head)

Triceps brachii (long head)

Latissimus dorsi

Triceps brachii tendon

Olecranon

Extensor carpi radialis longus (and brevis)

Extensor digitorum

Posterior view

Basilic vein

Extensor digitorum tendons

Metacarpophalangeal (MP) joint

Proximal interphalangeal (PIP) joint

Distal interphalangeal (DIP) joint

Extensor pollicis longus tendon

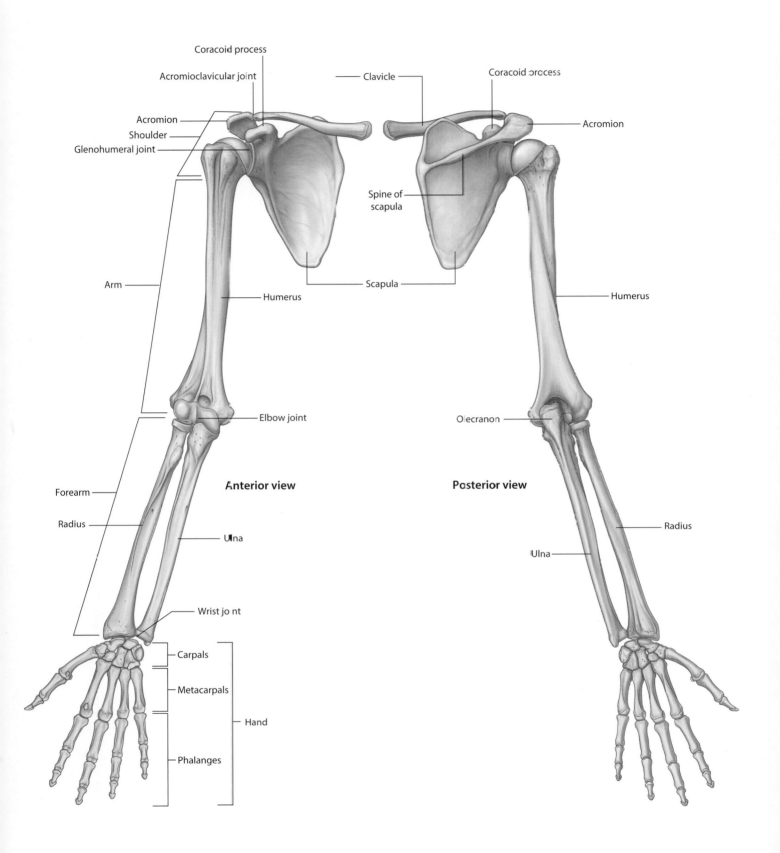

Coracoid process

Acromioclavicular joint

Clavicle

Coracoid process

Acromion

Acromion

Shoulder

Glenohumeral joint

Spine of
scapula

Arm

Humerus

Scapula

Humerus

Elbow joint

Olecranon

Anterior view

Posterior view

Forearm

Radius

Radius

Ulna

Ulna

Wrist joint

Carpals

Metacarpals

Hand

Phalanges

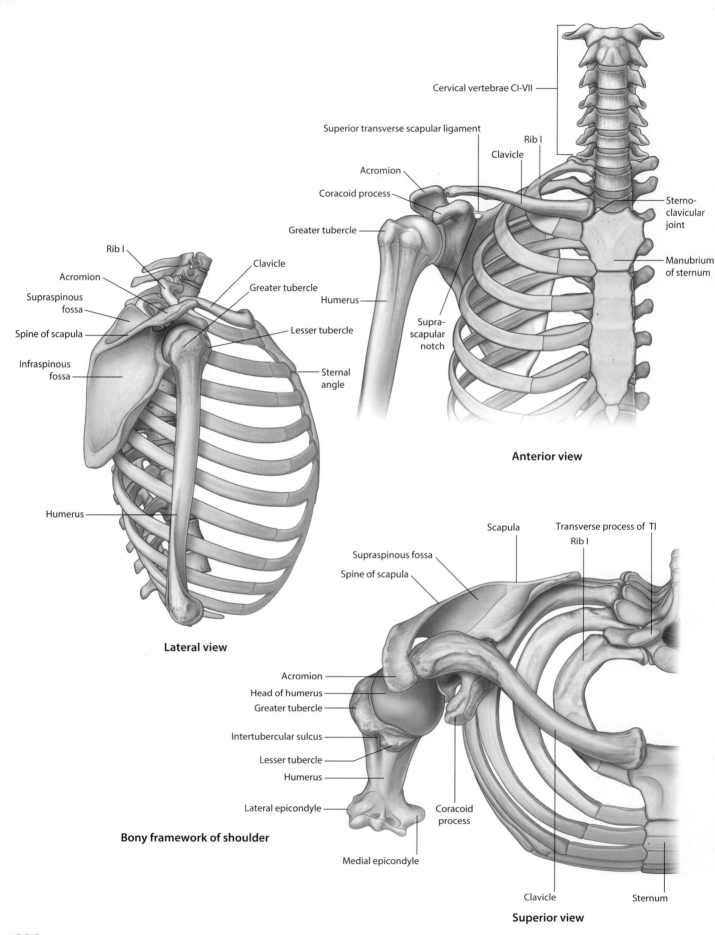

Cervical vertebrae CI-VII

Superior transverse scapular ligament

Rib I

Clavicle

Acromion

Coracoid process

Sterno-clavicular joint

Greater tubercle

Humerus

Manubrium of sternum

Supra-scapular notch

Anterior view

Rib I

Acromion

Clavicle

Supraspinous fossa

Greater tubercle

Spine of scapula

Lesser tubercle

Infraspinous fossa

Sternal angle

Humerus

Lateral view

Scapula

Supraspinous fossa

Transverse process of TI

Spine of scapula

Rib I

Acromion

Head of humerus

Greater tubercle

Intertubercular sulcus

Lesser tubercle

Humerus

Lateral epicondyle

Coracoid process

Bony framework of shoulder

Medial epicondyle

Clavicle

Sternum

Superior view

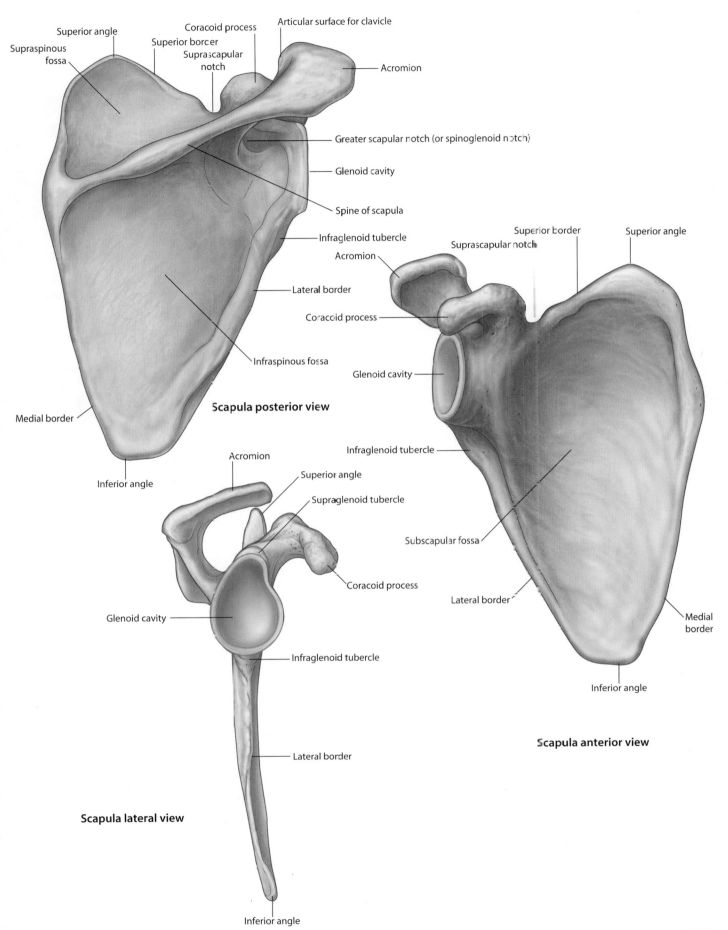

Superior angle

Supraspinous
fossa

Superior angle

Coracoid process

Superior border

Suprascapular
notch

Articular surface for clavicle

Acromion

Greater scapular notch (or spinoglenoid notch)

Glenoid cavity

Spine of scapula

Infraglenoid tubercle

Lateral border

Infraspinous fossa

Medial border

Inferior angle

Scapula posterior view

Superior border

Suprascapular notch

Superior angle

Acromion

Coracoid process

Glenoid cavity

Infraglenoid tubercle

Subscapular fossa

Lateral border

Medial
border

Inferior angle

Scapula anterior view

Acromion

Superior angle

Supraglenoid tubercle

Coracoid process

Glenoid cavity

Infraglenoid tubercle

Lateral border

Scapula lateral view

Inferior angle

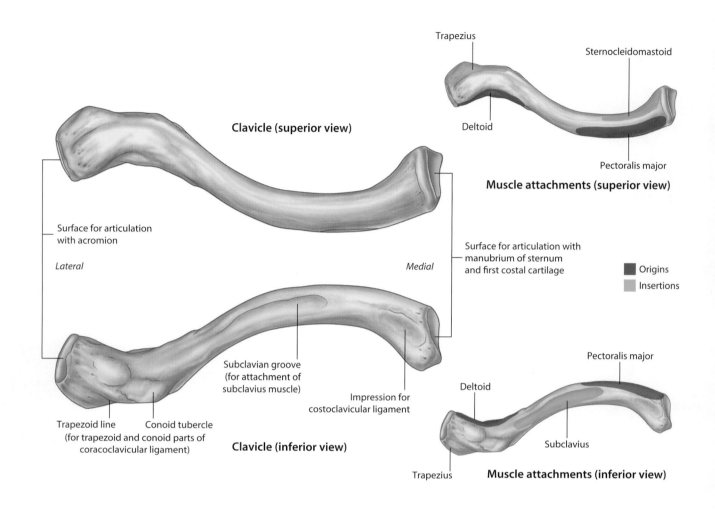

Trapezius

Sternocleidomastoid

Deltoid

Pectoralis major

Muscle attachments (superior view)

Clavicle (superior view)

Surface for articulation
with acromion

Lateral

Medial

Surface for articulation with
manubrium of sternum
and first costal cartilage

■ Origins
□ Insertions

Subclavian groove
(for attachment of
subclavius muscle)

Impression for
costoclavicular ligament

Pectoralis major

Deltoid

Trapezoid line
Conoid tubercle
(for trapezoid and conoid parts of
coracoclavicular ligament)

Clavicle (inferior view)

Subclavius

Trapezius

Muscle attachments (inferior view)

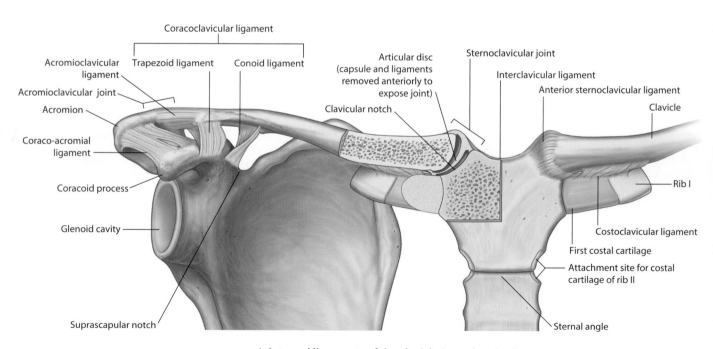

Coracoclavicular ligament

Acromioclavicular
ligament

Trapezoid ligament

Conoid ligament

Articular disc
(capsule and ligaments
removed anteriorly to
expose joint)

Sternoclavicular joint

Interclavicular ligament

Acromioclavicular joint

Anterior sternoclavicular ligament

Acromion

Clavicular notch

Clavicle

Coraco-acromial
ligament

Coracoid process

Rib I

Glenoid cavity

Costoclavicular ligament

First costal cartilage

Attachment site for costal
cartilage of rib II

Suprascapular notch

Sternal angle

Joints and ligaments of the clavicle (anterior view)

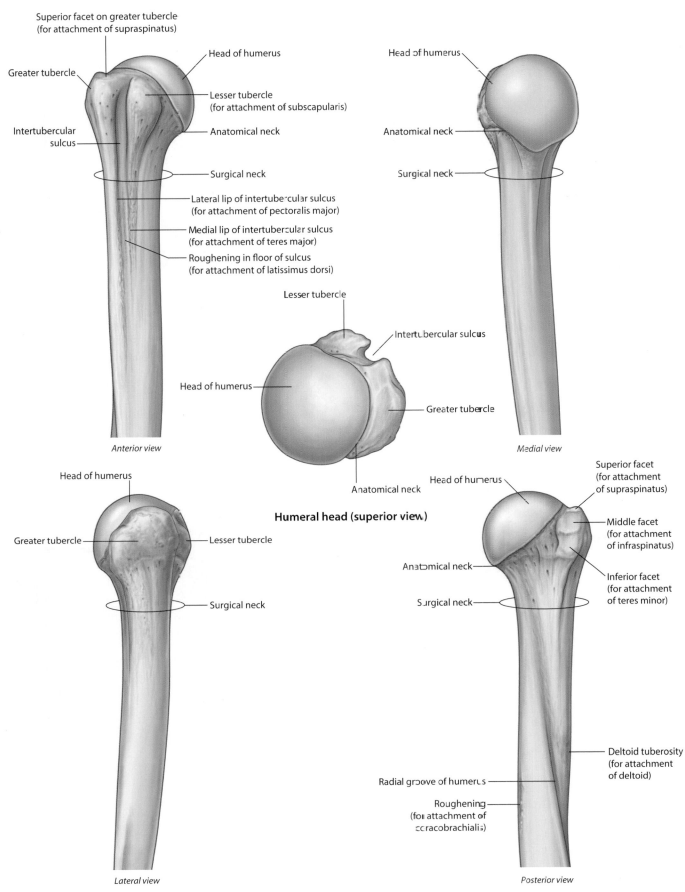

Superior facet on greater tubercle
(for attachment of supraspinatus)

Greater tubercle

Intertubercular
sulcus

Head of humerus

Lesser tubercle
(for attachment of subscapularis)

Anatomical neck

Surgical neck

Lateral lip of intertubercular sulcus
(for attachment of pectoralis major)

Medial lip of intertubercular sulcus
(for attachment of teres major)

Roughening in floor of sulcus
(for attachment of latissimus dorsi)

Anterior view

Head of humerus

Anatomical neck

Surgical neck

Medial view

Lesser tubercle

Intertubercular sulcus

Head of humerus

Greater tubercle

Anatomical neck

Humeral head (superior view)

Head of humerus

Greater tubercle

Lesser tubercle

Surgical neck

Lateral view

Head of humerus

Anatomical neck

Surgical neck

Superior facet
(for attachment
of supraspinatus)

Middle facet
(for attachment
of infraspinatus)

Inferior facet
(for attachment
of teres minor)

Deltoid tuberosity
(for attachment
of deltoid)

Radial groove of humerus

Roughening
(for attachment of
coracobrachialis)

Posterior view

Proximal end of humerus

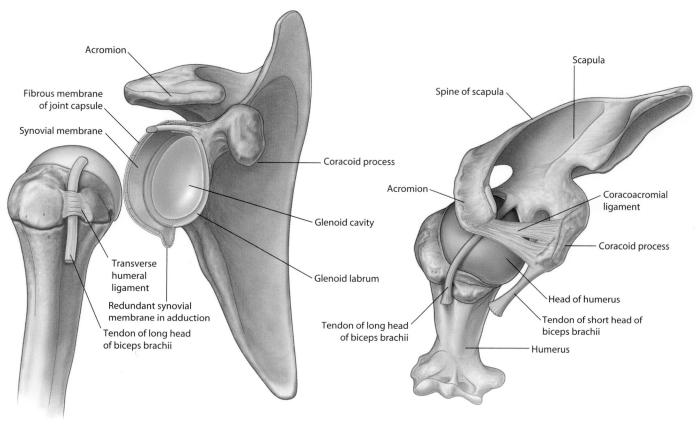

Acromion

Fibrous membrane
of joint capsule

Synovial membrane

Transverse
humeral
ligament

Redundant synovial
membrane in adduction

Tendon of long head
of biceps brachii

Coracoid process

Glenoid cavity

Glenoid labrum

Scapula

Spine of scapula

Acromion

Coracoacromial
ligament

Coracoid process

Head of humerus

Tendon of short head of
biceps brachii

Humerus

Tendon of long head
of biceps brachii

Origins of biceps brachii tendons (superior view)

Articular surfaces of glenohumeral joint (anterolateral oblique view)

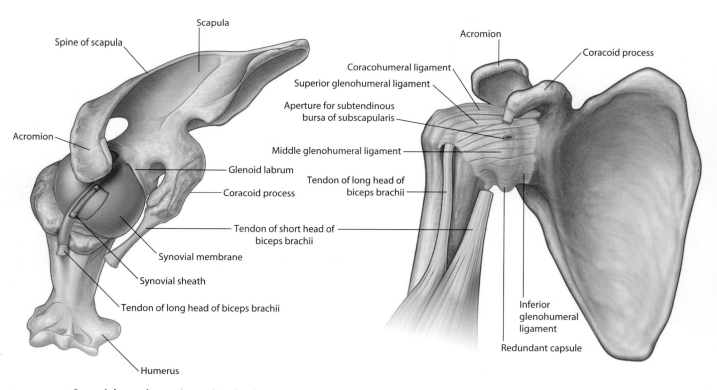

Spine of scapula

Scapula

Acromion

Glenoid labrum

Coracoid process

Tendon of short head of
biceps brachii

Synovial membrane

Synovial sheath

Tendon of long head of biceps brachii

Humerus

Synovial membrane (superior view)

Acromion

Coracohumeral ligament

Superior glenohumeral ligament

Aperture for subtendinous
bursa of subscapularis

Middle glenohumeral ligament

Tendon of long head of
biceps brachii

Coracoid process

Inferior
glenohumeral
ligament

Redundant capsule

Fibrous membrane of joint capsule (anterior view)

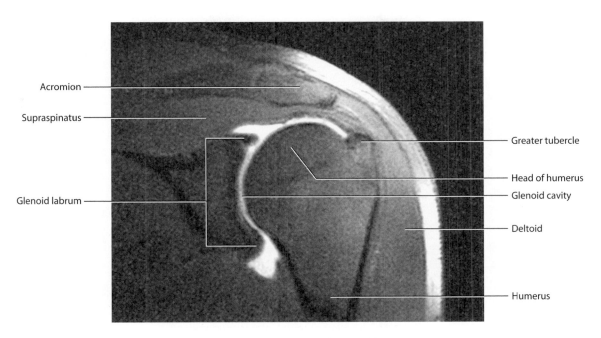

Acromion

Supraspinatus

Glenoid labrum

Greater tubercle

Head of humerus

Glenoid cavity

Deltoid

Humerus

Anterior view of the glenohumeral joint.
T1-weighted MR image in coronal plane

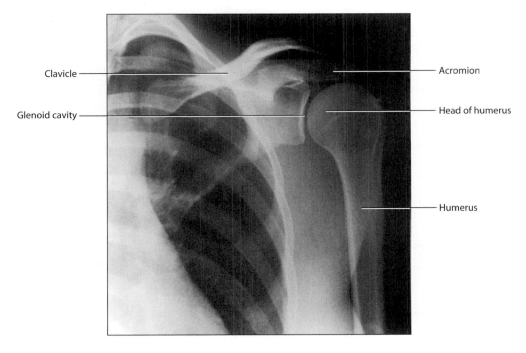

Clavicle

Glenoid cavity

Acromion

Head of humerus

Humerus

Normal glenohumeral joint.
Radiograph, AP view

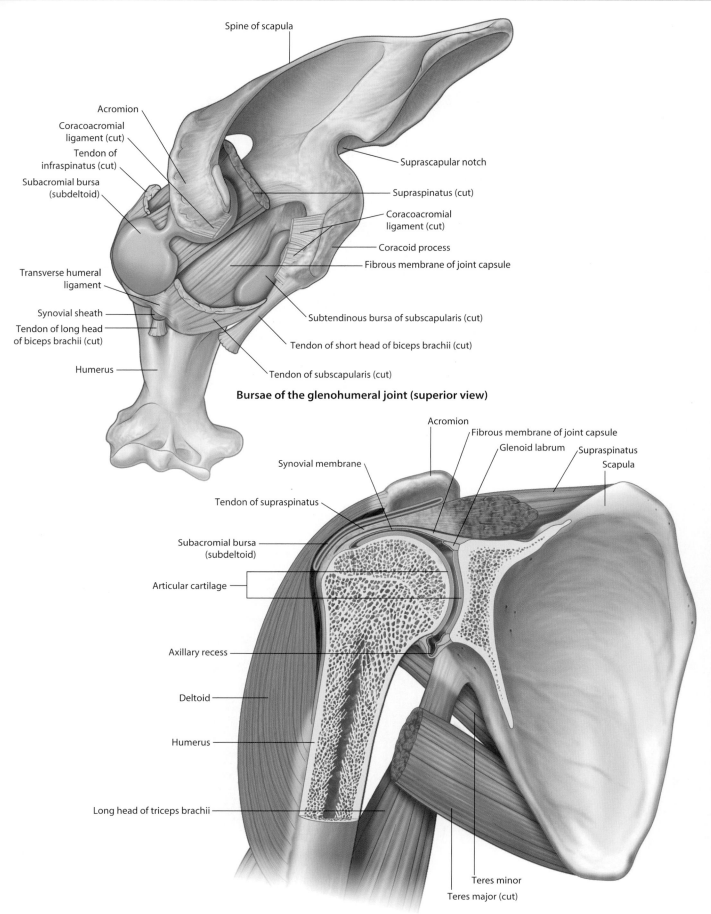

Spine of scapula

Acromion

Coracoacromial ligament (cut)

Tendon of infraspinatus (cut)

Subacromial bursa (subdeltoid)

Suprascapular notch

Supraspinatus (cut)

Coracoacromial ligament (cut)

Coracoid process

Fibrous membrane of joint capsule

Transverse humeral ligament

Synovial sheath

Tendon of long head of biceps brachii (cut)

Subtendinous bursa of subscapularis (cut)

Humerus

Tendon of short head of biceps brachii (cut)

Tendon of subscapularis (cut)

Bursae of the glenohumeral joint (superior view)

Acromion

Fibrous membrane of joint capsule

Glenoid labrum

Supraspinatus

Scapula

Synovial membrane

Tendon of supraspinatus

Subacromial bursa (subdeltoid)

Articular cartilage

Axillary recess

Deltoid

Humerus

Long head of triceps brachii

Teres minor

Teres major (cut)

Glenohumeral joint (anterior view)

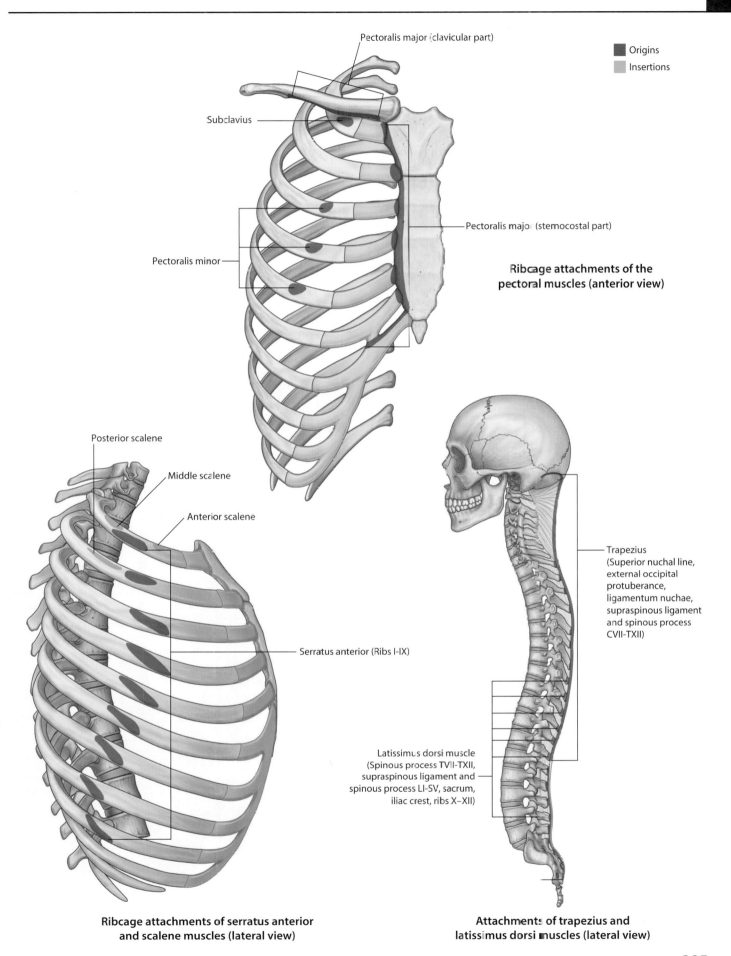

Pectoralis major (clavicular part)

Subclavius

Pectoralis minor

Pectoralis major (sternocostal part)

Origins
Insertions

Ribcage attachments of the pectoral muscles (anterior view)

Posterior scalene

Middle scalene

Anterior scalene

Serratus anterior (Ribs I–IX)

Trapezius
(Superior nuchal line, external occipital protuberance, ligamentum nuchae, supraspinous ligament and spinous process CVII–TXII)

Latissimus dorsi muscle
(Spinous process TVII–TXII, supraspinous ligament and spinous process LI–SV, sacrum, iliac crest, ribs X–XII)

Ribcage attachments of serratus anterior and scalene muscles (lateral view)

Attachments of trapezius and latissimus dorsi muscles (lateral view)

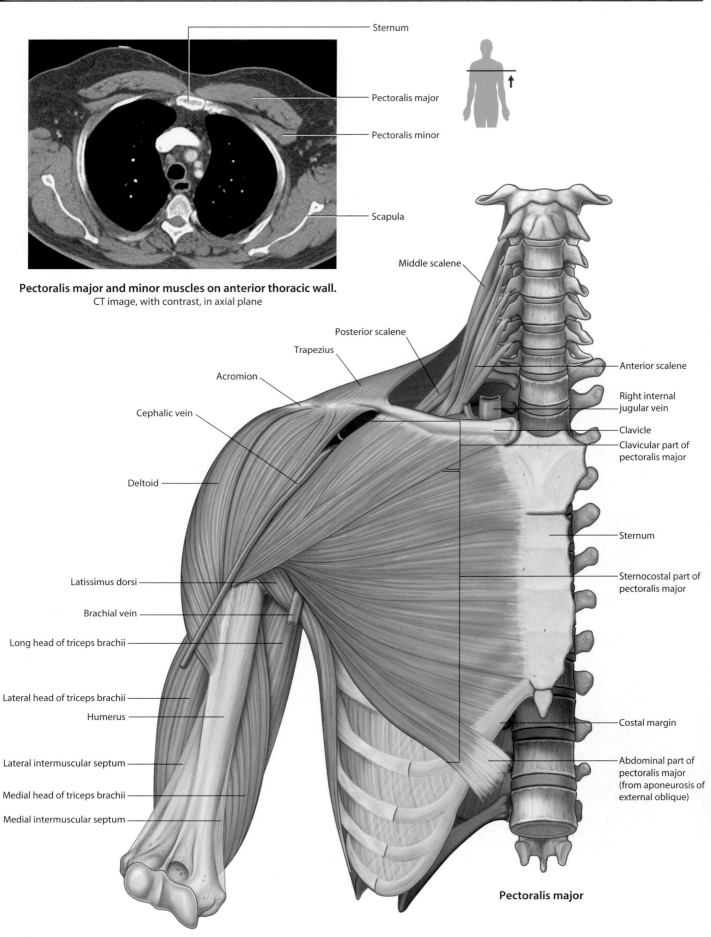

Sternum

Pectoralis major

Pectoralis minor

Scapula

Pectoralis major and minor muscles on anterior thoracic wall.
CT image, with contrast, in axial plane

Middle scalene

Posterior scalene

Trapezius

Acromion

Cephalic vein

Deltoid

Latissimus dorsi

Brachial vein

Long head of triceps brachii

Lateral head of triceps brachii

Humerus

Lateral intermuscular septum

Medial head of triceps brachii

Medial intermuscular septum

Anterior scalene

Right internal jugular vein

Clavicle

Clavicular part of pectoralis major

Sternum

Sternocostal part of pectoralis major

Costal margin

Abdominal part of pectoralis major (from aponeurosis of external oblique)

Pectoralis major

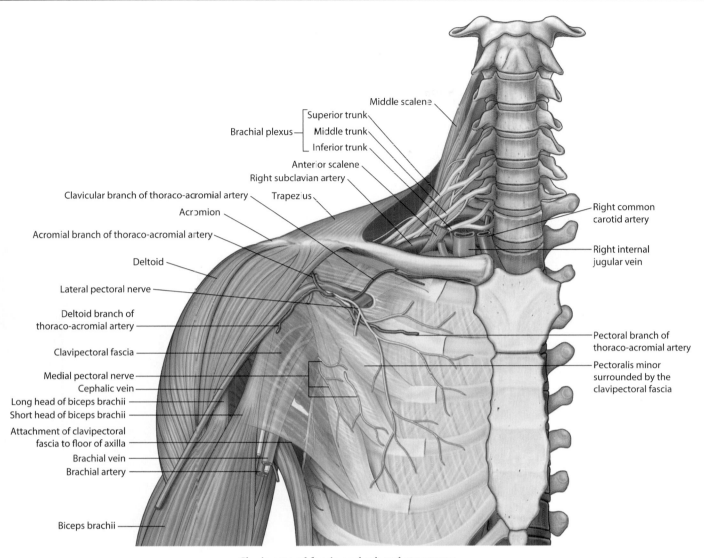

Middle scalene
Brachial plexus — Superior trunk
Middle trunk
Inferior trunk
Anterior scalene
Right subclavian artery
Clavicular branch of thoraco-acromial artery
Trapezius
Acromion
Acromial branch of thoraco-acromial artery
Deltoid
Lateral pectoral nerve
Deltoid branch of thoraco-acromial artery
Clavipectoral fascia
Medial pectoral nerve
Cephalic vein
Long head of biceps brachii
Short head of biceps brachii
Attachment of clavipectoral fascia to floor of axilla
Brachial vein
Brachial artery
Biceps brachii

Right common carotid artery
Right internal jugular vein
Pectoral branch of thoraco-acromial artery
Pectoralis minor surrounded by the clavipectoral fascia

Clavipectoral fascia and related structures

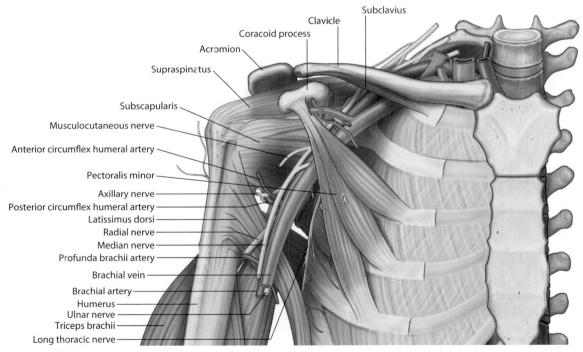

Subclavius
Clavicle
Coracoid process
Acromion
Supraspinatus
Subscapularis
Musculocutaneous nerve
Anterior circumflex humeral artery
Pectoralis minor
Axillary nerve
Posterior circumflex humeral artery
Latissimus dorsi
Radial nerve
Median nerve
Profunda brachii artery
Brachial vein
Brachial artery
Humerus
Ulnar nerve
Triceps brachii
Long thoracic nerve

Pectoralis minor

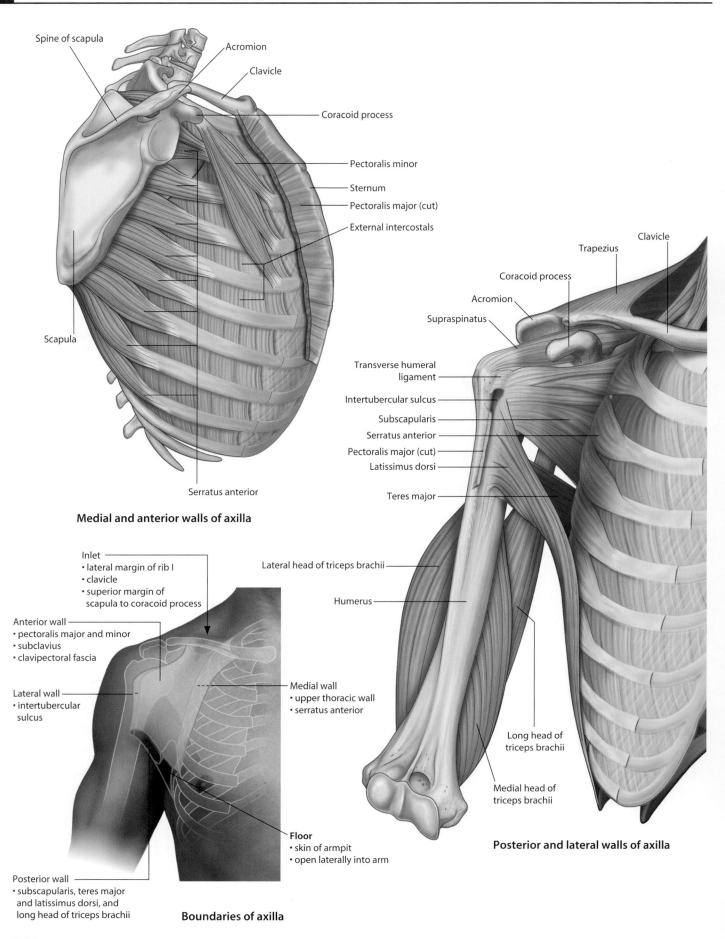

Spine of scapula

Acromion

Clavicle

Coracoid process

Pectoralis minor

Sternum

Pectoralis major (cut)

External intercostals

Scapula

Serratus anterior

Medial and anterior walls of axilla

Inlet
• lateral margin of rib I
• clavicle
• superior margin of
  scapula to coracoid process

Anterior wall
• pectoralis major and minor
• subclavius
• clavipectoral fascia

Lateral wall
• intertubercular
  sulcus

Medial wall
• upper thoracic wall
• serratus anterior

Posterior wall
• subscapularis, teres major
  and latissimus dorsi, and
  long head of triceps brachii

Floor
• skin of armpit
• open laterally into arm

Boundaries of axilla

Clavicle

Trapezius

Coracoid process

Acromion

Supraspinatus

Transverse humeral
ligament

Intertubercular sulcus

Subscapularis

Serratus anterior

Pectoralis major (cut)

Latissimus dorsi

Teres major

Lateral head of triceps brachii

Humerus

Long head of
triceps brachii

Medial head of
triceps brachii

Posterior and lateral walls of axilla

398

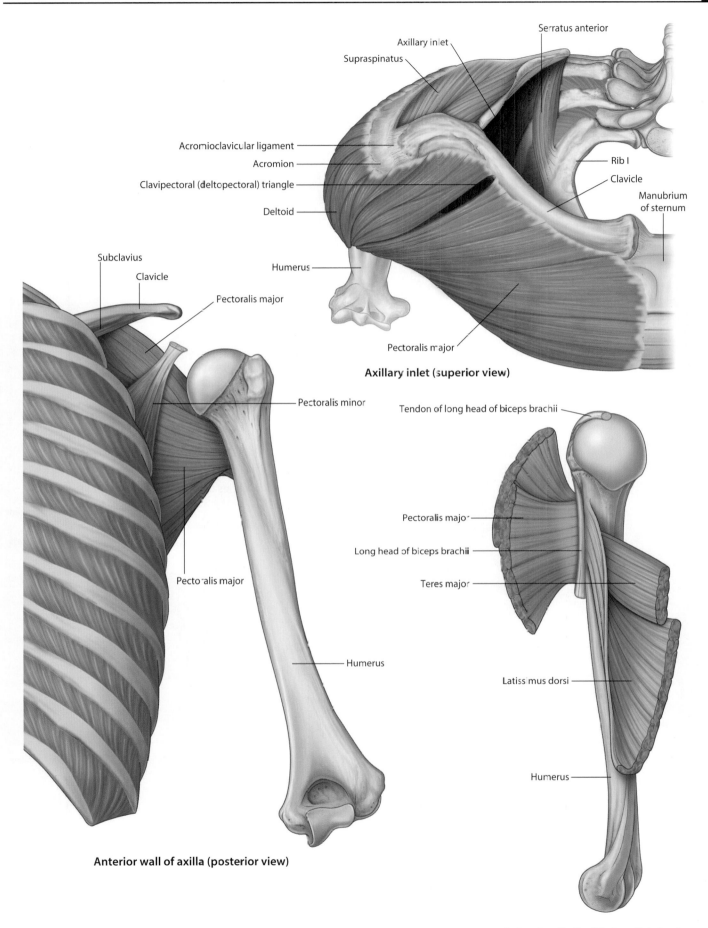

Axillary inlet
Supraspinatus
Serratus anterior
Axillary inlet
Acromioclavicular ligament
Acromion
Clavipectoral (deltopectoral) triangle
Deltoid
Rib I
Clavicle
Manubrium of sternum
Subclavius
Clavicle
Humerus
Pectoralis major
Pectoralis major

Axillary inlet (superior view)

Pectoralis minor
Tendon of long head of biceps brachii
Pectoralis major
Long head of biceps brachii
Teres major
Pectoralis major
Latissimus dorsi
Humerus
Humerus

Anterior wall of axilla (posterior view)

Lateral wall of axilla (medial view)

399

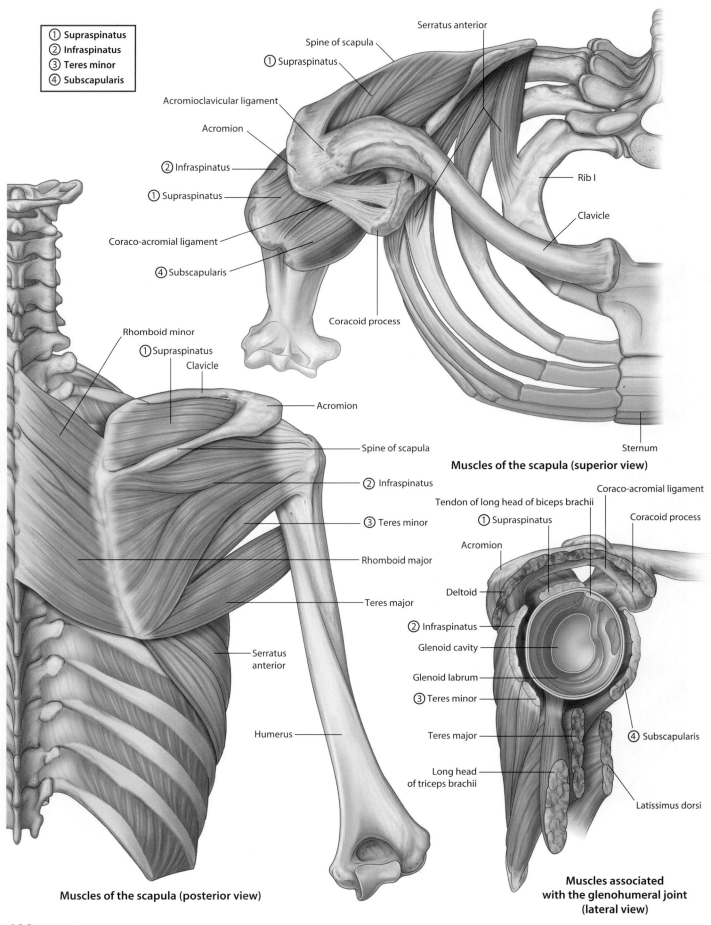

① Supraspinatus
② Infraspinatus
③ Teres minor
④ Subscapularis

Serratus anterior
Spine of scapula
① Supraspinatus
Acromioclavicular ligament
Acromion
② Infraspinatus
① Supraspinatus
Coraco-acromial ligament
④ Subscapularis
Coracoid process
Rib I
Clavicle
Sternum

Muscles of the scapula (superior view)

Rhomboid minor
① Supraspinatus
Clavicle
Acromion
Spine of scapula
② Infraspinatus
③ Teres minor
Rhomboid major
Teres major
Serratus anterior
Humerus

Muscles of the scapula (posterior view)

Coraco-acromial ligament
Tendon of long head of biceps brachii
Coracoid process
① Supraspinatus
Acromion
Deltoid
② Infraspinatus
Glenoid cavity
Glenoid labrum
③ Teres minor
Teres major
Long head of triceps brachii
④ Subscapularis
Latissimus dorsi

Muscles associated with the glenohumeral joint (lateral view)

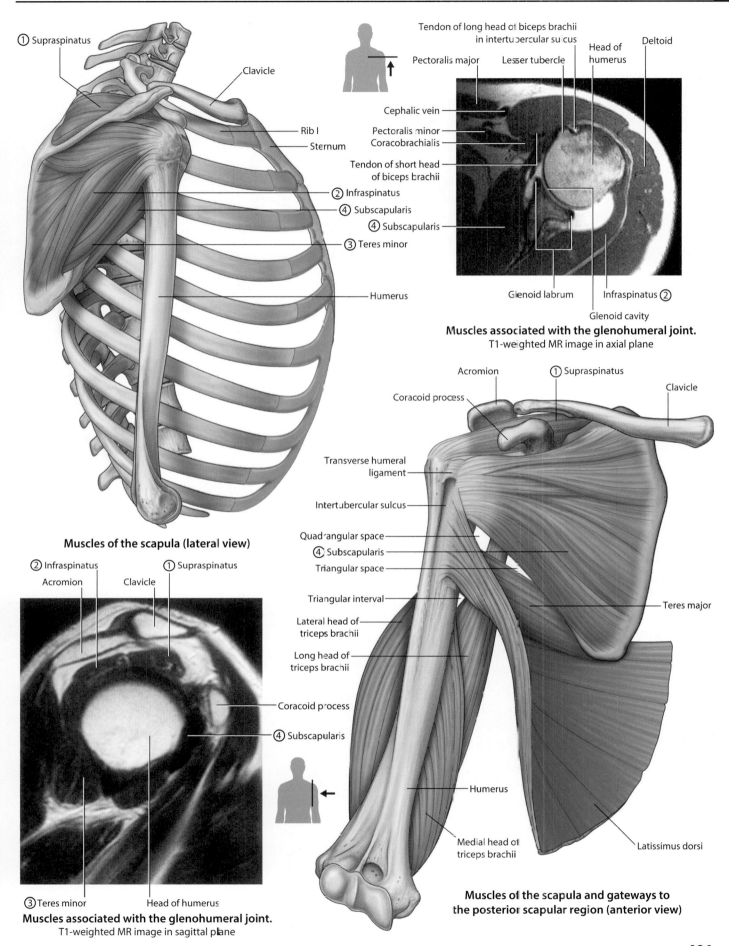

① Supraspinatus

Clavicle

Rib I

Sternum

② Infraspinatus

④ Subscapularis

③ Teres minor

Humerus

Muscles of the scapula (lateral view)

Tendon of long head of biceps brachii in intertubercular sulcus

Pectoralis major

Lesser tubercle

Head of humerus

Deltoid

Cephalic vein

Pectoralis minor

Coracobrachialis

Tendon of short head of biceps brachii

④ Subscapularis

Glenoid labrum

Infraspinatus ②

Glenoid cavity

Muscles associated with the glenohumeral joint.
T1-weighted MR image in axial plane

② Infraspinatus

Acromion

Clavicle

① Supraspinatus

③ Teres minor

Head of humerus

④ Subscapularis

Coracoid process

Muscles associated with the glenohumeral joint.
T1-weighted MR image in sagittal plane

Acromion

Coracoid process

① Supraspinatus

Clavicle

Transverse humeral ligament

Intertubercular sulcus

Quadrangular space

④ Subscapularis

Triangular space

Triangular interval

Lateral head of triceps brachii

Long head of triceps brachii

Humerus

Medial head of triceps brachii

Teres major

Latissimus dorsi

Muscles of the scapula and gateways to the posterior scapular region (anterior view)

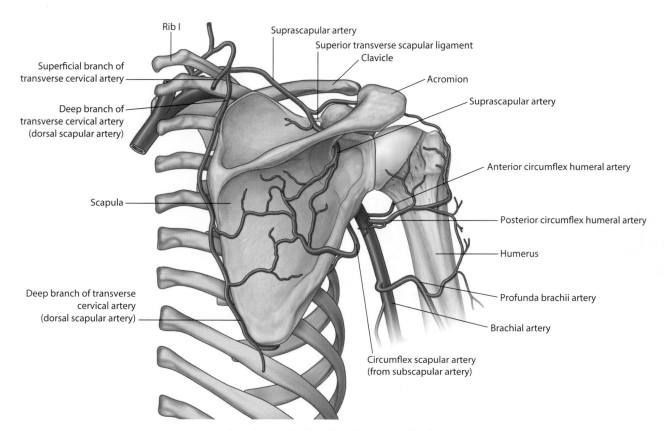

Rib I

Suprascapular artery

Superior transverse scapular ligament

Clavicle

Acromion

Superficial branch of transverse cervical artery

Deep branch of transverse cervical artery (dorsal scapular artery)

Suprascapular artery

Anterior circumflex humeral artery

Posterior circumflex humeral artery

Scapula

Humerus

Deep branch of transverse cervical artery (dorsal scapular artery)

Profunda brachii artery

Brachial artery

Circumflex scapular artery (from subscapular artery)

Arteries of the shoulder (posterior view)

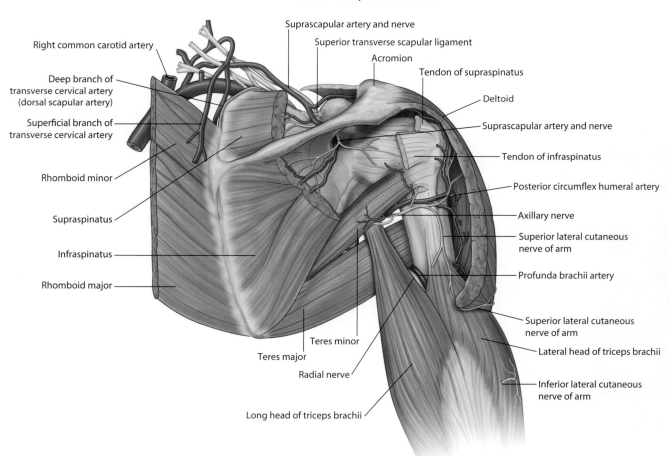

Suprascapular artery and nerve

Superior transverse scapular ligament

Acromion

Right common carotid artery

Tendon of supraspinatus

Deep branch of transverse cervical artery (dorsal scapular artery)

Deltoid

Superficial branch of transverse cervical artery

Suprascapular artery and nerve

Rhomboid minor

Tendon of infraspinatus

Posterior circumflex humeral artery

Supraspinatus

Axillary nerve

Infraspinatus

Superior lateral cutaneous nerve of arm

Rhomboid major

Profunda brachii artery

Superior lateral cutaneous nerve of arm

Lateral head of triceps brachii

Teres minor

Teres major

Inferior lateral cutaneous nerve of arm

Radial nerve

Long head of triceps brachii

Deep arteries and nerves of the shoulder (posterior view)

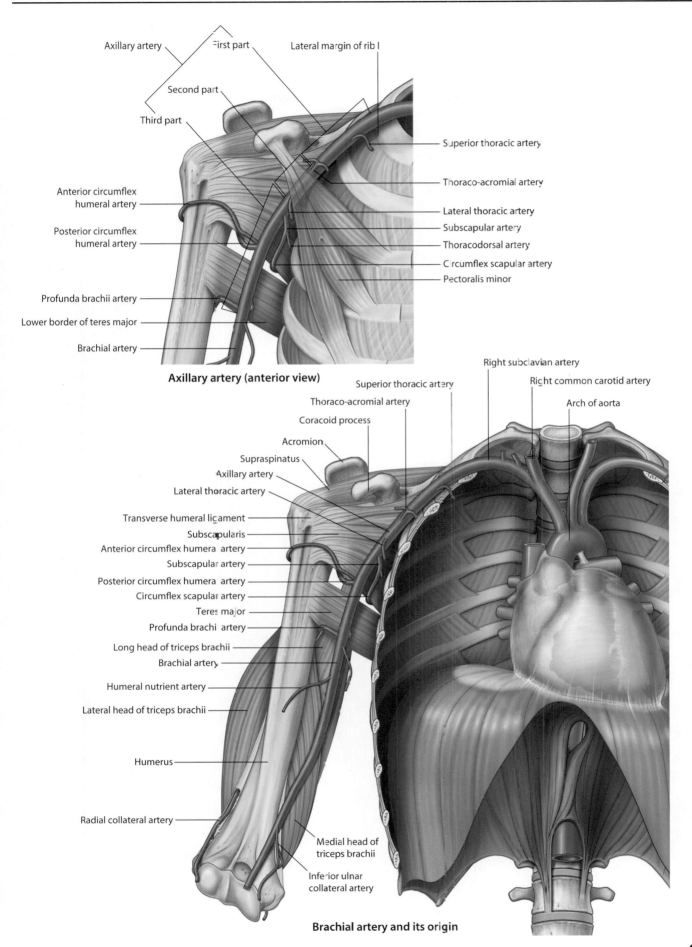

Axillary artery

First part

Second part

Third part

Lateral margin of rib I

Anterior circumflex humeral artery

Posterior circumflex humeral artery

Superior thoracic artery

Thoraco-acromial artery

Lateral thoracic artery

Subscapular artery

Thoracodorsal artery

Circumflex scapular artery

Pectoralis minor

Profunda brachii artery

Lower border of teres major

Brachial artery

Axillary artery (anterior view)

Superior thoracic artery

Thoraco-acromial artery

Coracoid process

Acromion

Supraspinatus

Axillary artery

Lateral thoracic artery

Transverse humeral ligament

Subscapularis

Anterior circumflex humeral artery

Subscapular artery

Posterior circumflex humeral artery

Circumflex scapular artery

Teres major

Profunda brachii artery

Long head of triceps brachii

Brachial artery

Humeral nutrient artery

Lateral head of triceps brachii

Humerus

Radial collateral artery

Medial head of triceps brachii

Inferior ulnar collateral artery

Right subclavian artery

Right common carotid artery

Arch of aorta

Brachial artery and its origin

403

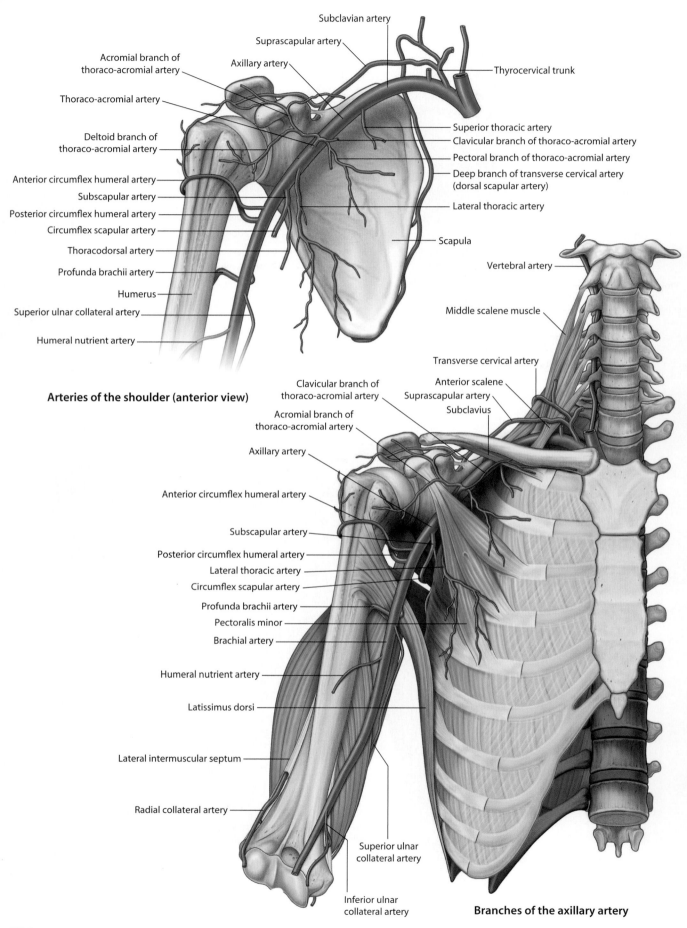

Subclavian artery

Suprascapular artery

Axillary artery

Acromial branch of
thoraco-acromial artery

Thoraco-acromial artery

Thyrocervical trunk

Deltoid branch of
thoraco-acromial artery

Superior thoracic artery

Clavicular branch of thoraco-acromial artery

Pectoral branch of thoraco-acromial artery

Deep branch of transverse cervical artery
(dorsal scapular artery)

Anterior circumflex humeral artery

Subscapular artery

Posterior circumflex humeral artery

Circumflex scapular artery

Thoracodorsal artery

Profunda brachii artery

Humerus

Superior ulnar collateral artery

Humeral nutrient artery

Lateral thoracic artery

Scapula

Vertebral artery

Middle scalene muscle

Arteries of the shoulder (anterior view)

Clavicular branch of
thoraco-acromial artery

Acromial branch of
thoraco-acromial artery

Axillary artery

Anterior circumflex humeral artery

Subscapular artery

Posterior circumflex humeral artery

Lateral thoracic artery

Circumflex scapular artery

Profunda brachii artery

Pectoralis minor

Brachial artery

Humeral nutrient artery

Latissimus dorsi

Lateral intermuscular septum

Radial collateral artery

Transverse cervical artery

Anterior scalene

Suprascapular artery

Subclavius

Superior ulnar
collateral artery

Inferior ulnar
collateral artery

Branches of the axillary artery

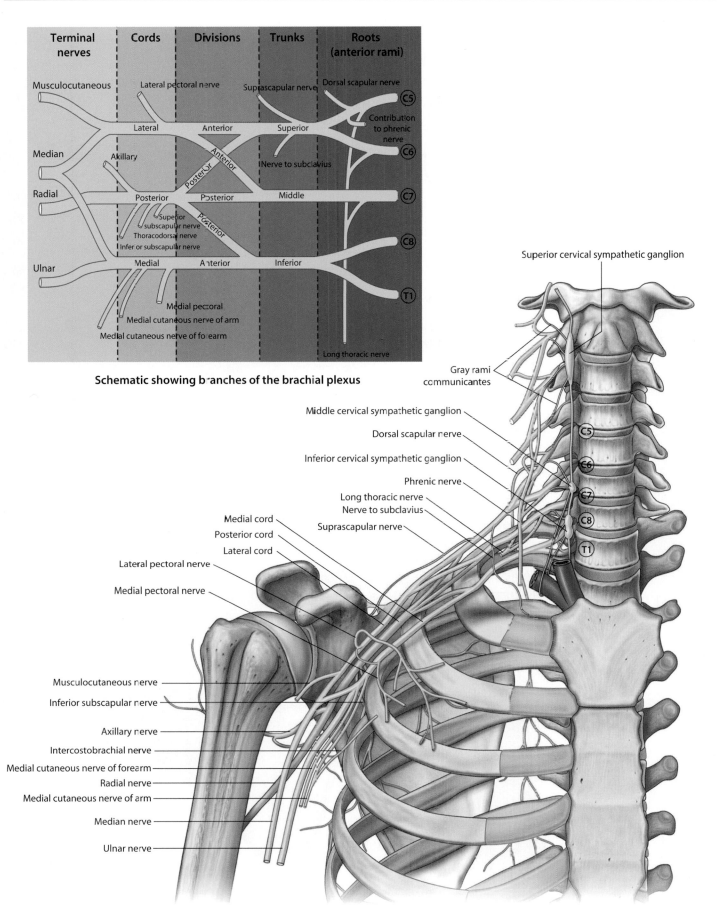

Terminal nerves	Cords	Divisions	Trunks	Roots (anterior rami)

Schematic showing branches of the brachial plexus

Superior cervical sympathetic ganglion

Gray rami communicantes

Middle cervical sympathetic ganglion

Dorsal scapular nerve

Inferior cervical sympathetic ganglion

Phrenic nerve

Long thoracic nerve

Nerve to subclavius

Suprascapular nerve

Medial cord

Posterior cord

Lateral cord

Lateral pectoral nerve

Medial pectoral nerve

Musculocutaneous nerve

Inferior subscapular nerve

Axillary nerve

Intercostobrachial nerve

Medial cutaneous nerve of forearm

Radial nerve

Medial cutaneous nerve of arm

Median nerve

Ulnar nerve

Brachial plexus

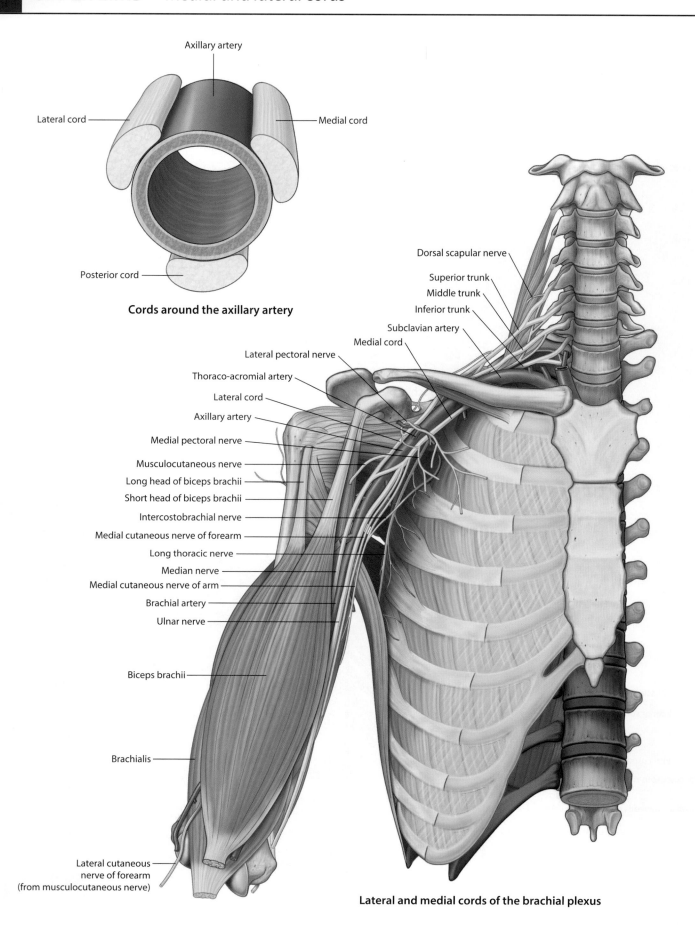

Axillary artery

Lateral cord

Medial cord

Posterior cord

Cords around the axillary artery

Dorsal scapular nerve

Superior trunk

Middle trunk

Inferior trunk

Subclavian artery

Medial cord

Lateral pectoral nerve

Thoraco-acromial artery

Lateral cord

Axillary artery

Medial pectoral nerve

Musculocutaneous nerve

Long head of biceps brachii

Short head of biceps brachii

Intercostobrachial nerve

Medial cutaneous nerve of forearm

Long thoracic nerve

Median nerve

Medial cutaneous nerve of arm

Brachial artery

Ulnar nerve

Biceps brachii

Brachialis

Lateral cutaneous
nerve of forearm
(from musculocutaneous nerve)

Lateral and medial cords of the brachial plexus

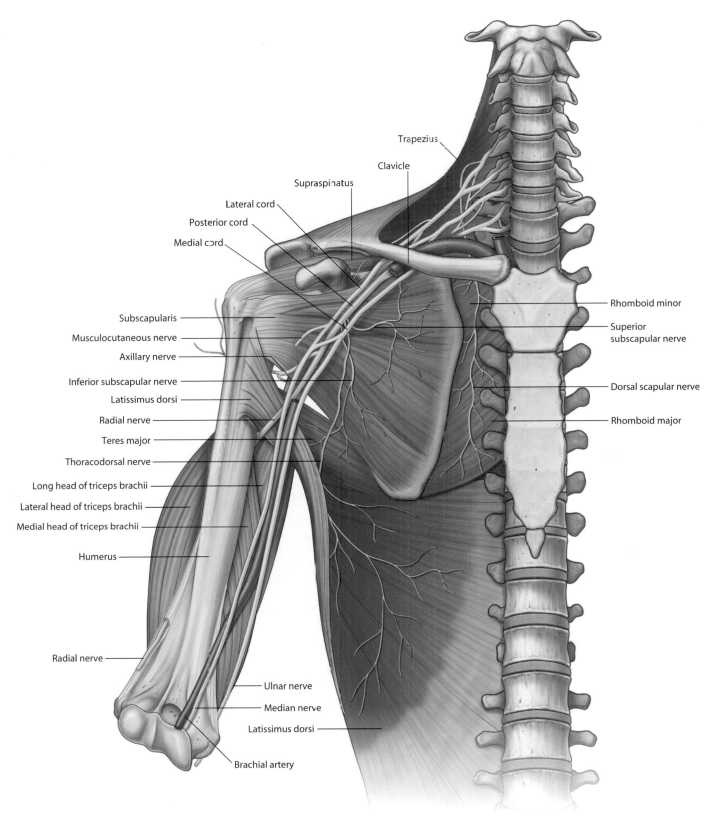

**Posterior cord of the brachial plexus
(ribs and associated muscles removed)**

Trapezius

Clavicle

Supraspinatus

Lateral cord

Posterior cord

Medial cord

Subscapularis

Musculocutaneous nerve

Axillary nerve

Inferior subscapular nerve

Latissimus dorsi

Radial nerve

Teres major

Thoracodorsal nerve

Long head of triceps brachii

Lateral head of triceps brachii

Medial head of triceps brachii

Humerus

Radial nerve

Ulnar nerve

Median nerve

Latissimus dorsi

Brachial artery

Rhomboid minor

Superior
subscapular nerve

Dorsal scapular nerve

Rhomboid major

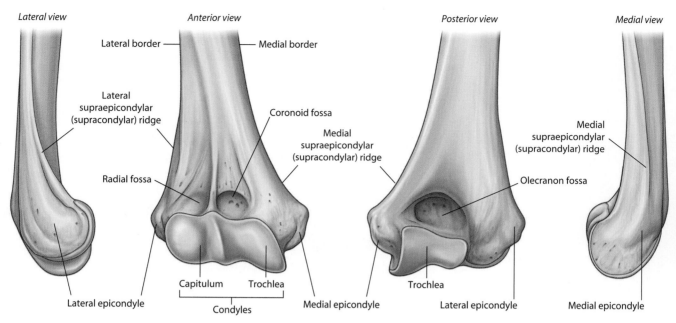

Lateral view   *Anterior view*   *Posterior view*   *Medial view*

Lateral border — — Medial border

Lateral supraepicondylar (supracondylar) ridge

Coronoid fossa

Medial supraepicondylar (supracondylar) ridge

Medial supraepicondylar (supracondylar) ridge

Radial fossa

Olecranon fossa

Capitulum   Trochlea

Trochlea

Lateral epicondyle   Condyles   Medial epicondyle   Lateral epicondyle   Medial epicondyle

Distal end of humerus

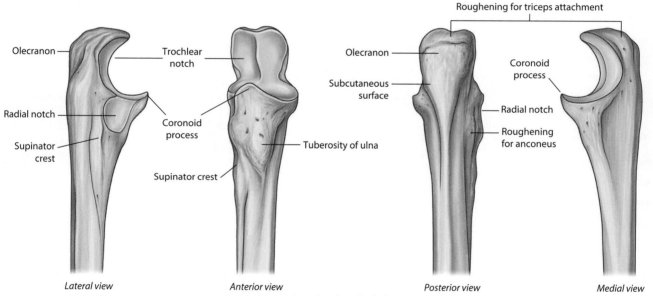

Roughening for triceps attachment

Olecranon — — Trochlear notch

Olecranon

Radial notch —

Coronoid process

Subcutaneous surface

Coronoid process

Supinator crest —

Coronoid process

Radial notch

Tuberosity of ulna

Roughening for anconeus

Supinator crest

Lateral view   *Anterior view*   *Posterior view*   *Medial view*

Proximal end of ulna

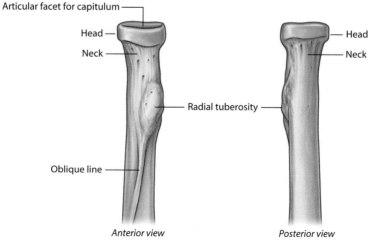

Articular facet for capitulum —

Head —

Head

Neck —

Neck

Radial tuberosity

Oblique line —

Anterior view   *Posterior view*

Proximal end of radius

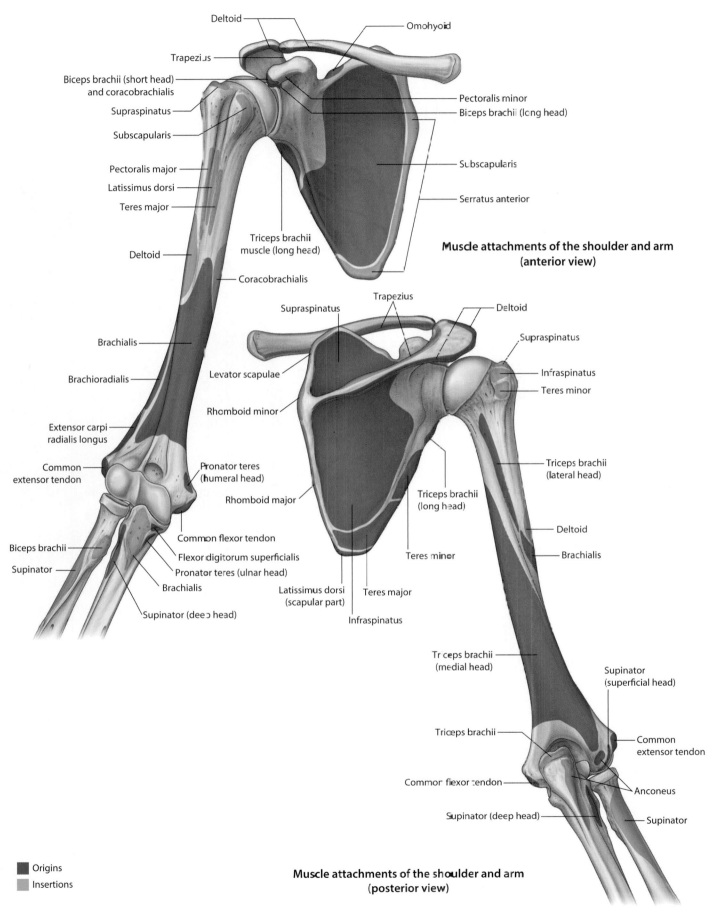

Deltoid

Trapezius

Biceps brachii (short head)
and coracobrachialis

Supraspinatus

Subscapularis

Pectoralis major

Latissimus dorsi

Teres major

Deltoid

Coracobrachialis

Brachialis

Brachioradialis

Extensor carpi
radialis longus

Common
extensor tendon

Biceps brachii

Supinator

Omohyoid

Pectoralis minor

Biceps brachii (long head)

Subscapularis

Serratus anterior

Triceps brachii
muscle (long head)

**Muscle attachments of the shoulder and arm
(anterior view)**

Trapezius

Supraspinatus

Deltoid

Supraspinatus

Infraspinatus

Teres minor

Levator scapulae

Rhomboid minor

Pronator teres
(humeral head)

Rhomboid major

Common flexor tendon

Flexor digitorum superficialis

Pronator teres (ulnar head)

Brachialis

Supinator (deep head)

Triceps brachii
(lateral head)

Triceps brachii
(long head)

Teres minor

Latissimus dorsi
(scapular part)

Teres major

Infraspinatus

Deltoid

Brachialis

Triceps brachii
(medial head)

Supinator
(superficial head)

Triceps brachii

Common
extensor tendon

Common flexor tendon

Anconeus

Supinator (deep head)

Supinator

■ Origins
■ Insertions

**Muscle attachments of the shoulder and arm
(posterior view)**

409

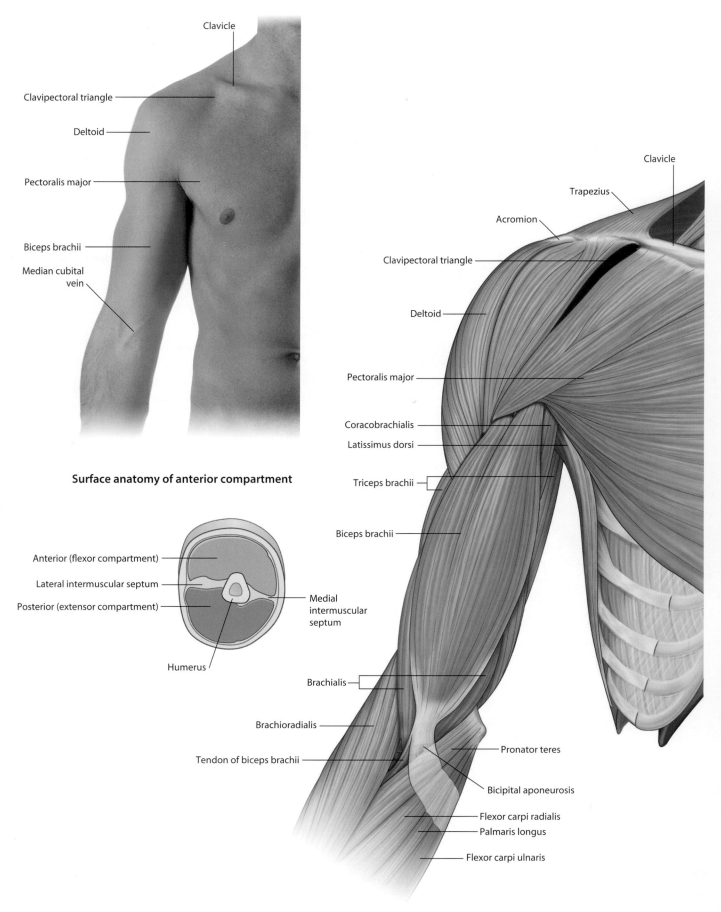

Clavicle

Clavipectoral triangle

Deltoid

Pectoralis major

Biceps brachii

Median cubital vein

Surface anatomy of anterior compartment

Anterior (flexor compartment)

Lateral intermuscular septum

Posterior (extensor compartment)

Medial intermuscular septum

Humerus

Clavicle

Trapezius

Acromion

Clavipectoral triangle

Deltoid

Pectoralis major

Coracobrachialis

Latissimus dorsi

Triceps brachii

Biceps brachii

Brachialis

Brachioradialis

Pronator teres

Tendon of biceps brachii

Bicipital aponeurosis

Flexor carpi radialis

Palmaris longus

Flexor carpi ulnaris

Muscles of anterior compartment of arm

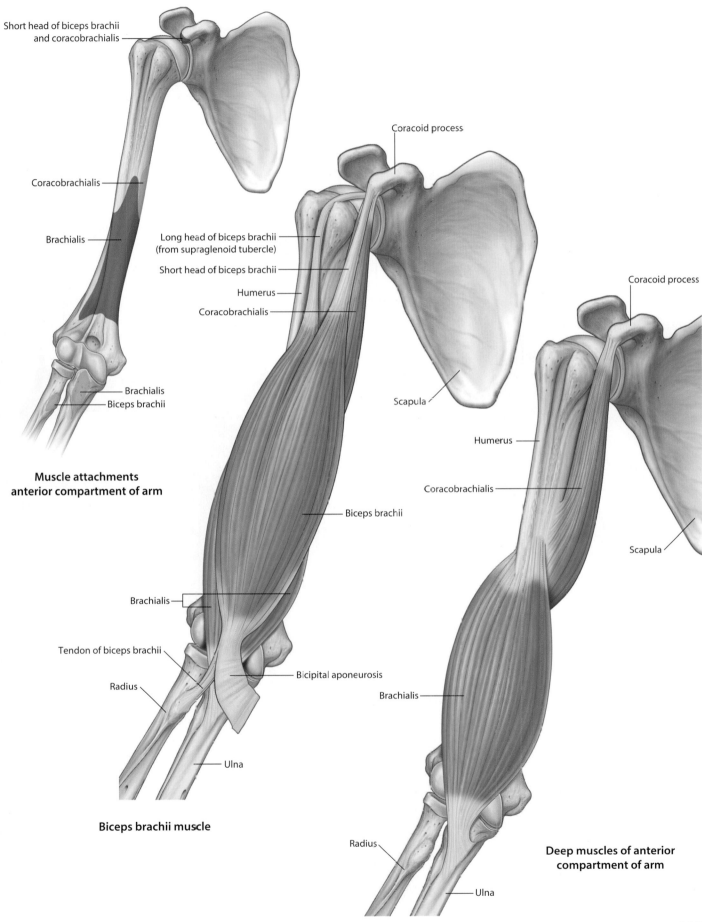

Short head of biceps brachii
and coracobrachialis

Coracoid process

Coracobrachialis

Brachialis

Long head of biceps brachii
(from supraglenoid tubercle)

Short head of biceps brachii

Humerus

Coracobrachialis

Coracoid process

Brachialis
Biceps brachii

Scapula

Humerus

**Muscle attachments
anterior compartment of arm**

Coracobrachialis

Biceps brachii

Scapula

Brachialis

Tendon of biceps brachii

Radius

Bicipital aponeurosis

Brachialis

Ulna

Radius

Biceps brachii muscle

Ulna

**Deep muscles of anterior
compartment of arm**

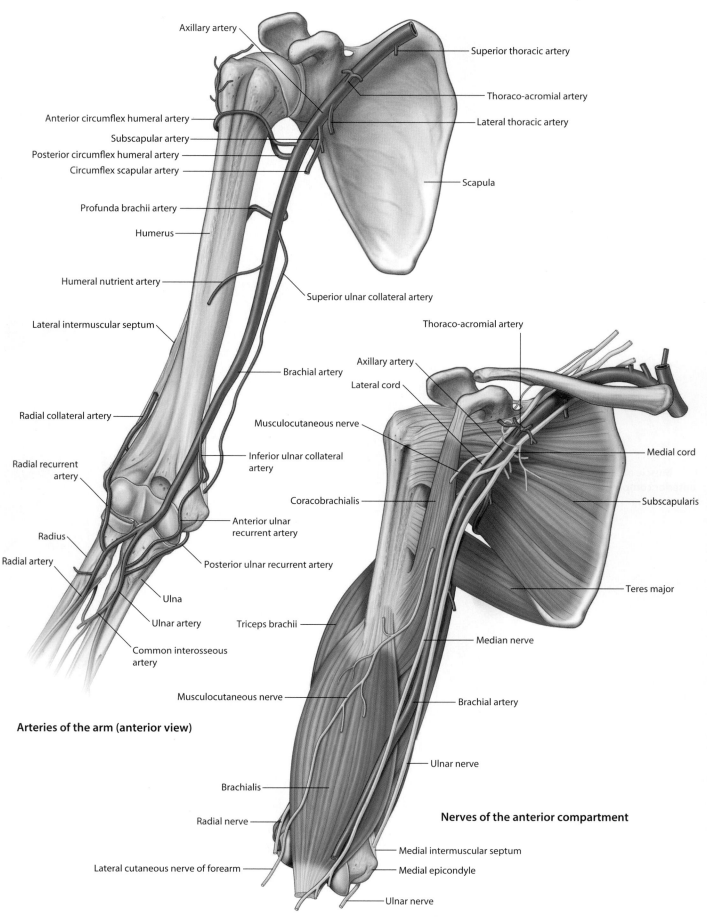

Axillary artery

Superior thoracic artery

Thoraco-acromial artery

Anterior circumflex humeral artery

Lateral thoracic artery

Subscapular artery

Posterior circumflex humeral artery

Circumflex scapular artery

Scapula

Profunda brachii artery

Humerus

Humeral nutrient artery

Superior ulnar collateral artery

Lateral intermuscular septum

Thoraco-acromial artery

Axillary artery

Lateral cord

Brachial artery

Musculocutaneous nerve

Medial cord

Radial collateral artery

Inferior ulnar collateral artery

Coracobrachialis

Subscapularis

Radial recurrent artery

Radius

Anterior ulnar recurrent artery

Radial artery

Posterior ulnar recurrent artery

Teres major

Ulna

Ulnar artery

Triceps brachii

Median nerve

Common interosseous artery

Musculocutaneous nerve

Brachial artery

Arteries of the arm (anterior view)

Ulnar nerve

Brachialis

Nerves of the anterior compartment

Radial nerve

Medial intermuscular septum

Medial epicondyle

Lateral cutaneous nerve of forearm

Ulnar nerve

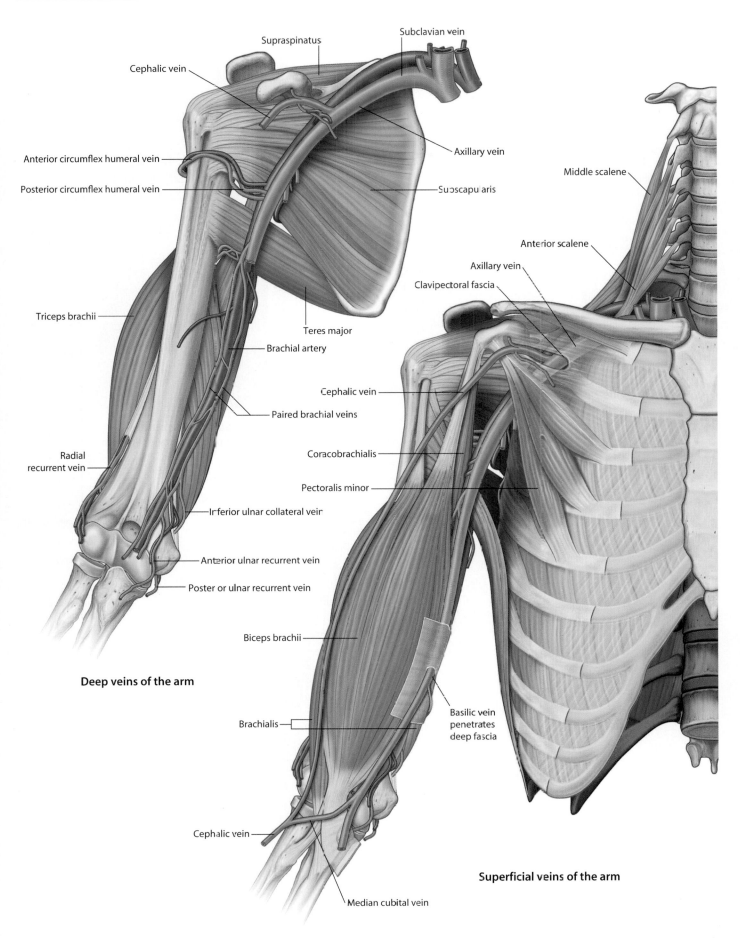

Supraspinatus

Subclavian vein

Cephalic vein

Axillary vein

Anterior circumflex humeral vein

Posterior circumflex humeral vein

Subscapularis

Middle scalene

Anterior scalene

Axillary vein

Clavipectoral fascia

Triceps brachii

Teres major

Brachial artery

Cephalic vein

Paired brachial veins

Coracobrachialis

Radial
recurrent vein

Pectoralis minor

Inferior ulnar collateral vein

Anterior ulnar recurrent vein

Posterior ulnar recurrent vein

Deep veins of the arm

Biceps brachii

Brachialis

Basilic vein
penetrates
deep fascia

Cephalic vein

Superficial veins of the arm

Median cubital vein

413

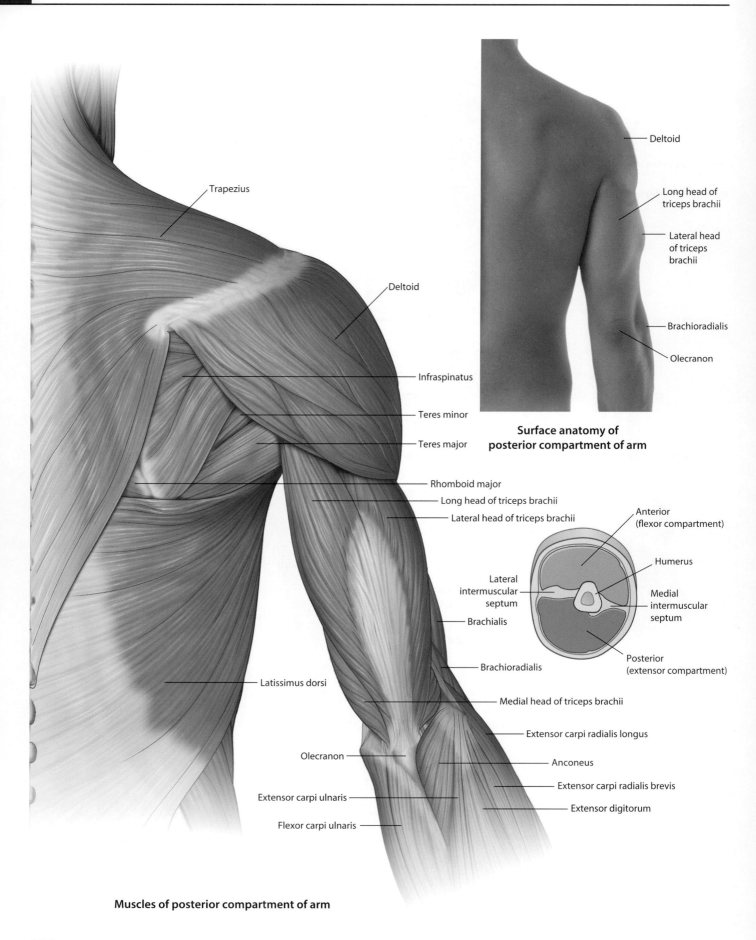

Trapezius

Deltoid

Infraspinatus

Teres minor

Teres major

Rhomboid major

Long head of triceps brachii

Lateral head of triceps brachii

Brachialis

Brachioradialis

Latissimus dorsi

Medial head of triceps brachii

Olecranon

Extensor carpi radialis longus

Anconeus

Extensor carpi ulnaris

Extensor carpi radialis brevis

Flexor carpi ulnaris

Extensor digitorum

Deltoid

Long head of triceps brachii

Lateral head of triceps brachii

Brachioradialis

Olecranon

Surface anatomy of posterior compartment of arm

Anterior (flexor compartment)

Humerus

Lateral intermuscular septum

Medial intermuscular septum

Posterior (extensor compartment)

Muscles of posterior compartment of arm

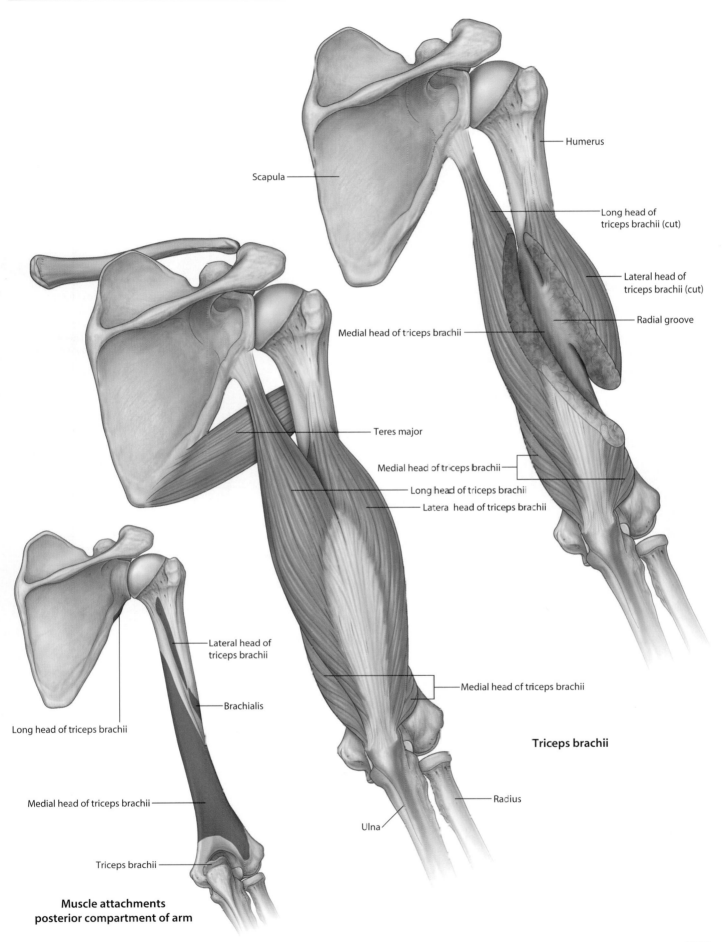

Humerus

Long head of
triceps brachii (cut)

Lateral head of
triceps brachii (cut)

Radial groove

Scapula

Medial head of triceps brachii

Teres major

Medial head of triceps brachii

Long head of triceps brachii

Lateral head of triceps brachii

Medial head of triceps brachii

Triceps brachii

Lateral head of
triceps brachii

Brachialis

Long head of triceps brachii

Radius

Medial head of triceps brachii

Ulna

Triceps brachii

**Muscle attachments
posterior compartment of arm**

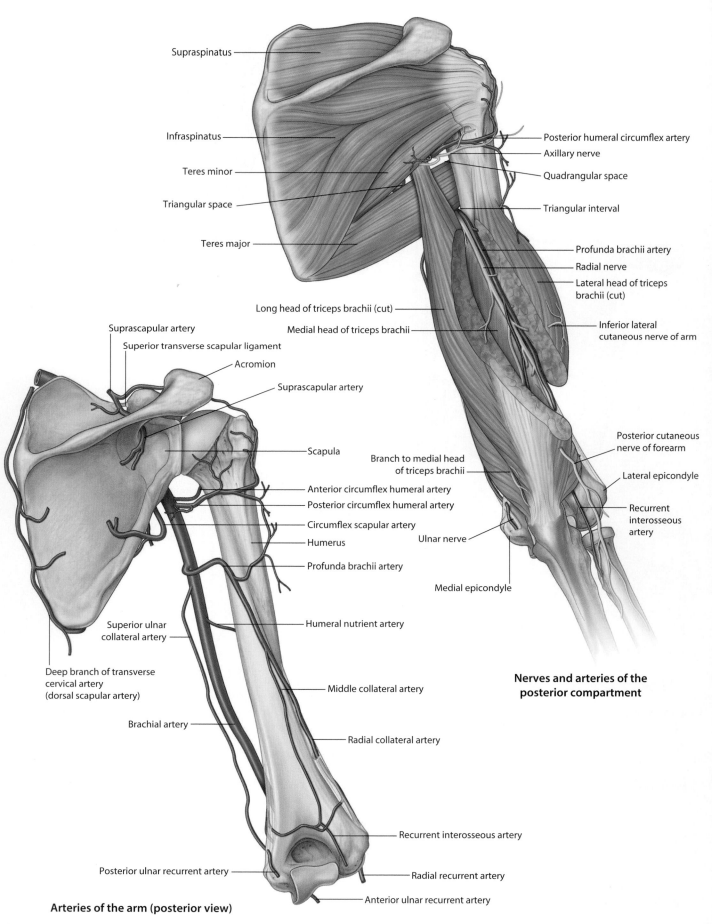

Supraspinatus

Infraspinatus

Teres minor

Triangular space

Teres major

Posterior humeral circumflex artery

Axillary nerve

Quadrangular space

Triangular interval

Profunda brachii artery

Radial nerve

Lateral head of triceps brachii (cut)

Long head of triceps brachii (cut)

Medial head of triceps brachii

Inferior lateral cutaneous nerve of arm

Suprascapular artery

Superior transverse scapular ligament

Acromion

Suprascapular artery

Scapula

Branch to medial head of triceps brachii

Anterior circumflex humeral artery

Posterior circumflex humeral artery

Circumflex scapular artery

Humerus

Profunda brachii artery

Ulnar nerve

Posterior cutaneous nerve of forearm

Lateral epicondyle

Recurrent interosseous artery

Medial epicondyle

Superior ulnar collateral artery

Humeral nutrient artery

Nerves and arteries of the posterior compartment

Deep branch of transverse cervical artery (dorsal scapular artery)

Middle collateral artery

Brachial artery

Radial collateral artery

Recurrent interosseous artery

Posterior ulnar recurrent artery

Radial recurrent artery

Anterior ulnar recurrent artery

Arteries of the arm (posterior view)

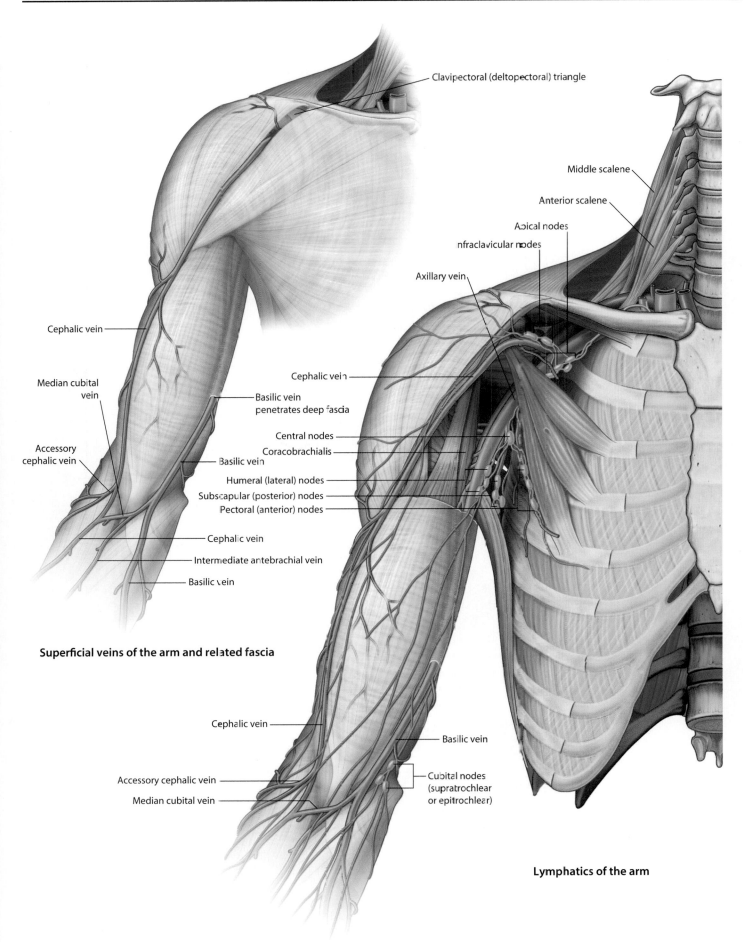

Clavipectoral (deltopectoral) triangle

Middle scalene

Anterior scalene

Apical nodes

Infraclavicular nodes

Axillary vein

Cephalic vein

Cephalic vein

Basilic vein
penetrates deep fascia

Central nodes

Coracobrachialis

Basilic vein

Humeral (lateral) nodes

Subscapular (posterior) nodes

Pectoral (anterior) nodes

Cephalic vein

Median cubital
vein

Accessory
cephalic vein

Cephalic vein

Intermediate antebrachial vein

Basilic vein

Superficial veins of the arm and related fascia

Cephalic vein

Basilic vein

Accessory cephalic vein

Median cubital vein

Cubital nodes
(supratrochlear
or epitrochlear)

Lymphatics of the arm

417

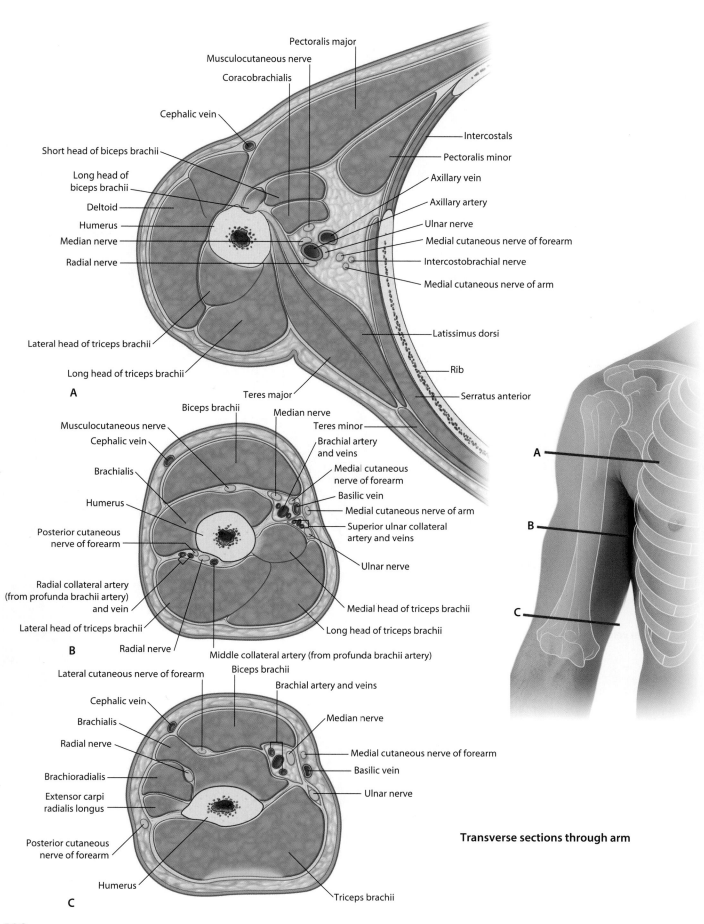

A

Pectoralis major
Musculocutaneous nerve
Coracobrachialis
Cephalic vein
Short head of biceps brachii
Long head of biceps brachii
Deltoid
Humerus
Median nerve
Radial nerve
Lateral head of triceps brachii
Long head of triceps brachii
Intercostals
Pectoralis minor
Axillary vein
Axillary artery
Ulnar nerve
Medial cutaneous nerve of forearm
Intercostobrachial nerve
Medial cutaneous nerve of arm
Latissimus dorsi
Rib
Serratus anterior
Teres major

B

Biceps brachii
Median nerve
Teres minor
Musculocutaneous nerve
Cephalic vein
Brachialis
Humerus
Posterior cutaneous nerve of forearm
Radial collateral artery (from profunda brachii artery) and vein
Lateral head of triceps brachii
Radial nerve
Brachial artery and veins
Medial cutaneous nerve of forearm
Basilic vein
Medial cutaneous nerve of arm
Superior ulnar collateral artery and veins
Ulnar nerve
Medial head of triceps brachii
Long head of triceps brachii
Middle collateral artery (from profunda brachii artery)

C

Lateral cutaneous nerve of forearm
Biceps brachii
Brachial artery and veins
Cephalic vein
Brachialis
Median nerve
Radial nerve
Brachioradialis
Medial cutaneous nerve of forearm
Extensor carpi radialis longus
Basilic vein
Ulnar nerve
Posterior cutaneous nerve of forearm
Humerus
Triceps brachii

Transverse sections through arm

A
B
C

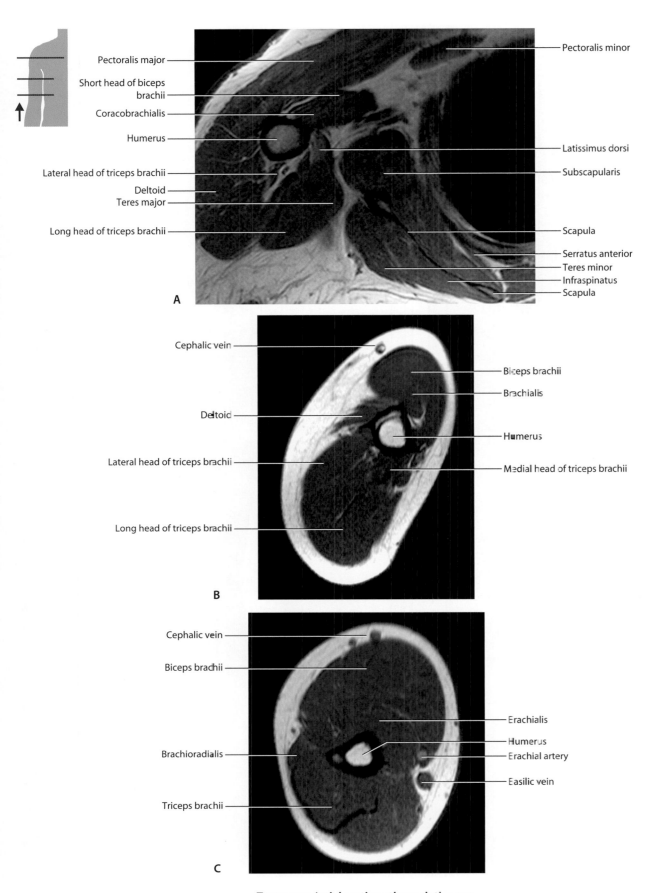

Pectoralis major

Short head of biceps brachii

Coracobrachialis

Humerus

Lateral head of triceps brachii

Deltoid

Teres major

Long head of triceps brachii

Pectoralis minor

Latissimus dorsi

Subscapularis

Scapula

Serratus anterior

Teres minor

Infraspinatus

Scapula

A

Cephalic vein

Deltoid

Lateral head of triceps brachii

Long head of triceps brachii

Biceps brachii

Brachialis

Humerus

Medial head of triceps brachii

B

Cephalic vein

Biceps brachii

Brachioradialis

Triceps brachii

Brachialis

Humerus

Brachial artery

Basilic vein

C

Transverse/axial sections through the arm.
A. Proximal/upper arm. B. Middle arm. C. Distal/lower arm.
T1-weighted MR image in axial plane

419

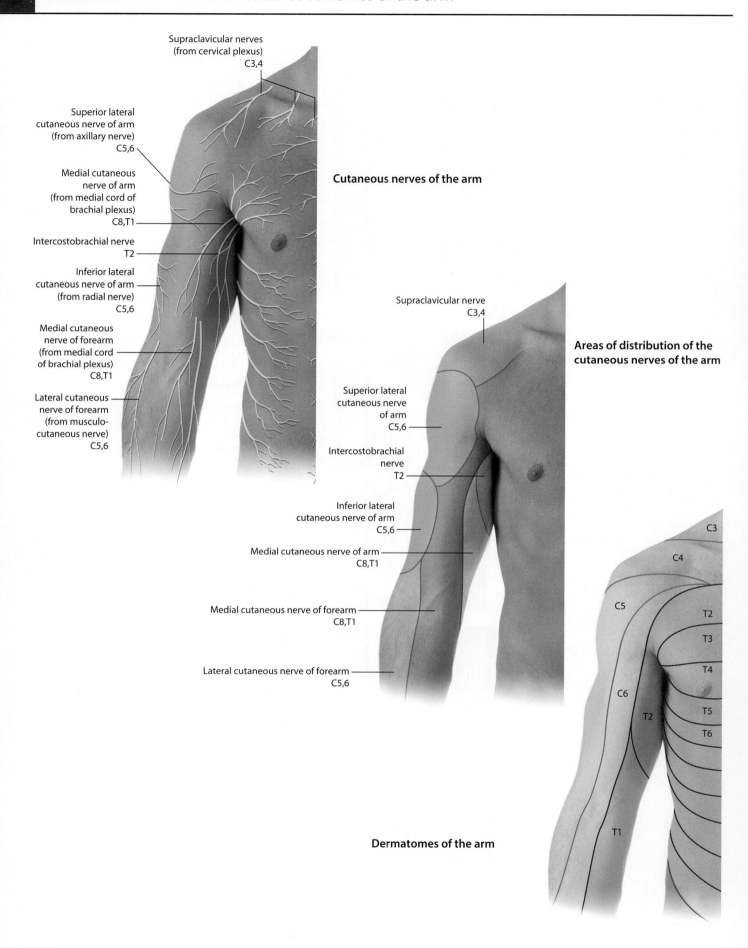

Supraclavicular nerves
(from cervical plexus)
C3,4

Superior lateral
cutaneous nerve of arm
(from axillary nerve)
C5,6

Medial cutaneous
nerve of arm
(from medial cord of
brachial plexus)
C8,T1

Intercostobrachial nerve
T2

Inferior lateral
cutaneous nerve of arm
(from radial nerve)
C5,6

Medial cutaneous
nerve of forearm
(from medial cord
of brachial plexus)
C8,T1

Lateral cutaneous
nerve of forearm
(from musculo-
cutaneous nerve)
C5,6

Cutaneous nerves of the arm

Supraclavicular nerve
C3,4

**Areas of distribution of the
cutaneous nerves of the arm**

Superior lateral
cutaneous nerve
of arm
C5,6

Intercostobrachial
nerve
T2

Inferior lateral
cutaneous nerve of arm
C5,6

Medial cutaneous nerve of arm
C8,T1

Medial cutaneous nerve of forearm
C8,T1

Lateral cutaneous nerve of forearm
C5,6

C3
C4
C5
T2
T3
T4
C6
T2
T5
T6
T1

Dermatomes of the arm

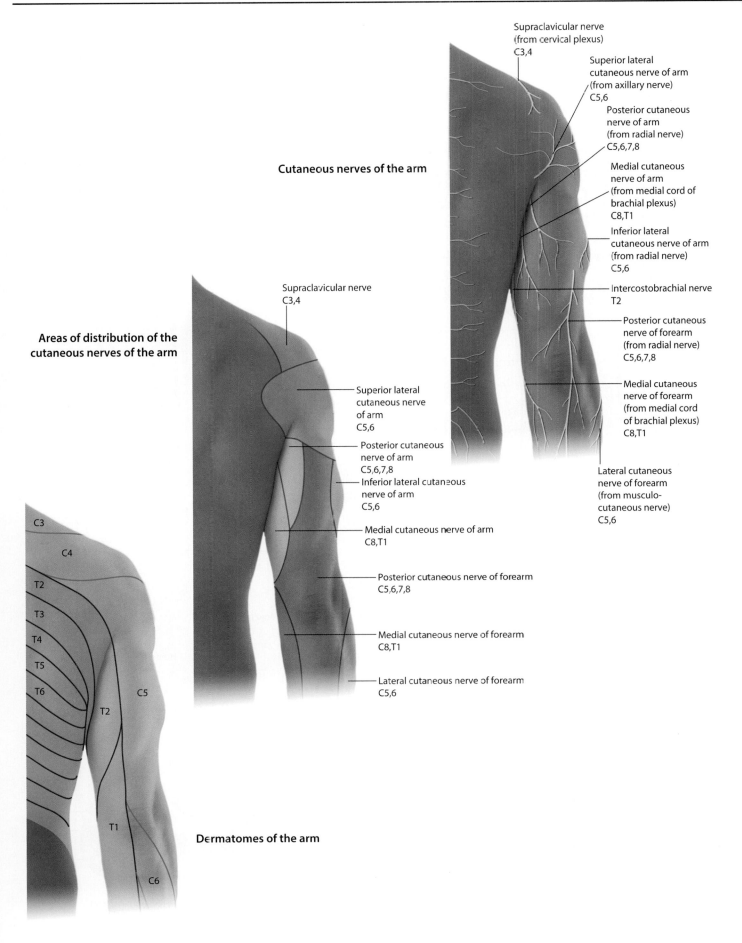

Cutaneous nerves of the arm

Supraclavicular nerve (from cervical plexus) C3,4

Superior lateral cutaneous nerve of arm (from axillary nerve) C5,6

Posterior cutaneous nerve of arm (from radial nerve) C5,6,7,8

Medial cutaneous nerve of arm (from medial cord of brachial plexus) C8,T1

Inferior lateral cutaneous nerve of arm (from radial nerve) C5,6

Intercostobrachial nerve T2

Posterior cutaneous nerve of forearm (from radial nerve) C5,6,7,8

Medial cutaneous nerve of forearm (from medial cord of brachial plexus) C8,T1

Lateral cutaneous nerve of forearm (from musculo-cutaneous nerve) C5,6

Areas of distribution of the cutaneous nerves of the arm

Supraclavicular nerve C3,4

Superior lateral cutaneous nerve of arm C5,6

Posterior cutaneous nerve of arm C5,6,7,8

Inferior lateral cutaneous nerve of arm C5,6

Medial cutaneous nerve of arm C8,T1

Posterior cutaneous nerve of forearm C5,6,7,8

Medial cutaneous nerve of forearm C8,T1

Lateral cutaneous nerve of forearm C5,6

C3

C4

T2

T3

T4

T5

T6

C5

T2

T1

C6

Dermatomes of the arm

421

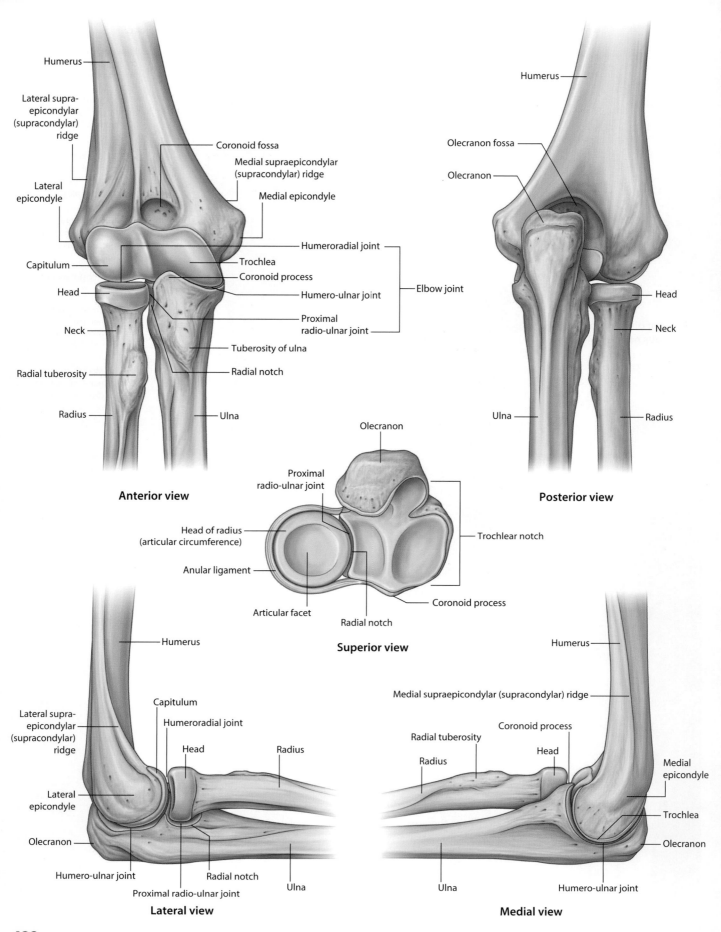

Anterior view

Humerus

Lateral supra-
epicondylar
(supracondylar)
ridge

Lateral
epicondyle

Capitulum

Head

Neck

Radial tuberosity

Radius

Coronoid fossa

Medial supraepicondylar
(supracondylar) ridge

Medial epicondyle

Humeroradial joint

Trochlea

Coronoid process

Humero-ulnar joint

Proximal
radio-ulnar joint

Tuberosity of ulna

Radial notch

Ulna

Elbow joint

Posterior view

Humerus

Olecranon fossa

Olecranon

Head

Neck

Ulna

Radius

Superior view

Olecranon

Proximal
radio-ulnar joint

Head of radius
(articular circumference)

Anular ligament

Articular facet

Radial notch

Trochlear notch

Coronoid process

Lateral view

Humerus

Lateral supra-
epicondylar
(supracondylar)
ridge

Lateral
epicondyle

Olecranon

Humero-ulnar joint

Proximal radio-ulnar joint

Capitulum

Humeroradial joint

Head

Radius

Radial notch

Ulna

Medial view

Humerus

Medial supraepicondylar (supracondylar) ridge

Radial tuberosity

Radius

Coronoid process

Head

Medial
epicondyle

Trochlea

Olecranon

Ulna

Humero-ulnar joint

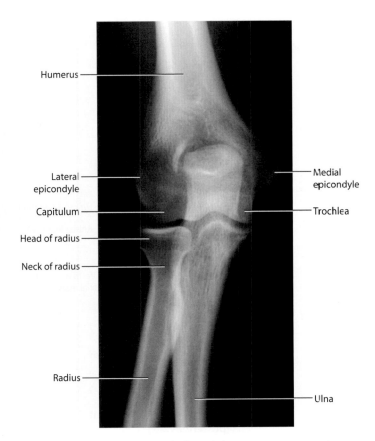

Normal elbow joint.
Radiograph, AP view

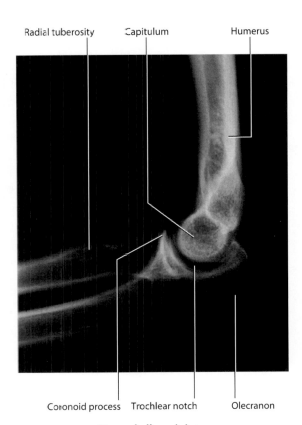

Normal elbow joint.
Radiograph, lateral view

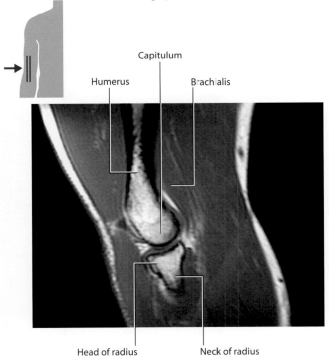

**Articulation of the capitulum of the humerus and the
head of the radius at the elbow joint.**
T2-weighted MR image in sagittal plane

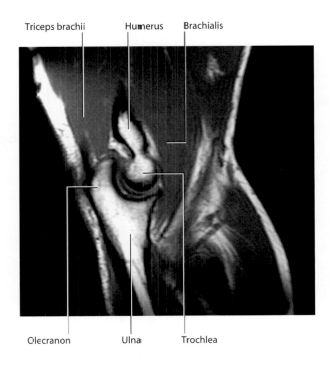

**Articulation of the trochlea of the humerus and the
trochlear notch of the ulna.**
T2-weighted MR image in sagittal plane

423

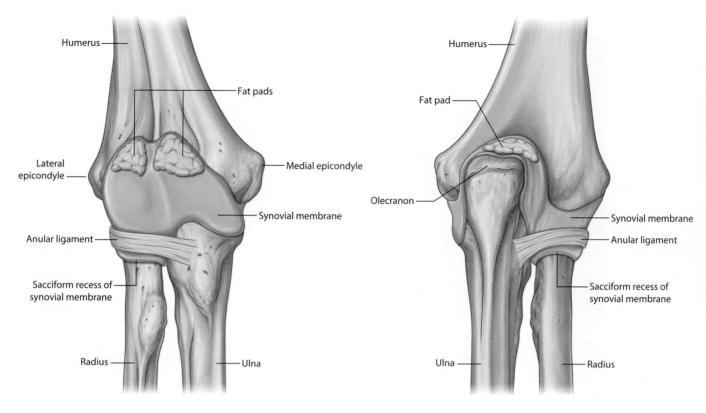

Synovial membrane of the elbow joint (anterior view)

Synovial membrane of the elbow joint (posterior view)

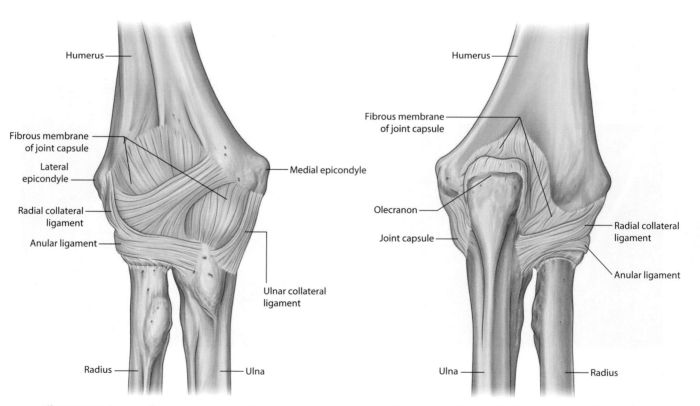

Fibrous membrane of joint capsule and ligaments of the elbow joint (anterior view)

Fibrous membrane of joint capsule and ligaments of the elbow joint (posterior view)

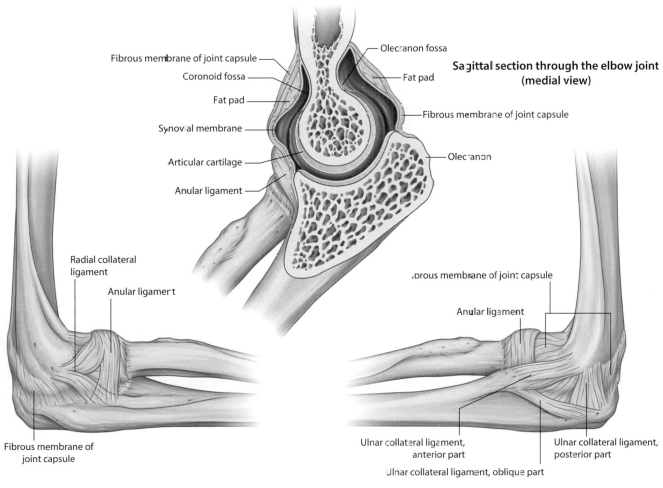

Fibrous membrane of joint capsule

Coronoid fossa

Fat pad

Synovial membrane

Articular cartilage

Anular ligament

Olecranon fossa

Fat pad

Sagittal section through the elbow joint (medial view)

Fibrous membrane of joint capsule

Olecranon

Radial collateral ligament

Anular ligament

Fibrous membrane of joint capsule

Fibrous membrane of joint capsule

Anular ligament

Ulnar collateral ligament, anterior part

Ulnar collateral ligament, oblique part

Ulnar collateral ligament, posterior part

Fibrous membrane of joint capsule and ligaments of the elbow joint (lateral view)

Fibrous membrane of joint capsule and ligaments of the elbow joint (medial view)

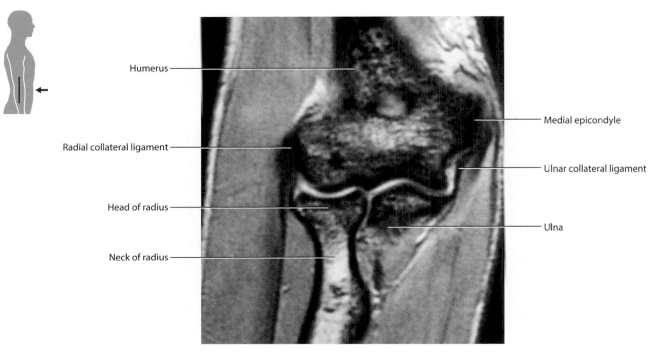

Humerus

Radial collateral ligament

Head of radius

Neck of radius

Medial epicondyle

Ulnar collateral ligament

Ulna

Normal elbow joint.
T2-weighted MR image in coronal plane

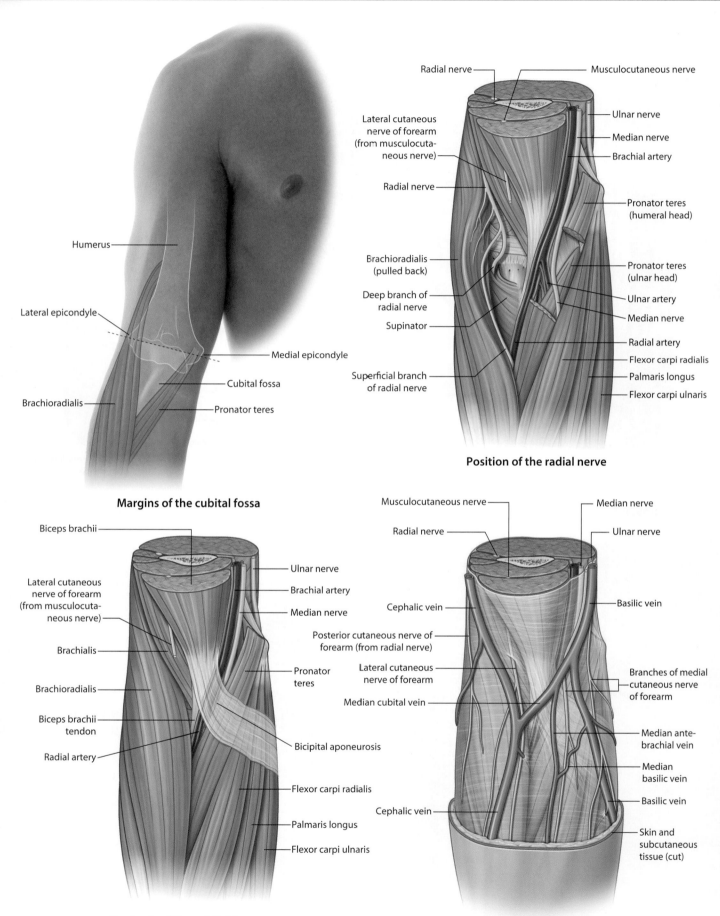

Humerus

Lateral epicondyle

Medial epicondyle

Cubital fossa

Brachioradialis

Pronator teres

Margins of the cubital fossa

Radial nerve

Musculocutaneous nerve

Lateral cutaneous nerve of forearm (from musculocutaneous nerve)

Ulnar nerve

Median nerve

Brachial artery

Radial nerve

Pronator teres (humeral head)

Brachioradialis (pulled back)

Pronator teres (ulnar head)

Deep branch of radial nerve

Ulnar artery

Supinator

Median nerve

Radial artery

Flexor carpi radialis

Palmaris longus

Superficial branch of radial nerve

Flexor carpi ulnaris

Position of the radial nerve

Biceps brachii

Ulnar nerve

Lateral cutaneous nerve of forearm (from musculocutaneous nerve)

Brachial artery

Median nerve

Brachialis

Brachioradialis

Pronator teres

Biceps brachii tendon

Radial artery

Bicipital aponeurosis

Flexor carpi radialis

Palmaris longus

Flexor carpi ulnaris

Contents of the cubital fossa

Musculocutaneous nerve

Median nerve

Radial nerve

Ulnar nerve

Cephalic vein

Basilic vein

Posterior cutaneous nerve of forearm (from radial nerve)

Lateral cutaneous nerve of forearm

Branches of medial cutaneous nerve of forearm

Median cubital vein

Median antebrachial vein

Median basilic vein

Cephalic vein

Basilic vein

Skin and subcutaneous tissue (cut)

Superficial structures

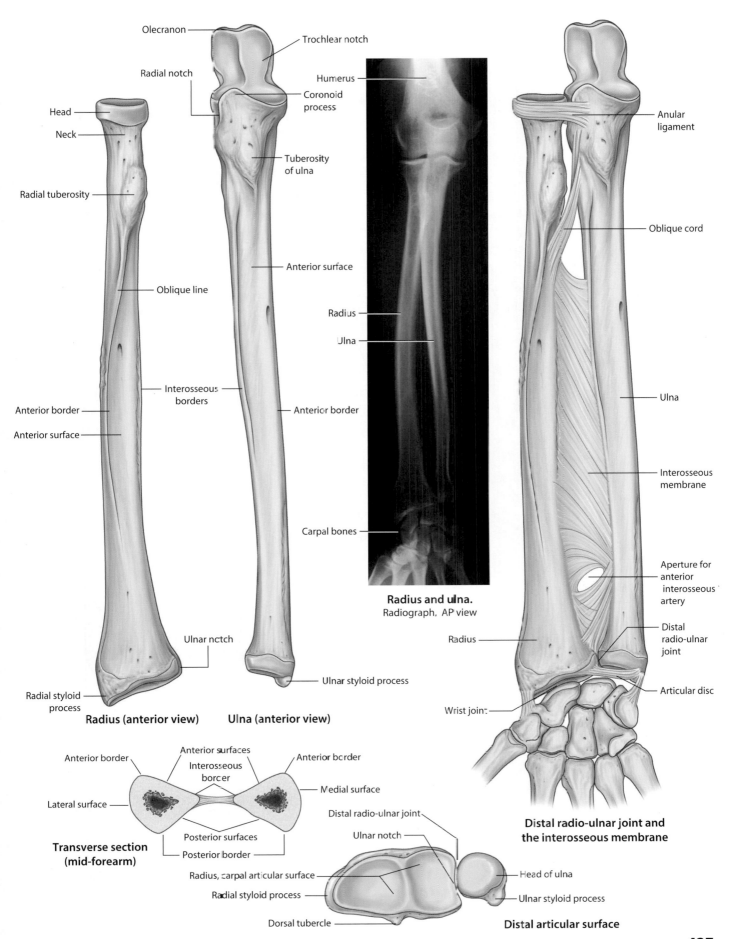

Olecranon

Trochlear notch

Radial notch

Humerus

Coronoid process

Head

Neck

Tuberosity of ulna

Radial tuberosity

Anular ligament

Anterior surface

Oblique cord

Oblique line

Radius

Ulna

Interosseous borders

Anterior border

Anterior border

Ulna

Anterior surface

Interosseous membrane

Carpal bones

Aperture for anterior interosseous artery

Distal radio-ulnar joint

Ulnar notch

Radius

Ulnar styloid process

Articular disc

Radial styloid process

Wrist joint

Radius (anterior view)   **Ulna (anterior view)**

Radius and ulna.
Radiograph, AP view

Distal radio-ulnar joint and the interosseous membrane

Anterior border

Anterior surfaces

Anterior border

Interosseous border

Distal radio-ulnar joint

Lateral surface

Medial surface

Ulnar notch

Posterior surfaces

Distal radio-ulnar joint

Head of ulna

Posterior border

Transverse section (mid-forearm)

Radius, carpal articular surface

Radial styloid process

Ulnar styloid process

Dorsal tubercle

Distal articular surface

427

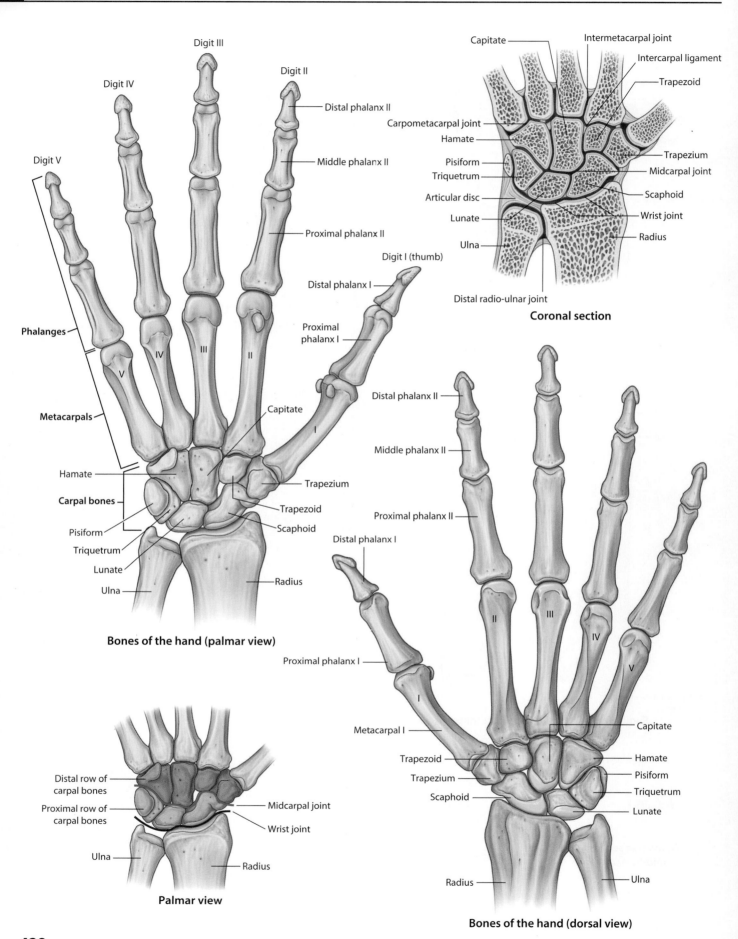

Digit III

Digit IV

Digit II

Distal phalanx II

Digit V

Middle phalanx II

Proximal phalanx II

Phalanges

Digit I (thumb)

Distal phalanx I

Proximal phalanx I

Metacarpals

Capitate

Hamate

Trapezium

Carpal bones

Trapezoid

Pisiform

Scaphoid

Triquetrum

Lunate

Ulna

Radius

Bones of the hand (palmar view)

Capitate

Intermetacarpal joint

Intercarpal ligament

Trapezoid

Carpometacarpal joint

Hamate

Pisiform

Trapezium

Triquetrum

Midcarpal joint

Articular disc

Scaphoid

Lunate

Wrist joint

Ulna

Radius

Distal radio-ulnar joint

Coronal section

Distal phalanx II

Middle phalanx II

Proximal phalanx II

Distal phalanx I

Proximal phalanx I

Metacarpal I

Capitate

Trapezoid

Hamate

Trapezium

Pisiform

Scaphoid

Triquetrum

Lunate

Radius

Ulna

Bones of the hand (dorsal view)

Distal row of carpal bones

Midcarpal joint

Proximal row of carpal bones

Wrist joint

Ulna

Radius

Palmar view

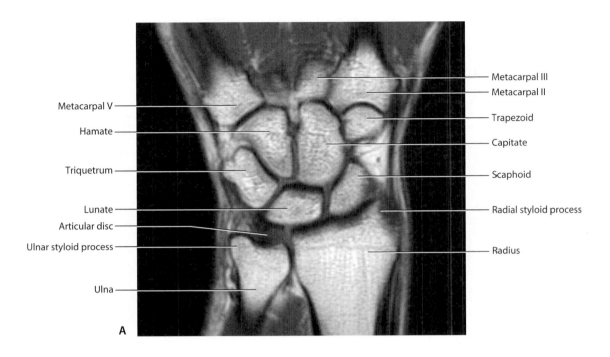

Metacarpal V

Hamate

Triquetrum

Lunate

Articular disc

Ulnar styloid process

Ulna

Metacarpal III

Metacarpal II

Trapezoid

Capitate

Scaphoid

Radial styloid process

Radius

A

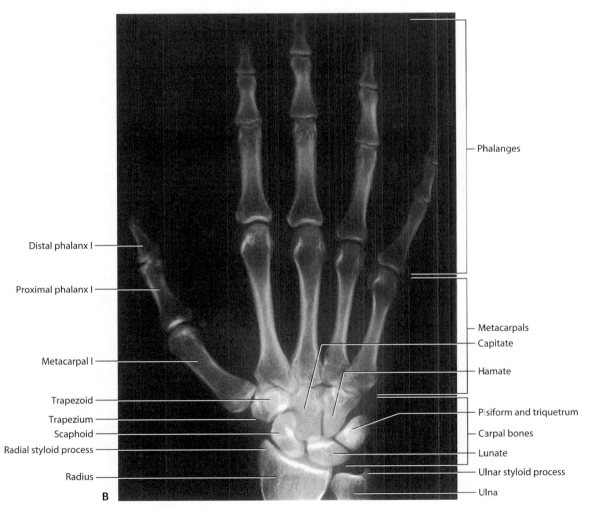

Distal phalanx I

Proximal phalanx I

Metacarpal I

Trapezoid

Trapezium

Scaphoid

Radial styloid process

Radius

Phalanges

Metacarpals

Capitate

Hamate

Pisiform and triquetrum

Carpal bones

Lunate

Ulnar styloid process

Ulna

B

Imaging of the wrist joint, the carpal bones, and the hand.
A. T1-weighted MR image in coronal plane
B. Radiograph, AP view

429

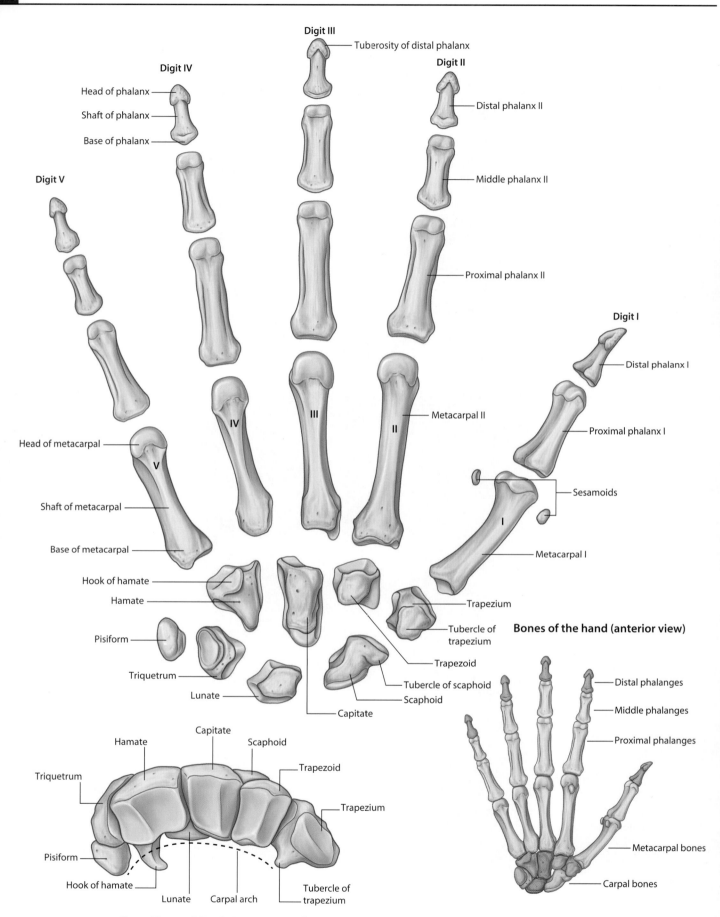

Digit III
Tuberosity of distal phalanx

Digit IV
Head of phalanx
Shaft of phalanx
Base of phalanx

Digit II
Distal phalanx II

Middle phalanx II

Digit V

Proximal phalanx II

Digit I
Distal phalanx I

Metacarpal II

Proximal phalanx I

Head of metacarpal

Sesamoids

Shaft of metacarpal

Base of metacarpal

Metacarpal I

Hook of hamate

Hamate

Trapezium

Pisiform

Tubercle of trapezium

Bones of the hand (anterior view)

Triquetrum

Trapezoid

Lunate

Tubercle of scaphoid

Scaphoid

Capitate

Distal phalanges

Middle phalanges

Hamate
Capitate
Scaphoid

Proximal phalanges

Triquetrum

Trapezoid

Pisiform

Trapezium

Metacarpal bones

Hook of hamate

Carpal bones

Lunate   Carpal arch

Tubercle of trapezium

Carpal bones (distal view; pronated)

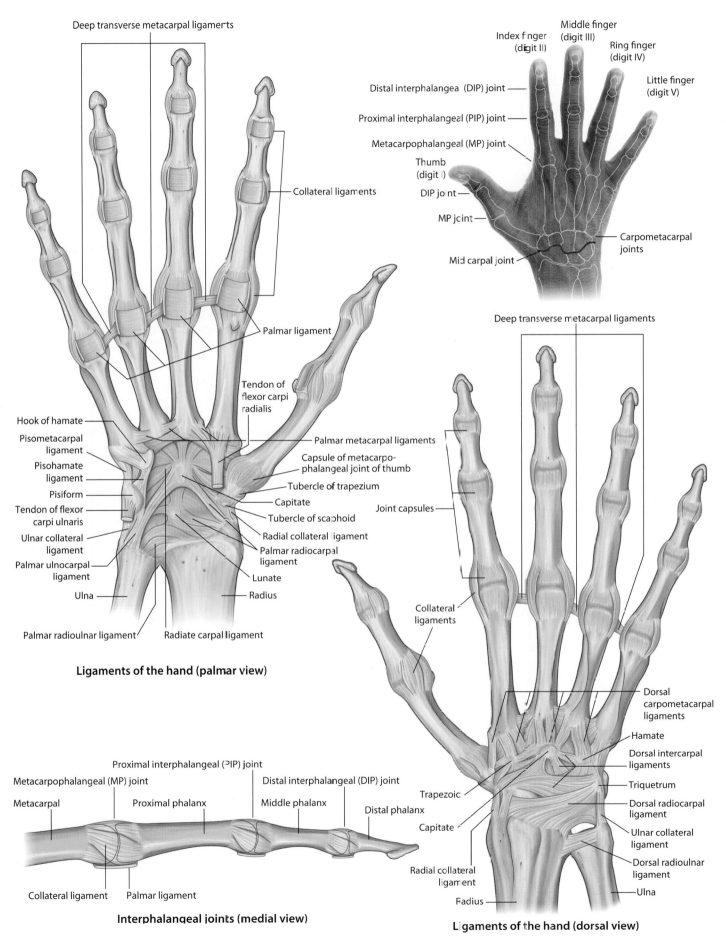

Deep transverse metacarpal ligaments

Collateral ligaments

Palmar ligament

Tendon of flexor carpi radialis

Hook of hamate
Pisometacarpal ligament
Pisohamate ligament
Pisiform
Tendon of flexor carpi ulnaris
Ulnar collateral ligament
Palmar ulnocarpal ligament
Ulna

Palmar radioulnar ligament

Palmar metacarpal ligaments
Capsule of metacarpo-phalangeal joint of thumb
Tubercle of trapezium
Capitate
Tubercle of scaphoid
Radial collateral ligament
Palmar radiocarpal ligament
Lunate
Radius

Radiate carpal ligament

Ligaments of the hand (palmar view)

Index finger (digit II)
Middle finger (digit III)
Ring finger (digit IV)
Little finger (digit V)

Distal interphalangeal (DIP) joint
Proximal interphalangeal (PIP) joint
Metacarpophalangeal (MP) joint
Thumb (digit I)
DIP joint
MP joint
Carpometacarpal joints
Mid carpal joint

Deep transverse metacarpal ligaments

Joint capsules

Collateral ligaments

Dorsal carpometacarpal ligaments
Hamate
Dorsal intercarpal ligaments
Triquetrum
Dorsal radiocarpal ligament
Ulnar collateral ligament
Dorsal radioulnar ligament
Ulna

Trapezoid
Capitate
Radial collateral ligament
Radius

Ligaments of the hand (dorsal view)

Metacarpophalangeal (MP) joint
Proximal interphalangeal (PIP) joint
Distal interphalangeal (DIP) joint
Metacarpal
Proximal phalanx
Middle phalanx
Distal phalanx

Collateral ligament
Palmar ligament

Interphalangeal joints (medial view)

431

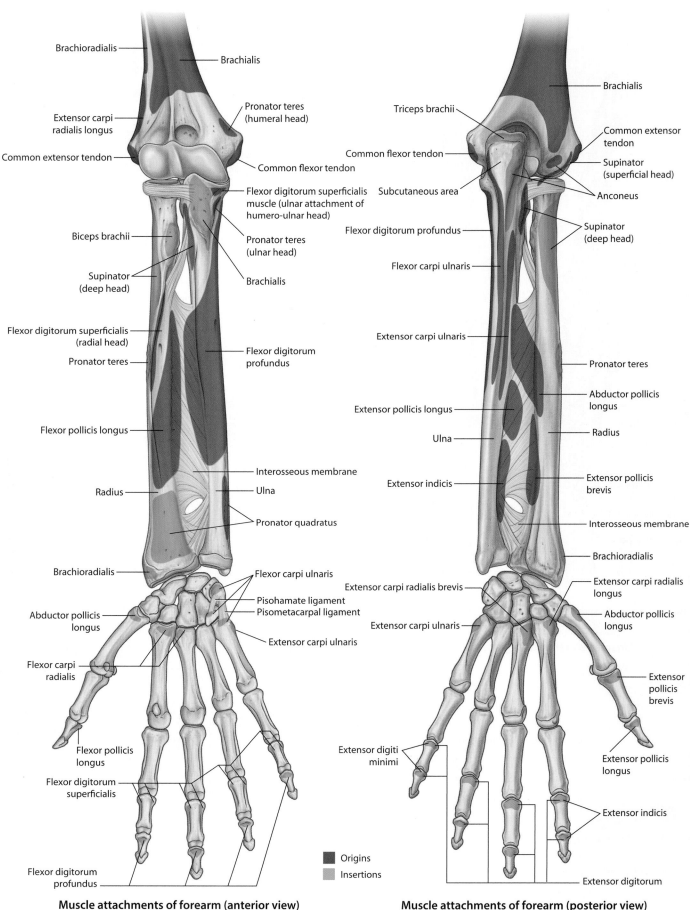

Brachioradialis

Brachialis

Extensor carpi radialis longus

Pronator teres (humeral head)

Common extensor tendon

Common flexor tendon

Flexor digitorum superficialis muscle (ulnar attachment of humero-ulnar head)

Biceps brachii

Pronator teres (ulnar head)

Supinator (deep head)

Brachialis

Flexor digitorum superficialis (radial head)

Flexor digitorum profundus

Pronator teres

Flexor pollicis longus

Interosseous membrane

Radius

Ulna

Pronator quadratus

Brachioradialis

Flexor carpi ulnaris

Pisohamate ligament

Pisometacarpal ligament

Abductor pollicis longus

Extensor carpi ulnaris

Flexor carpi radialis

Flexor pollicis longus

Flexor digitorum superficialis

Flexor digitorum profundus

Origins

Insertions

Muscle attachments of forearm (anterior view)

Triceps brachii

Brachialis

Common flexor tendon

Common extensor tendon

Supinator (superficial head)

Subcutaneous area

Anconeus

Flexor digitorum profundus

Supinator (deep head)

Flexor carpi ulnaris

Extensor carpi ulnaris

Pronator teres

Abductor pollicis longus

Extensor pollicis longus

Radius

Ulna

Extensor indicis

Extensor pollicis brevis

Interosseous membrane

Brachioradialis

Extensor carpi radialis brevis

Extensor carpi radialis longus

Extensor carpi ulnaris

Abductor pollicis longus

Extensor pollicis brevis

Extensor digiti minimi

Extensor pollicis longus

Extensor indicis

Extensor digitorum

Muscle attachments of forearm (posterior view)

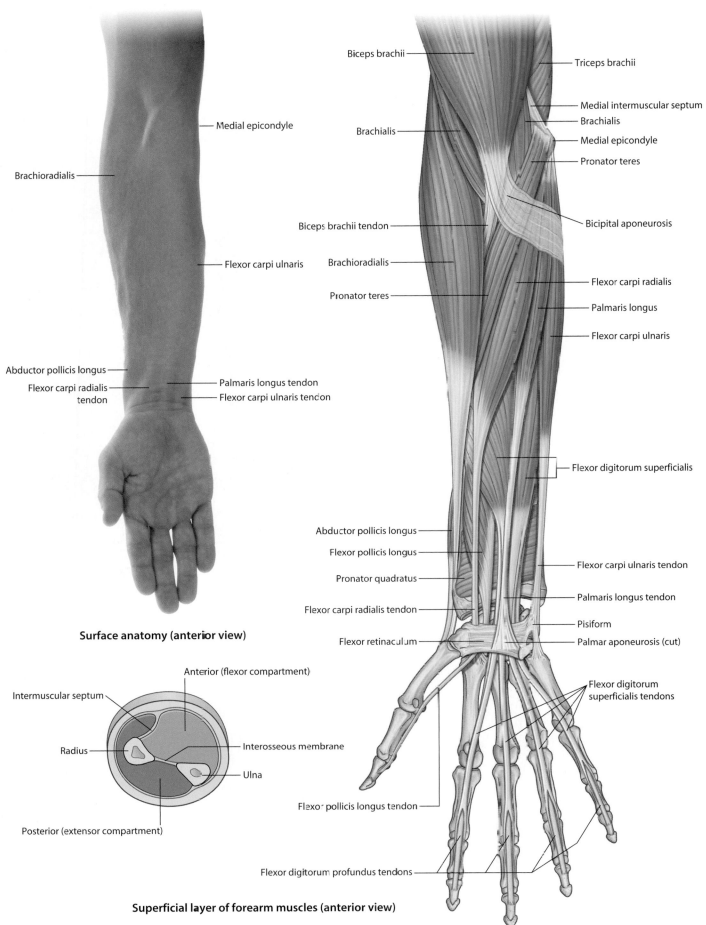

Surface anatomy (anterior view)

Brachioradialis

Medial epicondyle

Flexor carpi ulnaris

Abductor pollicis longus

Flexor carpi radialis tendon

Palmaris longus tendon

Flexor carpi ulnaris tendon

Biceps brachii

Triceps brachii

Medial intermuscular septum

Brachialis

Medial epicondyle

Pronator teres

Brachialis

Biceps brachii tendon

Bicipital aponeurosis

Brachioradialis

Flexor carpi radialis

Pronator teres

Palmaris longus

Flexor carpi ulnaris

Flexor digitorum superficialis

Abductor pollicis longus

Flexor pollicis longus

Flexor carpi ulnaris tendon

Pronator quadratus

Palmaris longus tendon

Flexor carpi radialis tendon

Pisiform

Flexor retinaculum

Palmar aponeurosis (cut)

Flexor digitorum superficialis tendons

Anterior (flexor compartment)

Intermuscular septum

Radius

Interosseous membrane

Ulna

Posterior (extensor compartment)

Flexor pollicis longus tendon

Flexor digitorum profundus tendons

Superficial layer of forearm muscles (anterior view)

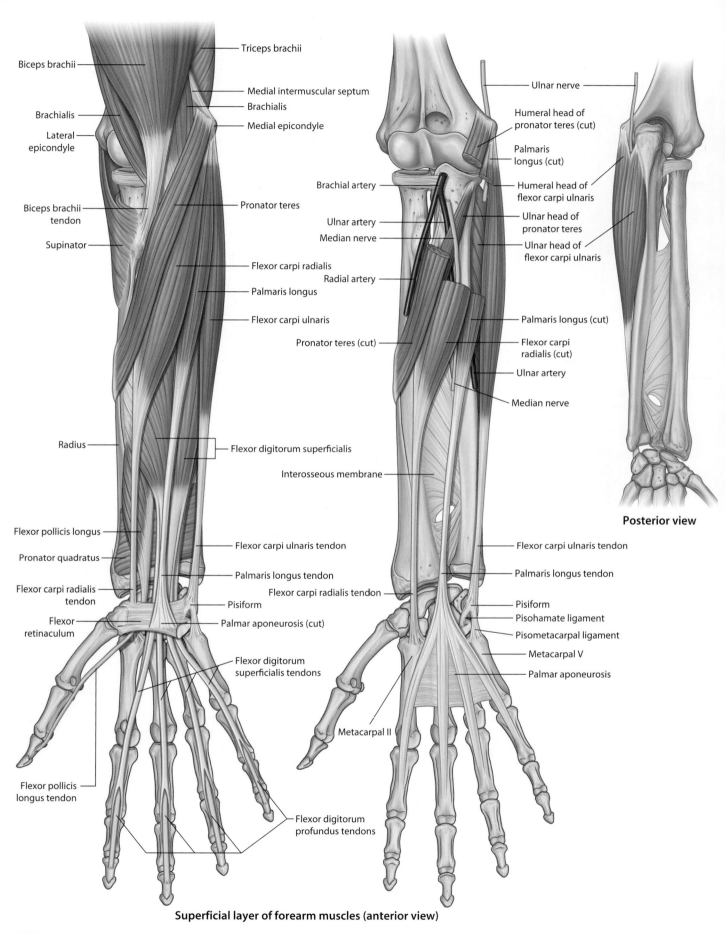

Biceps brachii

Triceps brachii

Brachialis

Medial intermuscular septum

Brachialis

Medial epicondyle

Lateral epicondyle

Biceps brachii tendon

Pronator teres

Supinator

Flexor carpi radialis

Palmaris longus

Flexor carpi ulnaris

Radius

Flexor digitorum superficialis

Flexor pollicis longus

Pronator quadratus

Flexor carpi radialis tendon

Flexor carpi ulnaris tendon

Palmaris longus tendon

Flexor carpi radialis tendon

Flexor retinaculum

Pisiform

Palmar aponeurosis (cut)

Flexor digitorum superficialis tendons

Flexor pollicis longus tendon

Flexor digitorum profundus tendons

Ulnar nerve

Humeral head of pronator teres (cut)

Palmaris longus (cut)

Humeral head of flexor carpi ulnaris

Brachial artery

Ulnar head of pronator teres

Ulnar artery

Median nerve

Ulnar head of flexor carpi ulnaris

Radial artery

Palmaris longus (cut)

Pronator teres (cut)

Flexor carpi radialis (cut)

Ulnar artery

Median nerve

Interosseous membrane

Flexor carpi ulnaris tendon

Palmaris longus tendon

Pisiform

Pisohamate ligament

Pisometacarpal ligament

Metacarpal V

Palmar aponeurosis

Metacarpal II

Posterior view

Superficial layer of forearm muscles (anterior view)

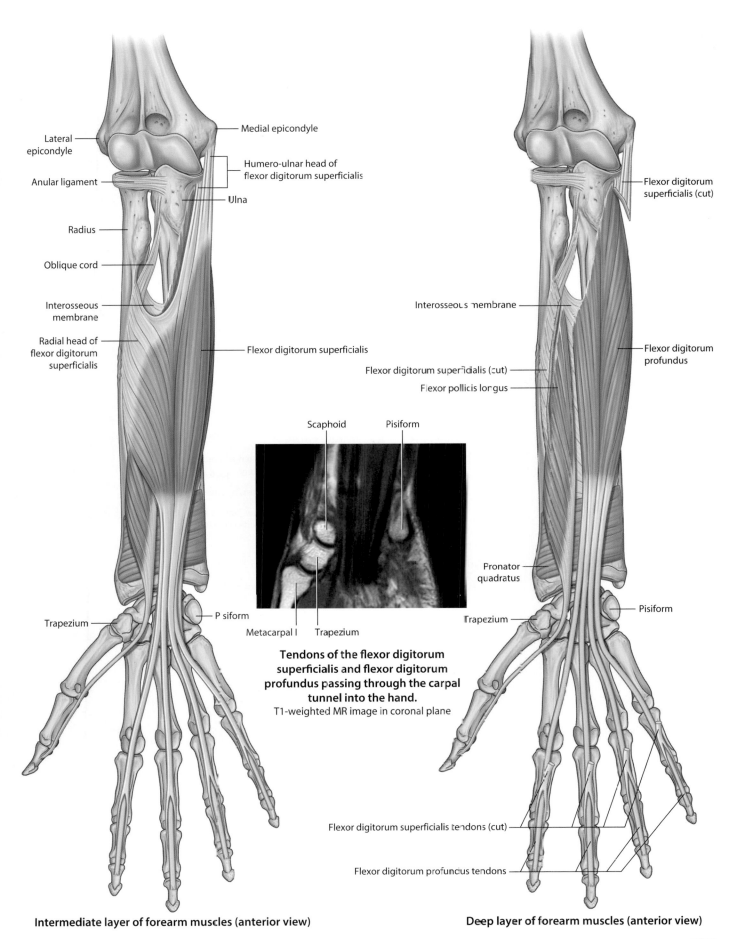

Lateral epicondyle

Medial epicondyle

Anular ligament

Humero-ulnar head of flexor digitorum superficialis

Ulna

Radius

Oblique cord

Interosseous membrane

Radial head of flexor digitorum superficialis

Flexor digitorum superficialis

Flexor digitorum superficialis (cut)

Interosseous membrane

Flexor digitorum profundus

Flexor digitorum superficialis (cut)

Flexor pollicis longus

Scaphoid

Pisiform

Trapezium

Pisiform

Pronator quadratus

Trapezium

Pisiform

Metacarpal I

Trapezium

Tendons of the flexor digitorum superficialis and flexor digitorum profundus passing through the carpal tunnel into the hand.
T1-weighted MR image in coronal plane

Flexor digitorum superficialis tendons (cut)

Flexor digitorum profundus tendons

Intermediate layer of forearm muscles (anterior view)

Deep layer of forearm muscles (anterior view)

435

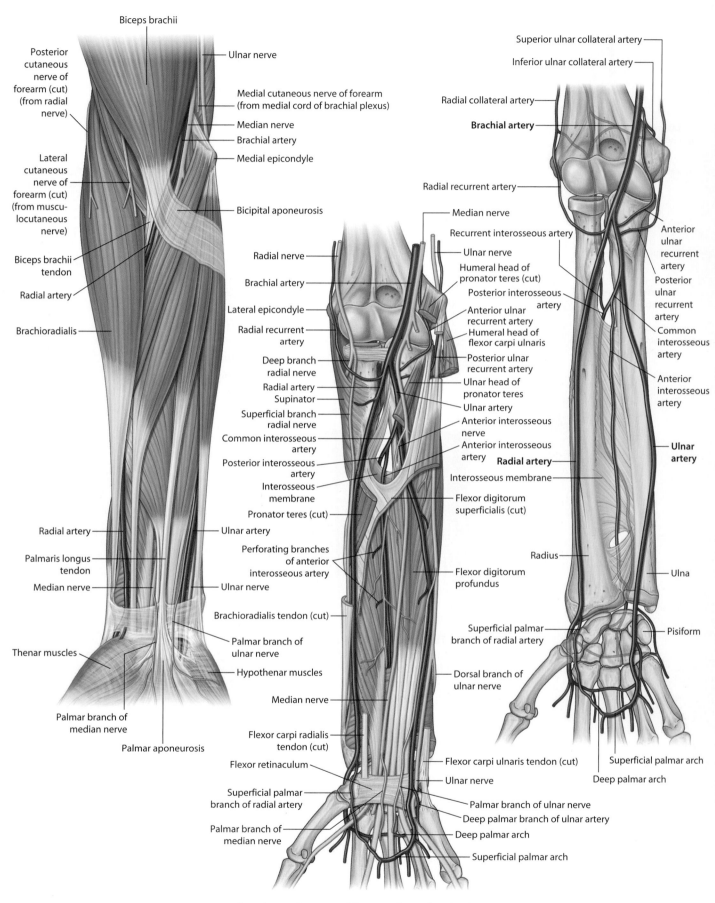

Biceps brachii

Posterior cutaneous nerve of forearm (cut) (from radial nerve)

Lateral cutaneous nerve of forearm (cut) (from musculo-cutaneous nerve)

Biceps brachii tendon

Radial artery

Brachioradialis

Radial artery

Palmaris longus tendon

Median nerve

Thenar muscles

Palmar branch of median nerve

Palmar aponeurosis

Ulnar nerve

Medial cutaneous nerve of forearm (from medial cord of brachial plexus)

Median nerve

Brachial artery

Medial epicondyle

Bicipital aponeurosis

Radial nerve

Brachial artery

Lateral epicondyle

Radial recurrent artery

Deep branch radial nerve

Radial artery

Supinator

Superficial branch radial nerve

Common interosseous artery

Posterior interosseous artery

Interosseous membrane

Pronator teres (cut)

Ulnar artery

Perforating branches of anterior interosseous artery

Brachioradialis tendon (cut)

Palmar branch of ulnar nerve

Hypothenar muscles

Median nerve

Flexor carpi radialis tendon (cut)

Flexor retinaculum

Superficial palmar branch of radial artery

Palmar branch of median nerve

Median nerve

Recurrent interosseous artery

Ulnar nerve

Humeral head of pronator teres (cut)

Posterior interosseous artery

Anterior ulnar recurrent artery

Humeral head of flexor carpi ulnaris

Posterior ulnar recurrent artery

Ulnar head of pronator teres

Ulnar artery

Anterior interosseous nerve

Anterior interosseous artery

Radial artery

Interosseous membrane

Flexor digitorum superficialis (cut)

Flexor digitorum profundus

Dorsal branch of ulnar nerve

Flexor carpi ulnaris tendon (cut)

Ulnar nerve

Palmar branch of ulnar nerve

Deep palmar branch of ulnar artery

Deep palmar arch

Superficial palmar arch

Superior ulnar collateral artery

Inferior ulnar collateral artery

Radial collateral artery

Brachial artery

Radial recurrent artery

Anterior ulnar recurrent artery

Posterior ulnar recurrent artery

Common interosseous artery

Anterior interosseous artery

Ulnar artery

Radius

Ulna

Superficial palmar branch of radial artery

Pisiform

Superficial palmar arch

Deep palmar arch

Arteries and nerves of forearm (anterior view)

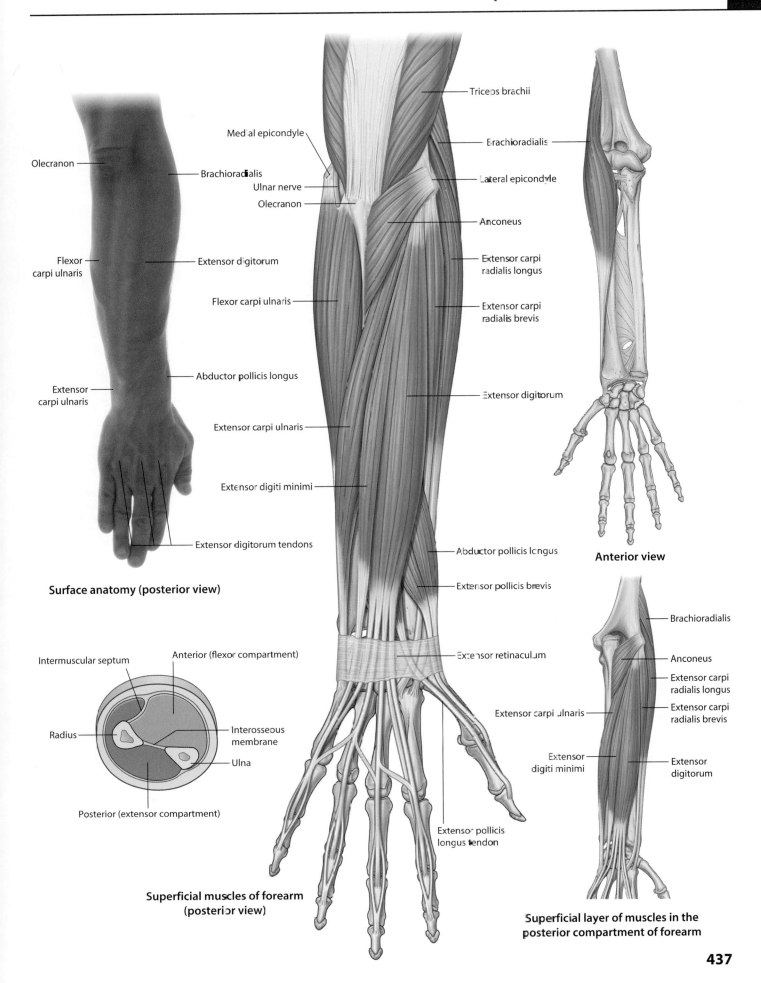

Olecranon

Flexor
carpi ulnaris

Extensor
carpi ulnaris

Surface anatomy (posterior view)

Medial epicondyle

Brachioradialis

Ulnar nerve

Olecranon

Extensor digitorum

Flexor carpi ulnaris

Abductor pollicis longus

Extensor carpi ulnaris

Extensor digiti minimi

Extensor digitorum tendons

Triceps brachii

Brachioradialis

Lateral epicondyle

Anconeus

Extensor carpi
radialis longus

Extensor carpi
radialis brevis

Extensor digitorum

Abductor pollicis longus

Extensor pollicis brevis

Extensor retinaculum

Extensor pollicis
longus tendon

Anterior view

Brachioradialis

Anconeus

Extensor carpi
radialis longus

Extensor carpi
radialis brevis

Extensor carpi ulnaris

Extensor
digiti minimi

Extensor
digitorum

**Superficial layer of muscles in the
posterior compartment of forearm**

Intermuscular septum

Anterior (flexor compartment)

Radius

Interosseous
membrane

Ulna

Posterior (extensor compartment)

**Superficial muscles of forearm
(posterior view)**

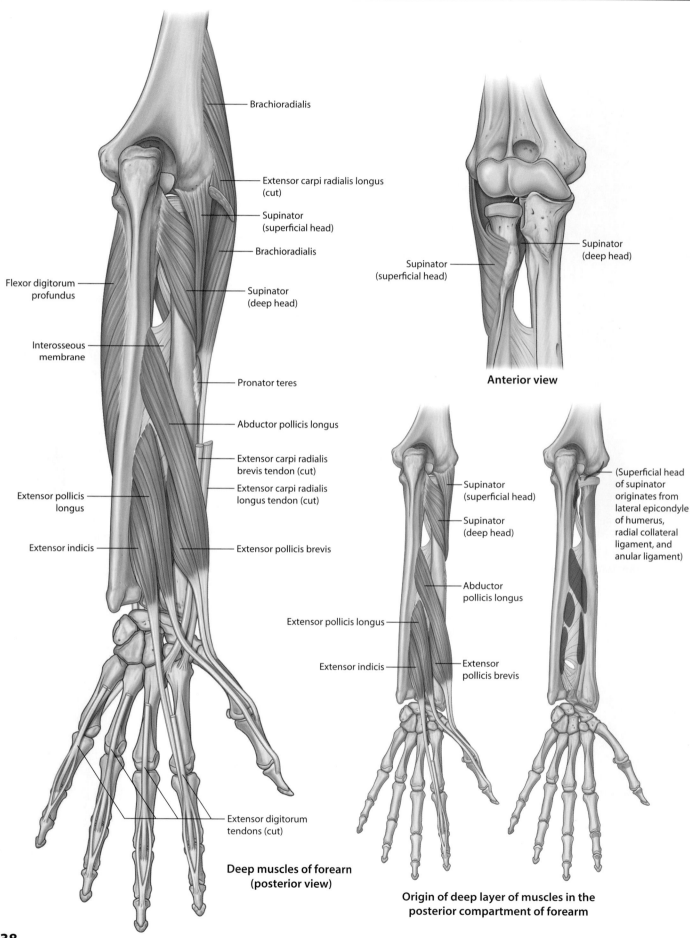

Brachioradialis

Extensor carpi radialis longus (cut)

Supinator (superficial head)

Brachioradialis

Flexor digitorum profundus

Supinator (deep head)

Interosseous membrane

Pronator teres

Abductor pollicis longus

Extensor carpi radialis brevis tendon (cut)

Extensor carpi radialis longus tendon (cut)

Extensor pollicis longus

Extensor indicis

Extensor pollicis brevis

Extensor digitorum tendons (cut)

Deep muscles of forearm (posterior view)

Anterior view

Supinator (superficial head)

Supinator (deep head)

Supinator (deep head)

Supinator (superficial head)

Abductor pollicis longus

Extensor pollicis longus

Extensor indicis

Extensor pollicis brevis

(Superficial head of supinator originates from lateral epicondyle of humerus, radial collateral ligament, and anular ligament)

Origin of deep layer of muscles in the posterior compartment of forearm

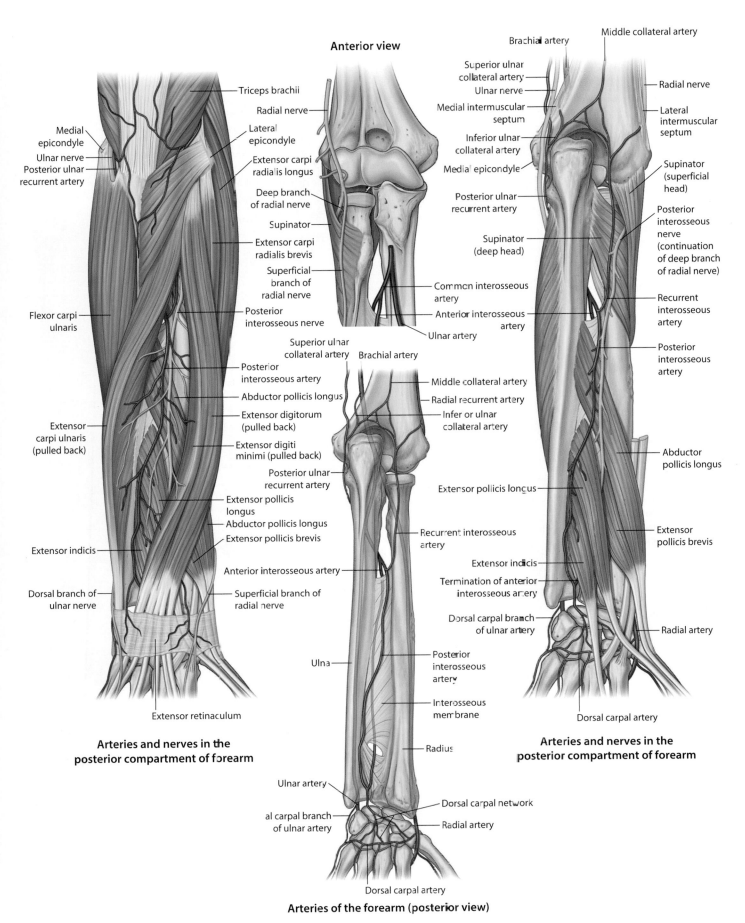

Anterior view

Triceps brachii

Medial epicondyle

Ulnar nerve

Posterior ulnar recurrent artery

Radial nerve

Lateral epicondyle

Extensor carpi radialis longus

Deep branch of radial nerve

Supinator

Extensor carpi radialis brevis

Superficial branch of radial nerve

Posterior interosseous nerve

Flexor carpi ulnaris

Superior ulnar collateral artery

Brachial artery

Posterior interosseous artery

Abductor pollicis longus

Extensor digitorum (pulled back)

Extensor carpi ulnaris (pulled back)

Extensor digiti minimi (pulled back)

Posterior ulnar recurrent artery

Extensor pollicis longus

Abductor pollicis longus

Extensor pollicis brevis

Extensor indicis

Dorsal branch of ulnar nerve

Superficial branch of radial nerve

Extensor retinaculum

Arteries and nerves in the posterior compartment of forearm

Brachial artery

Middle collateral artery

Superior ulnar collateral artery

Ulnar nerve

Medial intermuscular septum

Inferior ulnar collateral artery

Medial epicondyle

Posterior ulnar recurrent artery

Supinator (deep head)

Common interosseous artery

Anterior interosseous artery

Ulnar artery

Radial nerve

Lateral intermuscular septum

Supinator (superficial head)

Posterior interosseous nerve (continuation of deep branch of radial nerve)

Recurrent interosseous artery

Posterior interosseous artery

Abductor pollicis longus

Extensor pollicis brevis

Extensor indicis

Radial artery

Dorsal carpal artery

Arteries and nerves in the posterior compartment of forearm

Middle collateral artery

Radial recurrent artery

Inferior ulnar collateral artery

Extensor pollicis longus

Recurrent interosseous artery

Anterior interosseous artery

Termination of anterior interosseous artery

Dorsal carpal branch of ulnar artery

Ulna

Posterior interosseous artery

Interosseous membrane

Radius

Ulnar artery

al carpal branch of ulnar artery

Dorsal carpal network

Radial artery

Dorsal carpal artery

Arteries of the forearm (posterior view)

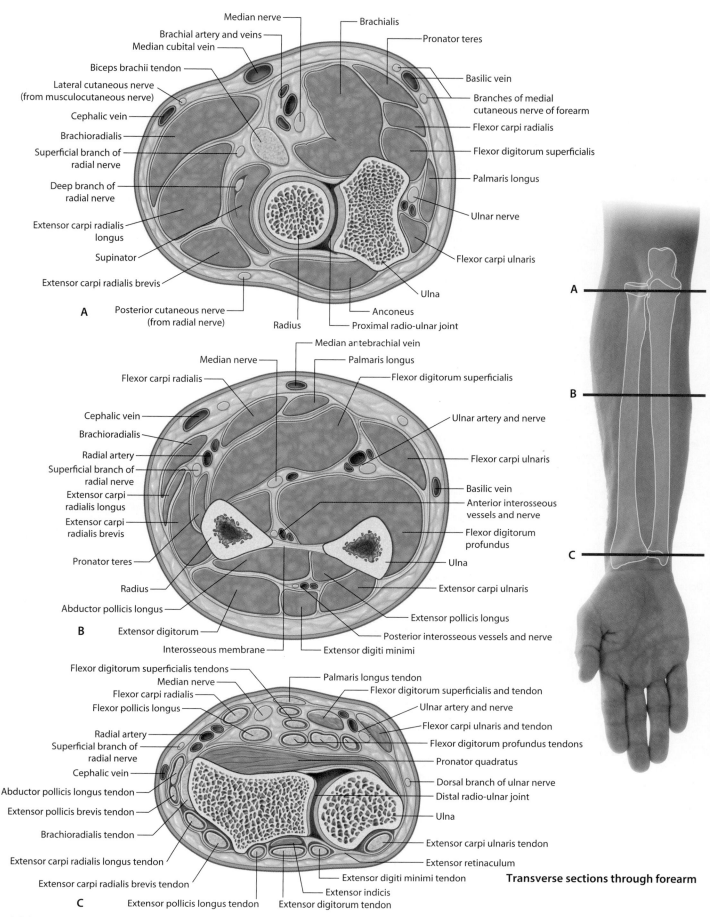

A

- Median nerve
- Brachial artery and veins
- Median cubital vein
- Biceps brachii tendon
- Lateral cutaneous nerve (from musculocutaneous nerve)
- Cephalic vein
- Brachioradialis
- Superficial branch of radial nerve
- Deep branch of radial nerve
- Extensor carpi radialis longus
- Supinator
- Extensor carpi radialis brevis
- Posterior cutaneous nerve (from radial nerve)
- Radius
- Brachialis
- Pronator teres
- Basilic vein
- Branches of medial cutaneous nerve of forearm
- Flexor carpi radialis
- Flexor digitorum superficialis
- Palmaris longus
- Ulnar nerve
- Flexor carpi ulnaris
- Ulna
- Anconeus
- Proximal radio-ulnar joint

B

- Median antebrachial vein
- Median nerve
- Palmaris longus
- Flexor carpi radialis
- Flexor digitorum superficialis
- Cephalic vein
- Brachioradialis
- Radial artery
- Superficial branch of radial nerve
- Extensor carpi radialis longus
- Extensor carpi radialis brevis
- Pronator teres
- Radius
- Abductor pollicis longus
- Extensor digitorum
- Interosseous membrane
- Ulnar artery and nerve
- Flexor carpi ulnaris
- Basilic vein
- Anterior interosseous vessels and nerve
- Flexor digitorum profundus
- Ulna
- Extensor carpi ulnaris
- Extensor pollicis longus
- Posterior interosseous vessels and nerve
- Extensor digiti minimi

C

- Flexor digitorum superficialis tendons
- Median nerve
- Flexor carpi radialis
- Flexor pollicis longus
- Radial artery
- Superficial branch of radial nerve
- Cephalic vein
- Abductor pollicis longus tendon
- Extensor pollicis brevis tendon
- Brachioradialis tendon
- Extensor carpi radialis longus tendon
- Extensor carpi radialis brevis tendon
- Extensor pollicis longus tendon
- Palmaris longus tendon
- Flexor digitorum superficialis and tendon
- Ulnar artery and nerve
- Flexor carpi ulnaris and tendon
- Flexor digitorum profundus tendons
- Pronator quadratus
- Dorsal branch of ulnar nerve
- Distal radio-ulnar joint
- Ulna
- Extensor carpi ulnaris tendon
- Extensor retinaculum
- Extensor digiti minimi tendon
- Extensor indicis
- Extensor digitorum tendon

Transverse sections through forearm

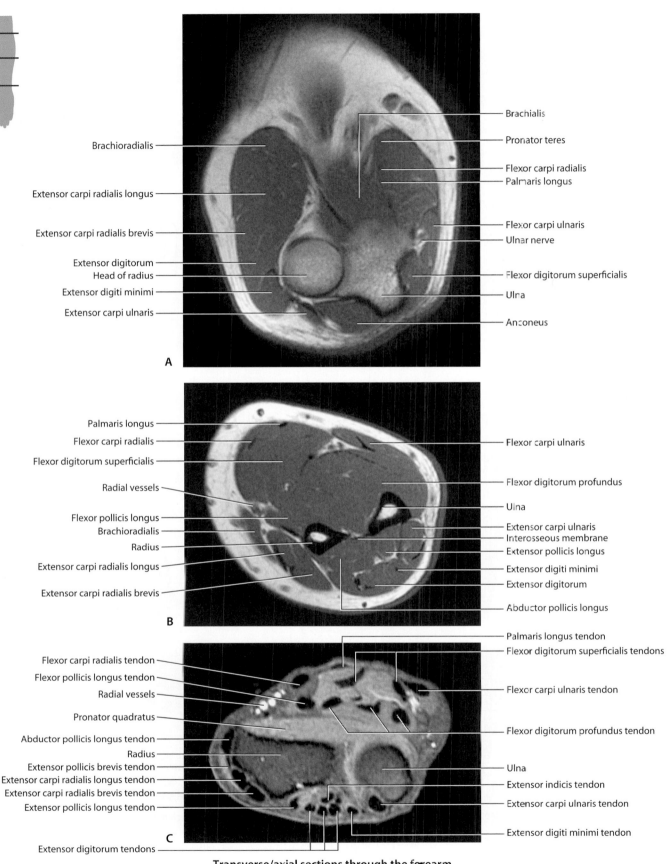

Brachioradialis

Extensor carpi radialis longus

Extensor carpi radialis brevis

Extensor digitorum
Head of radius
Extensor digiti minimi
Extensor carpi ulnaris

Brachialis

Pronator teres

Flexor carpi radialis
Palmaris longus

Flexor carpi ulnaris
Ulnar nerve

Flexor digitorum superficialis

Ulna

Anconeus

A

Palmaris longus

Flexor carpi radialis

Flexor digitorum superficialis

Radial vessels

Flexor pollicis longus
Brachioradialis
Radius

Extensor carpi radialis longus

Extensor carpi radialis brevis

Flexor carpi ulnaris

Flexor digitorum profundus

Ulna

Extensor carpi ulnaris
Interosseous membrane
Extensor pollicis longus
Extensor digiti minimi
Extensor digitorum

Abductor pollicis longus

B

Flexor carpi radialis tendon
Flexor pollicis longus tendon
Radial vessels
Pronator quadratus
Abductor pollicis longus tendon
Radius
Extensor pollicis brevis tendon
Extensor carpi radialis longus tendon
Extensor carpi radialis brevis tendon
Extensor pollicis longus tendon

Palmaris longus tendon
Flexor digitorum superficialis tendons

Flexor carpi ulnaris tendon

Flexor digitorum profundus tendon

Ulna

Extensor indicis tendon

Extensor carpi ulnaris tendon

Extensor digiti minimi tendon

C

Extensor digitorum tendons

Transverse/axial sections through the forearm.
A. Proximal/upper forearm.
B. Middle forearm.
C. Distal/lower forearm.
T1-weighted MR image in axial plane

441

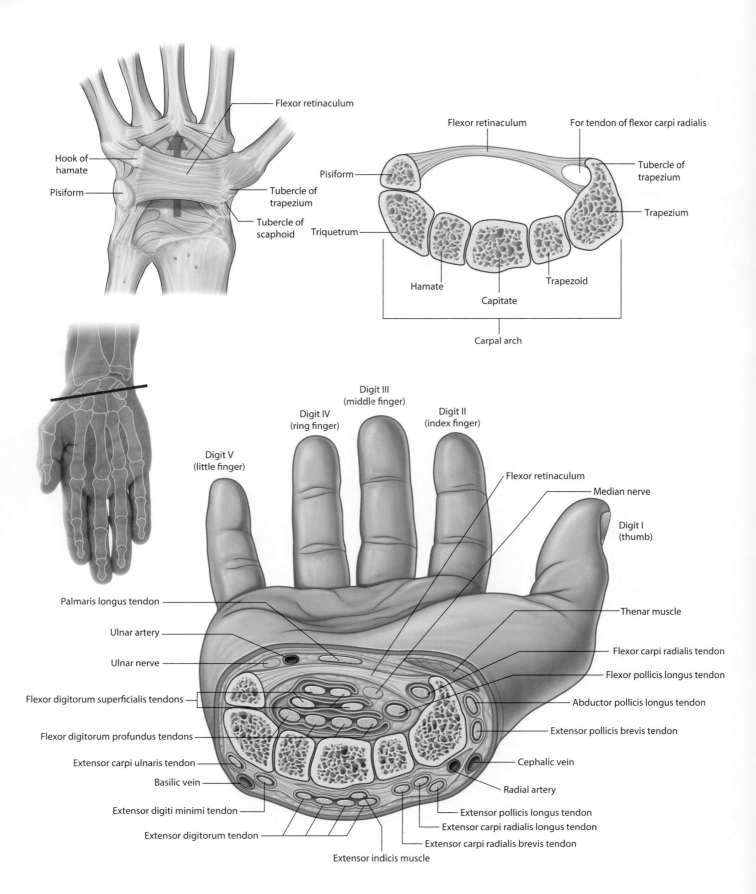

Flexor retinaculum

Hook of hamate

Pisiform

Tubercle of trapezium

Tubercle of scaphoid

Flexor retinaculum

For tendon of flexor carpi radialis

Pisiform

Tubercle of trapezium

Trapezium

Triquetrum

Hamate

Capitate

Trapezoid

Carpal arch

Digit III (middle finger)

Digit IV (ring finger)

Digit II (index finger)

Digit V (little finger)

Flexor retinaculum

Median nerve

Digit I (thumb)

Palmaris longus tendon

Ulnar artery

Ulnar nerve

Flexor digitorum superficialis tendons

Flexor digitorum profundus tendons

Extensor carpi ulnaris tendon

Basilic vein

Extensor digiti minimi tendon

Extensor digitorum tendon

Extensor indicis muscle

Thenar muscle

Flexor carpi radialis tendon

Flexor pollicis longus tendon

Abductor pollicis longus tendon

Extensor pollicis brevis tendon

Cephalic vein

Radial artery

Extensor pollicis longus tendon

Extensor carpi radialis longus tendon

Extensor carpi radialis brevis tendon

Carpal tunnel, structures and relations

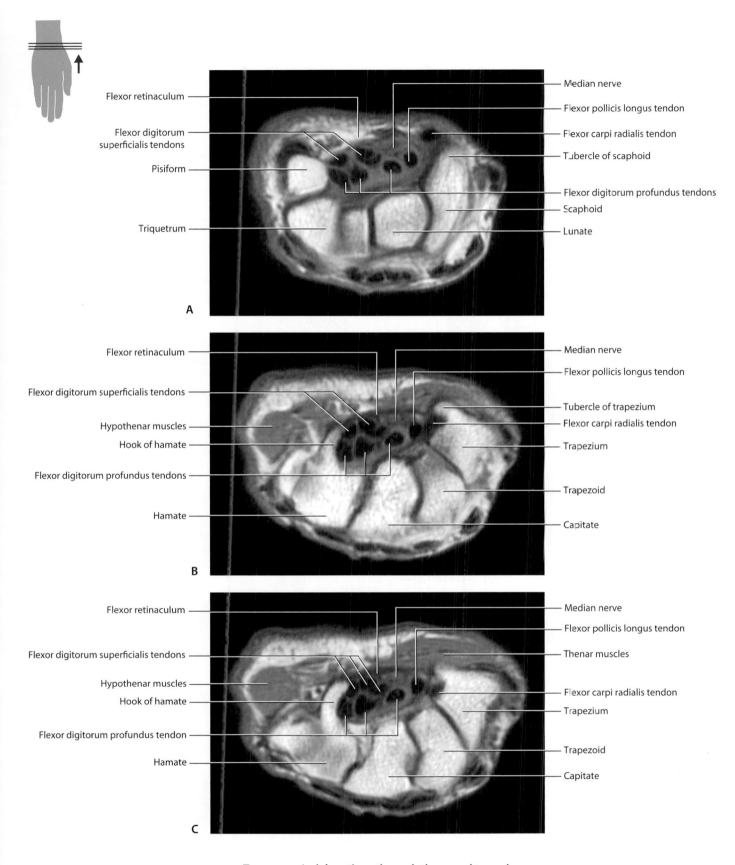

Flexor retinaculum

Flexor digitorum superficialis tendons

Pisiform

Triquetrum

Median nerve

Flexor pollicis longus tendon

Flexor carpi radialis tendon

Tubercle of scaphoid

Flexor digitorum profundus tendons

Scaphoid

Lunate

A

Flexor retinaculum

Flexor digitorum superficialis tendons

Hypothenar muscles

Hook of hamate

Flexor digitorum profundus tendons

Hamate

Median nerve

Flexor pollicis longus tendon

Tubercle of trapezium

Flexor carpi radialis tendon

Trapezium

Trapezoid

Capitate

B

Flexor retinaculum

Flexor digitorum superficialis tendons

Hypothenar muscles

Hook of hamate

Flexor digitorum profundus tendon

Hamate

Median nerve

Flexor pollicis longus tendon

Thenar muscles

Flexor carpi radialis tendon

Trapezium

Trapezoid

Capitate

C

Transverse/axial sections through the carpal tunnel.
A. Proximal end of carpal tunnel.
B. Middle portion of carpal tunnel.
C. Distal portion of carpal tunnel.
T1-weighted MR images in axial plane

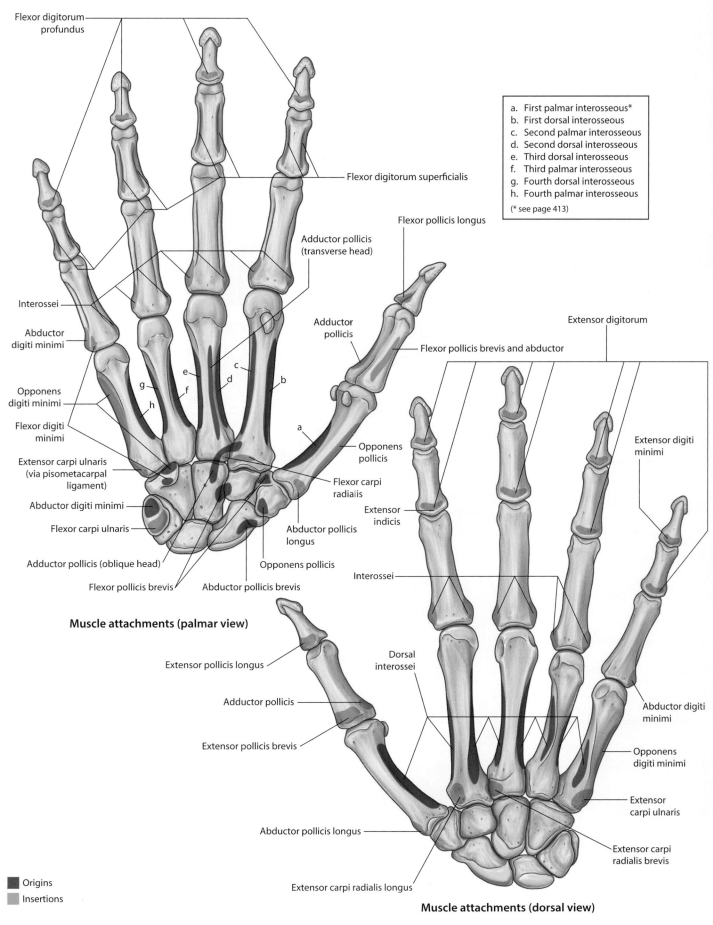

Flexor digitorum profundus

Flexor digitorum superficialis

Adductor pollicis (transverse head)

Flexor pollicis longus

a. First palmar interosseous*
b. First dorsal interosseous
c. Second palmar interosseous
d. Second dorsal interosseous
e. Third dorsal interosseous
f. Third palmar interosseous
g. Fourth dorsal interosseous
h. Fourth palmar interosseous
(* see page 413)

Adductor pollicis

Extensor digitorum

Flexor pollicis brevis and abductor

Interossei

Abductor digiti minimi

e d c b
g f h a

Extensor digiti minimi

Opponens digiti minimi

Opponens pollicis

Flexor digiti minimi

Extensor indicis

Extensor carpi ulnaris (via pisometacarpal ligament)

Flexor carpi radialis

Abductor digiti minimi

Extensor digiti minimi

Flexor carpi ulnaris

Abductor pollicis longus

Interossei

Abductor digiti minimi

Adductor pollicis (oblique head)

Opponens pollicis

Opponens digiti minimi

Flexor pollicis brevis

Abductor pollicis brevis

Muscle attachments (palmar view)

Extensor pollicis longus

Dorsal interossei

Adductor pollicis

Extensor pollicis brevis

Extensor carpi ulnaris

Opponens digiti minimi

Abductor pollicis longus

Extensor carpi radialis brevis

Extensor carpi radialis longus

Muscle attachments (dorsal view)

■ Origins
■ Insertions

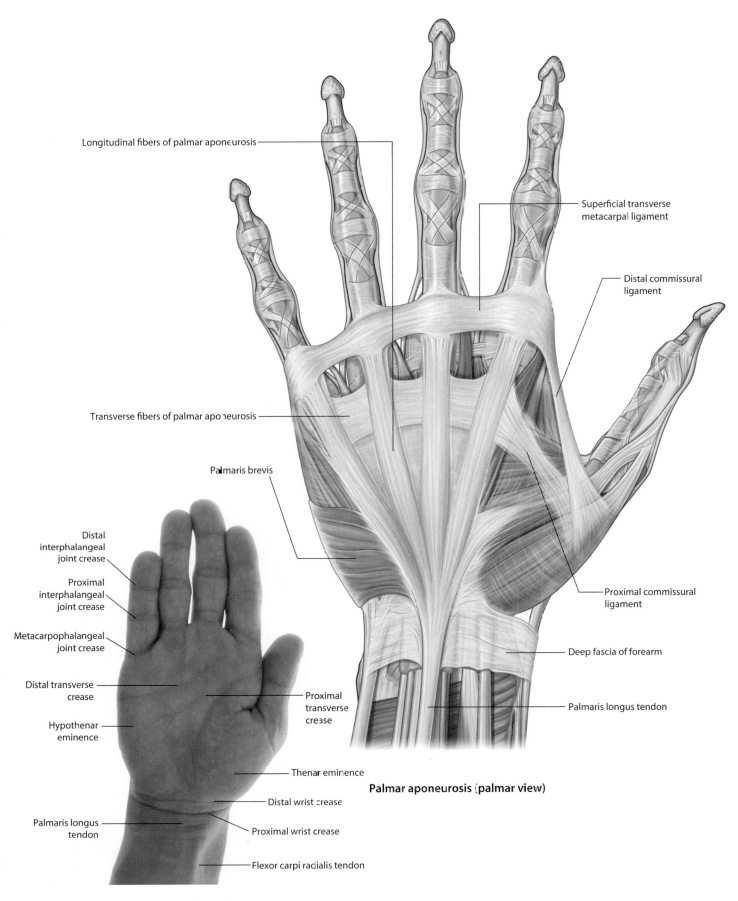

Longitudinal fibers of palmar aponeurosis

Superficial transverse metacarpal ligament

Distal commissural ligament

Transverse fibers of palmar aponeurosis

Palmaris brevis

Proximal commissural ligament

Deep fascia of forearm

Palmaris longus tendon

Palmar aponeurosis (palmar view)

Distal interphalangeal joint crease

Proximal interphalangeal joint crease

Metacarpophalangeal joint crease

Distal transverse crease

Hypothenar eminence

Palmaris longus tendon

Proximal transverse crease

Thenar eminence

Distal wrist crease

Proximal wrist crease

Flexor carpi radialis tendon

Surface anatomy (palmar view)

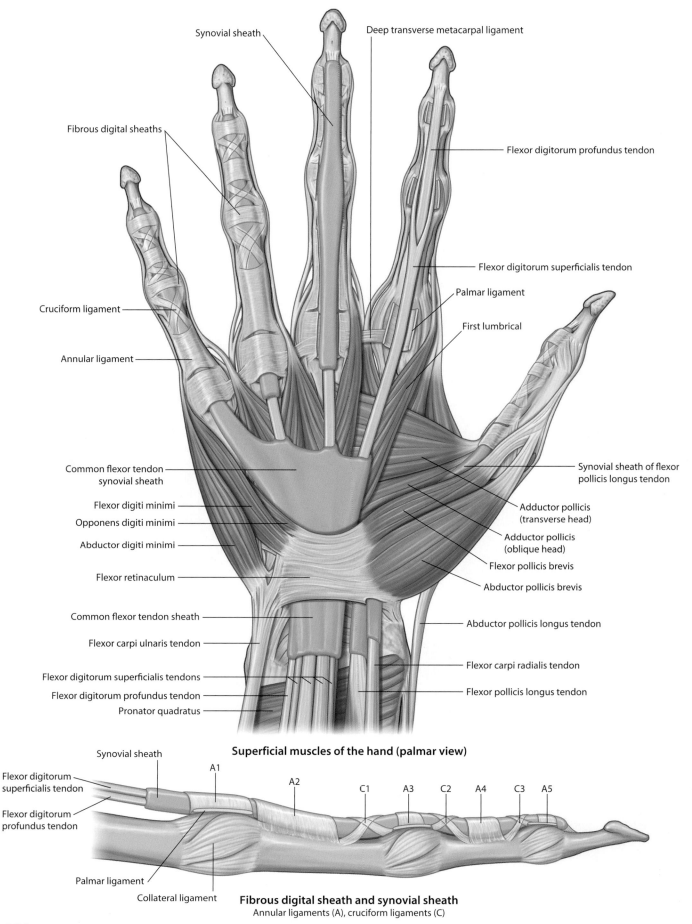

Synovial sheath

Deep transverse metacarpal ligament

Fibrous digital sheaths

Flexor digitorum profundus tendon

Flexor digitorum superficialis tendon

Cruciform ligament

Palmar ligament

First lumbrical

Annular ligament

Common flexor tendon synovial sheath

Synovial sheath of flexor pollicis longus tendon

Flexor digiti minimi

Adductor pollicis (transverse head)

Opponens digiti minimi

Adductor pollicis (oblique head)

Abductor digiti minimi

Flexor pollicis brevis

Flexor retinaculum

Abductor pollicis brevis

Common flexor tendon sheath

Abductor pollicis longus tendon

Flexor carpi ulnaris tendon

Flexor carpi radialis tendon

Flexor digitorum superficialis tendons

Flexor pollicis longus tendon

Flexor digitorum profundus tendon

Pronator quadratus

Superficial muscles of the hand (palmar view)

Synovial sheath

A1   A2   C1   A3   C2   A4   C3   A5

Flexor digitorum superficialis tendon

Flexor digitorum profundus tendon

Palmar ligament

Collateral ligament

Fibrous digital sheath and synovial sheath
Annular ligaments (A), cruciform ligaments (C)

446

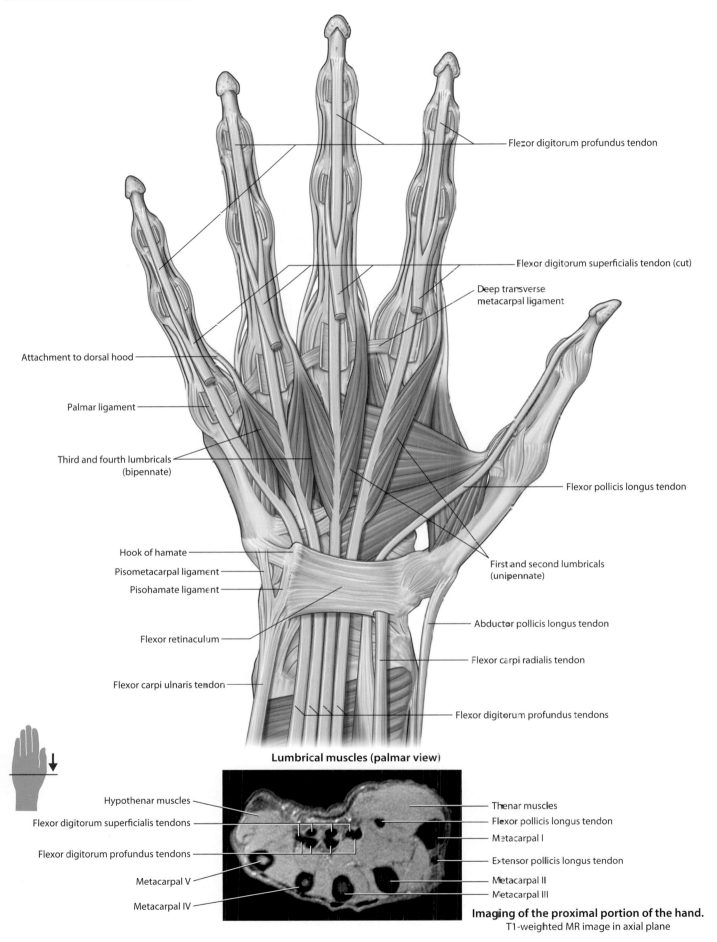

Flexor digitorum profundus tendon

Flexor digitorum superficialis tendon (cut)

Deep transverse
metacarpal ligament

Attachment to dorsal hood

Palmar ligament

Third and fourth lumbricals
(bipennate)

Flexor pollicis longus tendon

Hook of hamate

Pisometacarpal ligament

Pisohamate ligament

First and second lumbricals
(unipennate)

Flexor retinaculum

Abductor pollicis longus tendon

Flexor carpi radialis tendon

Flexor carpi ulnaris tendon

Flexor digitorum profundus tendons

Lumbrical muscles (palmar view)

Hypothenar muscles

Flexor digitorum superficialis tendons

Flexor digitorum profundus tendons

Metacarpal V

Metacarpal IV

Thenar muscles

Flexor pollicis longus tendon

Metacarpal I

Extensor pollicis longus tendon

Metacarpal II

Metacarpal III

Imaging of the proximal portion of the hand.
T1-weighted MR image in axial plane

447

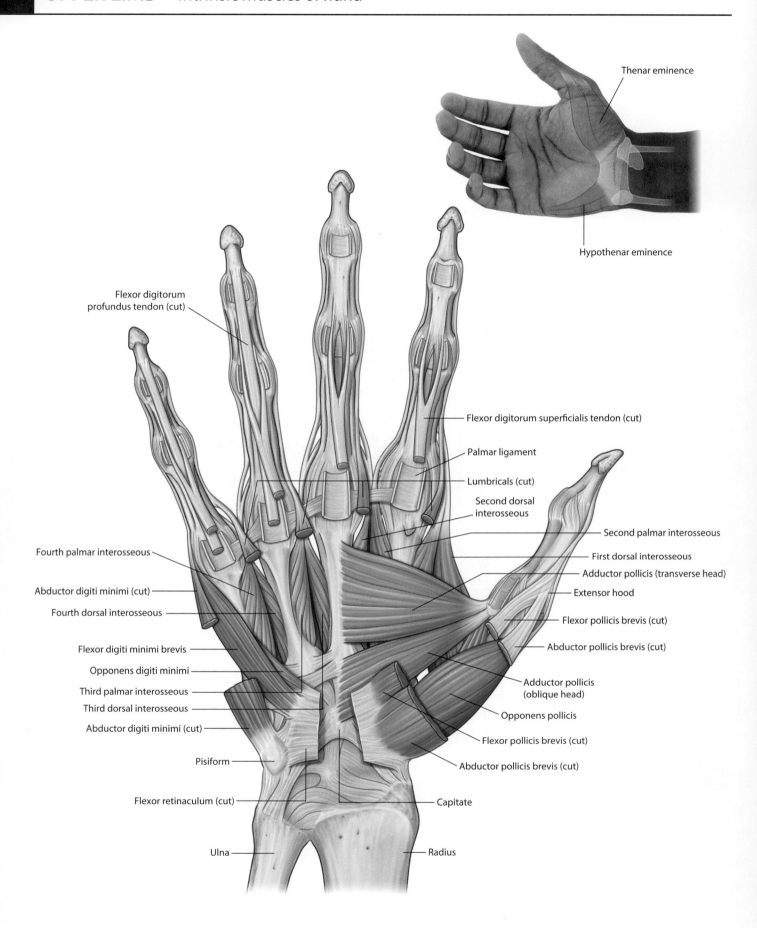

Thenar eminence

Hypothenar eminence

Flexor digitorum profundus tendon (cut)

Flexor digitorum superficialis tendon (cut)

Palmar ligament

Lumbricals (cut)

Second dorsal interosseous

Second palmar interosseous

First dorsal interosseous

Adductor pollicis (transverse head)

Extensor hood

Flexor pollicis brevis (cut)

Abductor pollicis brevis (cut)

Fourth palmar interosseous

Abductor digiti minimi (cut)

Fourth dorsal interosseous

Flexor digiti minimi brevis

Opponens digiti minimi

Third palmar interosseous

Third dorsal interosseous

Adductor pollicis (oblique head)

Opponens pollicis

Abductor digiti minimi (cut)

Flexor pollicis brevis (cut)

Pisiform

Abductor pollicis brevis (cut)

Flexor retinaculum (cut)

Capitate

Ulna

Radius

Deep muscles of the hand (palmar view)

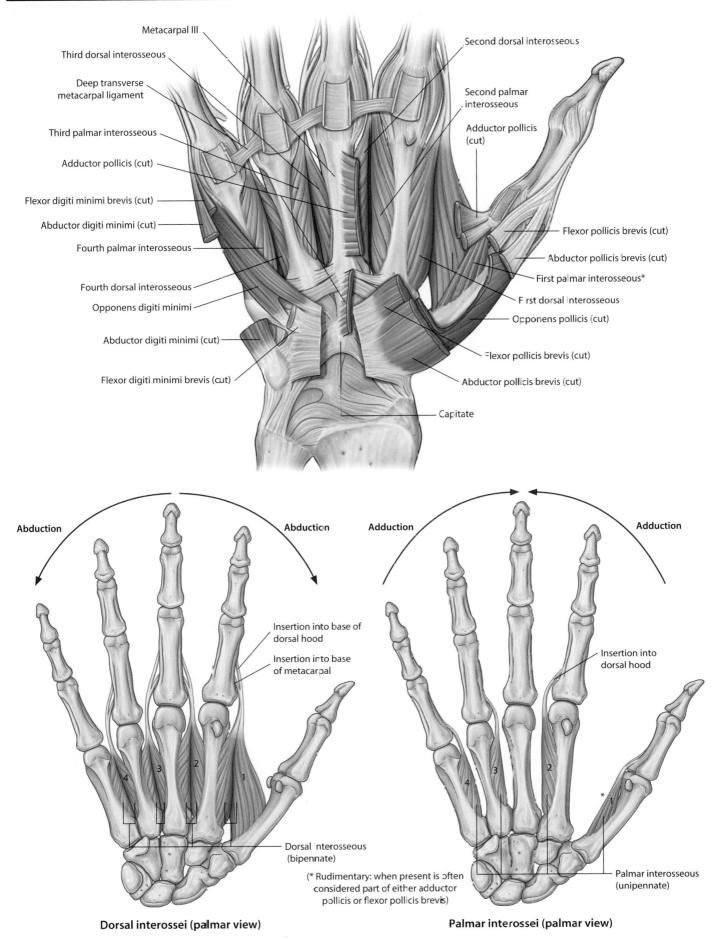

Metacarpal III

Third dorsal interosseous

Deep transverse metacarpal ligament

Third palmar interosseous

Adductor pollicis (cut)

Flexor digiti minimi brevis (cut)

Abductor digiti minimi (cut)

Fourth palmar interosseous

Fourth dorsal interosseous

Opponens digiti minimi

Abductor digiti minimi (cut)

Flexor digiti minimi brevis (cut)

Second dorsal interosseous

Second palmar interosseous

Adductor pollicis (cut)

Flexor pollicis brevis (cut)

Abductor pollicis brevis (cut)

First palmar interosseous*

First dorsal interosseous

Opponens pollicis (cut)

Flexor pollicis brevis (cut)

Abductor pollicis brevis (cut)

Capitate

Abduction

Abduction

Insertion into base of dorsal hood

Insertion into base of metacarpal

4 3 2 1

Dorsal interosseous (bipennate)

Dorsal interossei (palmar view)

Adduction

Adduction

Insertion into dorsal hood

4 3 2 1 *

(* Rudimentary: when present is often considered part of either adductor pollicis or flexor pollicis brevis)

Palmar interosseous (unipennate)

Palmar interossei (palmar view)

449

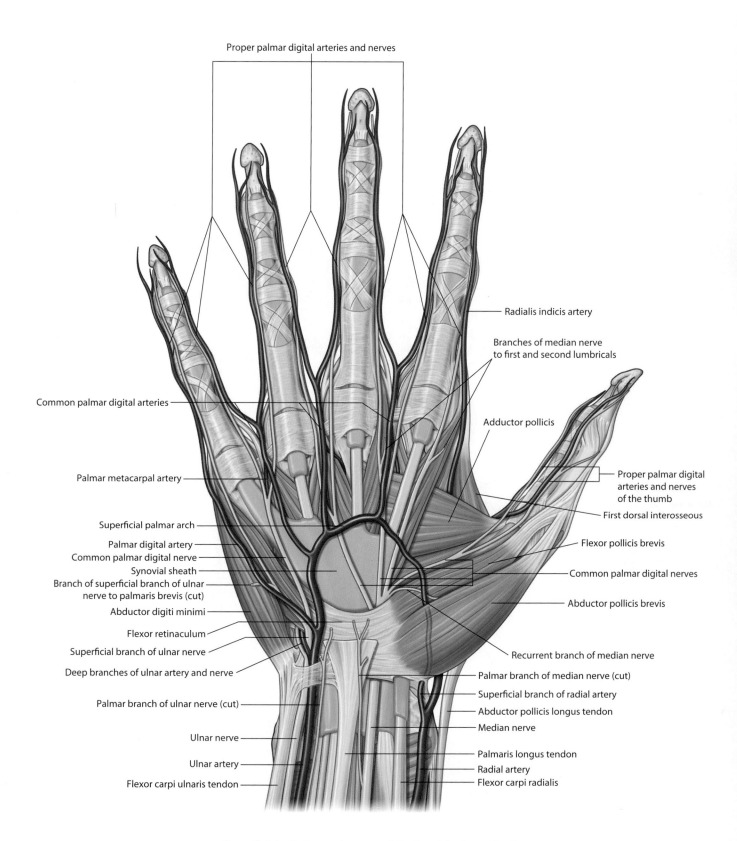

Proper palmar digital arteries and nerves

Radialis indicis artery

Branches of median nerve to first and second lumbricals

Common palmar digital arteries

Adductor pollicis

Palmar metacarpal artery

Proper palmar digital arteries and nerves of the thumb

First dorsal interosseous

Superficial palmar arch

Palmar digital artery

Common palmar digital nerve

Synovial sheath

Branch of superficial branch of ulnar nerve to palmaris brevis (cut)

Abductor digiti minimi

Flexor retinaculum

Superficial branch of ulnar nerve

Deep branches of ulnar artery and nerve

Palmar branch of ulnar nerve (cut)

Ulnar nerve

Ulnar artery

Flexor carpi ulnaris tendon

Flexor pollicis brevis

Common palmar digital nerves

Abductor pollicis brevis

Recurrent branch of median nerve

Palmar branch of median nerve (cut)

Superficial branch of radial artery

Abductor pollicis longus tendon

Median nerve

Palmaris longus tendon

Radial artery

Flexor carpi radialis

Superficial arteries and nerves of the hand (palmar view)

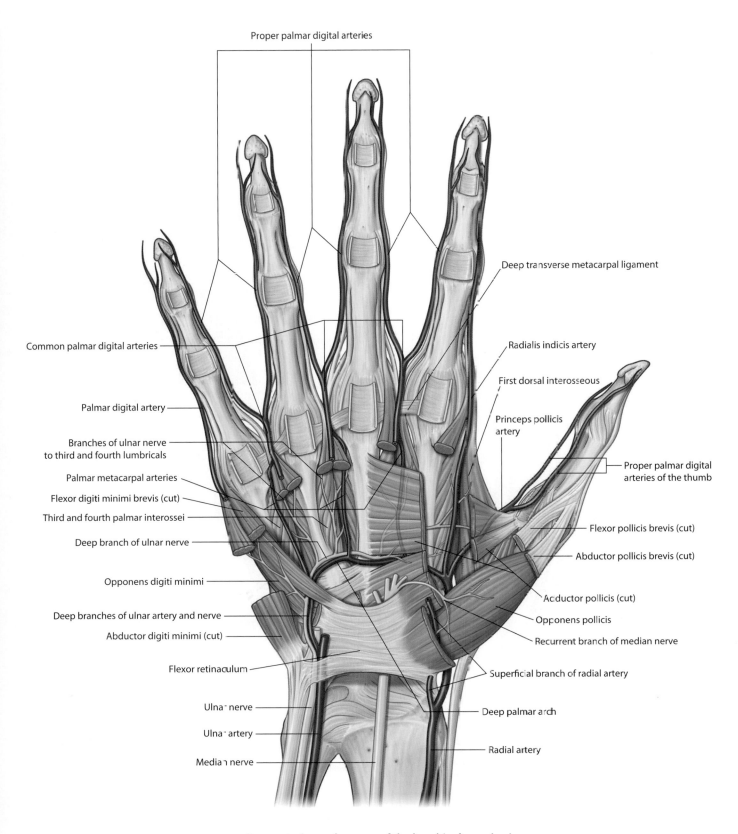

Proper palmar digital arteries

Deep transverse metacarpal ligament

Common palmar digital arteries

Radialis indicis artery

First dorsal interosseous

Palmar digital artery

Princeps pollicis artery

Branches of ulnar nerve to third and fourth lumbricals

Proper palmar digital arteries of the thumb

Palmar metacarpal arteries

Flexor digiti minimi brevis (cut)

Flexor pollicis brevis (cut)

Third and fourth palmar interossei

Abductor pollicis brevis (cut)

Deep branch of ulnar nerve

Opponens digiti minimi

Adductor pollicis (cut)

Opponens pollicis

Deep branches of ulnar artery and nerve

Recurrent branch of median nerve

Abductor digiti minimi (cut)

Flexor retinaculum

Superficial branch of radial artery

Ulnar nerve

Deep palmar arch

Ulnar artery

Radial artery

Median nerve

Deep arteries and nerves of the hand (palmar view)

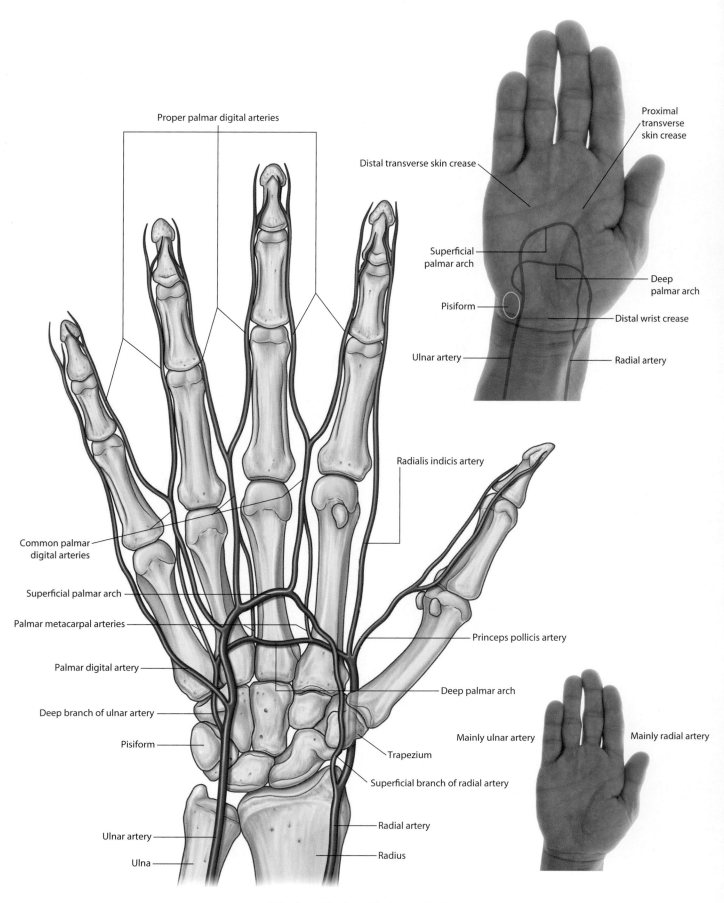

Proper palmar digital arteries

Distal transverse skin crease

Proximal transverse skin crease

Superficial palmar arch

Deep palmar arch

Pisiform

Distal wrist crease

Ulnar artery

Radial artery

Radialis indicis artery

Common palmar digital arteries

Superficial palmar arch

Palmar metacarpal arteries

Princeps pollicis artery

Palmar digital artery

Deep palmar arch

Deep branch of ulnar artery

Pisiform

Mainly ulnar artery

Mainly radial artery

Trapezium

Superficial branch of radial artery

Ulnar artery

Radial artery

Ulna

Radius

Arteries of the hand (palmar view)

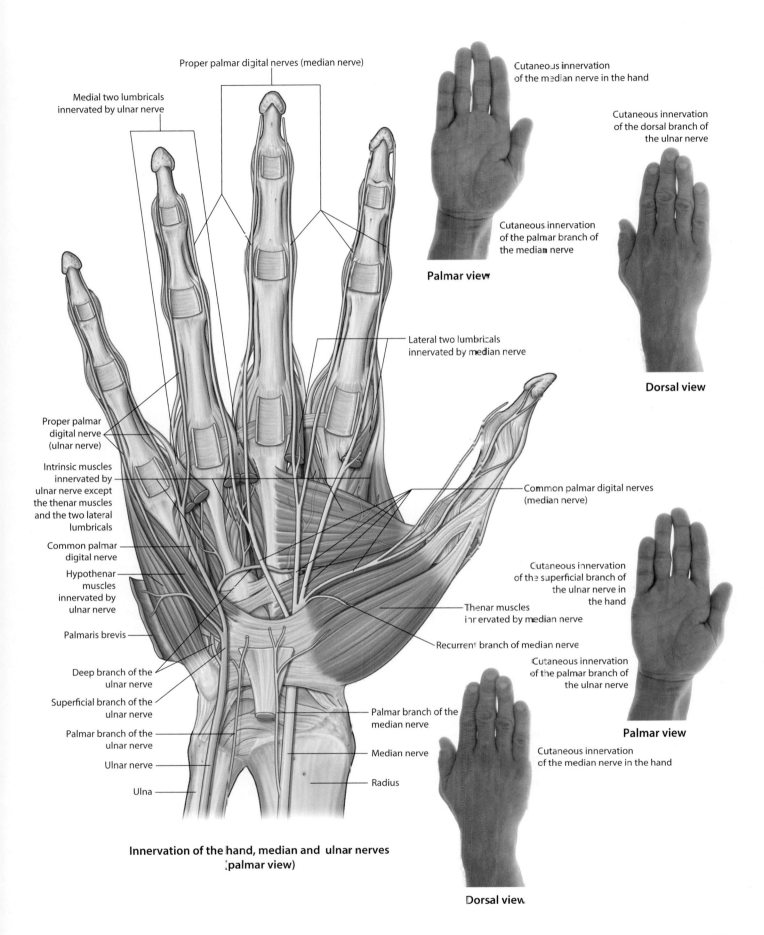

Proper palmar digital nerves (median nerve)

Medial two lumbricals innervated by ulnar nerve

Cutaneous innervation of the median nerve in the hand

Cutaneous innervation of the dorsal branch of the ulnar nerve

Cutaneous innervation of the palmar branch of the median nerve

Palmar view

Dorsal view

Lateral two lumbricals innervated by median nerve

Proper palmar digital nerve (ulnar nerve)

Intrinsic muscles innervated by ulnar nerve except the thenar muscles and the two lateral lumbricals

Common palmar digital nerve

Hypothenar muscles innervated by ulnar nerve

Palmaris brevis

Deep branch of the ulnar nerve

Superficial branch of the ulnar nerve

Palmar branch of the ulnar nerve

Ulnar nerve

Ulna

Common palmar digital nerves (median nerve)

Cutaneous innervation of the superficial branch of the ulnar nerve in the hand

Thenar muscles innervated by median nerve

Recurrent branch of median nerve

Cutaneous innervation of the palmar branch of the ulnar nerve

Palmar view

Palmar branch of the median nerve

Median nerve

Radius

Cutaneous innervation of the median nerve in the hand

Dorsal view

Innervation of the hand, median and ulnar nerves (palmar view)

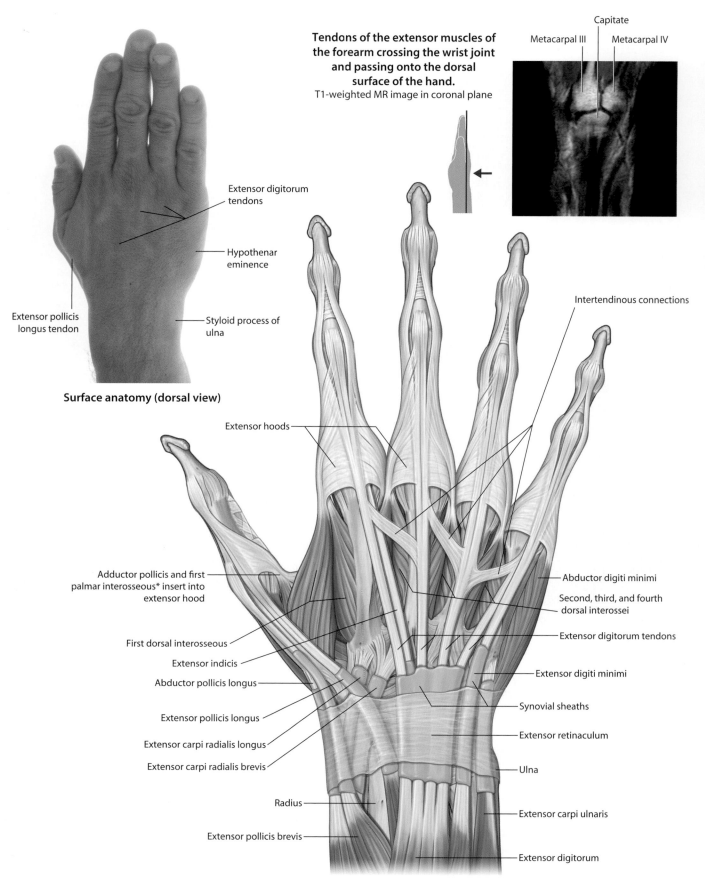

Surface anatomy (dorsal view)

Extensor digitorum tendons

Hypothenar eminence

Styloid process of ulna

Extensor pollicis longus tendon

Tendons of the extensor muscles of the forearm crossing the wrist joint and passing onto the dorsal surface of the hand.
T1-weighted MR image in coronal plane

Capitate

Metacarpal III

Metacarpal IV

Intertendinous connections

Extensor hoods

Adductor pollicis and first palmar interosseous* insert into extensor hood

First dorsal interosseous

Extensor indicis

Abductor pollicis longus

Extensor pollicis longus

Extensor carpi radialis longus

Extensor carpi radialis brevis

Radius

Extensor pollicis brevis

Abductor digiti minimi

Second, third, and fourth dorsal interossei

Extensor digitorum tendons

Extensor digiti minimi

Synovial sheaths

Extensor retinaculum

Ulna

Extensor carpi ulnaris

Extensor digitorum

Superficial structures of the hand (dorsal view)
(* see page 449)

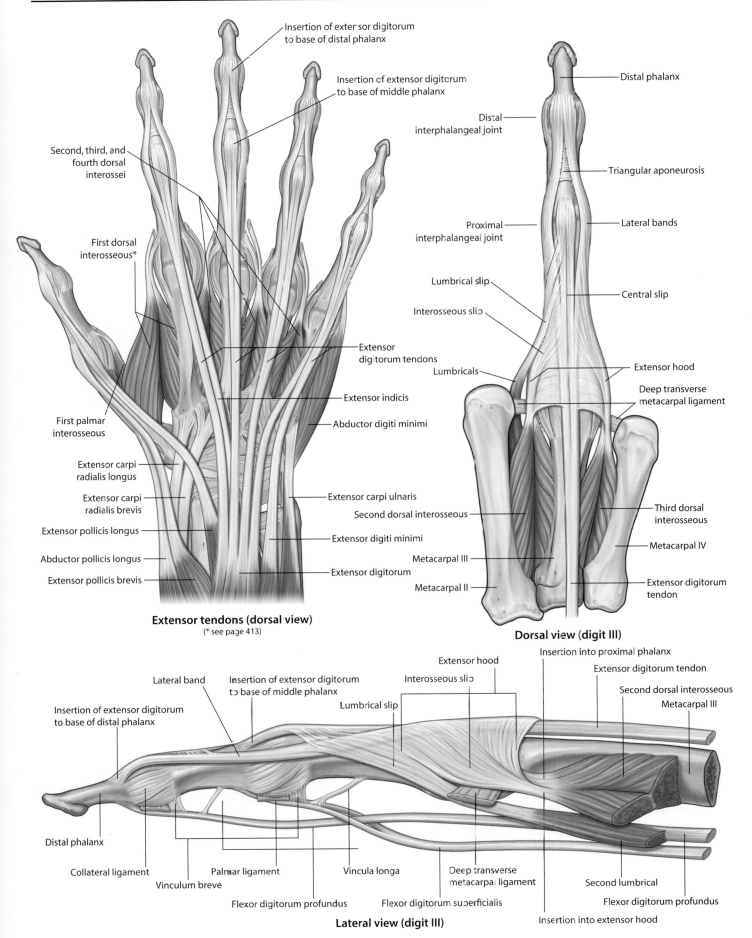

Insertion of extensor digitorum to base of distal phalanx

Insertion of extensor digitorum to base of middle phalanx

Second, third, and fourth dorsal interossei

First dorsal interosseous*

First palmar interosseous

Extensor carpi radialis longus

Extensor carpi radialis brevis

Extensor pollicis longus

Abductor pollicis longus

Extensor pollicis brevis

Extensor digitorum tendons

Extensor indicis

Abductor digiti minimi

Extensor carpi ulnaris

Second dorsal interosseous

Extensor digiti minimi

Extensor digitorum

Extensor tendons (dorsal view)
(* see page 413)

Distal phalanx

Distal interphalangeal joint

Triangular aponeurosis

Proximal interphalangeal joint

Lateral bands

Lumbrical slip

Interosseous slip

Central slip

Lumbricals

Extensor hood

Deep transverse metacarpal ligament

Third dorsal interosseous

Metacarpal IV

Metacarpal III

Metacarpal II

Extensor digitorum tendon

Dorsal view (digit III)

Lateral band

Insertion of extensor digitorum to base of middle phalanx

Insertion of extensor digitorum to base of distal phalanx

Extensor hood

Interosseous slip

Insertion into proximal phalanx

Extensor digitorum tendon

Second dorsal interosseous

Metacarpal III

Lumbrical slip

Distal phalanx

Collateral ligament

Vinculum breve

Palmar ligament

Flexor digitorum profundus

Vincula longa

Deep transverse metacarpal ligament

Flexor digitorum superficialis

Second lumbrical

Flexor digitorum profundus

Insertion into extensor hood

Lateral view (digit III)

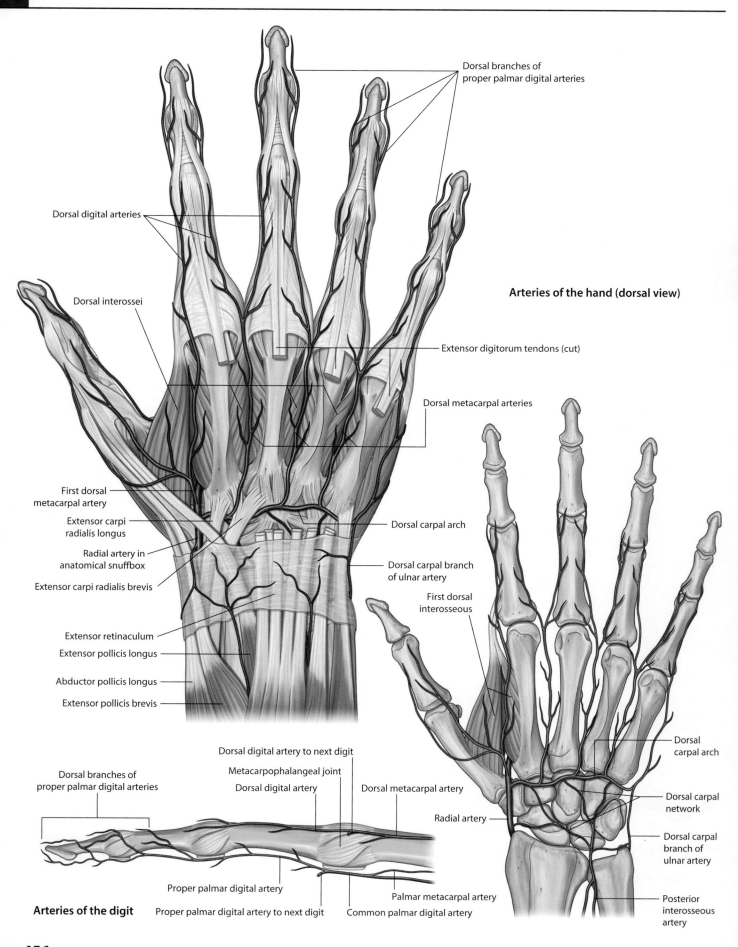

Dorsal branches of proper palmar digital arteries

Dorsal digital arteries

Dorsal interossei

Arteries of the hand (dorsal view)

Extensor digitorum tendons (cut)

Dorsal metacarpal arteries

First dorsal metacarpal artery

Extensor carpi radialis longus

Radial artery in anatomical snuffbox

Extensor carpi radialis brevis

Dorsal carpal arch

Dorsal carpal branch of ulnar artery

First dorsal interosseous

Extensor retinaculum

Extensor pollicis longus

Abductor pollicis longus

Extensor pollicis brevis

Dorsal carpal arch

Dorsal carpal network

Dorsal carpal branch of ulnar artery

Radial artery

Posterior interosseous artery

Dorsal branches of proper palmar digital arteries

Dorsal digital artery to next digit

Metacarpophalangeal joint

Dorsal digital artery

Dorsal metacarpal artery

Proper palmar digital artery

Arteries of the digit

Proper palmar digital artery to next digit

Common palmar digital artery

Palmar metacarpal artery

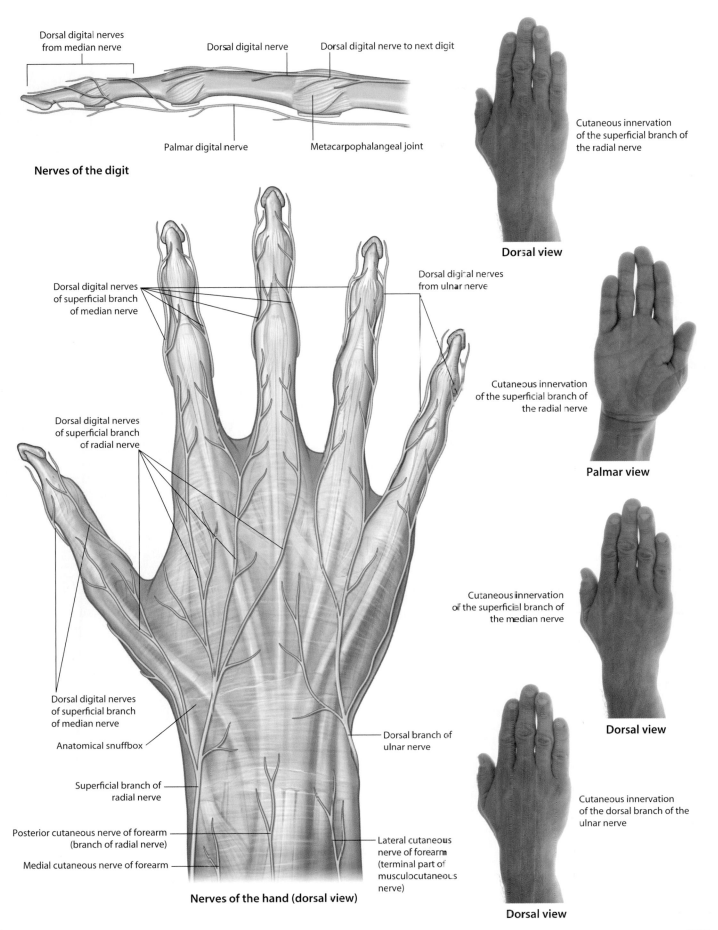

Dorsal digital nerves
from median nerve

Dorsal digital nerve

Dorsal digital nerve to next digit

Palmar digital nerve

Metacarpophalangeal joint

Nerves of the digit

Cutaneous innervation
of the superficial branch of
the radial nerve

Dorsal view

Dorsal digital nerves
of superficial branch
of median nerve

Dorsal digital nerves
from ulnar nerve

Dorsal digital nerves
of superficial branch
of radial nerve

Cutaneous innervation
of the superficial branch of
the radial nerve

Palmar view

Dorsal digital nerves
of superficial branch
of median nerve

Anatomical snuffbox

Dorsal branch of
ulnar nerve

Cutaneous innervation
of the superficial branch of
the median nerve

Superficial branch of
radial nerve

Dorsal view

Posterior cutaneous nerve of forearm
(branch of radial nerve)

Medial cutaneous nerve of forearm

Lateral cutaneous
nerve of forearm
(terminal part of
musculocutaneous
nerve)

Nerves of the hand (dorsal view)

Cutaneous innervation
of the dorsal branch of the
ulnar nerve

Dorsal view

457

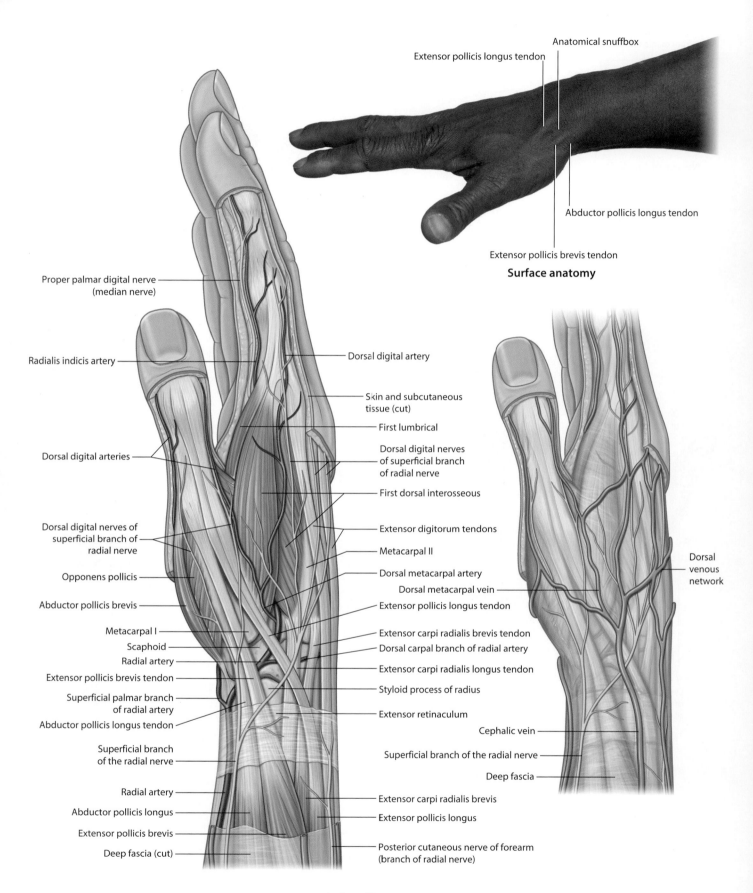

Anatomical snuffbox

Extensor pollicis longus tendon

Abductor pollicis longus tendon

Extensor pollicis brevis tendon

Surface anatomy

Proper palmar digital nerve (median nerve)

Radialis indicis artery

Dorsal digital arteries

Dorsal digital nerves of superficial branch of radial nerve

Opponens pollicis

Abductor pollicis brevis

Metacarpal I

Scaphoid

Radial artery

Extensor pollicis brevis tendon

Superficial palmar branch of radial artery

Abductor pollicis longus tendon

Superficial branch of the radial nerve

Radial artery

Abductor pollicis longus

Extensor pollicis brevis

Deep fascia (cut)

Dorsal digital artery

Skin and subcutaneous tissue (cut)

First lumbrical

Dorsal digital nerves of superficial branch of radial nerve

First dorsal interosseous

Extensor digitorum tendons

Metacarpal II

Dorsal metacarpal artery

Extensor pollicis longus tendon

Extensor carpi radialis brevis tendon

Dorsal carpal branch of radial artery

Extensor carpi radialis longus tendon

Styloid process of radius

Extensor retinaculum

Extensor carpi radialis brevis

Extensor pollicis longus

Posterior cutaneous nerve of forearm (branch of radial nerve)

Dorsal venous network

Dorsal metacarpal vein

Cephalic vein

Superficial branch of the radial nerve

Deep fascia

Anatomical snuffbox (lateral view)

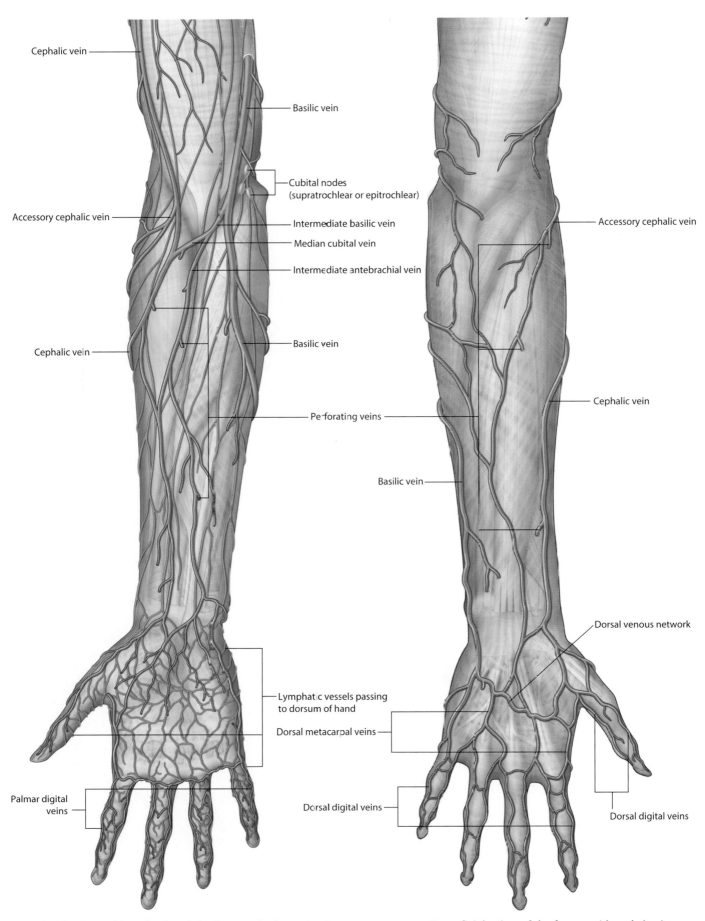

Cephalic vein

Basilic vein

Cubital nodes
(supratrochlear or epitrochlear)

Accessory cephalic vein

Intermediate basilic vein

Median cubital vein

Intermediate antebrachial vein

Cephalic vein

Basilic vein

Accessory cephalic vein

Cephalic vein

Perforating veins

Basilic vein

Dorsal venous network

Lymphatic vessels passing
to dorsum of hand

Dorsal metacarpal veins

Palmar digital
veins

Dorsal digital veins

Dorsal digital veins

Superficial veins and lymphatics of the forearm (palmar view)

Superficial veins of the forearm (dorsal view)

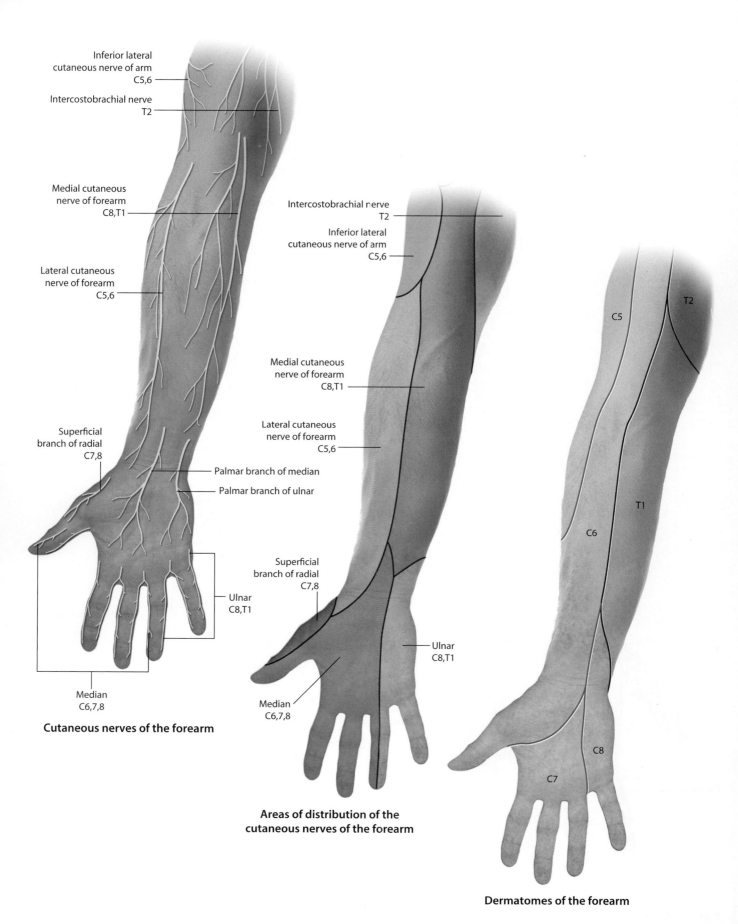

Inferior lateral
cutaneous nerve of arm
C5,6

Intercostobrachial nerve
T2

Medial cutaneous
nerve of forearm
C8,T1

Lateral cutaneous
nerve of forearm
C5,6

Superficial
branch of radial
C7,8

Palmar branch of median

Palmar branch of ulnar

Ulnar
C8,T1

Median
C6,7,8

Cutaneous nerves of the forearm

Intercostobrachial nerve
T2

Inferior lateral
cutaneous nerve of arm
C5,6

Medial cutaneous
nerve of forearm
C8,T1

Lateral cutaneous
nerve of forearm
C5,6

Superficial
branch of radial
C7,8

Ulnar
C8,T1

Median
C6,7,8

**Areas of distribution of the
cutaneous nerves of the forearm**

C5

T2

T1

C6

C8

C7

Dermatomes of the forearm

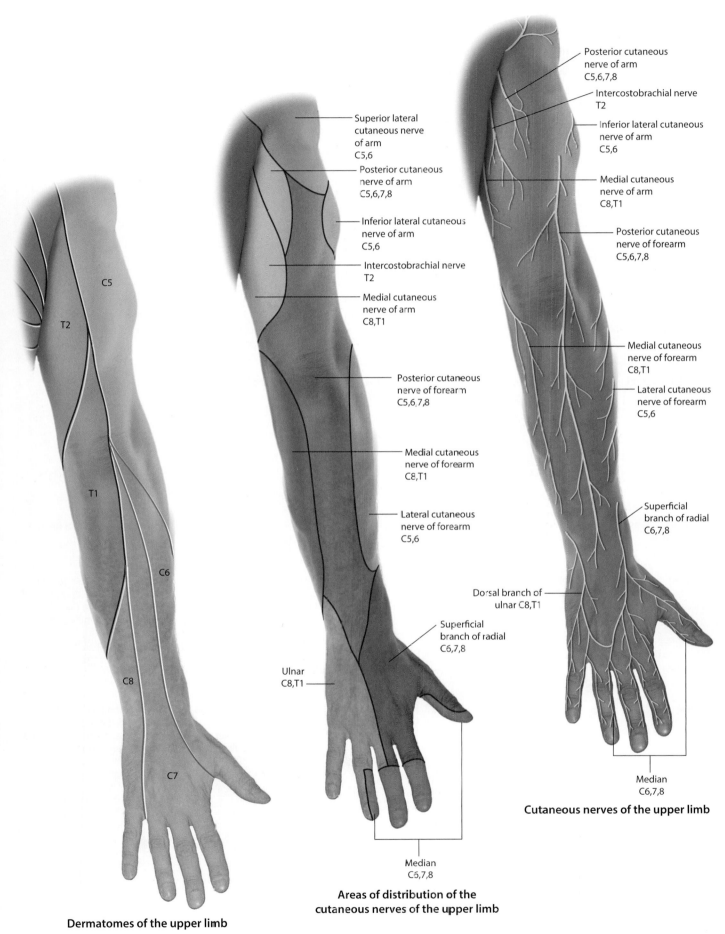

Superior lateral
cutaneous nerve
of arm
C5,6

Posterior cutaneous
nerve of arm
C5,6,7,8

Inferior lateral cutaneous
nerve of arm
C5,6

Intercostobrachial nerve
T2

Medial cutaneous
nerve of arm
C8,T1

Posterior cutaneous
nerve of forearm
C5,6,7,8

Medial cutaneous
nerve of forearm
C8,T1

Lateral cutaneous
nerve of forearm
C5,6

Superficial
branch of radial
C6,7,8

Ulnar
C8,T1

Superficial
branch of radial
C6,7,8

Dorsal branch of
ulnar C8,T1

Median
C6,7,8

Posterior cutaneous
nerve of arm
C5,6,7,8

Intercostobrachial nerve
T2

Inferior lateral cutaneous
nerve of arm
C5,6

Medial cutaneous
nerve of arm
C8,T1

Posterior cutaneous
nerve of forearm
C5,6,7,8

Medial cutaneous
nerve of forearm
C8,T1

Lateral cutaneous
nerve of forearm
C5,6

Cutaneous nerves of the upper limb

**Areas of distribution of the
cutaneous nerves of the upper limb**

Dermatomes of the upper limb

C5

T2

T1

C6

C8

C7

Branches of the brachial plexus

Branch		Origin	Spinal segments	Function: motor	Function: sensory
Dorsal scapular	1	C5 root	C5	Rhomboid major, rhomboid minor	
Long thoracic	2	C5 to C7 roots	C5 to C7	Serratus anterior	
Suprascapular	3	Superior trunk	C5, C6	Supraspinatus, infraspinatus	
Nerve to subclavius	4	Superior trunk	C5, C6	Subclavius	
Lateral pectoral	5	Lateral cord	C5 to C7	Pectoralis major	
Musculocutaneous	6	Lateral cord	C5 to C7	All muscles in the anterior compartment of the arm	Skin on lateral side of forearm
Medial pectoral	7	Medial cord	C8, T1 (also receives contributions from spinal segments C5 to C7 through a communication with the lateral pectoral nerve)	Pectoralis major, pectoralis minor	
Medial cutaneous of arm	8	Medial cord	Spinal segments: C8, T1		Skin on medial side of distal one-third of arm
Medial cutaneous of forearm	9	Medial cord	C8, T1		Skin on medial side of forearm
Median	10	Medial and lateral cords	(C5), C6 to T1	All muscles in the anterior compartment of the forearm (except flexor carpi ulnaris and medial half of flexor digitorum profundus), three thenar muscles of the thumb and two lateral lumbrical muscles	Skin over the palmar surface of the lateral three and one-half digits and over the lateral side of the palm and middle of the wrist
Ulnar	11	Medial cord	(C7), C8, T1	All intrinsic muscles of the hand (except three thenar muscles and two lateral lumbricals); also flexor carpi ulnaris and the medial half of flexor digitorum profundus in the forearm	Skin over the palmar surface of the medial one and one-half digits and associated palm and wrist, and skin over the dorsal surface of the medial one and one-half digits
Superior subscapular	12	Posterior cord	C5, C6	Subscapularis	
Thoracodorsal	13	Posterior cord	C6 to C8	Latissimus dorsi	

Branches of the brachial plexus

Branch		Origin	Spinal segments	Function: motor	Function: sensory
Inferior subscapular	14	Posterior cord	C5, C6	Subscapularis, teres major	
Axillary	15	Posterior cord	C5, C6	Deltoid, teres minor	Skin over upper lateral part of arm
Radial	16	Posterior cord	C5 to C8, (T1)	All muscles in the posterior compartments of arm and forearm	Skin on the posterior aspects of the arm and forearm, the lower lateral surface of the arm, and the dorsal lateral surface of the hand

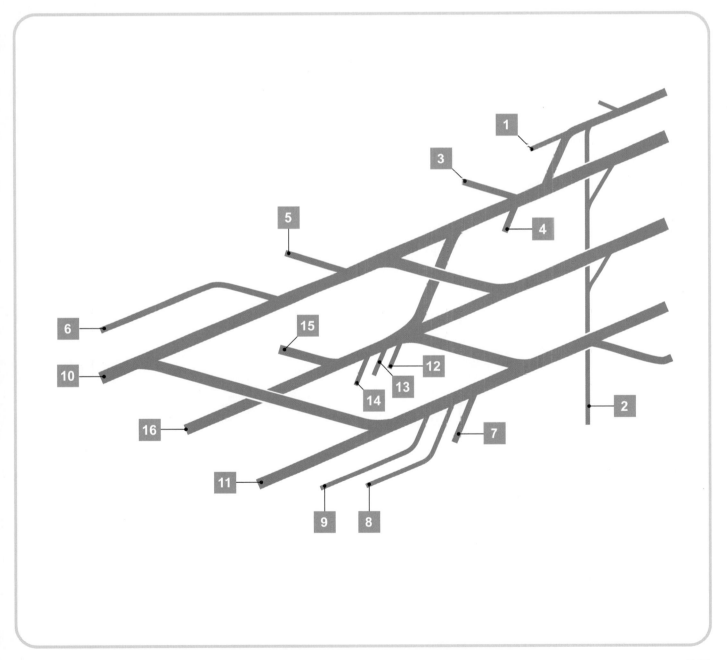

Muscles of the shoulder

(muscles of the shoulder spinal segments indicated in bold are the major segments innervating the muscle)

Muscle		Origin	Insertion	Innervation	Function
Trapezius	1	Superior nuchal line, external occipital protuberance, medial margin of the ligamentum nuchae, spinous processes of CVII to TXII and the related supraspinous ligaments	Superior edge of the crest of the spine of the scapula, acromion, posterior border of lateral one-third of clavicle	Motor spinal part of accessory nerve [XI]. Sensory (proprioception) anterior rami of C3 and C4	Powerful elevator of the scapula; rotates the scapula during abduction of humerus above horizontal; middle fibers retract scapula; lower fibers depress scapula
Deltoid	2	Inferior edge of the crest of the spine of the scapula, lateral margin of the acromion, anterior border of lateral one-third of clavicle	Deltoid tuberosity of humerus	Axillary nerve [**C5**, C6]	Major abductor of arm (abducts arm beyond initial 15° done by supraspinatus); clavicular fibers assist in flexing the arm; posterior fibers assist in extending the arm
Levator scapulae	3	Transverse processes of CI and CII vertebrae and posterior tubercles of transverse processes of CIII and CIV vertebrae	Posterior surface of medial border of scapula from superior angle to root of spine of the scapula	Branches directly from anterior rami of **C3** and **C4** spinal nerves and by branches [**C5**] from the dorsal scapular nerve	Elevates the scapula
Rhomboid minor	4	Lower end of ligamentum nuchae and spinous processes of CVII and TI vertebrae	Posterior surface of medial border of scapula at the root of the spine of the scapula	Dorsal scapular nerve [C4, **C5**]	Elevates and retracts the scapula
Rhomboid major	5	Spinous processes of TII–TV vertebrae and intervening supraspinous ligaments	Posterior surface of medial border of scapula from the root of the spine of the scapula to the inferior angle	Dorsal scapular nerve [**C4**, **C5**]	Elevates and retracts the scapula

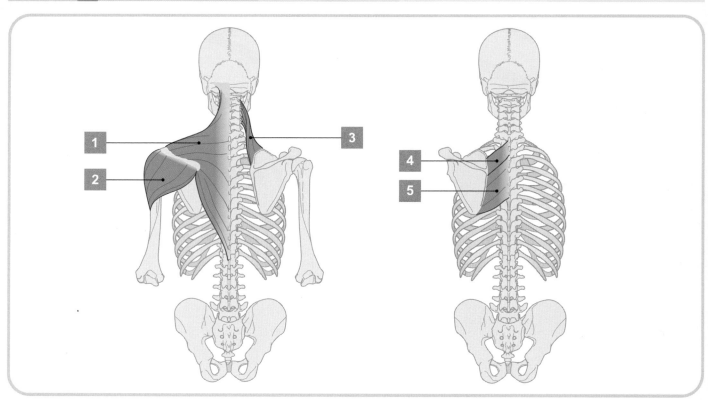

Muscles of the posterior scapular region

(spinal segments in bold are the major segments innervating the muscle)

Muscle		Origin	Insertion	Innervation	Function
Supraspinatus	1	Medial two-thirds of the supraspinous fossa of the scapula and the deep fascia that covers the muscle	Most superior facet on the greater tubercle of the humerus	Suprascapular nerve [**C5**, C6]	Rotator cuff muscle; participates in abduction of the glenohumeral joint; stabilization of glenohumeral joint
Infraspinatus	2	Medial two-thirds of the infraspinous fossa of the scapula and the deep fascia that covers the muscle	Middle facet on posterior surface of the greater tubercle of the humerus	Suprascapular nerve [**C5**, C6]	Rotator cuff muscle; lateral rotation of arm at the glenohumeral joint; stabilization of glenohumeral joint
Teres minor	3	Upper two-thirds of a flattened strip of bone on the posterior surface of the scapula immediately adjacent to the lateral border of the scapula	Inferior facet on the posterior surface of the greater tubercle of the humerus	Axillary nerve [**C5**, C6]	Rotator cuff muscle; lateral rotation of arm at the glenohumeral joint; stabilization of glenohumeral joint
Teres major	4	Elongate oval area on the posterior surface of the inferior angle of the scapula	Medial lip of the intertubercular sulcus on the anterior surface of the humerus	Inferior subscapular nerve [**C5**, **C6**, **C7**]	Medial rotation and extension of the arm at the glenohumeral joint
Long head of triceps brachii	5	Infraglenoid tubercle on scapula	Common tendon of insertion with medial and lateral heads on the olecranon process of ulna	Radial nerve [C6, **C7**, C8]	Extension of the forearm at the elbow joint; accessory adductor and extensor of the arm at the glenohumeral joint

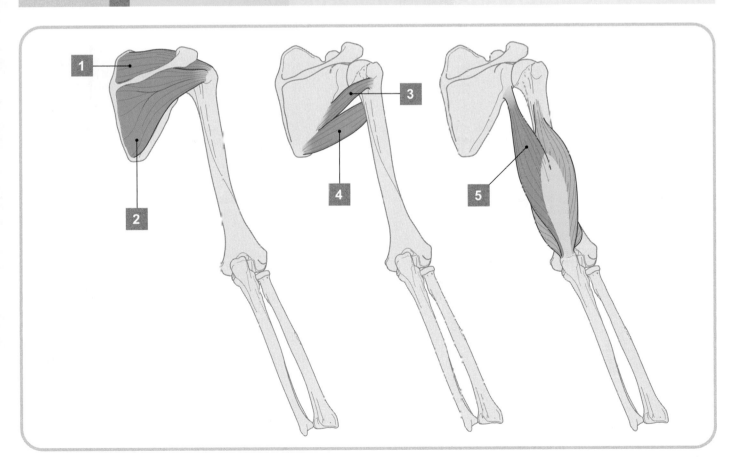

Muscles of the anterior wall of the axilla

(spinal segments in bold are the major segments innervating the muscle)

	Muscle	Origin	Insertion	Innervation	Function
1	Pectoralis major	Clavicular head—anterior surface of medial half of clavicle; sternocostal head-anterior surface of sternum; first seven costal cartilages; sternal end of sixth rib; aponeurosis of external obliqu	Lateral lip of intertubercular sulcus of humerus	Medial and lateral pectoral nerves; clavicular head [**C5**, C6]; sternocostal head [C6, C7, C8, T1]	Flexion, adduction, and medial rotation of arm at glenohumeral joint; clavicular head—flexion of extended arm; sternocostal head—extension of flexed arm
2	Subclavius	First rib at junction between rib and costal cartilage	Groove on inferior surface of middle one-third of clavicle	Nerve to subclavius [**C5, C6**]	Pulls tip of shoulder down; pulls clavicle medially to stabilize sternoclavicular joint
3	Pectoralis minor	Anterior surfaces and superior borders of ribs III to V; and from deep fascia overlying the related intercostal spaces	Coracoid process of scapula (medial border and upper surface)	Medial pectoral nerve [C5, C6, **C7**, **C8**, T1]	Pulls tip of shoulder down; protracts scapula

Muscles of the medial wall of the axilla

	Muscle	Origin	Insertion	Innervation	Function
4	Serratus anterior	Lateral surfaces of upper 8–9 ribs and deep fascia overlying the related intercostal spaces	Costal surface of medial border of scapula	Long thoracic nerve [**C5, C6, C7**]	Protraction and rotation of the scapula; keeps medial border and inferior angle of scapula opposed to thoracic wall

Muscles of the lateral and posterior wall of the axilla

(spinal segments enclosed in parentheses do not consistently innervate the muscle)

	Muscle	Origin	Insertion	Innervation	Function
5	Subscapularis	Medial two-thirds of subscapular fossa	Lesser tubercle of humerus	Upper and lower subscapular nerves [C5, **C6**, (C7)]	Rotator cuff muscle; medial rotation of the arm at the glenohumeral joint; stabilization of glenohumeral joint
6	Teres major	Elongate oval area on the posterior surface of the inferior angle of the scapula	Medial lip of the intertubercular sulcus on the anterior surface of the humerus	Lower subscapular nerve [C5, **C6, C7**]	Medial rotation and extension of the arm at the glenohumeral joint
7	Latissimus dorsi	Spinous processes of lower six thoracic vertebrae and related interspinous ligaments; via the thoracolumbar fascia to the spinous processes of the lumbar vertebrae, related interspinous ligaments, and iliac crest; lower 3–4 ribs	Floor of intertubercular sulcus	Thoracodorsal nerve [C6, **C7**, C8]	Adduction, medial rotation, and extension of the arm at the glenohumeral joint
8	Long head of triceps brachii	Infraglenoid tubercle on scapula	Common tendon of insertion with medial and lateral heads on the olecranon process of ulna	Radial nerve [C6, **C7**, C8]	Extension of the forearm at the elbow joint; accessory adductor and extensor of the arm at the glenohumeral joint

Muscles having parts that pass through the axilla

(spinal segments in bold are the major segments innervating the muscle)

Muscle		Origin	Insertion	Innervation	Function
Biceps brachii	9	Long head—supraglenoid tubercle of scapula; short head—apex of coracoid process	Tuberosity of radius	Musculocutaneous nerve [**C5**, **C6**]	Powerful flexor of the forearm at the elbow joint and supinator of the forearm; accessory flexor of the arm at the glenohumeral joint
Coracobrachialis	10	Apex of coracoid process	Linear roughening on midshaft of humerus on medial side	Musculocutaneous nerve [**C5**, **C6**, **C7**]	Flexor of the arm at the glenohumeral joint; adducts arm

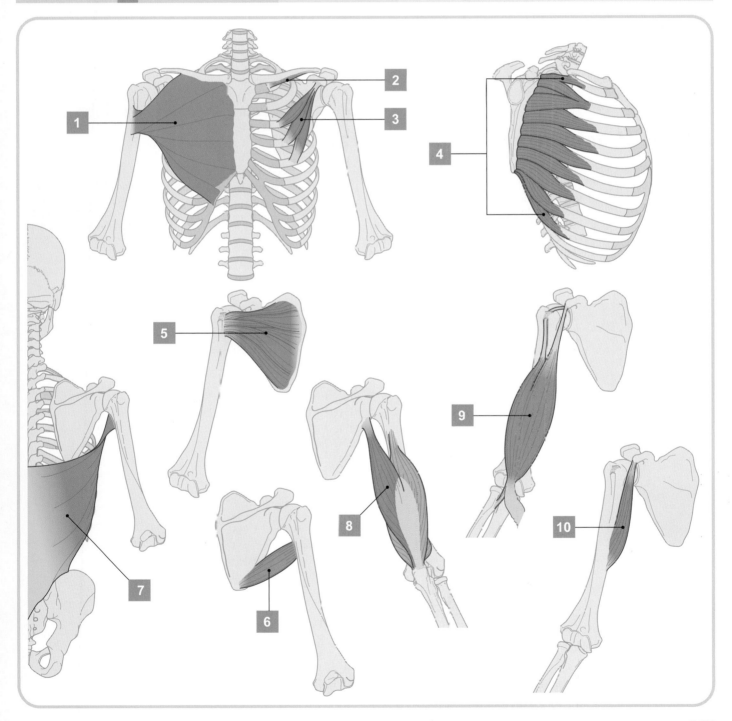

Muscles of the anterior compartment of the arm

(spinal segments in bold are the major segments innervating the muscle)

Muscle		Origin	Insertion	Innervation	Function
Coracobrachialis	1	Apex of coracoid process	Linear roughening on midshaft of humerus on medial side	Musculocutaneous nerve [**C5**, **C6**, **C7**]	Flexor of the arm at the glenohumeral joint
Biceps brachii	2	Long head-supraglenoid tubercle of scapula; short head-apex of coracoid process	Radial tuberosity	Musculocutaneous nerve [**C5**, **C6**]	Powerful flexor of the forearm at the elbow joint and supinator of the forearm; accessory flexor of the arm at the glenohumeral joint
Brachialis	3	Anterior aspect of humerus (medial and lateral surfaces) and adjacent intermuscular septae	Tuberosity of the ulna	Musculocutaneous nerve [C5, **C6**]; (small contribution by the radial nerve [C7] to lateral part of muscle)	Powerful flexor of the forearm at the elbow joint

Muscle of the posterior compartment of the arm

| Triceps brachii | 4 | Long head—infraglenoid tubercle of scapula; medial head—posterior surface of humerus;lateral head-posterior surface of humerus | Olecranon | Radial nerve [C6, **C7**, C8] | Extension of the forearm at the elbow joint. Long head can also extend and adduct the arm at the shoulder joint |

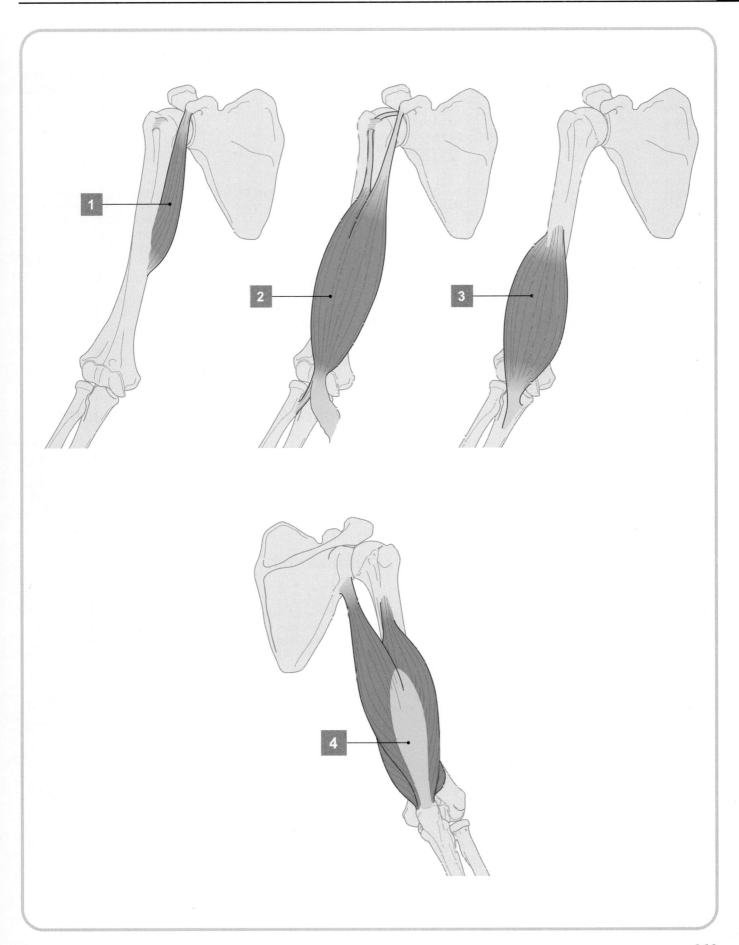

Superficial layer of muscles in the anterior compartment of the forearm

(spinal segments indicated in bold are the major segments innervating the muscle)

Muscle		Origin	Insertion	Innervation	Function
Flexor carpi ulnaris	1	Humeral head—medial epicondyle of humerus; ulnar head—olecranon and posterior border of ulna	Pisiform bone, and then via pisohamate and pisometacarpal ligaments into the hamate and base of metacarpal V	Ulnar nerve [C7, **C8**, T1]	Flexes and adducts the wrist joint
Palmaris longus	2	Medial epicondyle of humerus	Palmar aponeurosis of hand	Median nerve [**C7**, **C8**]	Flexes wrist joint; because the palmar aponeurosis anchors skin of the hand, contraction of the muscle resists shearing forces when gripping
Flexor carpi radialis	3	Medial epicondyle of humerus	Base of metacarpals II and III	Median nerve [**C6**, **C7**]	Flexes and abducts the wrist
Pronator teres	4	Humeral head—medial epicondyle and adjacent supraepicondylar ridge; ulnar head—medial side of coronoid process	Roughening on lateral surface, midshaft, of radius	Median nerve [**C6**, **C7**]	Pronation

Intermediate layer of muscles in the anterior compartment of the forearm

Muscle		Origin	Insertion	Innervation	Function
Flexor digitorum superficialis	5	Humero-ulnar head-medial epicondyle of humerus and adjacent margin of coronoid process; radial head—oblique line of radiu	Four tendons, which attach to the palmar surfaces of the middle phalanges of the index, middle, ring, and little fingers	Median nerve [**C8**, T1]	Flexes proximal interphalangeal joints of the index, middle, ring, and little fingers; can also flex metacarpophalangeal joints of the same fingers and the wrist joint

Deep layer of muscles in the anterior compartment of the forearm

Muscle		Origin	Insertion	Innervation	Function
Flexor digitorum profundus	6	Anterior and medial surfaces of ulna and anterior medial half of interosseous membrane	Four tendons, which attach to the palmar surfaces of the distal phalanges of the index, middle, ring, and little fingers	Lateral half by median nerve (anterior interosseous nerve); medial half by ulnar nerve [**C8**, T1]	Flexes distal interphalangeal joints of the index, middle, ring, and little fingers; can also flex metacarpophalangeal joints of the same fingers and the wrist joint
Flexor pollicis longus	7	Anterior surface of radius and radial half of interosseous membrane	Palmar surface of base of distal phalanx of thumb	Median nerve (anterior interosseous nerve) [C7, **C8**]	Flexes interphalangeal joint of the thumb; can also flex metacarpophalangeal joint of the thumb
Pronator quadratus	8	Linear ridge on distal anterior surface of ulna	Distal anterior surface of radius	Median nerve (anterior interosseous nerve) [C7, **C8**]	Pronation

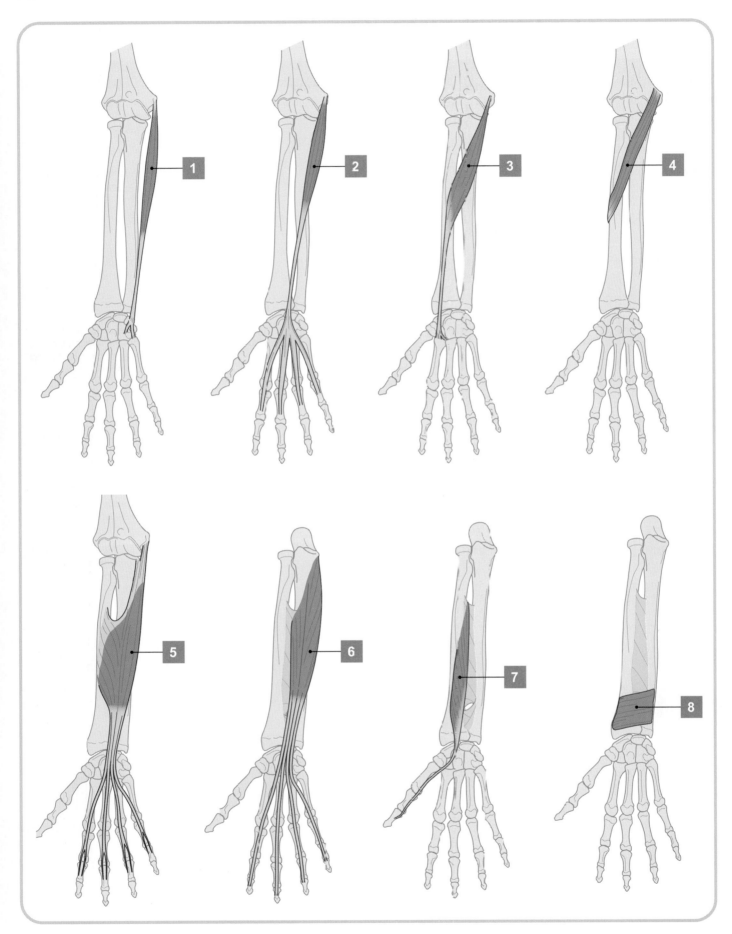

Superficial layer of muscles in the posterior compartment of the forearm

(spinal segments indicated in bold are the major segments innervating the muscle)

Muscle		Origin	Insertion	Innervation	Function
Brachioradialis	1	Proximal part of lateral supraepicondylar ridge of humerus and adjacent intermuscular septum	Lateral surface of distal end of radius	Radial nerve [C5, **C6**] before division into superficial and deep branches	Accessory flexor of elbow joint when forearm is midpronated
Extensor carpi radialis longus	2	Distal part of lateral supraepicondylar ridge of humerus and adjacent intermuscular septum	Dorsal surface of base of metacarpal II	Radial nerve [**C6**, C7] before division into superficial and deep branches	Extends and abducts the wrist
Extensor carpi radialis brevis	3	Lateral epicondyle of humerus and adjacent intermuscular septum	Dorsal surface of base of metacarpals II and III	Deep branch of radial nerve [**C7**, C8] before penetrating supinator muscle	Extends and abducts the wrist
Extensor digitorum	4	Lateral epicondyle of humerus and adjacent intermuscular septum and deep fascia	Four tendons, which insert via extensor hoods into the dorsal aspects of the bases of the middle and distal phalanges of the index, middle, ring, and little fingers	Posterior interosseous nerve [**C7**, C8]	Extends the index, middle, ring, and little fingers; can also extend the wrist
Extensor digiti minimi	5	Lateral epicondyle of humerus and adjacent intermuscular septum together with extensor digitorum	Extensor hood of the little finger	Posterior interosseous nerve [**C7**, C8]	Extends the little finger
Extensor carpi ulnaris	6	Lateral epicondyle of humerus and posterior border of ulna	Tubercle on the base of the medial side of metacarpal V	Posterior interosseous nerve [**C7**, C8]	Extends and adducts the wrist
Anconeus	7	Lateral epicondyle of humerus	Olecranon and proximal posterior surface of ulna	Radial nerve [**C6**, **C7**, **C8**] (via branch to medial head of triceps brachii)	Abduction of the ulna in pronation; accessory extensor of the elbow joint

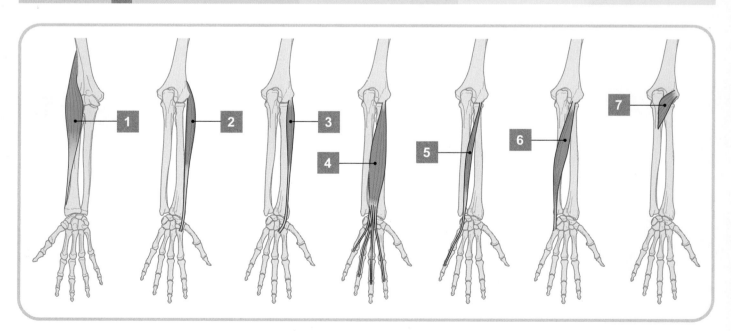

Deep layer of muscles in the posterior compartment of the forearm

(spinal segments indicated in bold are the major segments innervating the muscle)

Muscle		Origin	Insertion	Innervation	Function
Supinator	1	Superficial part—lateral epicondyle of humerus, radial collateral and anular ligaments; deep part-supinator crest of the ulna	Lateral surface of radius superior to the anterior oblique line	Posterior interosseous nerve [**C6**, C7]	Supination
Abductor pollicis longus	2	Posterior surfaces of ulna and radius (distal to the attachments of supinator and anconeus), and intervening interosseous membrane	Lateral side of base of metacarpal I	Posterior interosseous nerve [**C7**, C8]	Abducts carpometacarpal joint of thumb; accessory extensor of the thumb
Extensor pollicis brevis	3	Posterior surface of radius (distal to abductor pollicis longus) and the adjacent interosseous membrane	Dorsal surface of base of proximal phalanx of the thumb	Posterior interosseous nerve [**C7**, C8]	Extends metacarpophalangeal joint of the thumb; can also extend the carpometacarpal joint of the thumb
Extensor pollicis longus	4	Posterior surface of ulna (distal to the abductor pollicis longus) and the adjacent interosseous membrane	Dorsal surface of base of distal phalanx of thumb	Posterior interosseous nerve [**C7**, C8]	Extends interphalangeal joint of the thumb; can also extend carpometacarpal and metacarpophalangeal joints of the thumb
Extensor indicis	5	Posterior surface of ulna (distal to extensor pollicis longus) and adjacent interosseous membrane	Extensor hood of index finger	Posterior interosseous nerve [**C7**, C8]	Extends index finger

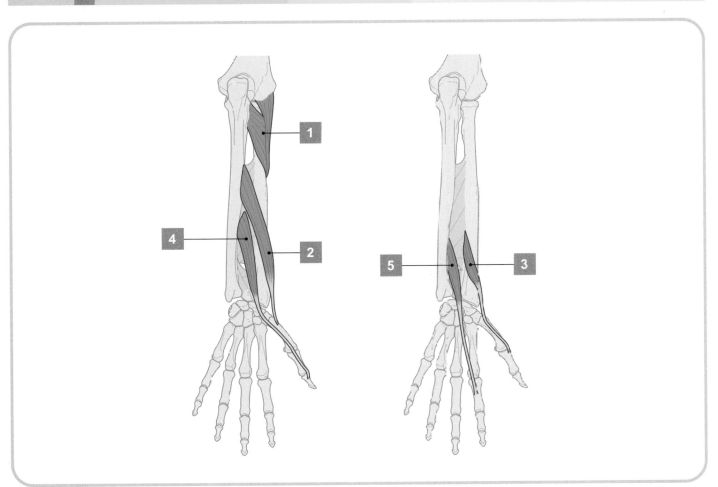

Intrinsic muscles of the hand

(spinal segments indicated in bold are the major segments innervating the muscle)

Muscle		Origin	Insertion	Innervation	Function
Palmaris brevis	1	Palmar aponeurosis and flexor retinaculum	Dermis of skin on the medial margin of the hand	Superficial branch of the ulnar nerve [C8, **T1**]	Improves grip
Dorsal interossei (four muscles)	2	Adjacent sides of metacarpals	Extensor hood and base of proximal phalanges of index, middle, and ring fingers	Deep branch of ulnar nerve [C8, **T1**]	Abduction of index, middle, and ring fingers at the metacarpophalangeal joints
Palmar interossei (four muscles: the first palmar interosseious associated with the thumb is rudimentary. When present it is often considered part of either adductor pollicics or flexor pollicis brevis)	3	Sides of metacarpals	Extensor hoods of the thumb, index, ring, and little fingers and the proximal phalanx of thumb	Deep branch of ulnar nerve [C8, **T1**]	Adduction of the thumb, index, ring, and little fingers at the metacarpophalangeal joints
Adductor pollicis	4	Transverse head—metacarpal III; oblique head—capitate and bases of metacarpals II and III	Base of proximal phalanx and extensor hood of thumb	Deep branch of ulnar nerve [C8, **T1**]	Adducts thumb
Lumbricals (four muscles)	5	Tendons of flexor digitorum profundus	Extensor hoods of index, ring, middle, and little fingers	Medial two by the deep branch of the ulnar nerve; lateral two by digital branches of the median nerve	Flex metacarpophalangeal joints while extending interphalangeal joints

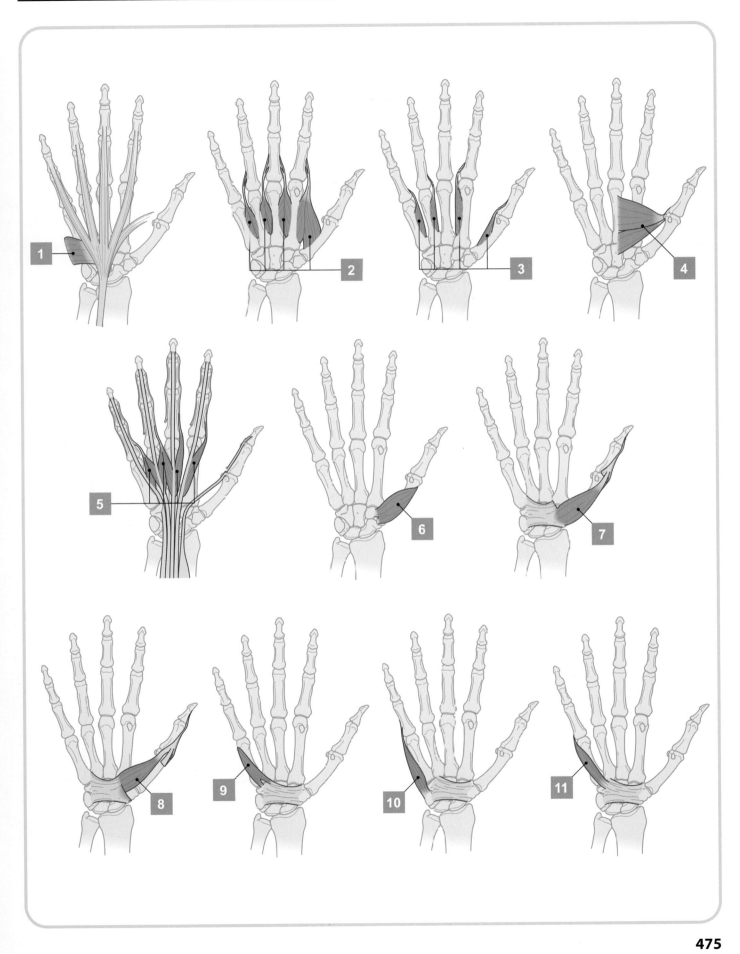

HEAD AND NECK

8

CONTENTS

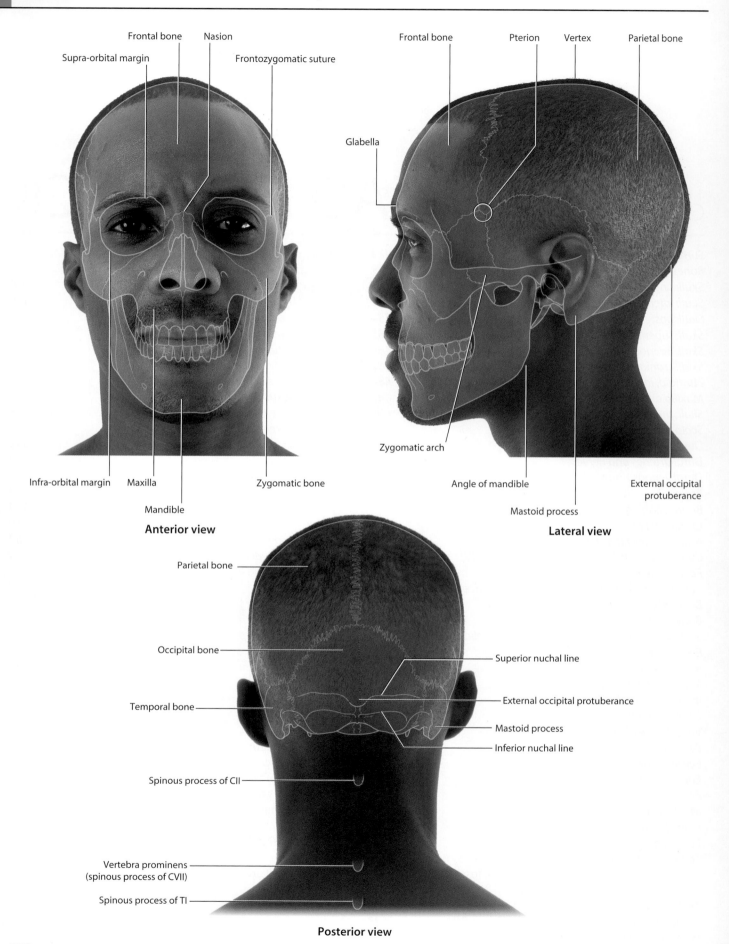

Frontal bone

Supra-orbital margin

Nasion

Frontozygomatic suture

Infra-orbital margin

Maxilla

Mandible

Zygomatic bone

Anterior view

Frontal bone

Pterion

Vertex

Parietal bone

Glabella

Zygomatic arch

Angle of mandible

Mastoid process

External occipital protuberance

Lateral view

Parietal bone

Occipital bone

Superior nuchal line

Temporal bone

External occipital protuberance

Mastoid process

Inferior nuchal line

Spinous process of CII

Vertebra prominens (spinous process of CVII)

Spinous process of TI

Posterior view

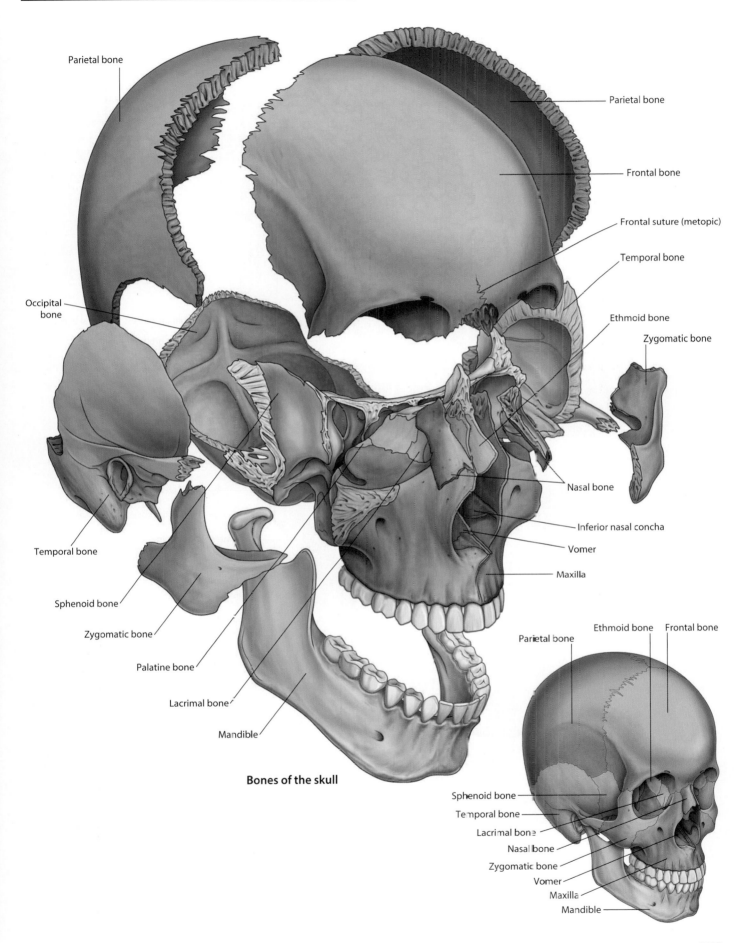

Parietal bone

Parietal bone

Frontal bone

Frontal suture (metopic)

Temporal bone

Ethmoid bone

Zygomatic bone

Occipital bone

Nasal bone

Inferior nasal concha

Vomer

Maxilla

Temporal bone

Sphenoid bone

Zygomatic bone

Palatine bone

Lacrimal bone

Mandible

Bones of the skull

Parietal bone

Ethmoid bone

Frontal bone

Sphenoid bone

Temporal bone

Lacrimal bone

Nasal bone

Zygomatic bone

Vomer

Maxilla

Mandible

479

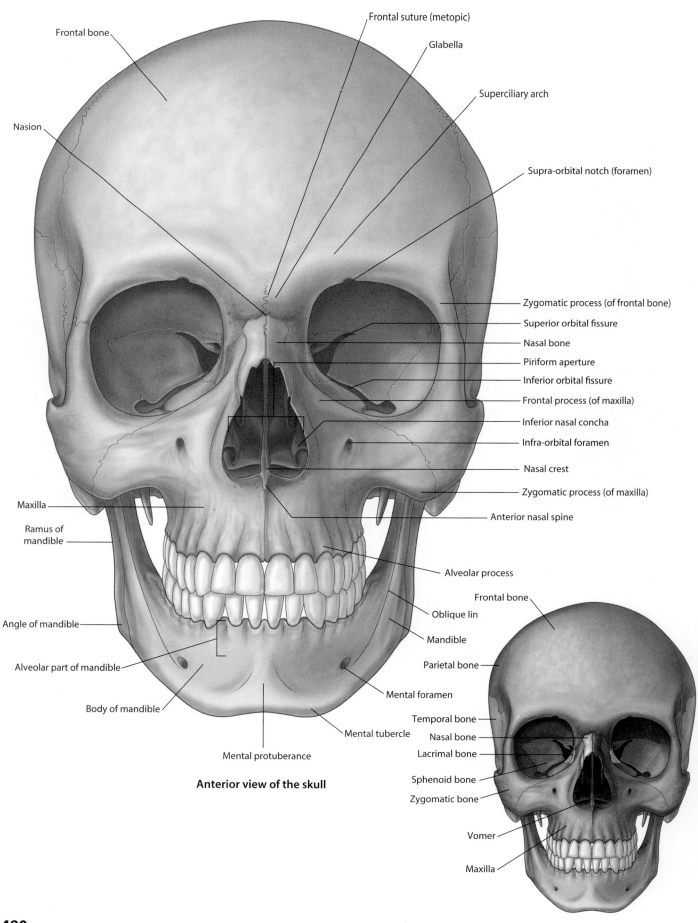

Frontal suture (metopic)

Glabella

Superciliary arch

Frontal bone

Nasion

Supra-orbital notch (foramen)

Zygomatic process (of frontal bone)

Superior orbital fissure

Nasal bone

Piriform aperture

Inferior orbital fissure

Frontal process (of maxilla)

Inferior nasal concha

Infra-orbital foramen

Nasal crest

Zygomatic process (of maxilla)

Anterior nasal spine

Maxilla

Ramus of mandible

Alveolar process

Oblique lin

Mandible

Angle of mandible

Alveolar part of mandible

Frontal bone

Parietal bone

Mental foramen

Body of mandible

Temporal bone

Nasal bone

Lacrimal bone

Sphenoid bone

Zygomatic bone

Vomer

Maxilla

Mental tubercle

Mental protuberance

Anterior view of the skull

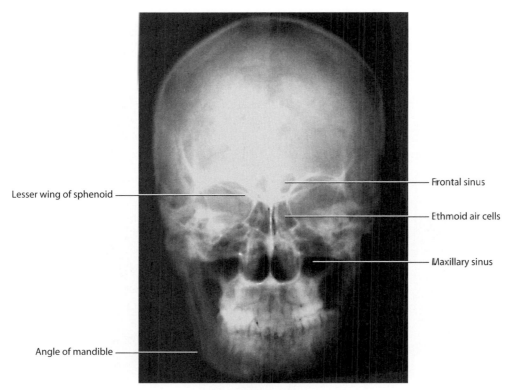

Frontal sinus

Ethmoid air cells

Maxillary sinus

Lesser wing of sphenoid

Angle of mandible

Anterior view of the skull.
Radiograph, AP view

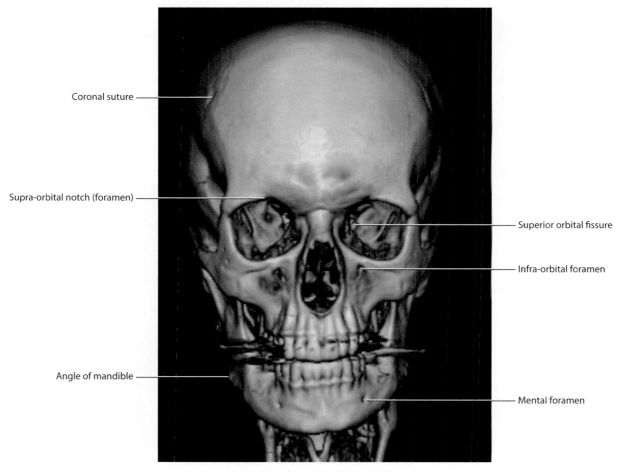

Coronal suture

Supra-orbital notch (foramen)

Angle of mandible

Superior orbital fissure

Infra-orbital foramen

Mental foramen

Anterior view of the skull.
Volume-rendered anterior view using multidetector computed tomography

481

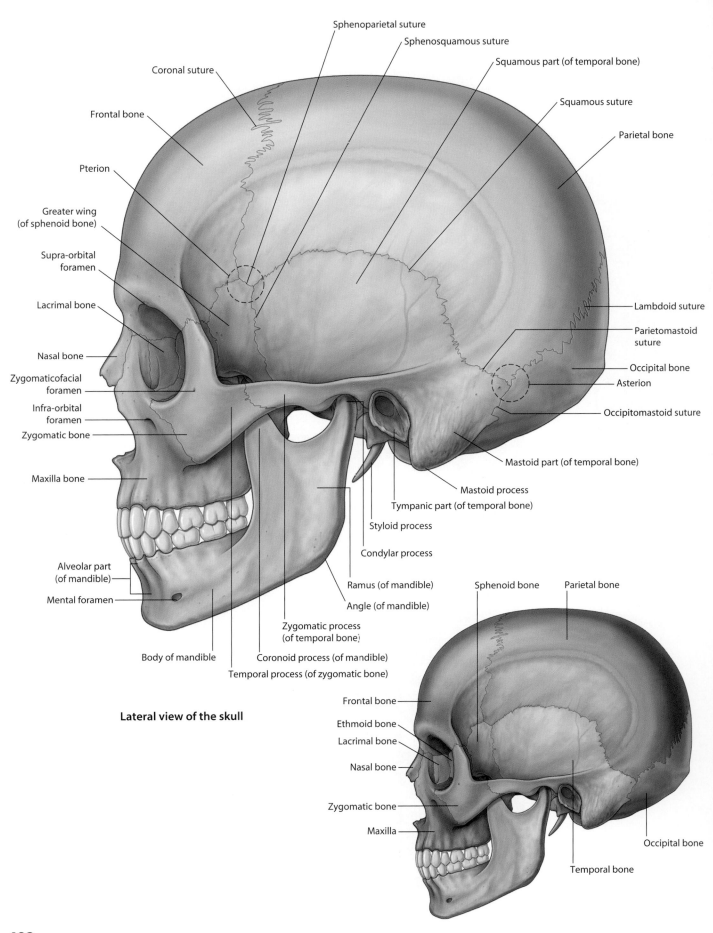

Sphenoparietal suture

Sphenosquamous suture

Squamous part (of temporal bone)

Coronal suture

Squamous suture

Frontal bone

Parietal bone

Pterion

Greater wing
(of sphenoid bone)

Supra-orbital
foramen

Lacrimal bone

Lambdoid suture

Parietomastoid
suture

Nasal bone

Zygomaticofacial
foramen

Occipital bone

Asterion

Infra-orbital
foramen

Occipitomastoid suture

Zygomatic bone

Maxilla bone

Mastoid part (of temporal bone)

Mastoid process

Tympanic part (of temporal bone)

Styloid process

Condylar process

Alveolar part
(of mandible)

Ramus (of mandible)

Mental foramen

Angle (of mandible)

Zygomatic process
(of temporal bone)

Body of mandible

Coronoid process (of mandible)

Temporal process (of zygomatic bone)

Lateral view of the skull

Sphenoid bone

Parietal bone

Frontal bone

Ethmoid bone

Lacrimal bone

Nasal bone

Zygomatic bone

Maxilla

Occipital bone

Temporal bone

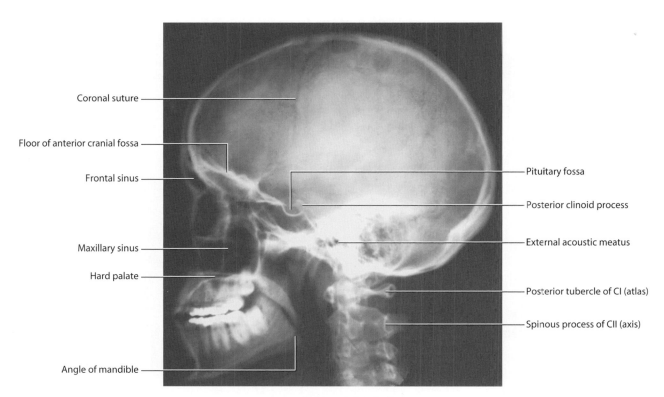

Coronal suture

Floor of anterior cranial fossa

Frontal sinus

Maxillary sinus

Hard palate

Angle of mandible

Pituitary fossa

Posterior clinoid process

External acoustic meatus

Posterior tubercle of CI (atlas)

Spinous process of CII (axis)

Lateral view of the skull.
Radiograph, lateral view

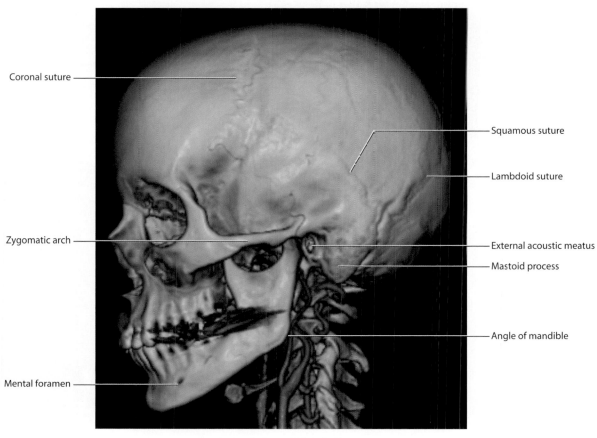

Coronal suture

Zygomatic arch

Mental foramen

Squamous suture

Lambdoid suture

External acoustic meatus

Mastoid process

Angle of mandible

Lateral view of the skull.
Volume-rendered lateral view using multidetector computed tomography

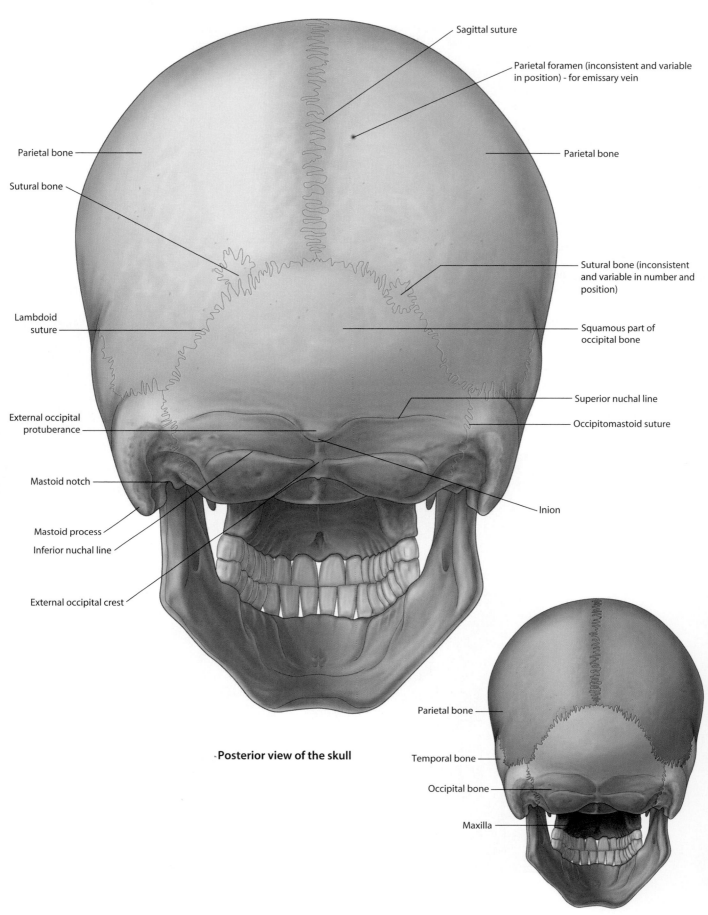

Sagittal suture

Parietal foramen (inconsistent and variable in position) - for emissary vein

Parietal bone

Parietal bone

Sutural bone

Sutural bone (inconsistent and variable in number and position)

Lambdoid suture

Squamous part of occipital bone

External occipital protuberance

Superior nuchal line

Occipitomastoid suture

Mastoid notch

Inion

Mastoid process

Inferior nuchal line

External occipital crest

Posterior view of the skull

Parietal bone

Temporal bone

Occipital bone

Maxilla

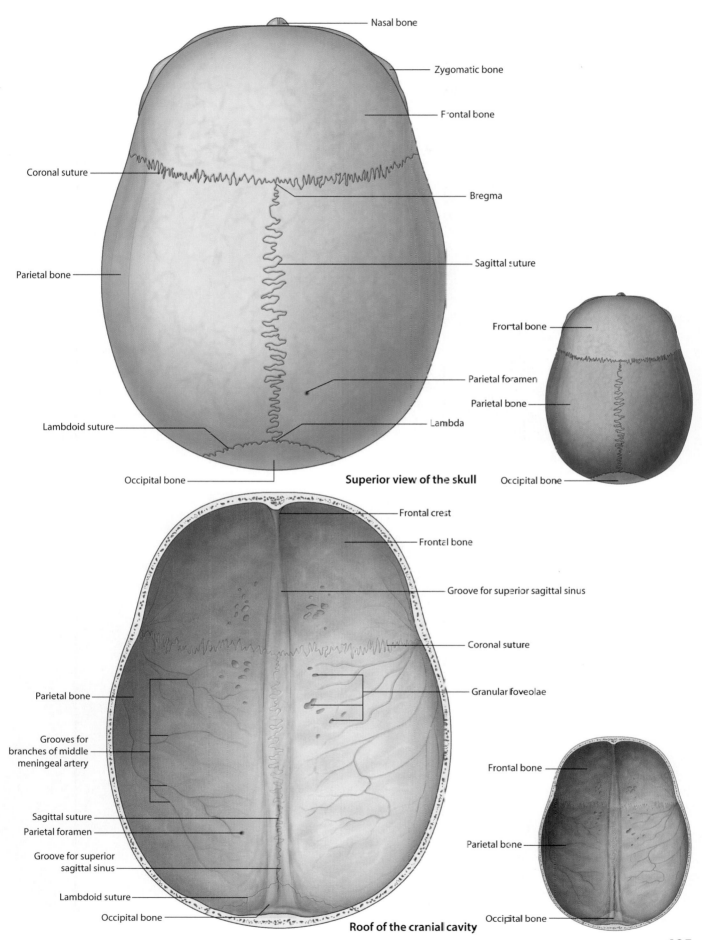

Superior view of the skull

Nasal bone

Zygomatic bone

Frontal bone

Coronal suture

Bregma

Sagittal suture

Parietal bone

Frontal bone

Parietal foramen

Parietal bone

Lambdoid suture

Lambda

Occipital bone

Occipital bone

Roof of the cranial cavity

Frontal crest

Frontal bone

Groove for superior sagittal sinus

Coronal suture

Parietal bone

Granular foveolae

Grooves for branches of middle meningeal artery

Frontal bone

Sagittal suture

Parietal foramen

Parietal bone

Groove for superior sagittal sinus

Lambdoid suture

Occipital bone

Occipital bone

485

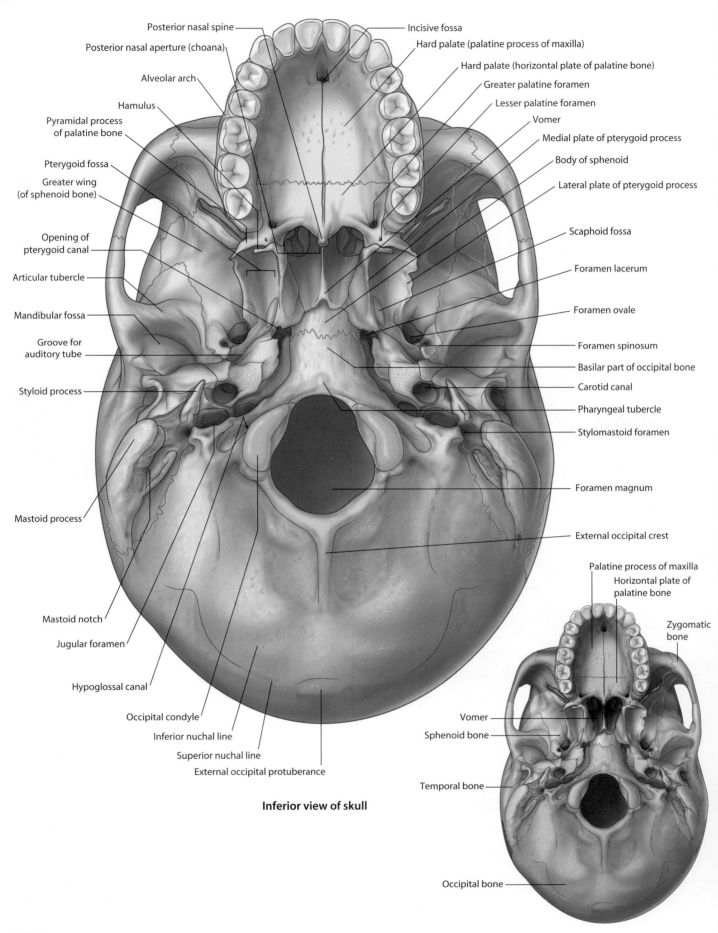

Posterior nasal spine

Posterior nasal aperture (choana)

Alveolar arch

Hamulus

Pyramidal process of palatine bone

Pterygoid fossa

Greater wing (of sphenoid bone)

Opening of pterygoid canal

Articular tubercle

Mandibular fossa

Groove for auditory tube

Styloid process

Mastoid process

Mastoid notch

Jugular foramen

Hypoglossal canal

Occipital condyle

Inferior nuchal line

Superior nuchal line

External occipital protuberance

Incisive fossa

Hard palate (palatine process of maxilla)

Hard palate (horizontal plate of palatine bone)

Greater palatine foramen

Lesser palatine foramen

Vomer

Medial plate of pterygoid process

Body of sphenoid

Lateral plate of pterygoid process

Scaphoid fossa

Foramen lacerum

Foramen ovale

Foramen spinosum

Basilar part of occipital bone

Carotid canal

Pharyngeal tubercle

Stylomastoid foramen

Foramen magnum

External occipital crest

Palatine process of maxilla

Horizontal plate of palatine bone

Zygomatic bone

Vomer

Sphenoid bone

Temporal bone

Occipital bone

Inferior view of skull

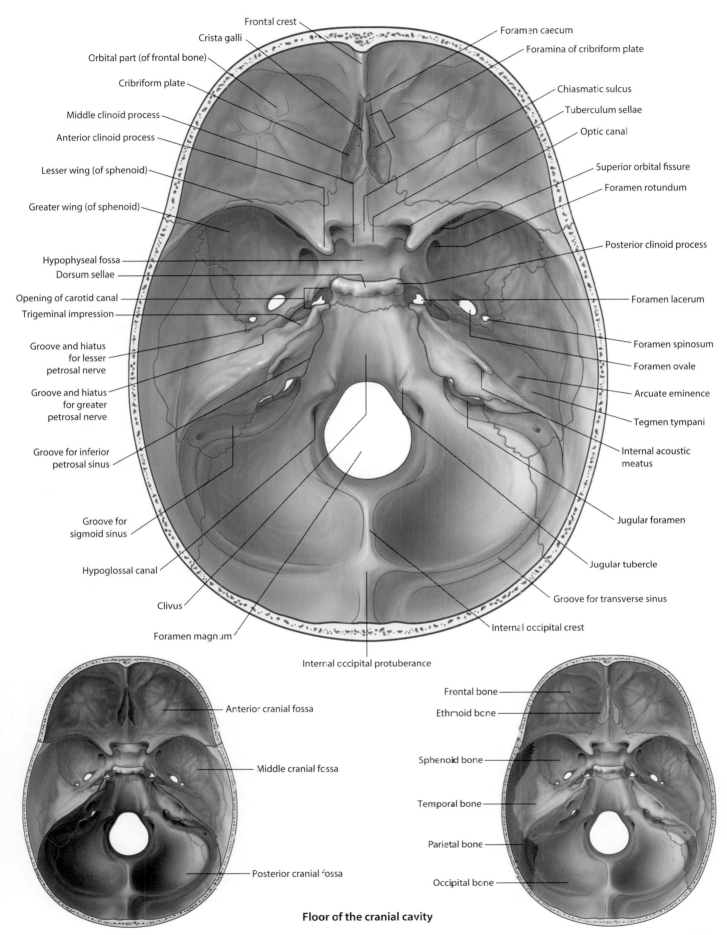

Frontal crest

Crista galli

Orbital part (of frontal bone)

Cribriform plate

Middle clinoid process

Anterior clinoid process

Lesser wing (of sphenoid)

Greater wing (of sphenoid)

Hypophyseal fossa

Dorsum sellae

Opening of carotid canal

Trigeminal impression

Groove and hiatus for lesser petrosal nerve

Groove and hiatus for greater petrosal nerve

Groove for inferior petrosal sinus

Groove for sigmoid sinus

Hypoglossal canal

Clivus

Foramen magnum

Foramen caecum

Foramina of cribriform plate

Chiasmatic sulcus

Tuberculum sellae

Optic canal

Superior orbital fissure

Foramen rotundum

Posterior clinoid process

Foramen lacerum

Foramen spinosum

Foramen ovale

Arcuate eminence

Tegmen tympani

Internal acoustic meatus

Jugular foramen

Jugular tubercle

Groove for transverse sinus

Internal occipital crest

Internal occipital protuberance

Anterior cranial fossa

Middle cranial fossa

Posterior cranial fossa

Frontal bone

Ethmoid bone

Sphenoid bone

Temporal bone

Parietal bone

Occipital bone

Floor of the cranial cavity

487

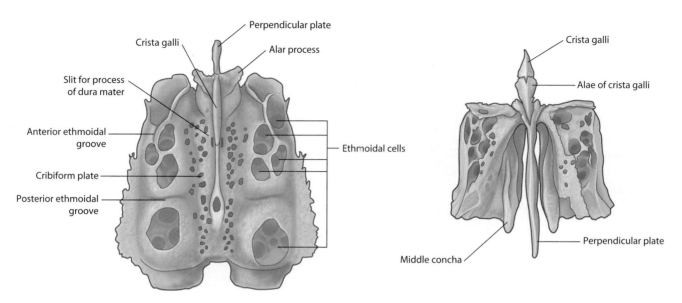

Perpendicular plate

Crista galli

Alar process

Slit for process
of dura mater

Anterior ethmoidal
groove

Ethmoidal cells

Cribiform plate

Posterior ethmoidal
groove

Ethmoid bone (superior view)

Crista galli

Alae of crista galli

Perpendicular plate

Middle concha

Ethmoid bone (posterior view)

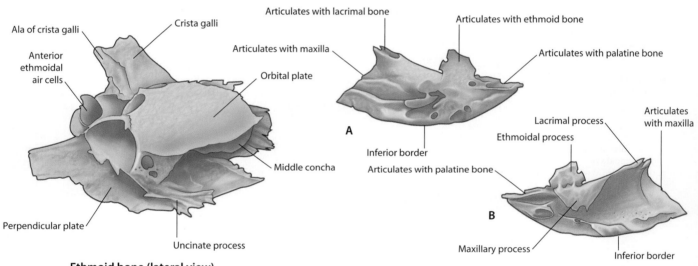

Ala of crista galli

Crista galli

Anterior
ethmoidal
air cells

Orbital plate

Middle concha

Perpendicular plate

Uncinate process

Ethmoid bone (lateral view)

Articulates with lacrimal bone

Articulates with ethmoid bone

Articulates with maxilla

Articulates with palatine bone

Orbital plate

A

Inferior border

Articulates with palatine bone

Lacrimal process

Ethmoidal process

Articulates
with maxilla

B

Maxillary process

Inferior border

**Right inferior concha
A. Medial view B. Lateral view**

Articulates with frontal bone

Orbital surface

Lacrimal groove (for lacrimal sac)

Articulates
with ethmoid
bone

Articulates
with
maxilla

Nasal surface

Posterior
lacrimal crest

Lacrimal
hamulus

A

B

Descending process
for inferior nasal
concha

**Right lacrimal bone
A. Lateral view B. Medial view**

Articulates with ethmoid bone

Articlates with
sphenoid bone

Articulates with
septal cartilage

Alae

Articulates with maxillae and palatine bones

Vomer (lateral view)

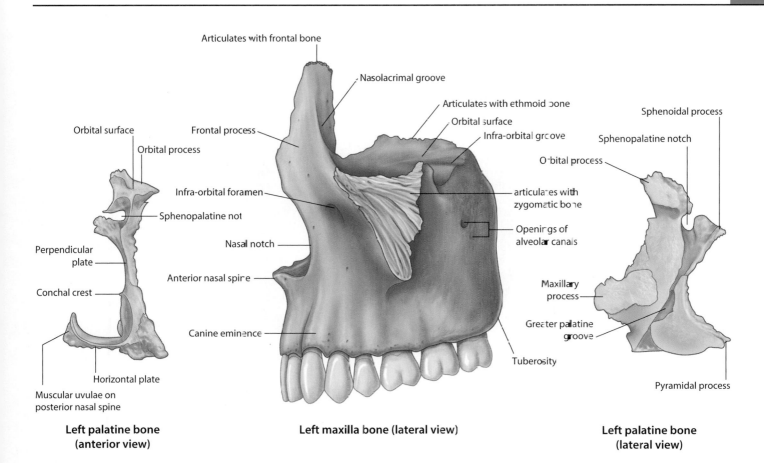

Left palatine bone
(anterior view)

- Orbital surface
- Orbital process
- Perpendicular plate
- Conchal crest
- Horizontal plate
- Muscular uvulae on posterior nasal spine
- Infra-orbital foramen
- Sphenopalatine not
- Frontal process
- Nasal notch
- Anterior nasal spire
- Canine eminence

Left maxilla bone (lateral view)

- Articulates with frontal bone
- Nasolacrimal groove
- Articulates with ethmoid bone
- Orbital surface
- Infra-orbital groove
- articulates with zygomatic bone
- Openings of alveolar canals
- Tuberosity

Left palatine bone
(lateral view)

- Sphenoidal process
- Sphenopalatine notch
- Orbital process
- Maxillary process
- Greater palatine groove
- Pyramidal process

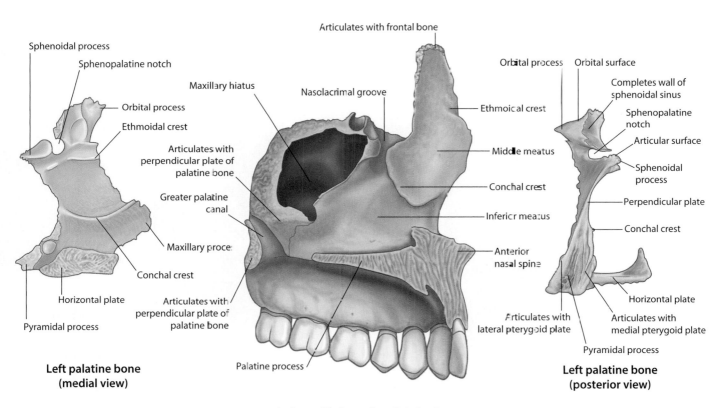

Left palatine bone
(medial view)

- Sphenoidal process
- Sphenopalatine notch
- Orbital process
- Ethmoidal crest
- Articulates with perpendicular plate of palatine bone
- Greater palatine canal
- Maxillary proces
- Conchal crest
- Horizontal plate
- Pyramidal process
- Articulates with perpendicular plate of palatine bone

Left maxilla bone (medial view)

- Articulates with frontal bone
- Maxillary hiatus
- Nasolacrimal groove
- Palatine process

Left palatine bone
(posterior view)

- Orbital process
- Orbital surface
- Completes wall of sphenoidal sinus
- Ethmoidal crest
- Middle meatus
- Sphenopalatine notch
- Articular surface
- Conchal crest
- Sphenoidal process
- Inferior meatus
- Perpendicular plate
- Conchal crest
- Anterior nasal spine
- Horizontal plate
- Articulates with lateral pterygoid plate
- Articulates with medial pterygoid plate
- Pyramidal process

489

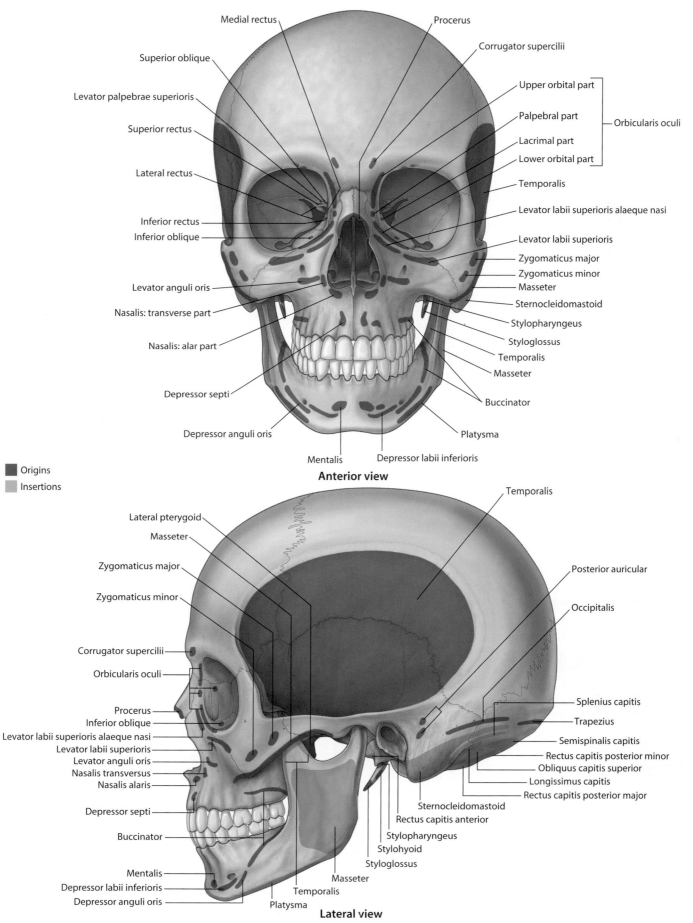

Anterior view

Medial rectus

Superior oblique

Levator palpebrae superioris

Superior rectus

Lateral rectus

Inferior rectus

Inferior oblique

Levator anguli oris

Nasalis: transverse part

Nasalis: alar part

Depressor septi

Depressor anguli oris

Mentalis

Procerus

Corrugator supercilii

Upper orbital part

Palpebral part

Lacrimal part

Lower orbital part

Orbicularis oculi

Temporalis

Levator labii superioris alaeque nasi

Levator labii superioris

Zygomaticus major

Zygomaticus minor

Masseter

Sternocleidomastoid

Stylopharyngeus

Styloglossus

Temporalis

Masseter

Buccinator

Platysma

Depressor labii inferioris

Origins

Insertions

Lateral view

Lateral pterygoid

Masseter

Zygomaticus major

Zygomaticus minor

Corrugator supercilii

Orbicularis oculi

Procerus

Inferior oblique

Levator labii superioris alaeque nasi

Levator labii superioris

Levator anguli oris

Nasalis transversus

Nasalis alaris

Depressor septi

Buccinator

Mentalis

Depressor labii inferioris

Depressor anguli oris

Platysma

Temporalis

Masseter

Stylopharyngeus

Stylohyoid

Styloglossus

Rectus capitis anterior

Sternocleidomastoid

Temporalis

Posterior auricular

Occipitalis

Splenius capitis

Trapezius

Semispinalis capitis

Rectus capitis posterior minor

Obliquus capitis superior

Longissimus capitis

Rectus capitis posterior major

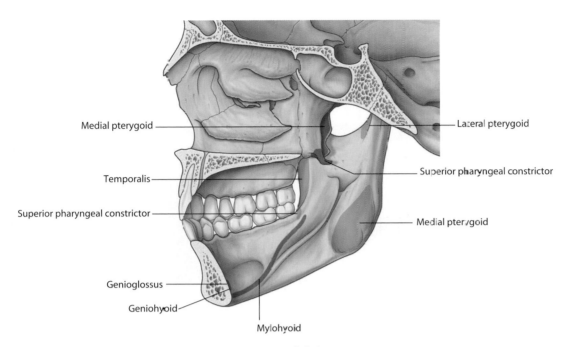

Medial pterygoid

Temporalis

Superior pharyngeal constrictor

Genioglossus

Geniohyoid

Mylohyoid

Lateral pterygoid

Superior pharyngeal constrictor

Medial pterygoid

Medial view

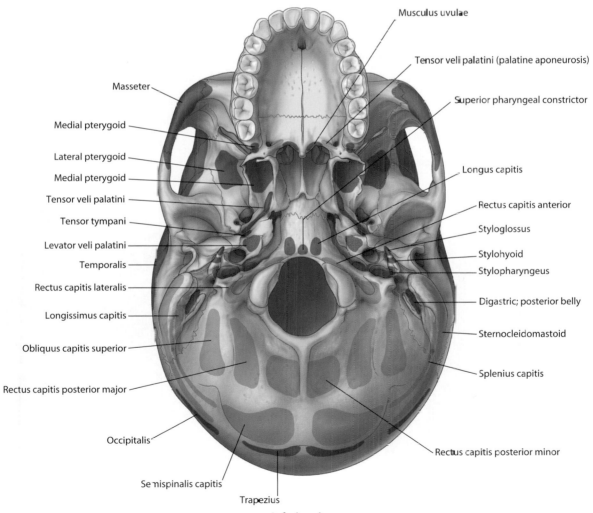

Musculus uvulae

Tensor veli palatini (palatine aponeurosis)

Superior pharyngeal constrictor

Masseter

Medial pterygoid

Lateral pterygoid

Medial pterygoid

Tensor veli palatini

Tensor tympani

Levator veli palatini

Temporalis

Rectus capitis lateralis

Longissimus capitis

Obliquus capitis superior

Rectus capitis posterior major

Occipitalis

Semispinalis capitis

Trapezius

Longus capitis

Rectus capitis anterior

Styloglossus

Stylohyoid

Stylopharyngeus

Digastric; posterior belly

Sternocleidomastoid

Splenius capitis

Rectus capitis posterior minor

Inferior view

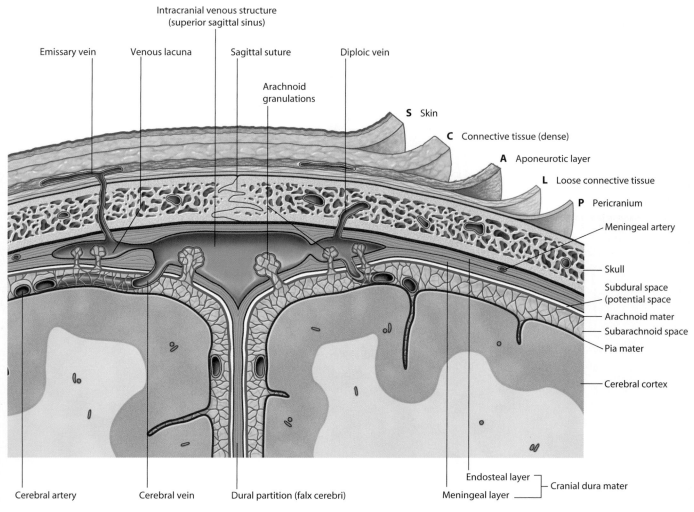

Intracranial venous structure (superior sagittal sinus)

Emissary vein

Venous lacuna

Sagittal suture

Diploic vein

Arachnoid granulations

S Skin

C Connective tissue (dense)

A Aponeurotic layer

L Loose connective tissue

P Pericranium

Meningeal artery

Skull

Subdural space (potential space

Arachnoid mater

Subarachnoid space

Pia mater

Cerebral cortex

Cerebral artery

Cerebral vein

Dural partition (falx cerebri)

Endosteal layer ⎤ Cranial dura mater
Meningeal layer ⎦

Scalp and cranial meninges

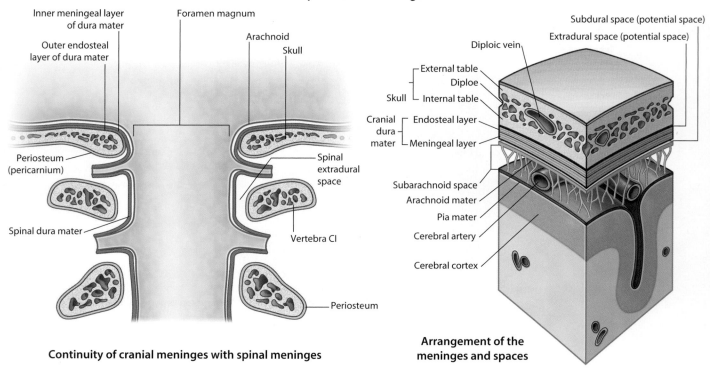

Inner meningeal layer of dura mater

Outer endosteal layer of dura mater

Foramen magnum

Arachnoid

Skull

Periosteum (pericarnium)

Spinal dura mater

Spinal extradural space

Vertebra CI

Periosteum

Continuity of cranial meninges with spinal meninges

Subdural space (potential space)

Extradural space (potential space)

Diploic vein

External table

Diploe

Skull ⎡ Internal table

Cranial dura mater ⎡ Endosteal layer
⎣ Meningeal layer

Subarachnoid space

Arachnoid mater

Pia mater

Cerebral artery

Cerebral cortex

Arrangement of the meninges and spaces

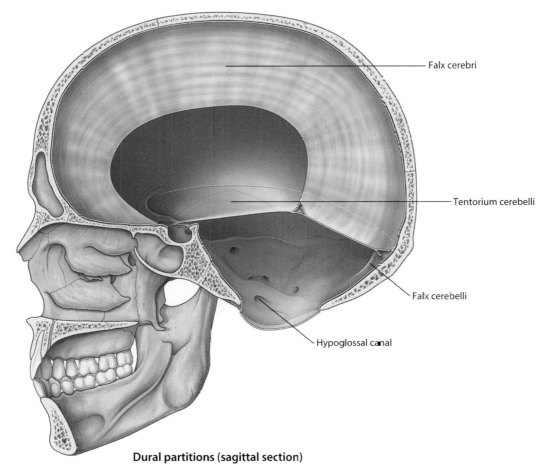

Dural partitions (sagittal section)

Falx cerebri

Tentorium cerebelli

Falx cerebelli

Hypoglossal canal

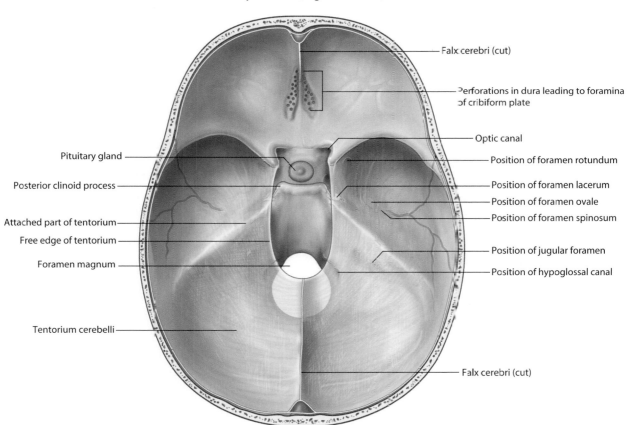

Falx cerebri (cut)

Perforations in dura leading to foramina of cribiform plate

Optic canal

Position of foramen rotundum

Position of foramen lacerum

Position of foramen ovale

Position of foramen spinosum

Position of jugular foramen

Position of hypoglossal canal

Falx cerebri (cut)

Pituitary gland

Posterior clinoid process

Attached part of tentorium

Free edge of tentorium

Foramen magnum

Tentorium cerebelli

Cranial cavity (superior view)

493

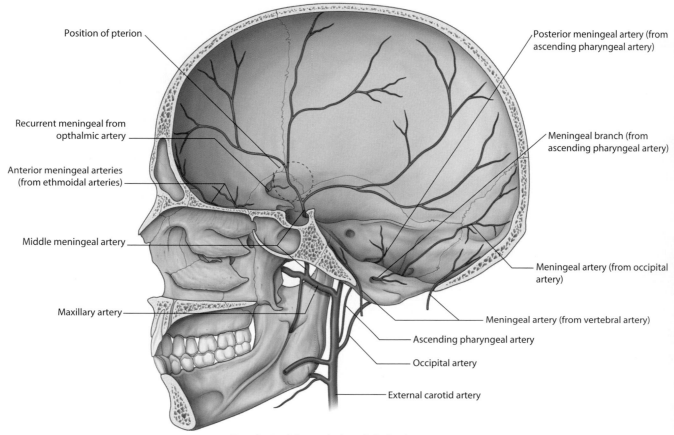

Position of pterion

Recurrent meningeal from opthalmic artery

Anterior meningeal arteries (from ethmoidal arteries)

Middle meningeal artery

Maxillary artery

Posterior meningeal artery (from ascending pharyngeal artery)

Meningeal branch (from ascending pharyngeal artery)

Meningeal artery (from occipital artery)

Meningeal artery (from vertebral artery)

Ascending pharyngeal artery

Occipital artery

External carotid artery

Dural arterial supply (medial view)

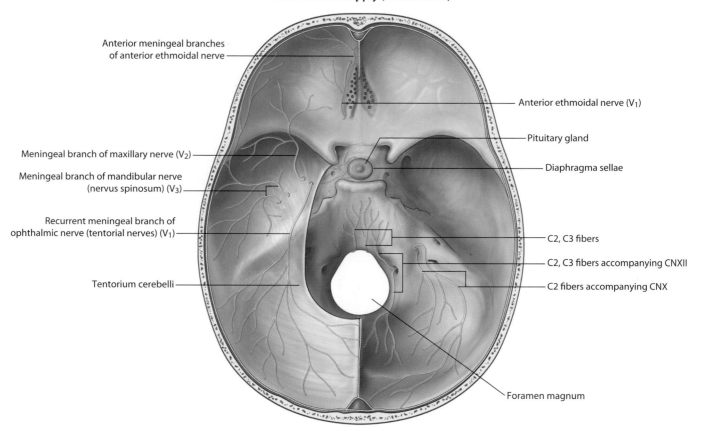

Anterior meningeal branches of anterior ethmoidal nerve

Meningeal branch of maxillary nerve (V_2)

Meningeal branch of mandibular nerve (nervus spinosum) (V_3)

Recurrent meningeal branch of ophthalmic nerve (tentorial nerves) (V_1)

Tentorium cerebelli

Anterior ethmoidal nerve (V_1)

Pituitary gland

Diaphragma sellae

C2, C3 fibers

C2, C3 fibers accompanying CNXII

C2 fibers accompanying CNX

Foramen magnum

Dural innervation (superior view)

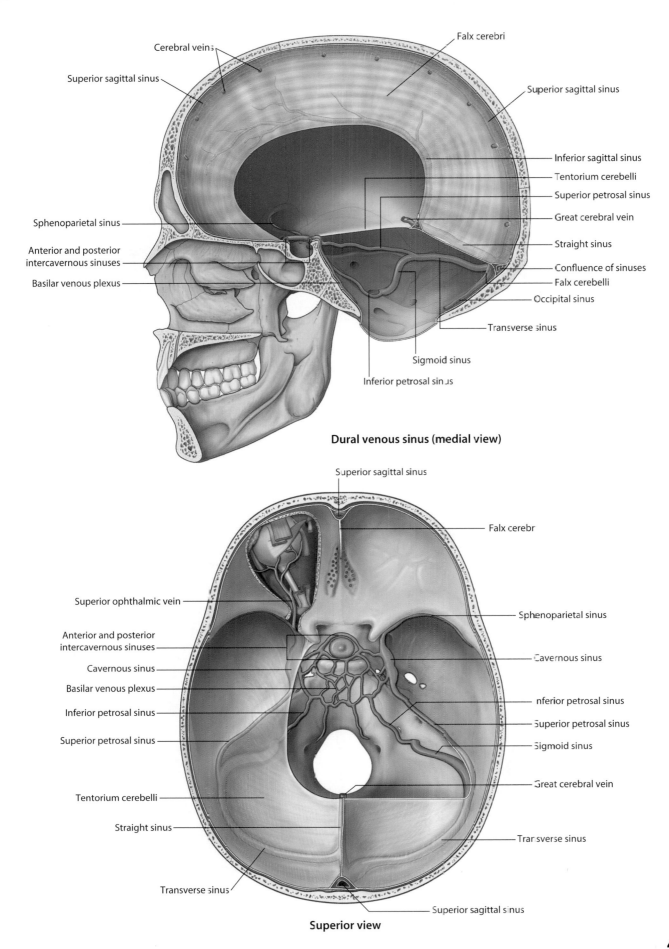

Dural venous sinus (medial view)

Cerebral veins
Superior sagittal sinus
Falx cerebri
Superior sagittal sinus
Inferior sagittal sinus
Tentorium cerebelli
Superior petrosal sinus
Great cerebral vein
Straight sinus
Confluence of sinuses
Falx cerebelli
Occipital sinus
Transverse sinus
Sphenoparietal sinus
Anterior and posterior intercavernous sinuses
Basilar venous plexus
Sigmoid sinus
Inferior petrosal sinus

Superior view

Superior sagittal sinus
Falx cerebri
Superior ophthalmic vein
Sphenoparietal sinus
Anterior and posterior intercavernous sinuses
Cavernous sinus
Cavernous sinus
Basilar venous plexus
Inferior petrosal sinus
Inferior petrosal sinus
Superior petrosal sinus
Superior petrosal sinus
Sigmoid sinus
Tentorium cerebelli
Great cerebral vein
Straight sinus
Transverse sinus
Transverse sinus
Superior sagittal sinus

495

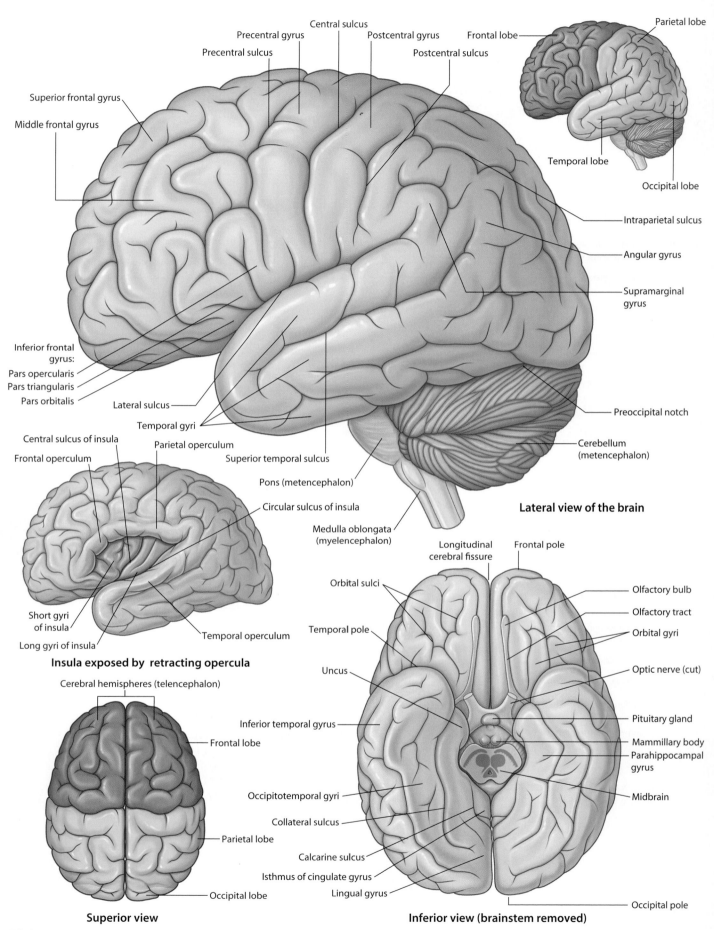

Precentral gyrus

Central sulcus

Precentral sulcus

Postcentral gyrus

Postcentral sulcus

Frontal lobe

Parietal lobe

Superior frontal gyrus

Middle frontal gyrus

Temporal lobe

Occipital lobe

Intraparietal sulcus

Angular gyrus

Supramarginal gyrus

Inferior frontal gyrus:

Pars opercularis

Pars triangularis

Pars orbitalis

Lateral sulcus

Temporal gyri

Preoccipital notch

Cerebellum (metencephalon)

Central sulcus of insula

Frontal operculum

Parietal operculum

Superior temporal sulcus

Circular sulcus of insula

Pons (metencephalon)

Lateral view of the brain

Short gyri of insula

Long gyri of insula

Temporal operculum

Medulla oblongata (myelencephalon)

Longitudinal cerebral fissure

Frontal pole

Insula exposed by retracting opercula

Orbital sulci

Temporal pole

Uncus

Olfactory bulb

Olfactory tract

Orbital gyri

Optic nerve (cut)

Cerebral hemispheres (telencephalon)

Inferior temporal gyrus

Frontal lobe

Pituitary gland

Mammillary body

Parahippocampal gyrus

Occipitotemporal gyri

Collateral sulcus

Midbrain

Parietal lobe

Calcarine sulcus

Isthmus of cingulate gyrus

Lingual gyrus

Occipital lobe

Occipital pole

Superior view

Inferior view (brainstem removed)

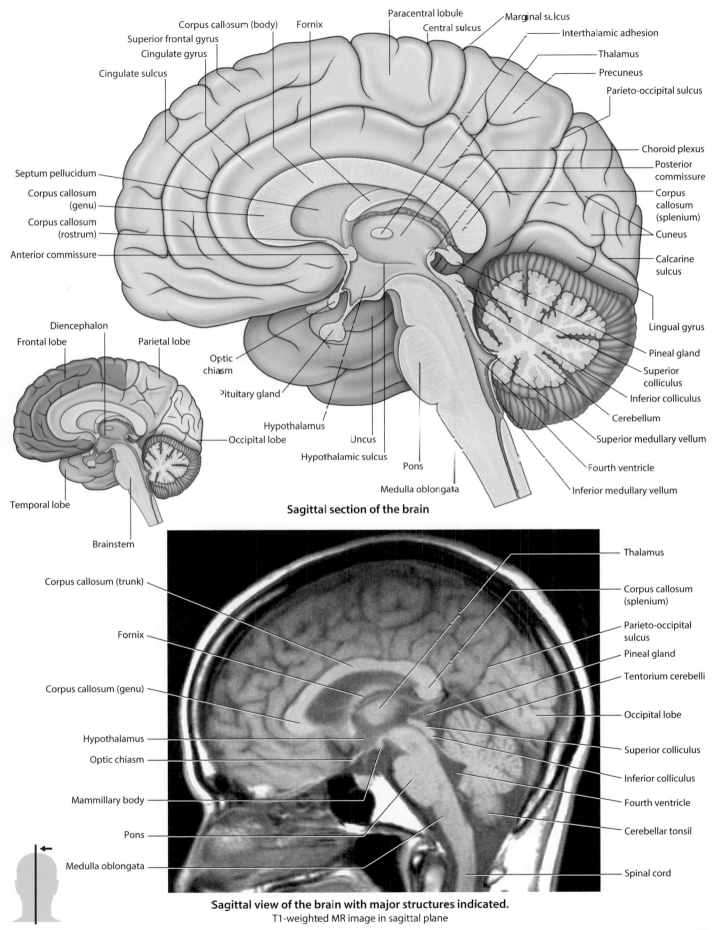

Corpus callosum (body)   Fornix   Paracentral lobule   Marginal sulcus

Superior frontal gyrus   Central sulcus   Interthalamic adhesion

Cingulate gyrus   Thalamus

Cingulate sulcus   Precuneus

Parieto-occipital sulcus

Choroid plexus

Posterior commissure

Septum pellucidum

Corpus callosum (genu)   Corpus callosum (splenium)

Corpus callosum (rostrum)   Cuneus

Anterior commissure   Calcarine sulcus

Diencephalon   Lingual gyrus

Frontal lobe   Parietal lobe   Pineal gland

Optic chiasm   Superior colliculus

Pituitary gland   Inferior colliculus

Cerebellum

Hypothalamus   Superior medullary vellum

Occipital lobe   Uncus   Fourth ventricle

Hypothalamic sulcus   Inferior medullary vellum

Pons

Temporal lobe   Medulla oblongata

Brainstem

Sagittal section of the brain

Thalamus

Corpus callosum (trunk)   Corpus callosum (splenium)

Fornix   Parieto-occipital sulcus

Pineal gland

Corpus callosum (genu)   Tentorium cerebelli

Occipital lobe

Hypothalamus   Superior colliculus

Optic chiasm   Inferior colliculus

Mammillary body   Fourth ventricle

Pons   Cerebellar tonsil

Medulla oblongata   Spinal cord

Sagittal view of the brain with major structures indicated.
T1-weighted MR image in sagittal plane

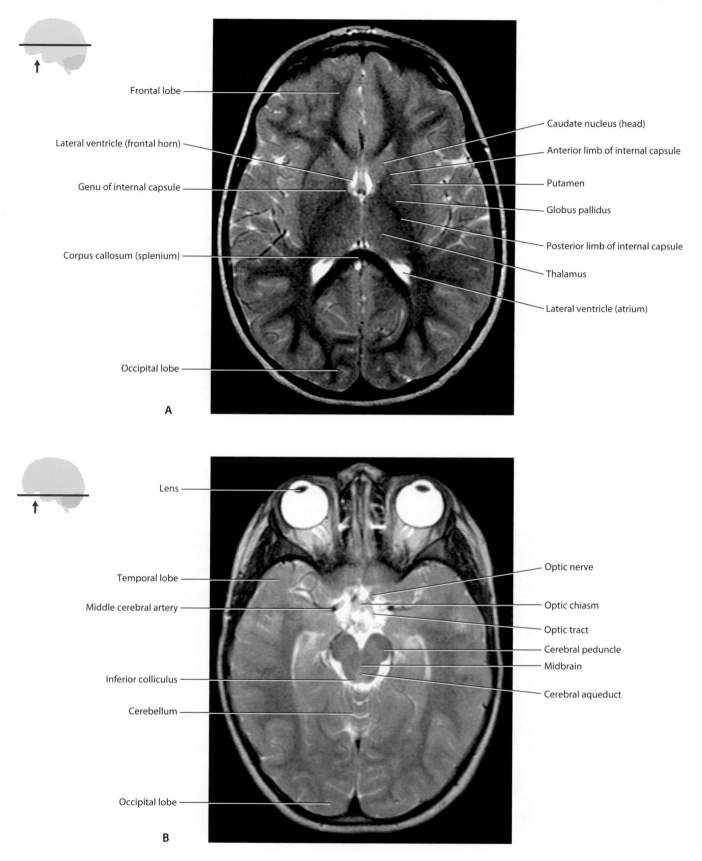

Frontal lobe

Lateral ventricle (frontal horn)

Genu of internal capsule

Corpus callosum (splenium)

Occipital lobe

Caudate nucleus (head)

Anterior limb of internal capsule

Putamen

Globus pallidus

Posterior limb of internal capsule

Thalamus

Lateral ventricle (atrium)

A

Lens

Temporal lobe

Middle cerebral artery

Inferior colliculus

Cerebellum

Occipital lobe

Optic nerve

Optic chiasm

Optic tract

Cerebral peduncle

Midbrain

Cerebral aqueduct

B

Axial or horizontal sections through the brain with major structures indicated.
A. Section showing structures related to the internal capsule.
B. Section showing structures related to the midbrain.
T1-weighted MR image in axial plane

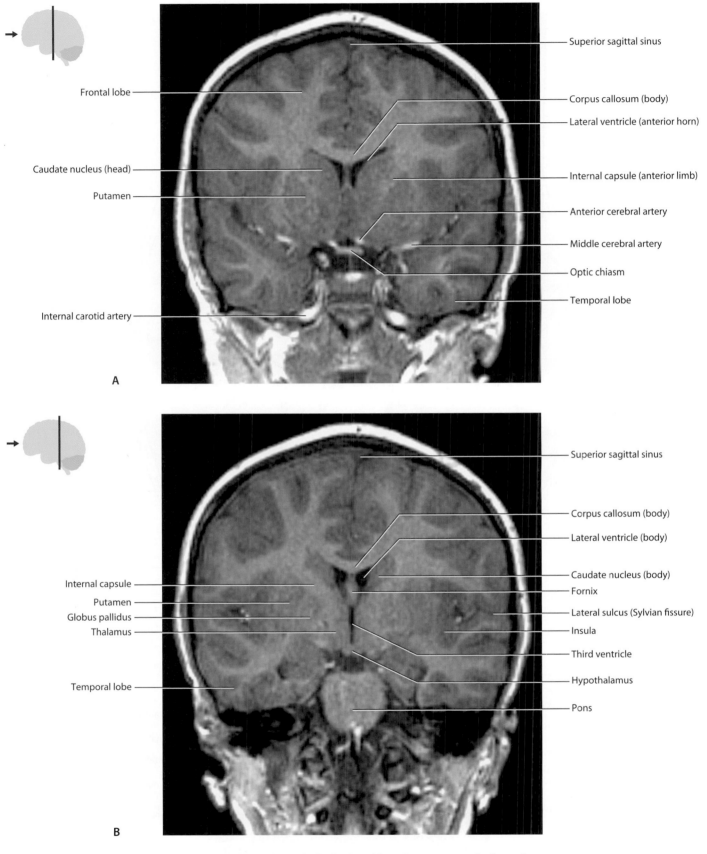

Frontal lobe

Caudate nucleus (head)

Putamen

Internal carotid artery

Superior sagittal sinus

Corpus callosum (body)

Lateral ventricle (anterior horn)

Internal capsule (anterior limb)

Anterior cerebral artery

Middle cerebral artery

Optic chiasm

Temporal lobe

A

Internal capsule

Putamen

Globus pallidus

Thalamus

Temporal lobe

Superior sagittal sinus

Corpus callosum (body)

Lateral ventricle (body)

Caudate nucleus (body)

Fornix

Lateral sulcus (Sylvian fissure)

Insula

Third ventricle

Hypothalamus

Pons

B

Coronal sections through the brain with major structures indicated.
A. Section showing structures related to the optic chiasm.
B. Section showing structures related to the third ventricle.
T1-weighted MR image in coronal plane

499

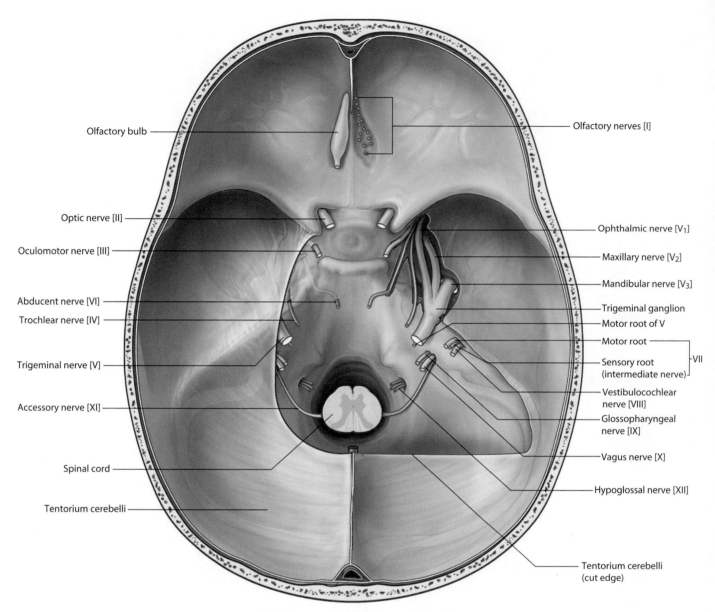

Olfactory bulb

Olfactory nerves [I]

Optic nerve [II]

Ophthalmic nerve [V₁]

Oculomotor nerve [III]

Maxillary nerve [V₂]

Mandibular nerve [V₃]

Trigeminal ganglion

Abducent nerve [VI]

Motor root of V

Trochlear nerve [IV]

Motor root

Sensory root
(intermediate nerve)

VII

Trigeminal nerve [V]

Vestibulocochlear
nerve [VIII]

Accessory nerve [XI]

Glossopharyngeal
nerve [IX]

Vagus nerve [X]

Spinal cord

Hypoglossal nerve [XII]

Tentorium cerebelli

Tentorium cerebelli
(cut edge)

Cranial nerves exiting the cranial cavity

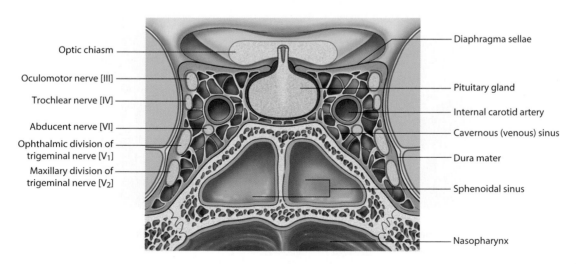

Optic chiasm

Diaphragma sellae

Oculomotor nerve [III]

Pituitary gland

Trochlear nerve [IV]

Abducent nerve [VI]

Internal carotid artery

Cavernous (venous) sinus

Ophthalmic division of
trigeminal nerve [V₁]

Dura mater

Maxillary division of
trigeminal nerve [V₂]

Sphenoidal sinus

Nasopharynx

Cranial nerves in the cavernous sinus

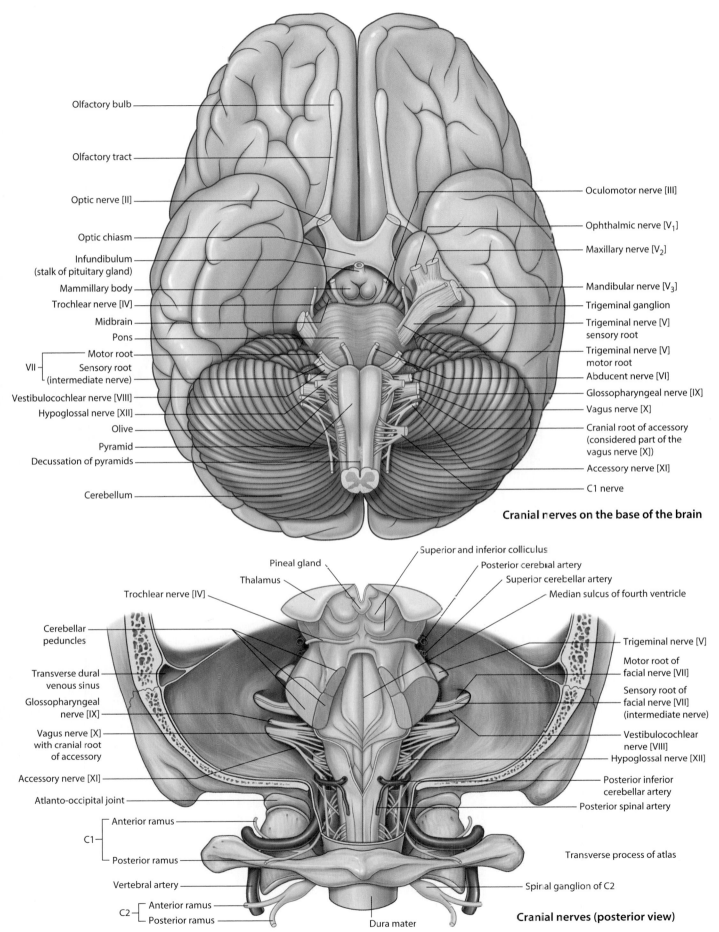

Olfactory bulb

Olfactory tract

Optic nerve [II]

Optic chiasm

Infundibulum
(stalk of pituitary gland)

Mammillary body

Trochlear nerve [IV]

Midbrain

Pons

VII ⎰ Motor root
      ⎱ Sensory root
        (intermediate nerve)

Vestibulocochlear nerve [VIII]

Hypoglossal nerve [XII]

Olive

Pyramid

Decussation of pyramids

Cerebellum

Oculomotor nerve [III]

Ophthalmic nerve [V_1]

Maxillary nerve [V_2]

Mandibular nerve [V_3]

Trigeminal ganglion

Trigeminal nerve [V]
sensory root

Trigeminal nerve [V]
motor root

Abducent nerve [VI]

Glossopharyngeal nerve [IX]

Vagus nerve [X]

Cranial root of accessory
(considered part of the
vagus nerve [X])

Accessory nerve [XI]

C1 nerve

Cranial nerves on the base of the brain

Pineal gland

Thalamus

Trochlear nerve [IV]

Cerebellar
peduncles

Transverse dural
venous sinus

Glossopharyngeal
nerve [IX]

Vagus nerve [X]
with cranial root
of accessory

Accessory nerve [XI]

Atlanto-occipital joint

⎰ Anterior ramus
C1 ⎱
  ⎱ Posterior ramus

Vertebral artery

C2 ⎰ Anterior ramus
     ⎱ Posterior ramus

Superior and inferior colliculus

Posterior cerebral artery

Superior cerebellar artery

Median sulcus of fourth ventricle

Trigeminal nerve [V]

Motor root of
facial nerve [VII]

Sensory root of
facial nerve [VII]
(intermediate nerve)

Vestibulocochlear
nerve [VIII]

Hypoglossal nerve [XII]

Posterior inferior
cerebellar artery

Posterior spinal artery

Transverse process of atlas

Spinal ganglion of C2

Dura mater

Cranial nerves (posterior view)

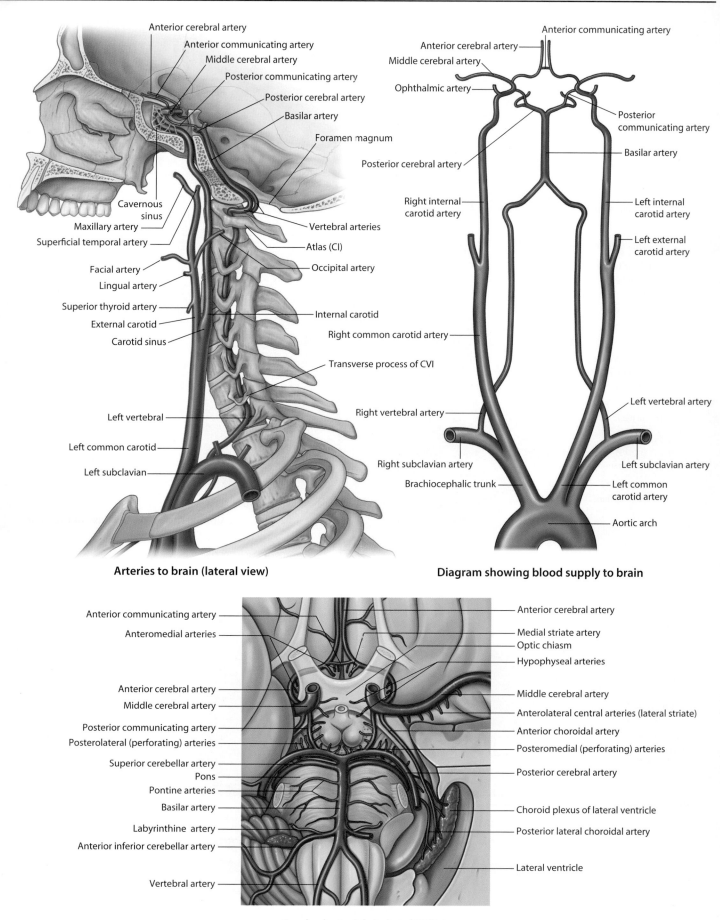

Arteries to brain (lateral view)

Anterior cerebral artery
Anterior communicating artery
Middle cerebral artery
Posterior communicating artery
Posterior cerebral artery
Basilar artery
Foramen magnum
Vertebral arteries
Atlas (CI)
Occipital artery
Cavernous sinus
Maxillary artery
Superficial temporal artery
Facial artery
Lingual artery
Superior thyroid artery
External carotid
Carotid sinus
Internal carotid
Transverse process of CVI
Left vertebral
Left common carotid
Left subclavian

Diagram showing blood supply to brain

Anterior communicating artery
Anterior cerebral artery
Middle cerebral artery
Ophthalmic artery
Posterior cerebral artery
Right internal carotid artery
Posterior communicating artery
Basilar artery
Left internal carotid artery
Left external carotid artery
Right common carotid artery
Right vertebral artery
Left vertebral artery
Right subclavian artery
Left subclavian artery
Brachiocephalic trunk
Left common carotid artery
Aortic arch

Cerebral arterial circle (of Willis)

Anterior communicating artery
Anteromedial arteries
Anterior cerebral artery
Middle cerebral artery
Posterior communicating artery
Posterolateral (perforating) arteries
Superior cerebellar artery
Pons
Pontine arteries
Basilar artery
Labyrinthine artery
Anterior inferior cerebellar artery
Vertebral artery
Anterior cerebral artery
Medial striate artery
Optic chiasm
Hypophyseal arteries
Middle cerebral artery
Anterolateral central arteries (lateral striate)
Anterior choroidal artery
Posteromedial (perforating) arteries
Posterior cerebral artery
Choroid plexus of lateral ventricle
Posterior lateral choroidal artery
Lateral ventricle

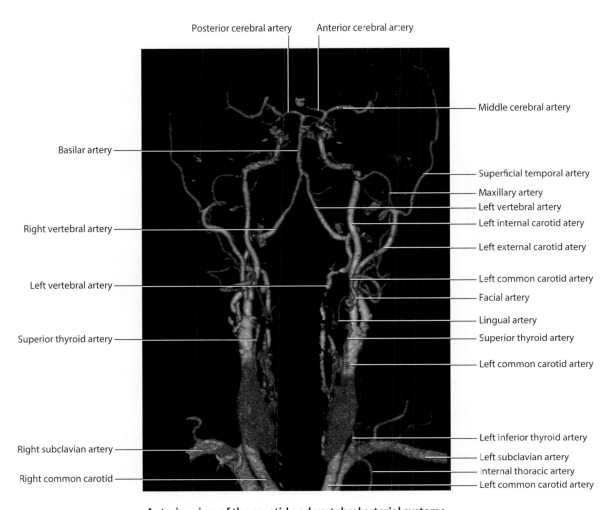

Posterior cerebral artery
Anterior cerebral artery
Middle cerebral artery
Basilar artery
Superficial temporal artery
Maxillary artery
Left vertebral artery
Left internal carotid atery
Left external carotid atery
Right vertebral artery
Left common carotid artery
Facial artery
Lingual artery
Left vertebral artery
Superior thyroid artery
Superior thyroid artery
Left common carotid artery
Left inferior thyroid artery
Right subclavian artery
Left subclavian artery
Internal thoracic artery
Right common carotid
Left common carotid artery

Anterior view of the carotid and vertebral arterial systems.
Volume-rendered anterior view using multidetector computed tomography

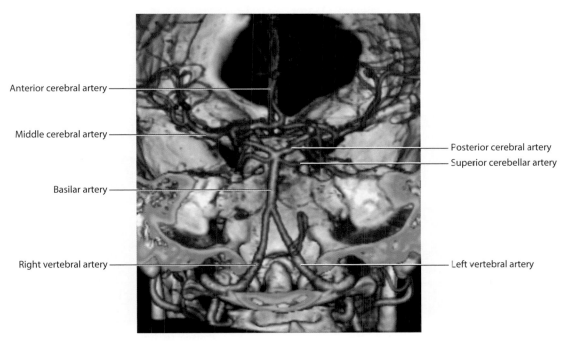

Anterior cerebral artery
Middle cerebral artery
Posterior cerebral artery
Superior cerebellar artery
Basilar artery
Right vertebral artery
Left vertebral artery

Posterior view of the cerebral arterial circle (of Willis).
Volume-rendered posterior view using multidetector computed tomography

503

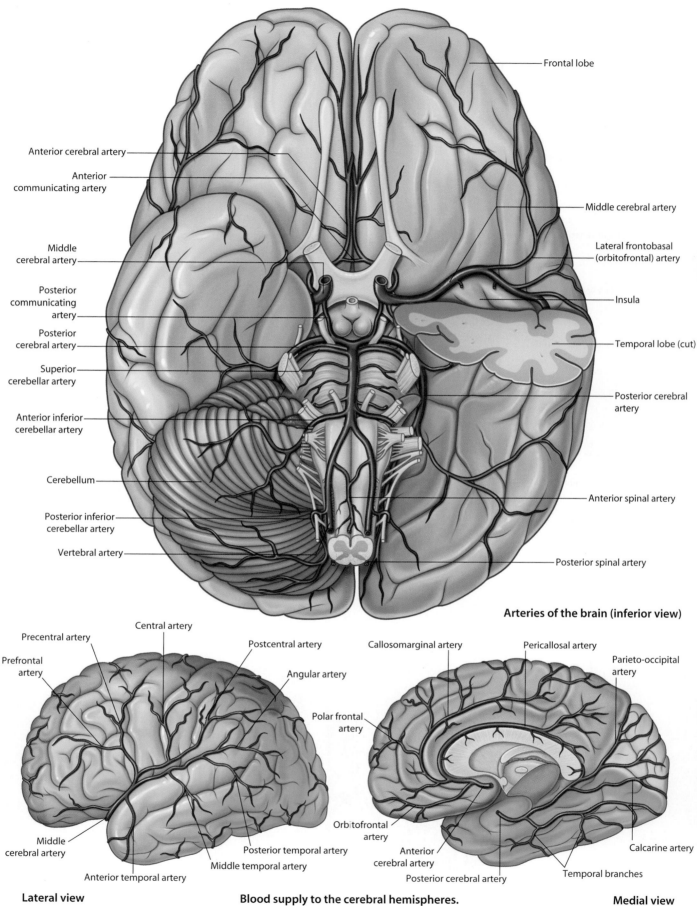

Anterior cerebral artery

Anterior communicating artery

Middle cerebral artery

Posterior communicating artery

Posterior cerebral artery

Superior cerebellar artery

Anterior inferior cerebellar artery

Cerebellum

Posterior inferior cerebellar artery

Vertebral artery

Frontal lobe

Middle cerebral artery

Lateral frontobasal (orbitofrontal) artery

Insula

Temporal lobe (cut)

Posterior cerebral artery

Anterior spinal artery

Posterior spinal artery

Arteries of the brain (inferior view)

Precentral artery

Central artery

Postcentral artery

Prefrontal artery

Angular artery

Polar frontal artery

Middle cerebral artery

Anterior temporal artery

Middle temporal artery

Posterior temporal artery

Callosomarginal artery

Pericallosal artery

Parieto-occipital artery

Orbitofrontal artery

Anterior cerebral artery

Posterior cerebral artery

Temporal branches

Calcarine artery

Lateral view

Blood supply to the cerebral hemispheres.
Anterior cerebral artery (pink), middle cerebral artery (blue), posterior cerebral artery (green)

Medial view

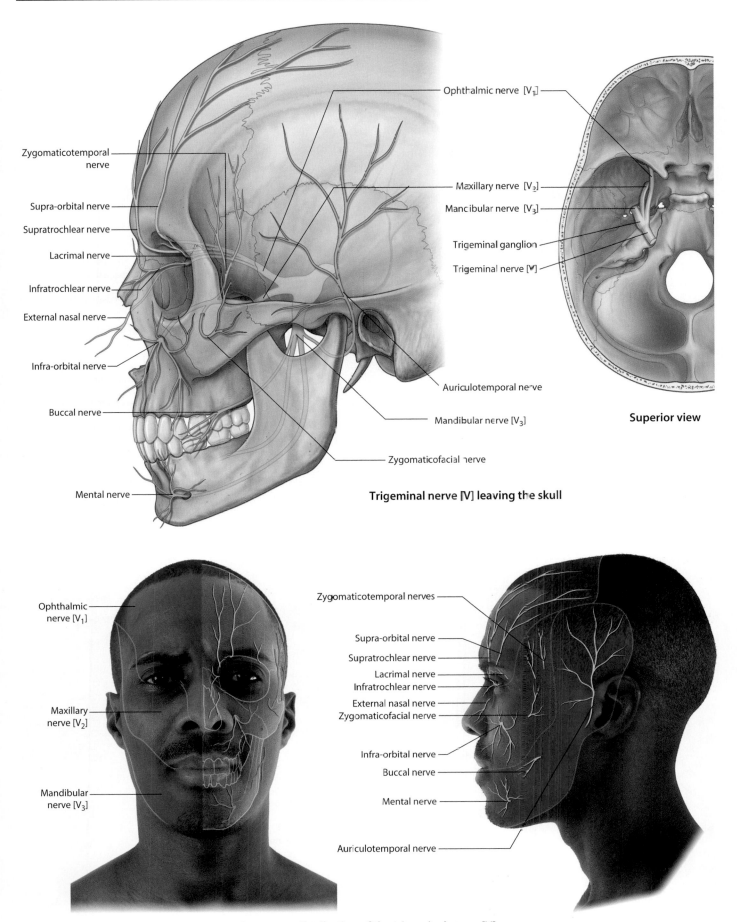

Ophthalmic nerve [V₁]

Zygomaticotemporal nerve

Supra-orbital nerve

Supratrochlear nerve

Lacrimal nerve

Infratrochlear nerve

External nasal nerve

Infra-orbital nerve

Buccal nerve

Mental nerve

Maxillary nerve [V₂]

Mandibular nerve [V₃]

Trigeminal ganglion

Trigeminal nerve [V]

Auriculotemporal nerve

Mandibular nerve [V₃]

Zygomaticofacial nerve

Superior view

Trigeminal nerve [V] leaving the skull

Ophthalmic nerve [V₁]

Maxillary nerve [V₂]

Mandibular nerve [V₃]

Zygomaticotemporal nerves

Supra-orbital nerve

Supratrochlear nerve

Lacrimal nerve

Infratrochlear nerve

External nasal nerve

Zygomaticofacial nerve

Infra-orbital nerve

Buccal nerve

Mental nerve

Auriculotemporal nerve

Cutaneous distribution of the trigeminal nerve [V]

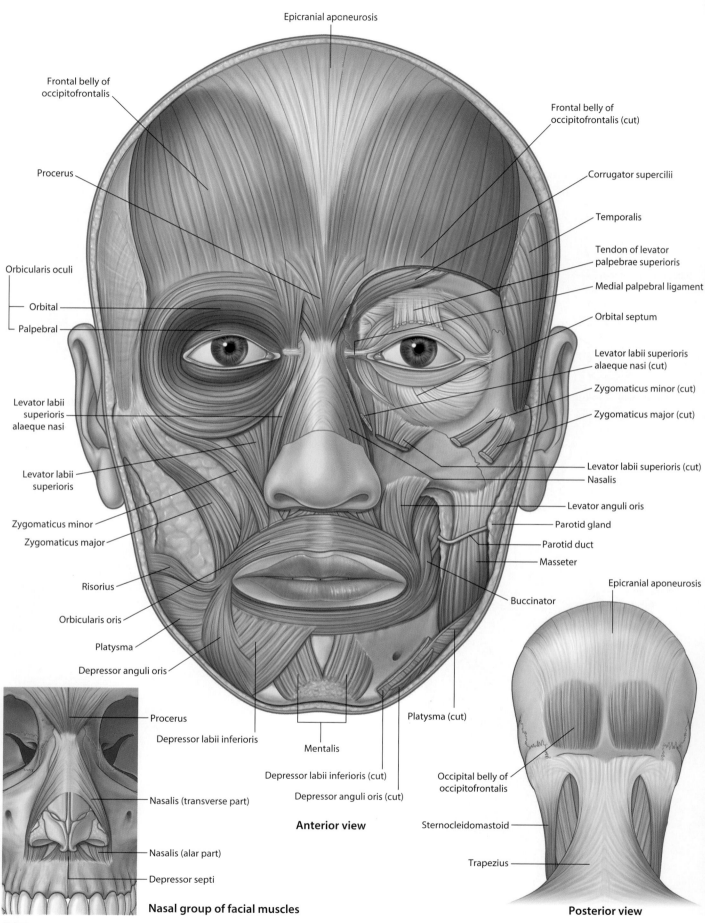

Epicranial aponeurosis

Frontal belly of occipitofrontalis

Procerus

Orbicularis oculi

Orbital

Palpebral

Levator labii superioris alaeque nasi

Levator labii superioris

Zygomaticus minor

Zygomaticus major

Risorius

Orbicularis oris

Platysma

Depressor anguli oris

Frontal belly of occipitofrontalis (cut)

Corrugator supercilii

Temporalis

Tendon of levator palpebrae superioris

Medial palpebral ligament

Orbital septum

Levator labii superioris alaeque nasi (cut)

Zygomaticus minor (cut)

Zygomaticus major (cut)

Levator labii superioris (cut)

Nasalis

Levator anguli oris

Parotid gland

Parotid duct

Masseter

Buccinator

Procerus

Depressor labii inferioris

Mentalis

Depressor labii inferioris (cut)

Depressor anguli oris (cut)

Platysma (cut)

Anterior view

Nasalis (transverse part)

Nasalis (alar part)

Depressor septi

Nasal group of facial muscles

Epicranial aponeurosis

Occipital belly of occipitofrontalis

Sternocleidomastoid

Trapezius

Posterior view

506

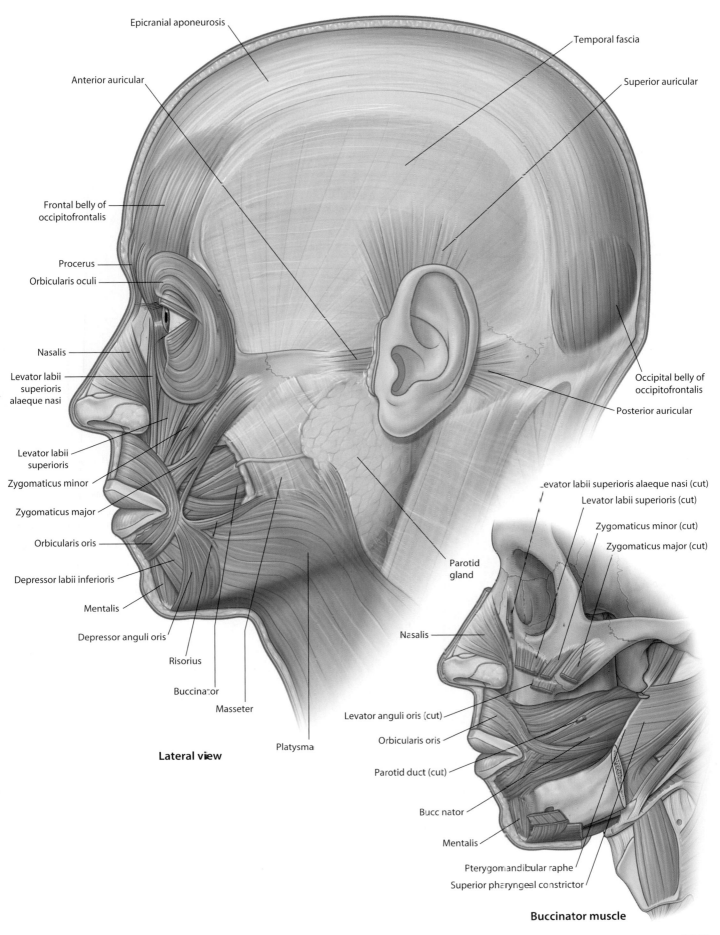

Epicranial aponeurosis

Anterior auricular

Frontal belly of occipitofrontalis

Procerus

Orbicularis oculi

Nasalis

Levator labii superioris alaeque nasi

Levator labii superioris

Zygomaticus minor

Zygomaticus major

Orbicularis oris

Depressor labii inferioris

Mentalis

Depressor anguli oris

Risorius

Buccinator

Masseter

Platysma

Lateral view

Temporal fascia

Superior auricular

Occipital belly of occipitofrontalis

Posterior auricular

Parotid gland

Levator labii superioris alaeque nasi (cut)

Levator labii superioris (cut)

Zygomaticus minor (cut)

Zygomaticus major (cut)

Nasalis

Levator anguli oris (cut)

Orbicularis oris

Parotid duct (cut)

Buccinator

Mentalis

Pterygomandibular raphe

Superior pharyngeal constrictor

Buccinator muscle

507

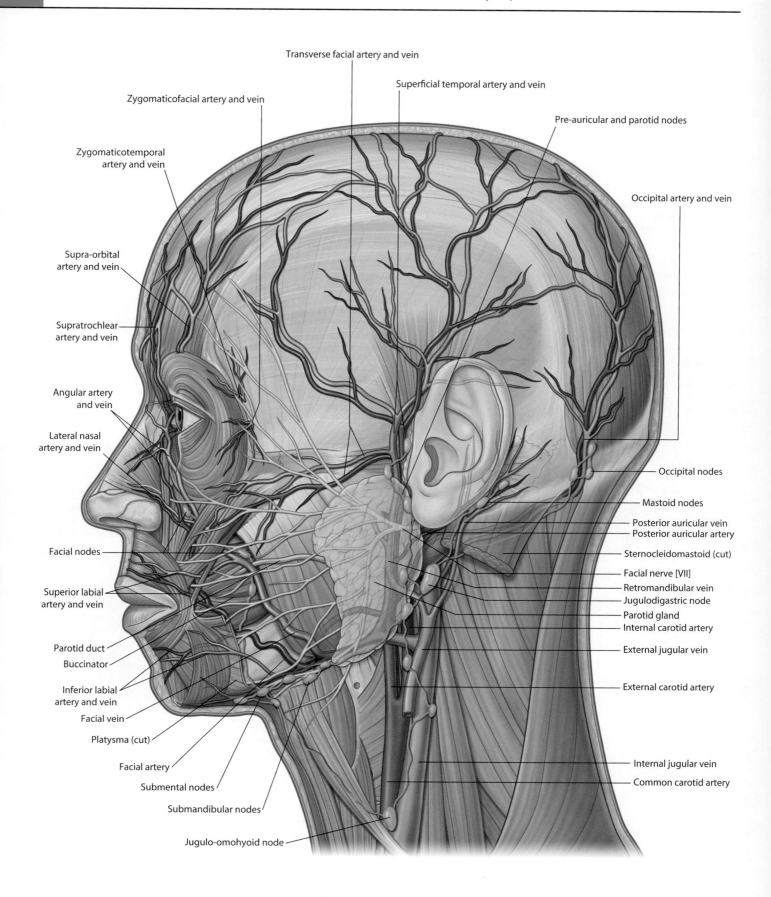

Transverse facial artery and vein

Superficial temporal artery and vein

Zygomaticofacial artery and vein

Pre-auricular and parotid nodes

Zygomaticotemporal artery and vein

Occipital artery and vein

Supra-orbital artery and vein

Supratrochlear artery and vein

Angular artery and vein

Lateral nasal artery and vein

Occipital nodes

Mastoid nodes

Posterior auricular vein
Posterior auricular artery

Facial nodes

Sternocleidomastoid (cut)

Facial nerve [VII]

Superior labial artery and vein

Retromandibular vein
Jugulodigastric node
Parotid gland
Internal carotid artery

Parotid duct

External jugular vein

Buccinator

Inferior labial artery and vein

External carotid artery

Facial vein

Platysma (cut)

Facial artery

Internal jugular vein

Submental nodes

Common carotid artery

Submandibular nodes

Jugulo-omohyoid node

Vasculature, facial nerve [VII] and lymphatics of the face

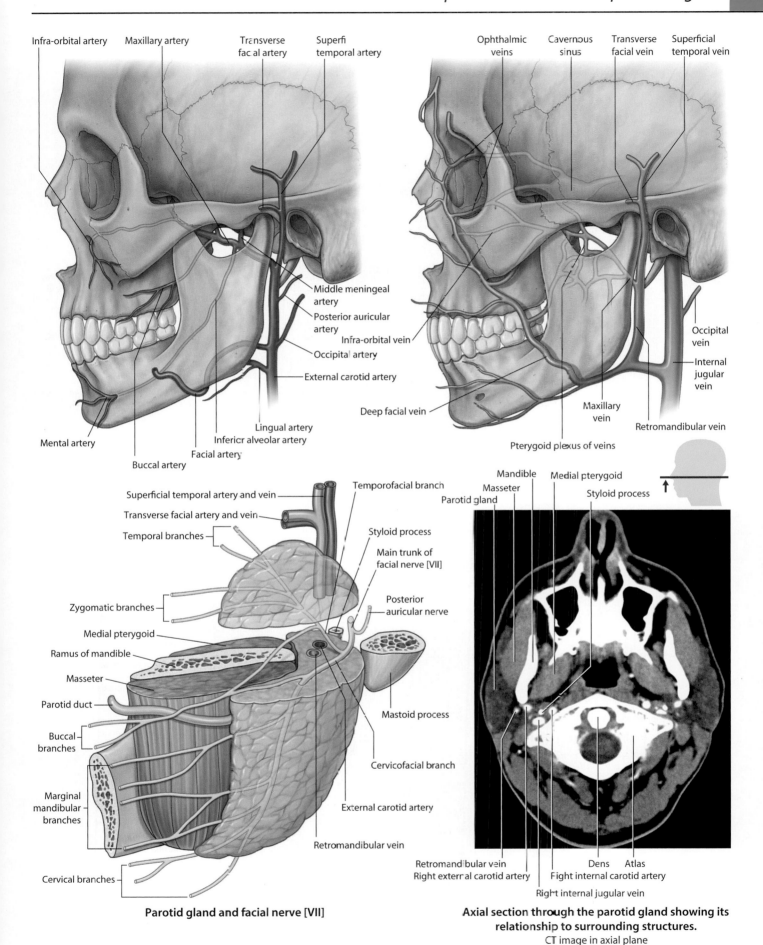

Infra-orbital artery   Maxillary artery   Transverse facial artery   Superficial temporal artery

Middle meningeal artery

Posterior auricular artery

Infra-orbital vein

Occipital artery

External carotid artery

Mental artery

Lingual artery

Inferior alveolar artery

Facial artery

Buccal artery

Ophthalmic veins   Cavernous sinus   Transverse facial vein   Superficial temporal vein

Occipital vein

Internal jugular vein

Deep facial vein

Maxillary vein

Retromandibular vein

Pterygoid plexus of veins

Superficial temporal artery and vein

Transverse facial artery and vein

Temporal branches

Zygomatic branches

Medial pterygoid

Ramus of mandible

Masseter

Parotid duct

Buccal branches

Marginal mandibular branches

Cervical branches

Temporofacial branch

Styloid process

Main trunk of facial nerve [VII]

Posterior auricular nerve

Mastoid process

Cervicofacial branch

External carotid artery

Retromandibular vein

Parotid gland and facial nerve [VII]

Mandible   Medial pterygoid

Masseter   Styloid process

Parotid gland

Retromandibular vein

Right external carotid artery

Dens   Atlas

Right internal carotid artery

Right internal jugular vein

Axial section through the parotid gland showing its relationship to surrounding structures.
CT image in axial plane

509

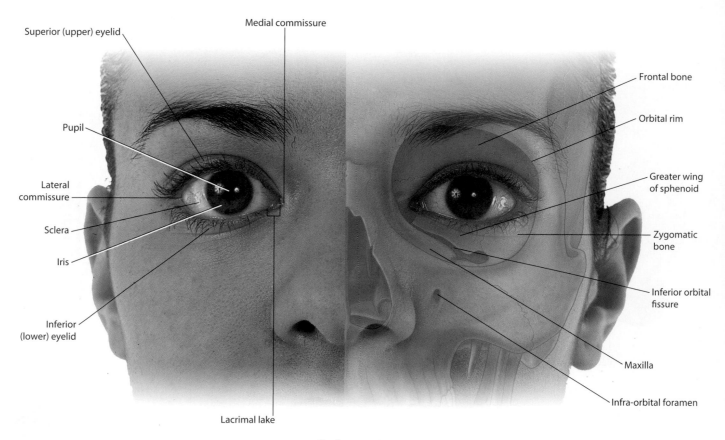

Superior (upper) eyelid

Medial commissure

Frontal bone

Orbital rim

Pupil

Greater wing
of sphenoid

Lateral
commissure

Zygomatic
bone

Sclera

Iris

Inferior orbital
fissure

Inferior
(lower) eyelid

Maxilla

Infra-orbital foramen

Lacrimal lake

Surface anatomy

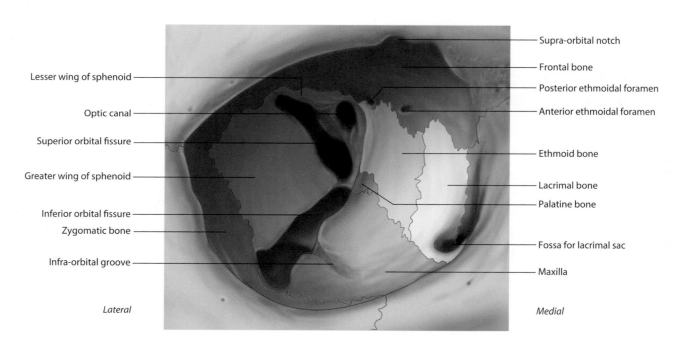

Lesser wing of sphenoid

Supra-orbital notch

Frontal bone

Optic canal

Posterior ethmoidal foramen

Anterior ethmoidal foramen

Superior orbital fissure

Greater wing of sphenoid

Ethmoid bone

Inferior orbital fissure

Lacrimal bone

Zygomatic bone

Palatine bone

Infra-orbital groove

Fossa for lacrimal sac

Maxilla

Lateral

Medial

Bones of the right orbit

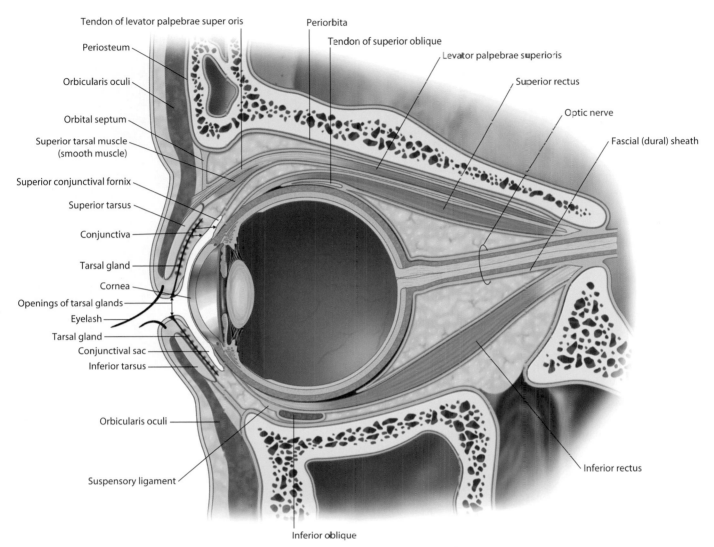

Tendon of levator palpebrae super oris

Periosteum

Orbicularis oculi

Orbital septum

Superior tarsal muscle
(smooth muscle)

Superior conjunctival fornix

Superior tarsus

Conjunctiva

Tarsal gland

Cornea

Openings of tarsal glands

Eyelash

Tarsal gland

Conjunctival sac

Inferior tarsus

Orbicularis oculi

Suspensory ligament

Periorbita

Tendon of superior oblique

Levator palpebrae superioris

Superior rectus

Optic nerve

Fascial (dural) sheath

Inferior rectus

Inferior oblique

Sagittal section through orbit and eyeball

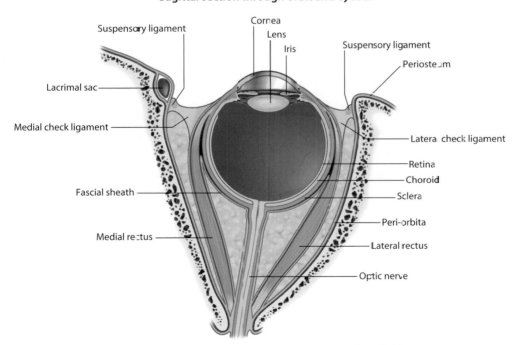

Suspensory ligament

Lacrimal sac

Medial check ligament

Fascial sheath

Medial rectus

Cornea

Lens

Iris

Suspensory ligament

Periosteum

Lateral check ligament

Retina

Choroid

Sclera

Peri-orbita

Lateral rectus

Optic nerve

Horizontal (axial) section through orbit and eyeball

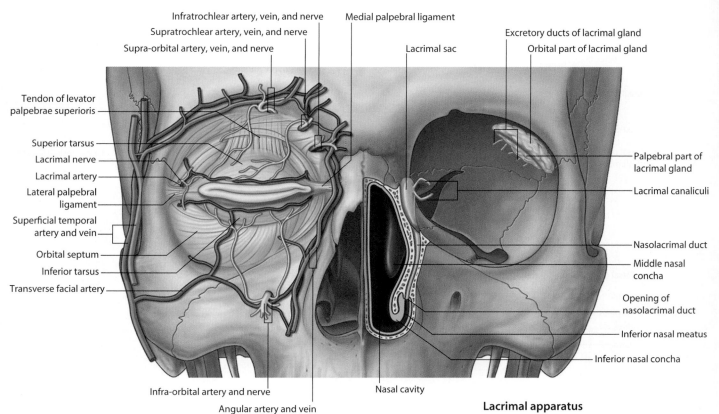

Infratrochlear artery, vein, and nerve
Supratrochlear artery, vein, and nerve
Supra-orbital artery, vein, and nerve

Medial palpebral ligament

Lacrimal sac

Excretory ducts of lacrimal gland
Orbital part of lacrimal gland

Tendon of levator palpebrae superioris

Superior tarsus
Lacrimal nerve
Lacrimal artery
Lateral palpebral ligament
Superficial temporal artery and vein
Orbital septum
Inferior tarsus
Transverse facial artery

Palpebral part of lacrimal gland
Lacrimal canaliculi
Nasolacrimal duct
Middle nasal concha
Opening of nasolacrimal duct
Inferior nasal meatus
Inferior nasal concha

Infra-orbital artery and nerve

Angular artery and vein

Nasal cavity

Vasculature and nerves of the eyelids

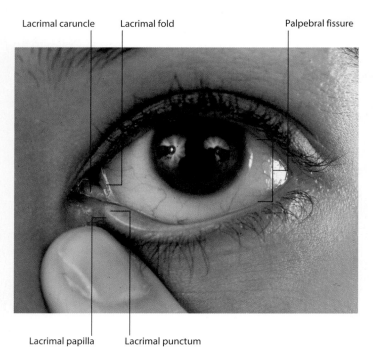

Lacrimal caruncle
Lacrimal fold
Palpebral fissure

Lacrimal papilla
Lacrimal punctum

Lacrimal papilla and punctum of left eye

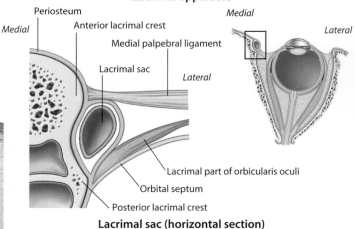

Periosteum
Anterior lacrimal crest
Medial palpebral ligament
Lacrimal sac

Medial
Lateral

Medial
Lateral

Lacrimal apparatus

Lacrimal part of orbicularis oculi
Orbital septum
Posterior lacrimal crest

Lacrimal sac (horizontal section)

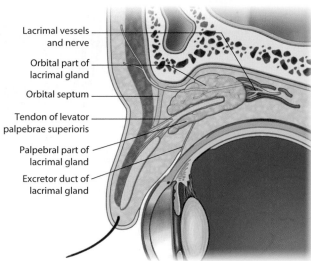

Lacrimal vessels and nerve
Orbital part of lacrimal gland
Orbital septum
Tendon of levator palpebrae superioris
Palpebral part of lacrimal gland
Excretor duct of lacrimal gland

Lacrimal gland and levator palpebrae superioris (parasagittal section)

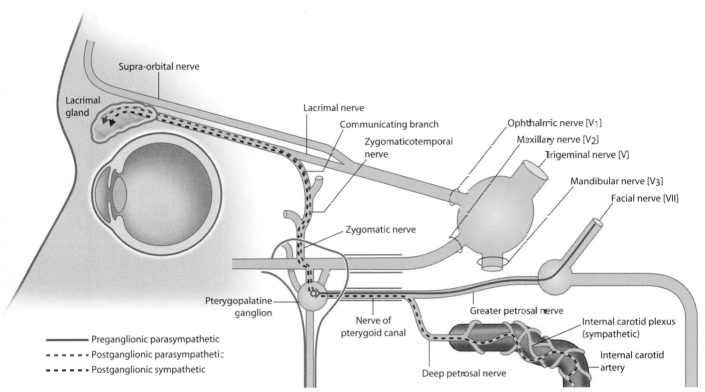

Supra-orbital nerve

Lacrimal gland

Lacrimal nerve

Communicating branch

Zygomaticotemporal nerve

Ophthalmic nerve [V₁]

Maxillary nerve [V₂]

Trigeminal nerve [V]

Mandibular nerve [V₃]

Facial nerve [VII]

Zygomatic nerve

Pterygopalatine ganglion

Nerve of pterygoid canal

Greater petrosal nerve

Internal carotid plexus (sympathetic)

Internal carotid artery

Deep petrosal nerve

———— Preganglionic parasympathetic

- - - - - Postganglionic parasympathetic

▪ ▪ ▪ ▪ ▪ Postganglionic sympathetic

Visceral efferent (motor) innervation of the lacrimal gland

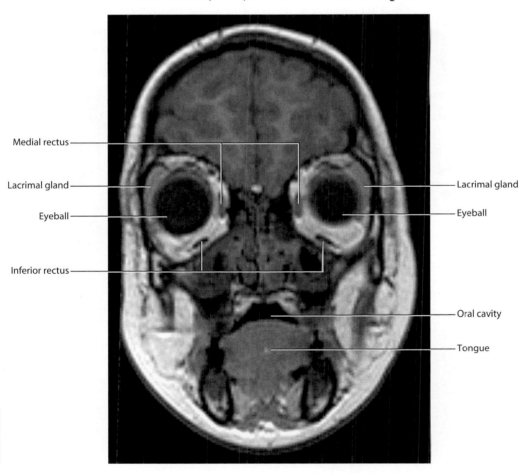

Medial rectus

Lacrimal gland

Eyeball

Inferior rectus

Lacrimal gland

Eyeball

Oral cavity

Tongue

**Coronal section through the orbit showing the lacrimal gland
and its relationship to surrounding structures.**
T1-weighted MR image in coronal plane

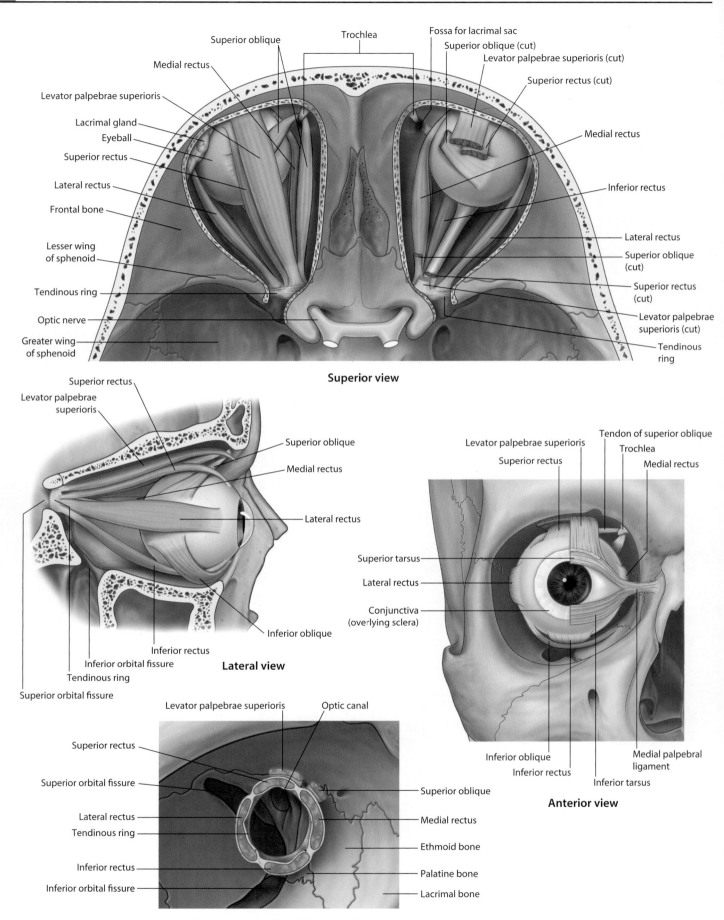

Superior view

Lateral view

Anterior view

Origins of muscles of the eyeball

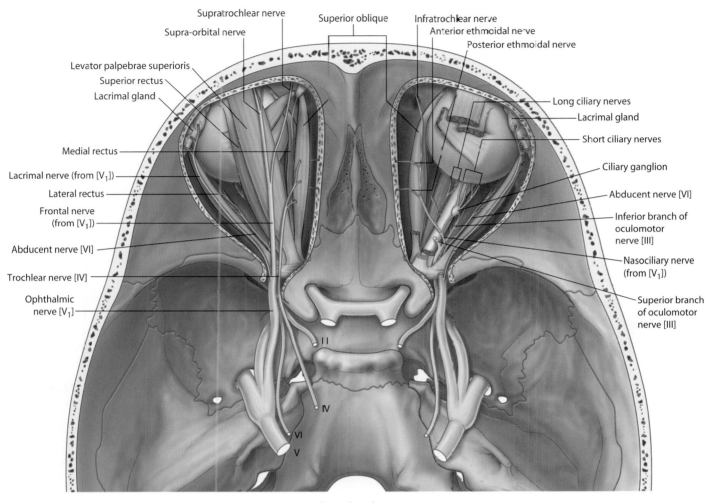

Supratrochlear nerve
Superior oblique
Infratrochlear nerve
Supra-orbital nerve
Anterior ethmoidal nerve
Posterior ethmoidal nerve
Levator palpebrae superioris
Superior rectus
Lacrimal gland
Long ciliary nerves
Lacrimal gland
Short ciliary nerves
Medial rectus
Lacrimal nerve (from [V₁])
Ciliary ganglion
Lateral rectus
Abducent nerve [VI]
Frontal nerve (from [V₁])
Inferior branch of oculomotor nerve [III]
Abducent nerve [VI]
Trochlear nerve [IV]
Nasociliary nerve (from [V₁])
Ophthalmic nerve [V₁]
Superior branch of oculomotor nerve [III]

II
IV
VI
V

Superior view

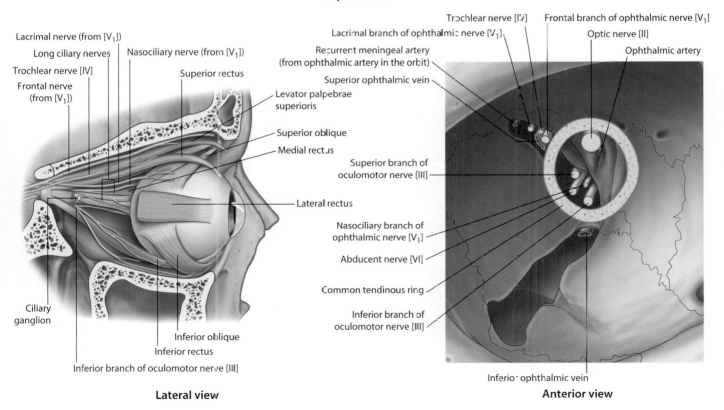

Lacrimal nerve (from [V₁])
Trochlear nerve [IV]
Frontal branch of ophthalmic nerve [V₁]
Long ciliary nerves
Nasociliary nerve (from [V₁])
Lacrimal branch of ophthalmic nerve [V₁]
Optic nerve [II]
Trochlear nerve [IV]
Recurrent meningeal artery (from ophthalmic artery in the orbit)
Ophthalmic artery
Frontal nerve (from [V₁])
Superior rectus
Superior ophthalmic vein
Levator palpebrae superioris
Superior oblique
Superior branch of oculomotor nerve [III]
Medial rectus
Lateral rectus
Nasociliary branch of ophthalmic nerve [V₁]
Abducent nerve [VI]
Ciliary ganglion
Common tendinous ring
Inferior branch of oculomotor nerve [III]
Inferior oblique
Inferior rectus
Inferior branch of oculomotor nerve [III]
Inferior ophthalmic vein

Lateral view
Anterior view

515

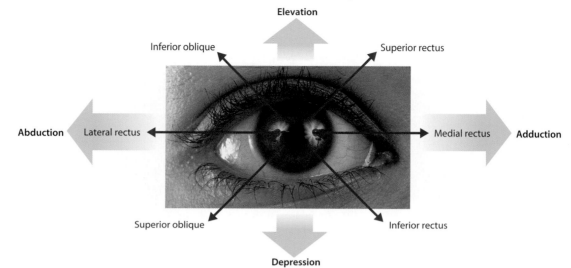

Elevation

Inferior oblique | Superior rectus

Abduction | Lateral rectus | Medial rectus | Adduction

Superior oblique | Inferior rectus

Depression

Actions of individual muscles (anatomical action)

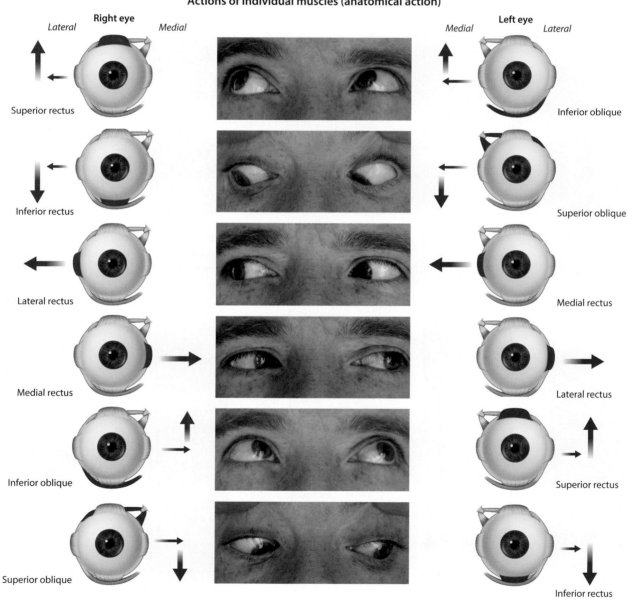

Right eye

Lateral | *Medial*

Superior rectus

Inferior rectus

Lateral rectus

Medial rectus

Inferior oblique

Superior oblique

Left eye

Medial | *Lateral*

Inferior oblique

Superior oblique

Medial rectus

Lateral rectus

Superior rectus

Inferior rectus

Movement of eyes when testing specific muscle (clinical testing).

For testing some muscles, a patient is "asked" to first move the eye into a position (small arrow) where the indicated muscle can best be tested. The large arrow indicates the direction the patient is then "asked" to move the eye to test the muscle

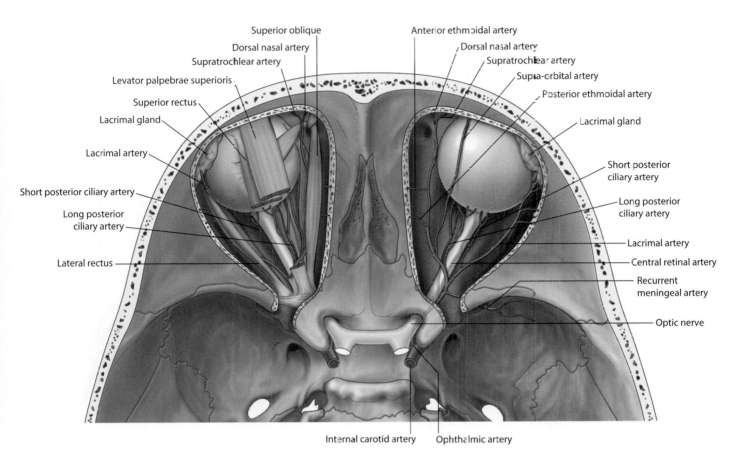

Superior oblique
Dorsal nasal artery
Supratrochlear artery
Levator palpebrae superioris
Superior rectus
Lacrimal gland
Lacrimal artery
Short posterior ciliary artery
Long posterior ciliary artery
Lateral rectus

Anterior ethmoidal artery
Dorsal nasal artery
Supratrochlear artery
Supra-orbital artery
Posterior ethmoidal artery
Lacrimal gland
Short posterior ciliary artery
Long posterior ciliary artery
Lacrimal artery
Central retinal artery
Recurrent meningeal artery
Optic nerve

Internal carotid artery   Ophthalmic artery

Arteries of the orbit and eyeball (superior view)

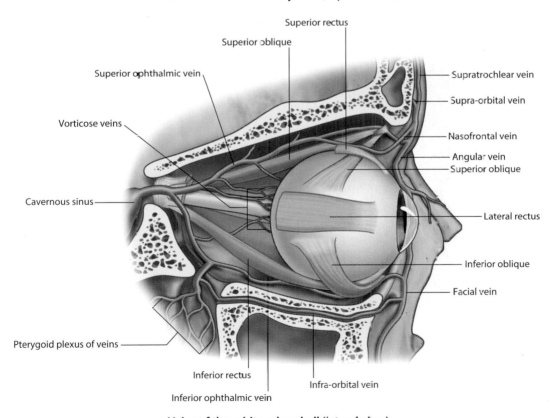

Superior rectus
Superior oblique
Superior ophthalmic vein
Vorticose veins
Cavernous sinus
Pterygoid plexus of veins

Supratrochlear vein
Supra-orbital vein
Nasofrontal vein
Angular vein
Superior oblique
Lateral rectus
Inferior oblique
Facial vein

Inferior rectus
Inferior ophthalmic vein
Infra-orbital vein

Veins of the orbit and eyeball (lateral view)

517

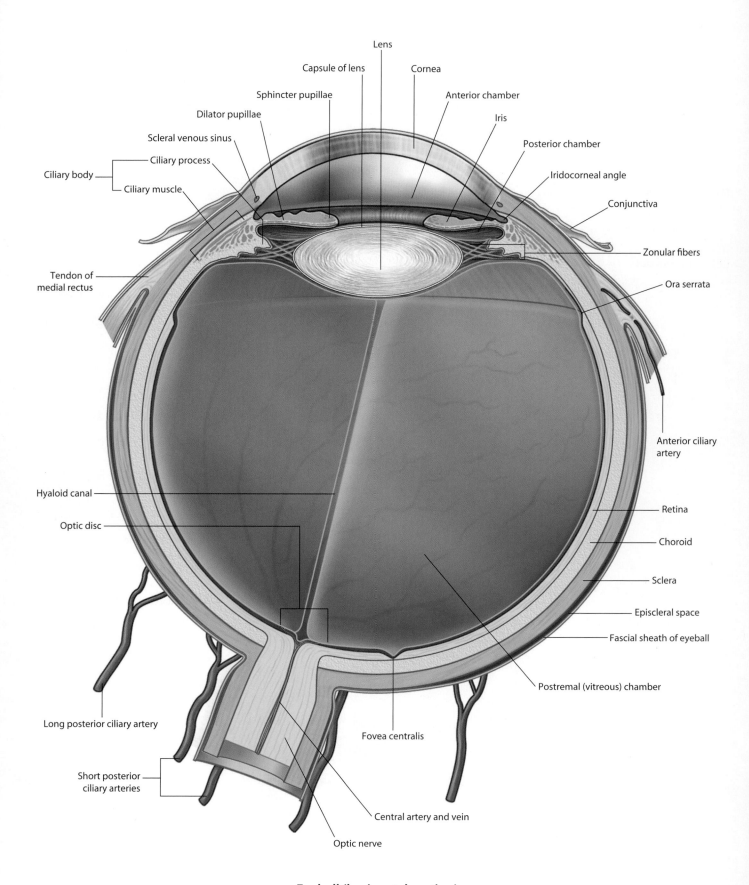

Lens

Capsule of lens

Cornea

Sphincter pupillae

Anterior chamber

Dilator pupillae

Iris

Scleral venous sinus

Posterior chamber

Ciliary process

Iridocorneal angle

Ciliary body

Conjunctiva

Ciliary muscle

Zonular fibers

Tendon of
medial rectus

Ora serrata

Anterior ciliary
artery

Hyaloid canal

Retina

Optic disc

Choroid

Sclera

Episcleral space

Fascial sheath of eyeball

Postremal (vitreous) chamber

Long posterior ciliary artery

Short posterior
ciliary arteries

Fovea centralis

Central artery and vein

Optic nerve

Eyeball (horizontal section)

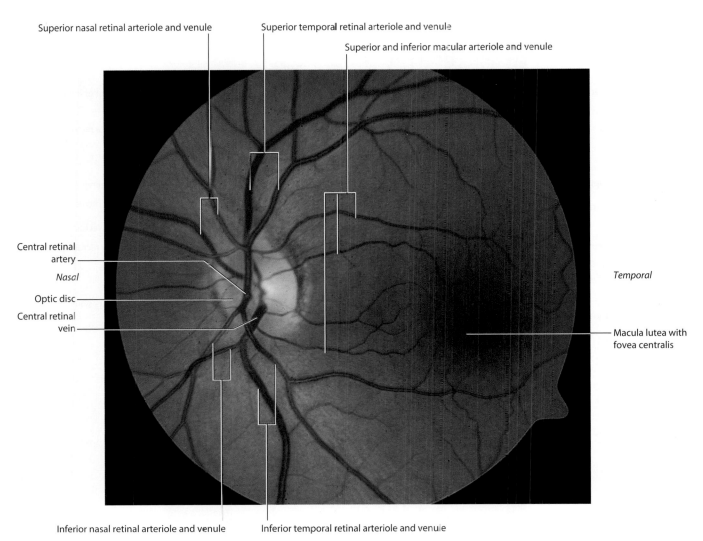

Superior nasal retinal arteriole and venule

Superior temporal retinal arteriole and venule

Superior and inferior macular arteriole and venule

Central retinal artery

Nasal

Optic disc

Central retinal vein

Temporal

Macula lutea with fovea centralis

Inferior nasal retinal arteriole and venule

Inferior temporal retinal arteriole and venule

Ophthalmoscopic view of the left retina showing the optic disc, the macula lutea, and the retinal vasculature.

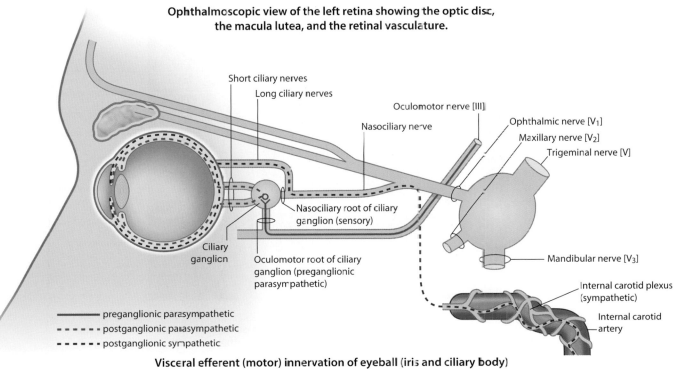

Short ciliary nerves

Long ciliary nerves

Oculomotor nerve [III]

Nasociliary nerve

Ophthalmic nerve [V₁]

Maxillary nerve [V₂]

Trigeminal nerve [V]

Nasociliary root of ciliary ganglion (sensory)

Ciliary ganglion

Oculomotor root of ciliary ganglion (preganglionic parasympathetic)

Mandibular nerve [V₃]

Internal carotid plexus (sympathetic)

Internal carotid artery

preganglionic parasympathetic

postganglionic parasympathetic

postganglionic sympathetic

Visceral efferent (motor) innervation of eyeball (iris and ciliary body)

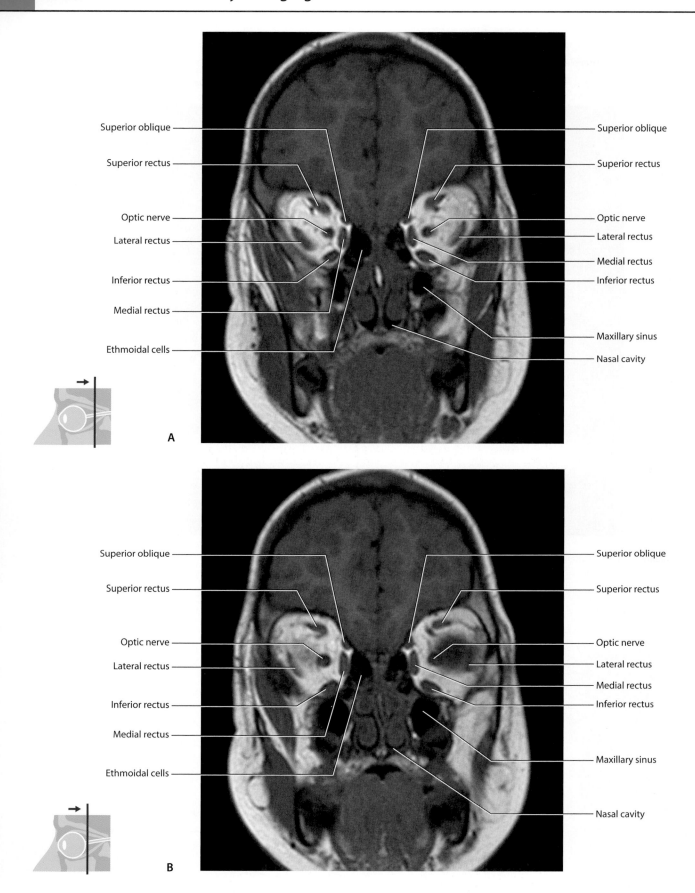

Superior oblique

Superior rectus

Optic nerve

Lateral rectus

Inferior rectus

Medial rectus

Ethmoidal cells

Superior oblique

Superior rectus

Optic nerve

Lateral rectus

Medial rectus

Inferior rectus

Maxillary sinus

Nasal cavity

A

Superior oblique

Superior rectus

Optic nerve

Lateral rectus

Inferior rectus

Medial rectus

Ethmoidal cells

Superior oblique

Superior rectus

Optic nerve

Lateral rectus

Medial rectus

Inferior rectus

Maxillary sinus

Nasal cavity

B

A through D – Coronal sections that pass through the orbit from posterior to anterior showing the extrinsic (extra-ocular) muscles and their relationships with each other and with other structures.
T1-weighted MR images in coronal plane

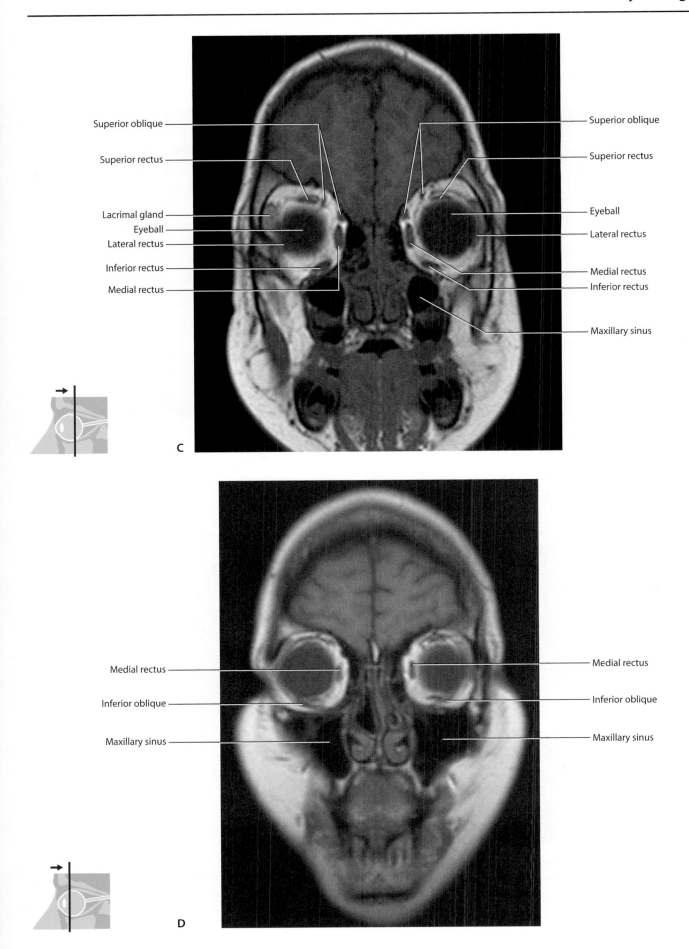

Superior oblique
Superior rectus
Lacrimal gland
Eyeball
Lateral rectus
Inferior rectus
Medial rectus

Superior oblique
Superior rectus
Eyeball
Lateral rectus
Medial rectus
Inferior rectus
Maxillary sinus

C

Medial rectus
Inferior oblique
Maxillary sinus

Medial rectus
Inferior oblique
Maxillary sinus

D

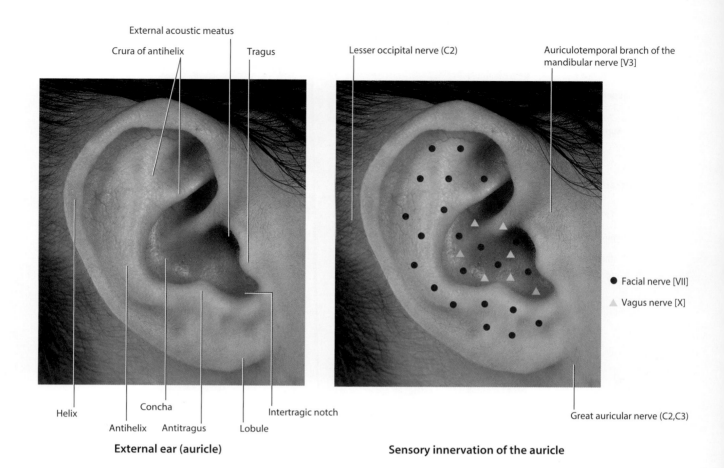

External acoustic meatus

Crura of antihelix

Tragus

Lesser occipital nerve (C2)

Auriculotemporal branch of the mandibular nerve [V3]

● Facial nerve [VII]

▲ Vagus nerve [X]

Great auricular nerve (C2,C3)

Helix

Concha

Antihelix   Antitragus   Lobule

Intertragic notch

External ear (auricle)

Sensory innervation of the auricle

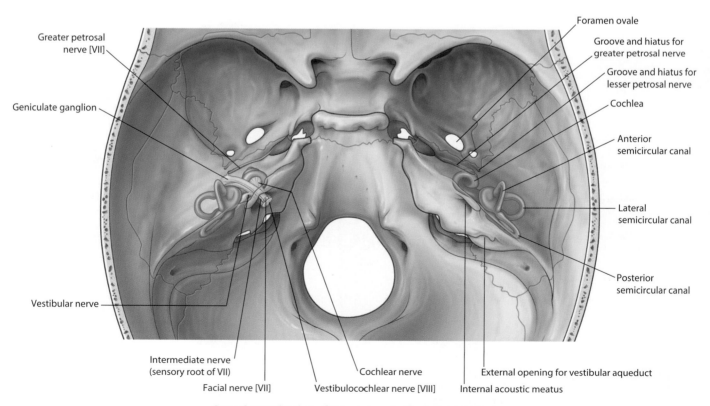

Greater petrosal nerve [VII]

Geniculate ganglion

Foramen ovale

Groove and hiatus for greater petrosal nerve

Groove and hiatus for lesser petrosal nerve

Cochlea

Anterior semicircular canal

Lateral semicircular canal

Posterior semicircular canal

Vestibular nerve

Intermediate nerve (sensory root of VII)

Facial nerve [VII]

Vestibulocochlear nerve [VIII]

Cochlear nerve

External opening for vestibular aqueduct

Internal acoustic meatus

Superior projection of internal ear in the temporal bone

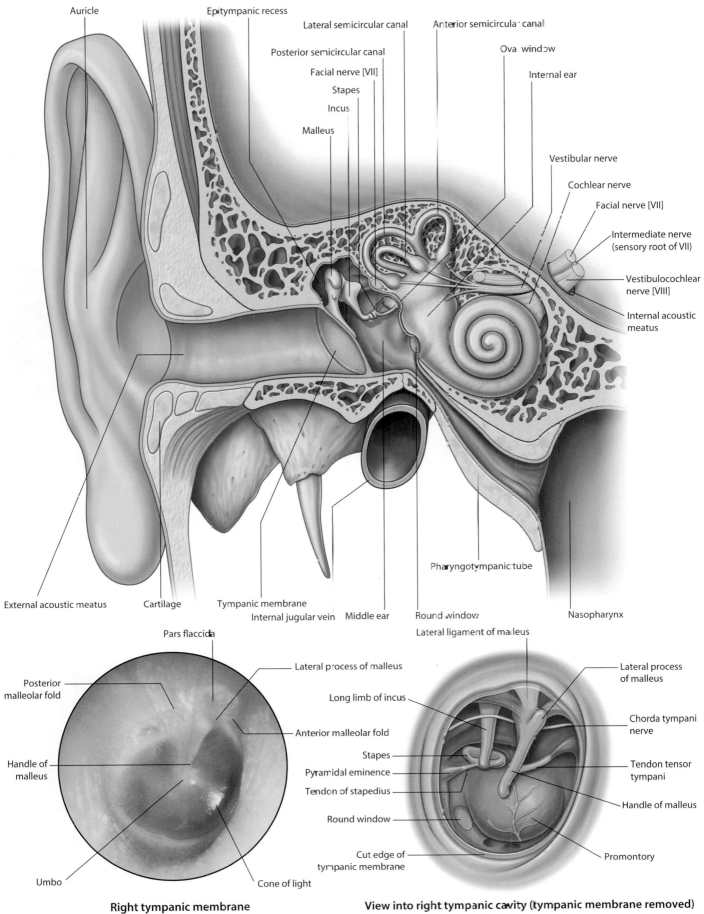

Auricle
Epitympanic recess
Lateral semicircular canal
Anterior semicircular canal
Posterior semicircular canal
Oval window
Facial nerve [VII]
Internal ear
Stapes
Incus
Malleus

Vestibular nerve
Cochlear nerve
Facial nerve [VII]
Intermediate nerve (sensory root of VII)
Vestibulocochlear nerve [VIII]
Internal acoustic meatus

Pharyngotympanic tube

External acoustic meatus
Cartilage
Tympanic membrane
Internal jugular vein
Middle ear
Round window
Nasopharynx

Pars flaccida
Lateral ligament of malleus

Lateral process of malleus
Posterior malleolar fold
Lateral process of malleus

Long limb of incus
Chorda tympani nerve
Anterior malleolar fold
Handle of malleus
Stapes
Tendon tensor tympani
Pyramidal eminence
Tendon of stapedius
Handle of malleus
Round window
Cut edge of tympanic membrane
Promontory
Umbo
Cone of light

Right tympanic membrane

View into right tympanic cavity (tympanic membrane removed)

523

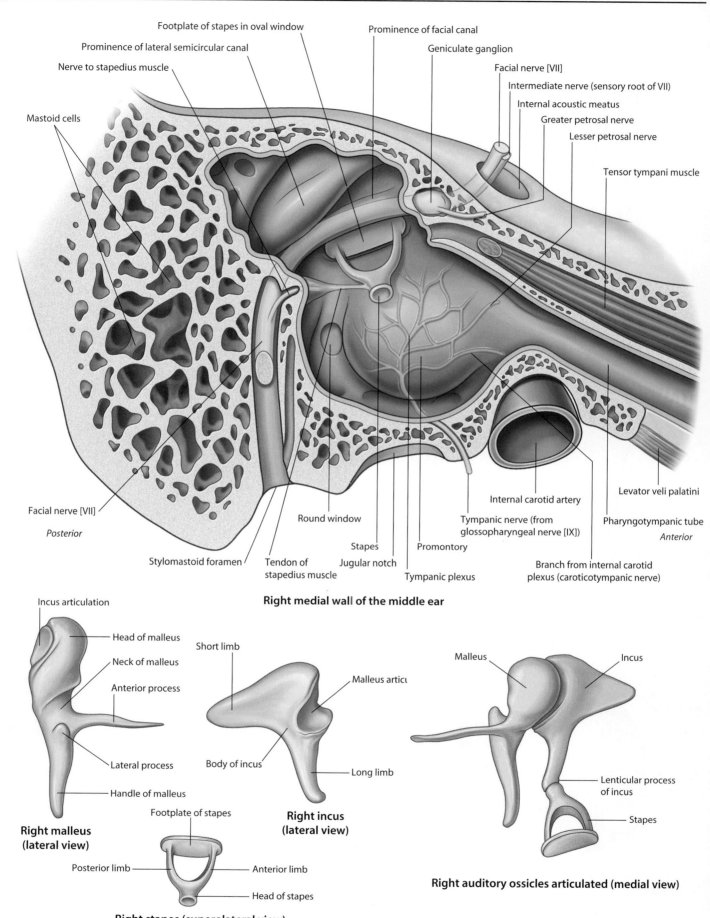

Footplate of stapes in oval window

Prominence of lateral semicircular canal

Nerve to stapedius muscle

Prominence of facial canal

Geniculate ganglion

Facial nerve [VII]

Intermediate nerve (sensory root of VII)

Internal acoustic meatus

Greater petrosal nerve

Lesser petrosal nerve

Tensor tympani muscle

Mastoid cells

Facial nerve [VII]

Posterior

Stylomastoid foramen

Tendon of stapedius muscle

Jugular notch

Round window

Stapes

Promontory

Tympanic plexus

Tympanic nerve (from glossopharyngeal nerve [IX])

Internal carotid artery

Branch from internal carotid plexus (caroticotympanic nerve)

Levator veli palatini

Pharyngotympanic tube

Anterior

Right medial wall of the middle ear

Incus articulation

Head of malleus

Neck of malleus

Anterior process

Lateral process

Handle of malleus

Right malleus (lateral view)

Short limb

Malleus articu

Body of incus

Long limb

Right incus (lateral view)

Footplate of stapes

Posterior limb

Anterior limb

Head of stapes

Right stapes (superolateral view)

Malleus

Incus

Lenticular process of incus

Stapes

Right auditory ossicles articulated (medial view)

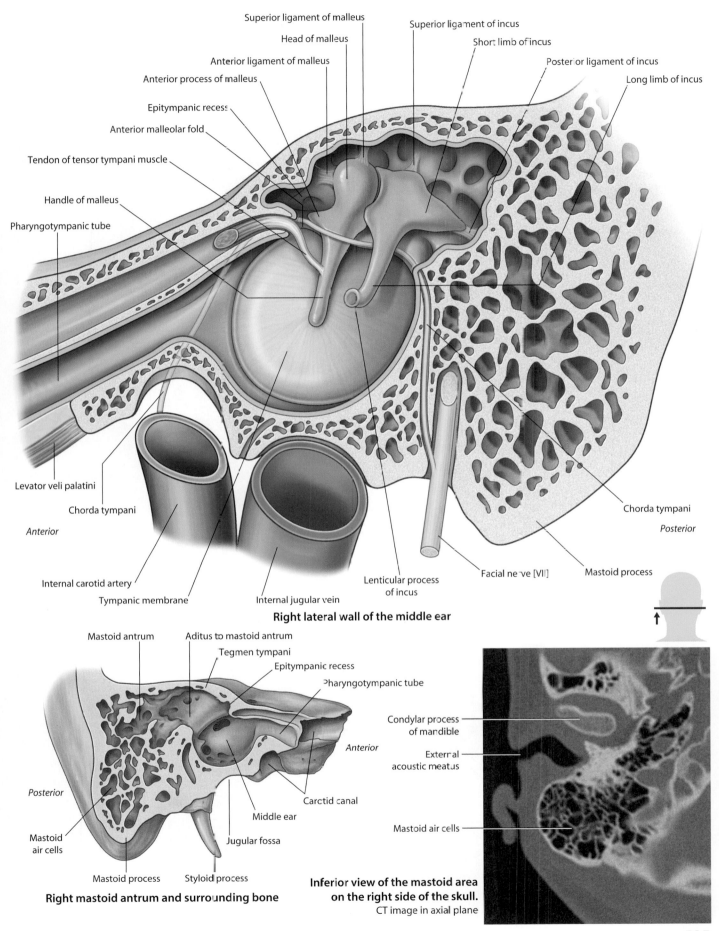

Superior ligament of malleus

Head of malleus

Superior ligament of incus

Anterior ligament of malleus

Short limb of incus

Anterior process of malleus

Posterior ligament of incus

Epitympanic recess

Long limb of incus

Anterior malleolar fold

Tendon of tensor tympani muscle

Handle of malleus

Pharyngotympanic tube

Levator veli palatini

Chorda tympani

Anterior

Internal carotid artery

Tympanic membrane

Internal jugular vein

Lenticular process of incus

Facial nerve [VII]

Mastoid process

Chorda tympani

Posterior

Right lateral wall of the middle ear

Mastoid antrum

Aditus to mastoid antrum

Tegmen tympani

Epitympanic recess

Pharyngotympanic tube

Anterior

Posterior

Mastoid air cells

Mastoid process

Styloid process

Carotid canal

Middle ear

Jugular fossa

Right mastoid antrum and surrounding bone

Condylar process of mandible

External acoustic meatus

Mastoid air cells

Inferior view of the mastoid area on the right side of the skull.
CT image in axial plane

525

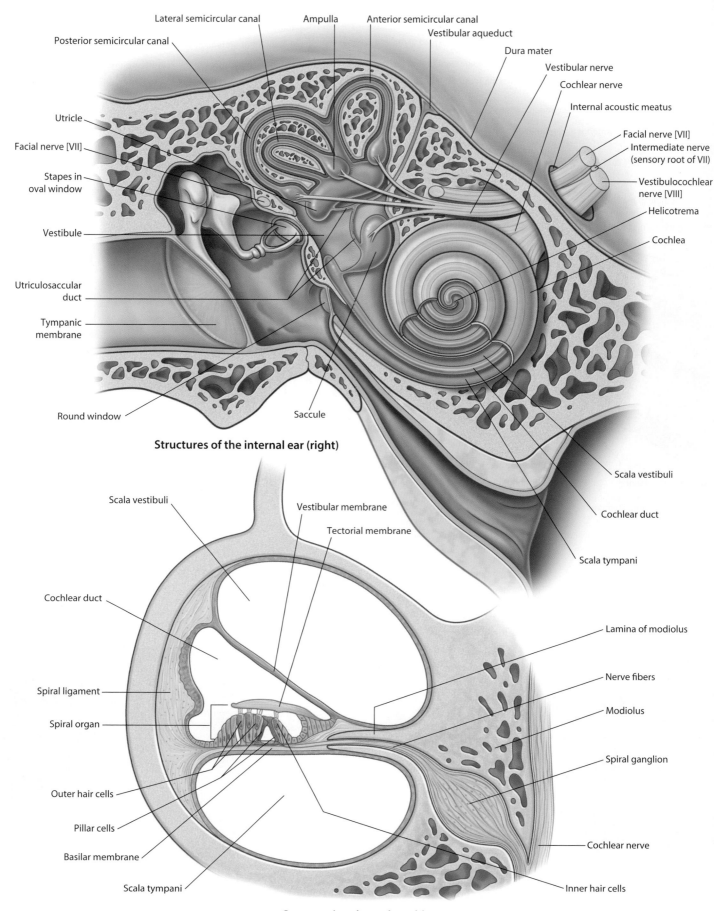

Lateral semicircular canal

Posterior semicircular canal

Ampulla

Anterior semicircular canal

Vestibular aqueduct

Dura mater

Vestibular nerve

Cochlear nerve

Internal acoustic meatus

Utricle

Facial nerve [VII]

Stapes in oval window

Vestibule

Utriculosaccular duct

Tympanic membrane

Round window

Saccule

Facial nerve [VII]

Intermediate nerve (sensory root of VII)

Vestibulocochlear nerve [VIII]

Helicotrema

Cochlea

Scala vestibuli

Cochlear duct

Scala tympani

Structures of the internal ear (right)

Scala vestibuli

Vestibular membrane

Tectorial membrane

Cochlear duct

Spiral ligament

Spiral organ

Outer hair cells

Pillar cells

Basilar membrane

Scala tympani

Lamina of modiolus

Nerve fibers

Modiolus

Spiral ganglion

Cochlear nerve

Inner hair cells

Cross section through cochlea

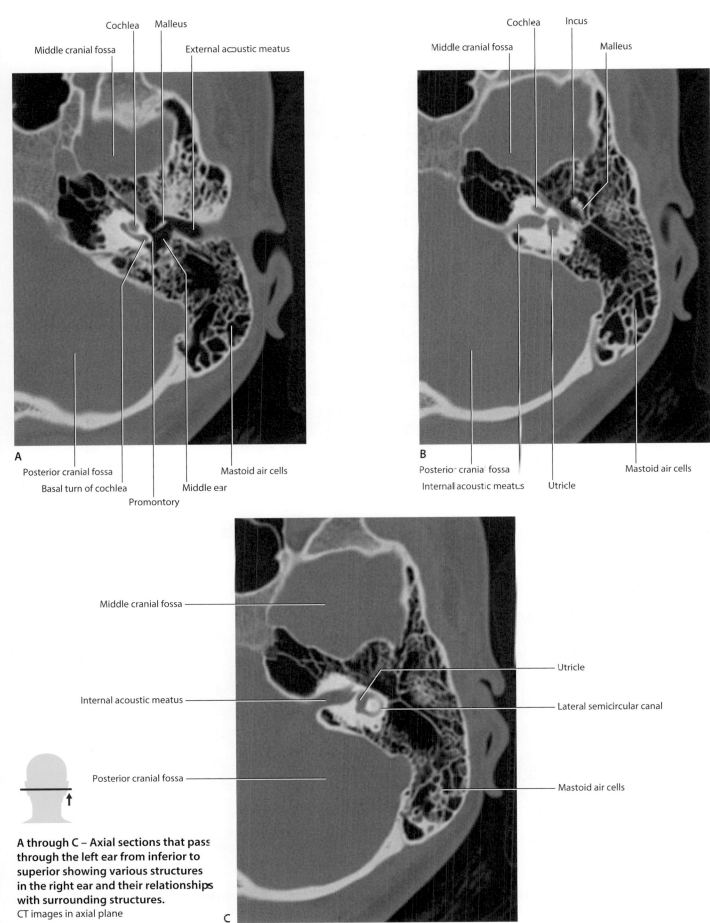

A — Cochlea, Malleus, Middle cranial fossa, External acoustic meatus, Posterior cranial fossa, Basal turn of cochlea, Promontory, Middle ear, Mastoid air cells

B — Cochlea, Incus, Malleus, Middle cranial fossa, Posterior cranial fossa, Internal acoustic meatus, Utricle, Mastoid air cells

C — Middle cranial fossa, Internal acoustic meatus, Posterior cranial fossa, Utricle, Lateral semicircular canal, Mastoid air cells

A through C – Axial sections that pass through the left ear from inferior to superior showing various structures in the right ear and their relationships with surrounding structures.
CT images in axial plane

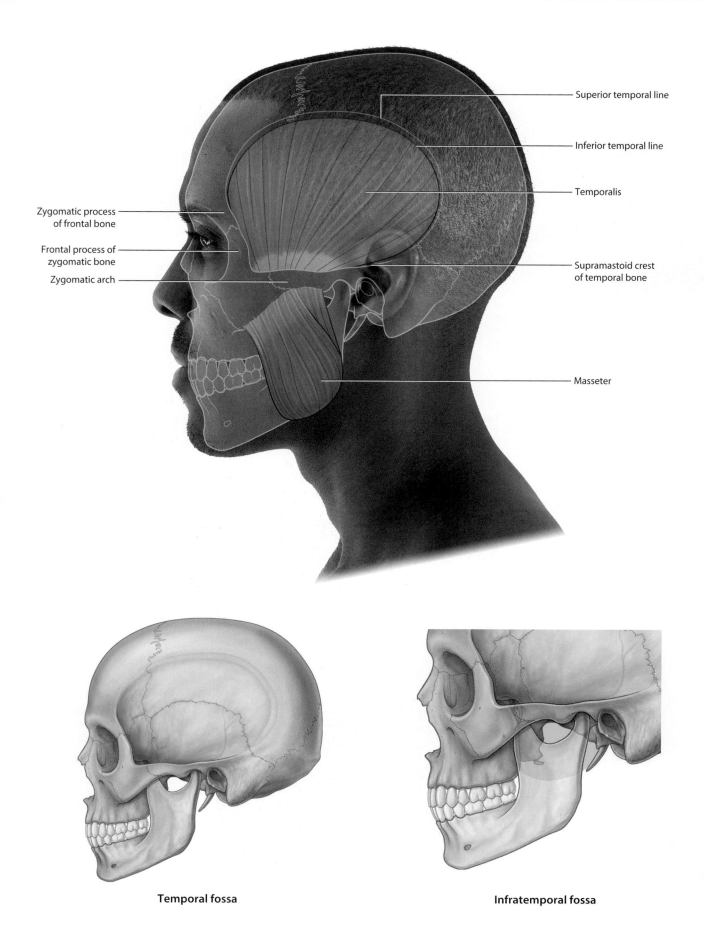

Superior temporal line

Inferior temporal line

Temporalis

Zygomatic process of frontal bone

Frontal process of zygomatic bone

Zygomatic arch

Supramastoid crest of temporal bone

Masseter

Temporal fossa

Infratemporal fossa

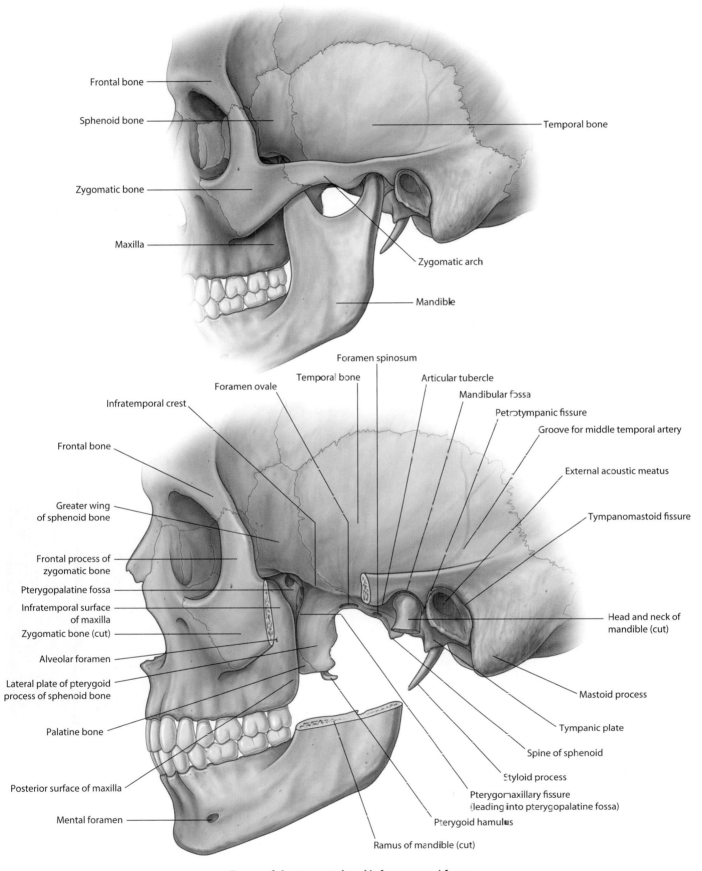

Frontal bone

Sphenoid bone

Zygomatic bone

Maxilla

Temporal bone

Zygomatic arch

Mandible

Foramen spinosum

Temporal bone

Foramen ovale

Articular tubercle

Mandibular fossa

Infratemporal crest

Petrotympanic fissure

Groove for middle temporal artery

Frontal bone

External acoustic meatus

Greater wing
of sphenoid bone

Tympanomastoid fissure

Frontal process of
zygomatic bone

Pterygopalatine fossa

Infratemporal surface
of maxilla

Zygomatic bone (cut)

Alveolar foramen

Head and neck of
mandible (cut)

Lateral plate of pterygoid
process of sphenoid bone

Palatine bone

Mastoid process

Tympanic plate

Posterior surface of maxilla

Spine of sphenoid

Styloid process

Mental foramen

Pterygomaxillary fissure
(leading into pterygopalatine fossa)

Pterygoid hamulus

Ramus of mandible (cut)

Bones of the temporal and infratemporal fossae

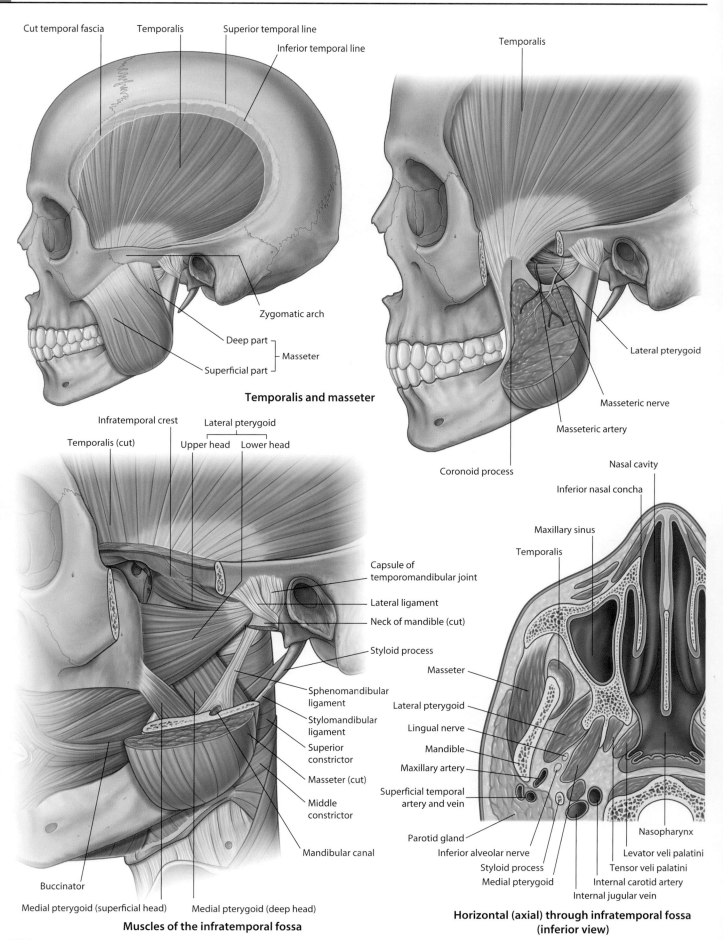

Cut temporal fascia

Temporalis

Superior temporal line

Inferior temporal line

Zygomatic arch

Deep part
} Masseter
Superficial part

Temporalis and masseter

Temporalis

Lateral pterygoid

Masseteric nerve

Masseteric artery

Coronoid process

Infratemporal crest

Lateral pterygoid

Temporalis (cut)

Upper head   Lower head

Capsule of
temporomandibular joint

Lateral ligament

Neck of mandible (cut)

Styloid process

Sphenomandibular
ligament

Stylomandibular
ligament

Superior
constrictor

Masseter (cut)

Middle
constrictor

Mandibular canal

Buccinator

Medial pterygoid (superficial head)

Medial pterygoid (deep head)

Muscles of the infratemporal fossa

Nasal cavity

Inferior nasal concha

Maxillary sinus

Temporalis

Masseter

Lateral pterygoid

Lingual nerve

Mandible

Maxillary artery

Superficial temporal
artery and vein

Parotid gland

Inferior alveolar nerve

Styloid process

Medial pterygoid

Nasopharynx

Levator veli palatini

Tensor veli palatini

Internal carotid artery

Internal jugular vein

**Horizontal (axial) through infratemporal fossa
(inferior view)**

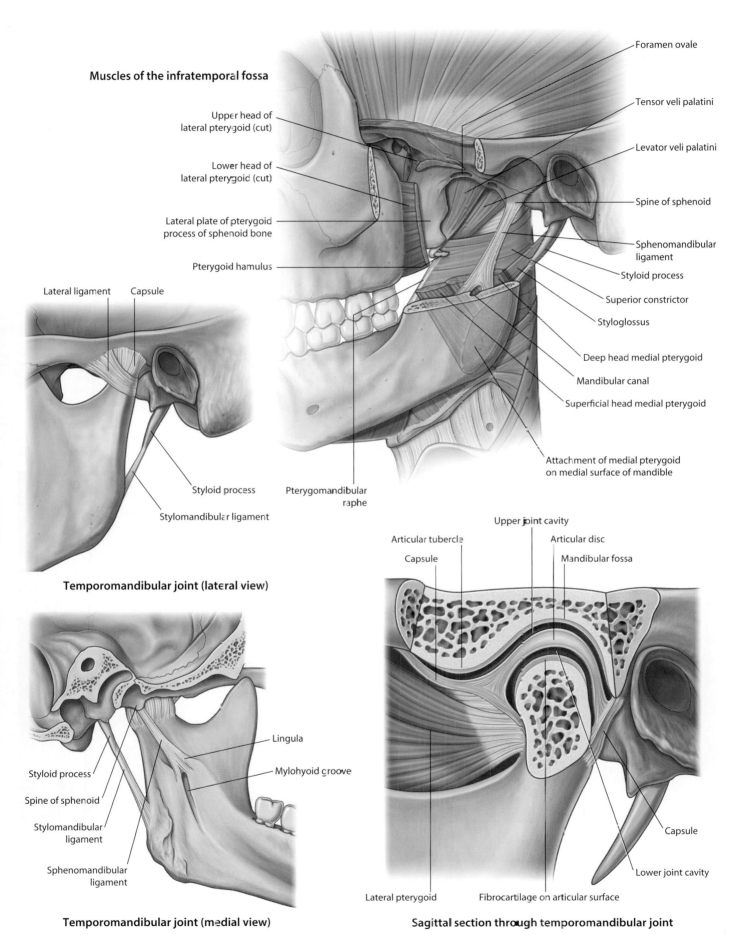

Muscles of the infratemporal fossa

Upper head of lateral pterygoid (cut)

Lower head of lateral pterygoid (cut)

Lateral plate of pterygoid process of sphenoid bone

Pterygoid hamulus

Foramen ovale

Tensor veli palatini

Levator veli palatini

Spine of sphenoid

Sphenomandibular ligament

Styloid process

Superior constrictor

Styloglossus

Deep head medial pterygoid

Mandibular canal

Superficial head medial pterygoid

Attachment of medial pterygoid on medial surface of mandible

Lateral ligament

Capsule

Styloid process

Stylomandibular ligament

Pterygomandibular raphe

Temporomandibular joint (lateral view)

Styloid process

Spine of sphenoid

Stylomandibular ligament

Sphenomandibular ligament

Lingula

Mylohyoid groove

Temporomandibular joint (medial view)

Articular tubercle

Capsule

Upper joint cavity

Articular disc

Mandibular fossa

Capsule

Lower joint cavity

Lateral pterygoid

Fibrocartilage on articular surface

Sagittal section through temporomandibular joint

531

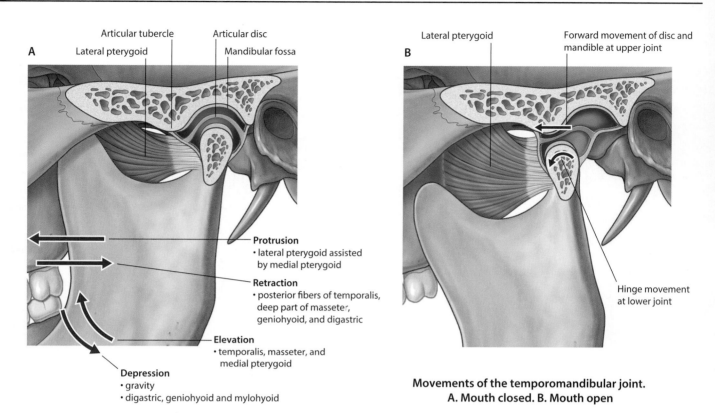

A
Lateral pterygoid — Articular tubercle — Articular disc — Mandibular fossa

Protrusion
• lateral pterygoid assisted by medial pterygoid

Retraction
• posterior fibers of temporalis, deep part of masseter, geniohyoid, and digastric

Elevation
• temporalis, masseter, and medial pterygoid

Depression
• gravity
• digastric, geniohyoid and mylohyoid

B
Lateral pterygoid — Forward movement of disc and mandible at upper joint

Hinge movement at lower joint

Movements of the temporomandibular joint.
A. Mouth closed. B. Mouth open

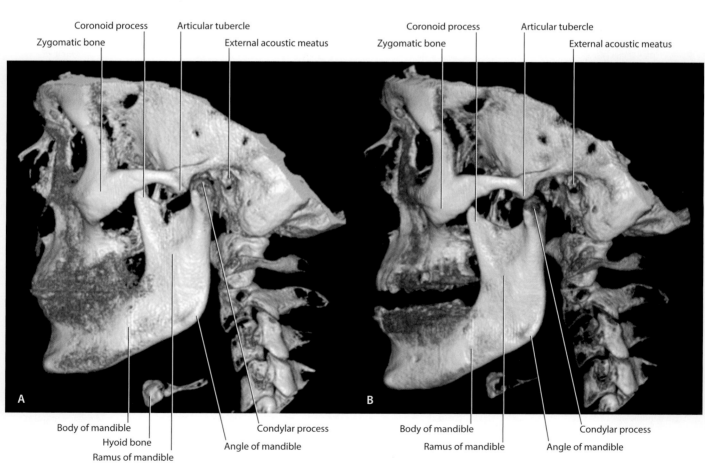

Zygomatic bone — Coronoid process — Articular tubercle — External acoustic meatus

Zygomatic bone — Coronoid process — Articular tubercle — External acoustic meatus

A

B

Body of mandible — Hyoid bone — Ramus of mandible — Angle of mandible — Condylar process

Body of mandible — Ramus of mandible — Angle of mandible — Condylar process

Lateral view of the right temporomandibular joint.
A. Mouth closed. B. Mouth open.
Image taken with Cone Beam Computerized Tomography (CBCT)
technology viewed in the radiographic mode

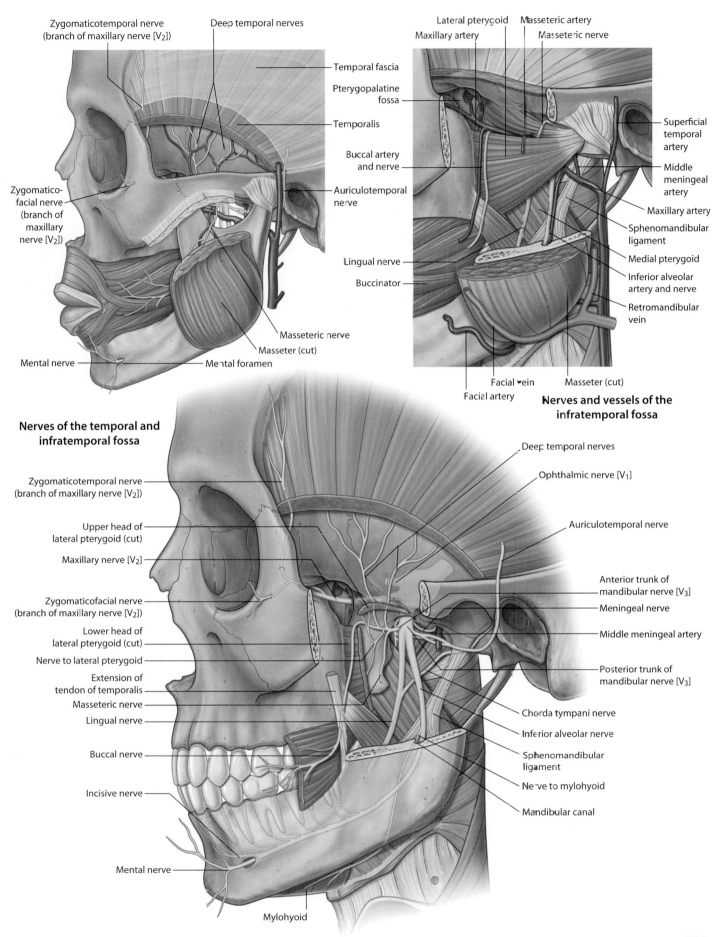

Zygomaticotemporal nerve (branch of maxillary nerve [V₂])

Deep temporal nerves

Temporal fascia

Pterygopalatine fossa

Temporalis

Buccal artery and nerve

Auriculotemporal nerve

Zygomatico-facial nerve (branch of maxillary nerve [V₂])

Mental nerve

Masseteric nerve

Masseter (cut)

Mental foramen

Nerves of the temporal and infratemporal fossa

Lateral pterygoid

Maxillary artery

Masseteric artery

Masseteric nerve

Superficial temporal artery

Middle meningeal artery

Maxillary artery

Sphenomandibular ligament

Medial pterygoid

Inferior alveolar artery and nerve

Retromandibular vein

Lingual nerve

Buccinator

Facial vein

Facial artery

Masseter (cut)

Nerves and vessels of the infratemporal fossa

Zygomaticotemporal nerve (branch of maxillary nerve [V₂])

Upper head of lateral pterygoid (cut)

Maxillary nerve [V₂]

Zygomaticofacial nerve (branch of maxillary nerve [V₂])

Lower head of lateral pterygoid (cut)

Nerve to lateral pterygoid

Extension of tendon of temporalis

Masseteric nerve

Lingual nerve

Buccal nerve

Incisive nerve

Mental nerve

Mylohyoid

Deep temporal nerves

Ophthalmic nerve [V₁]

Auriculotemporal nerve

Anterior trunk of mandibular nerve [V₃]

Meningeal nerve

Middle meningeal artery

Posterior trunk of mandibular nerve [V₃]

Chorda tympani nerve

Inferior alveolar nerve

Sphenomandibular ligament

Nerve to mylohyoid

Mandibular canal

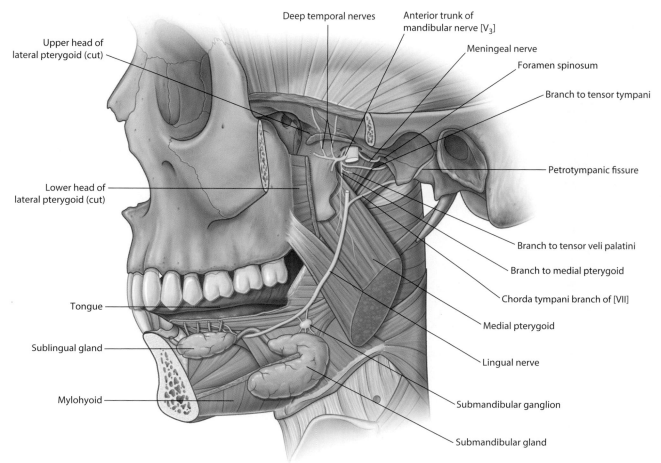

Deep temporal nerves

Anterior trunk of mandibular nerve [V₃]

Upper head of lateral pterygoid (cut)

Meningeal nerve

Foramen spinosum

Branch to tensor tympani

Lower head of lateral pterygoid (cut)

Petrotympanic fissure

Branch to tensor veli palatini

Branch to medial pterygoid

Chorda tympani branch of [VII]

Tongue

Medial pterygoid

Sublingual gland

Lingual nerve

Mylohyoid

Submandibular ganglion

Submandibular gland

Nerves of the infratemporal fossa

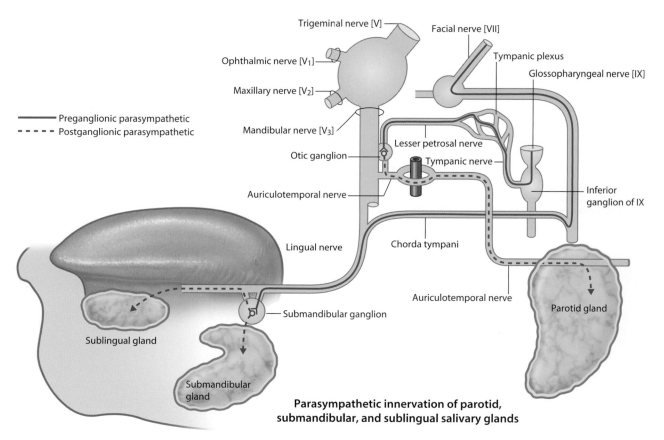

Trigeminal nerve [V]

Facial nerve [VII]

Ophthalmic nerve [V₁]

Tympanic plexus

Glossopharyngeal nerve [IX]

Maxillary nerve [V₂]

—— Preganglionic parasympathetic
‑ ‑ ‑ Postganglionic parasympathetic

Mandibular nerve [V₃]

Lesser petrosal nerve

Otic ganglion

Tympanic nerve

Auriculotemporal nerve

Inferior ganglion of IX

Lingual nerve

Chorda tympani

Auriculotemporal nerve

Parotid gland

Submandibular ganglion

Sublingual gland

Submandibular gland

Parasympathetic innervation of parotid, submandibular, and sublingual salivary glands

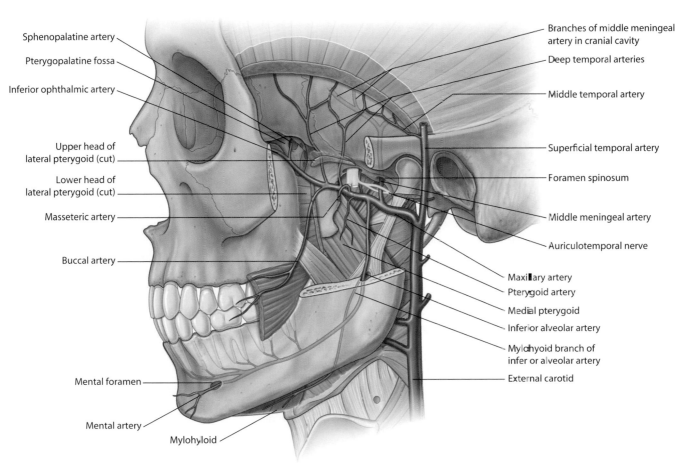

Sphenopalatine artery

Pterygopalatine fossa

Inferior ophthalmic artery

Upper head of
lateral pterygoid (cut)

Lower head of
lateral pterygoid (cut)

Masseteric artery

Buccal artery

Mental foramen

Mental artery

Mylohyloid

Branches of middle meningeal
artery in cranial cavity

Deep temporal arteries

Middle temporal artery

Superficial temporal artery

Foramen spinosum

Middle meningeal artery

Auriculotemporal nerve

Maxillary artery

Pterygoid artery

Medial pterygoid

Inferior alveolar artery

Mylohyoid branch of
inferior alveolar artery

External carotid

Arteries of the temporal and infratemporal fossae

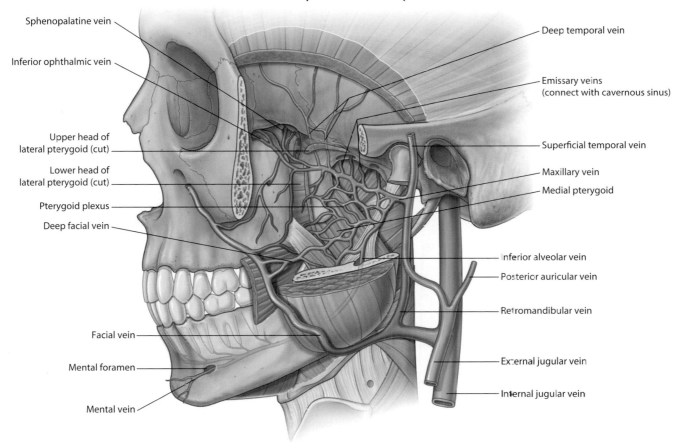

Sphenopalatine vein

Inferior ophthalmic vein

Upper head of
lateral pterygoid (cut)

Lower head of
lateral pterygoid (cut)

Pterygoid plexus

Deep facial vein

Facial vein

Mental foramen

Mental vein

Deep temporal vein

Emissary veins
(connect with cavernous sinus)

Superficial temporal vein

Maxillary vein

Medial pterygoid

Inferior alveolar vein

Posterior auricular vein

Retromandibular vein

External jugular vein

Internal jugular vein

Veins of the temporal and infratemporal fossae

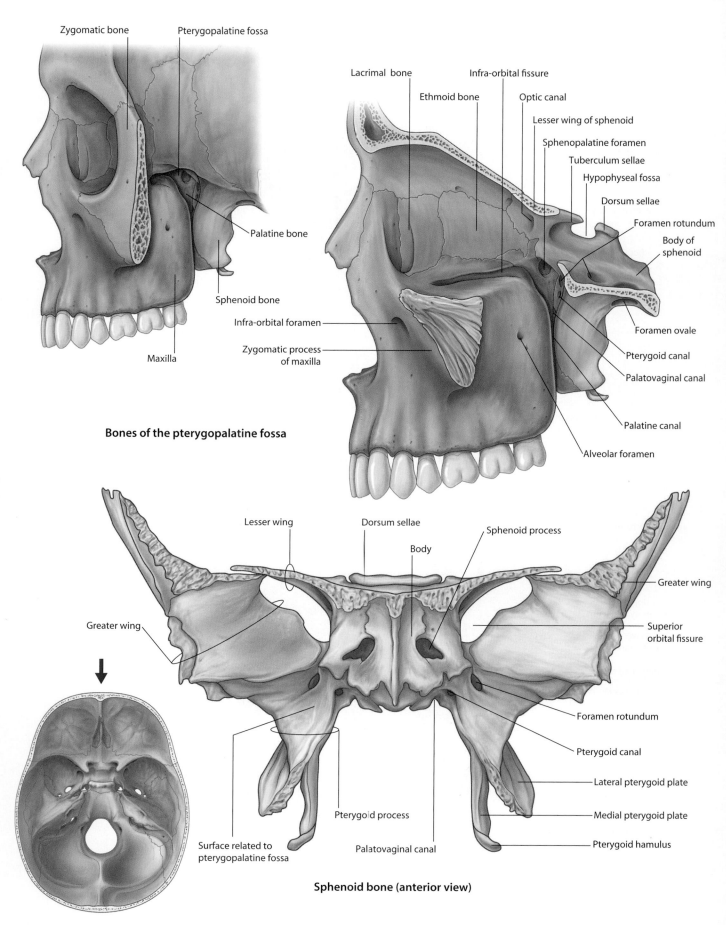

Zygomatic bone

Pterygopalatine fossa

Palatine bone

Sphenoid bone

Infra-orbital foramen

Zygomatic process of maxilla

Maxilla

Bones of the pterygopalatine fossa

Lacrimal bone

Ethmoid bone

Infra-orbital fissure

Optic canal

Lesser wing of sphenoid

Sphenopalatine foramen

Tuberculum sellae

Hypophyseal fossa

Dorsum sellae

Foramen rotundum

Body of sphenoid

Foramen ovale

Pterygoid canal

Palatovaginal canal

Palatine canal

Alveolar foramen

Lesser wing

Dorsum sellae

Body

Sphenoid process

Greater wing

Greater wing

Superior orbital fissure

Foramen rotundum

Pterygoid canal

Lateral pterygoid plate

Medial pterygoid plate

Pterygoid hamulus

Surface related to pterygopalatine fossa

Pterygoid process

Palatovaginal canal

Sphenoid bone (anterior view)

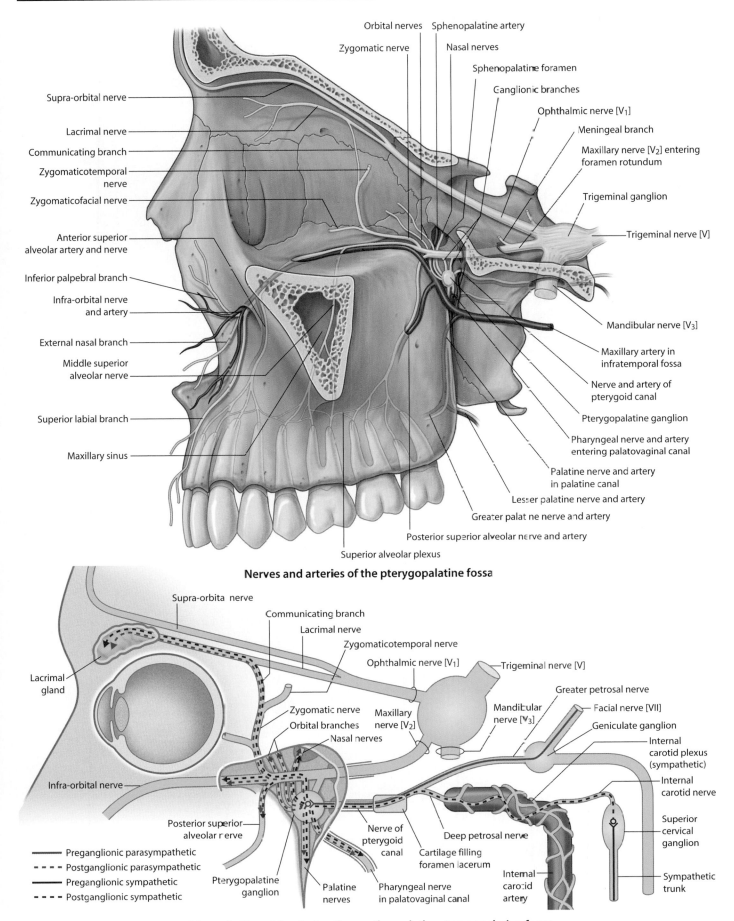

Supra-orbital nerve

Lacrimal nerve

Communicating branch

Zygomaticotemporal nerve

Zygomaticofacial nerve

Anterior superior alveolar artery and nerve

Inferior palpebral branch

Infra-orbital nerve and artery

External nasal branch

Middle superior alveolar nerve

Superior labial branch

Maxillary sinus

Orbital nerves

Zygomatic nerve

Sphenopalatine artery

Nasal nerves

Sphenopalatine foramen

Ganglionic branches

Ophthalmic nerve [V₁]

Meningeal branch

Maxillary nerve [V₂] entering foramen rotundum

Trigeminal ganglion

Trigeminal nerve [V]

Mandibular nerve [V₃]

Maxillary artery in infratemporal fossa

Nerve and artery of pterygoid canal

Pterygopalatine ganglion

Pharyngeal nerve and artery entering palatovaginal canal

Palatine nerve and artery in palatine canal

Lesser palatine nerve and artery

Greater palatine nerve and artery

Posterior superior alveolar nerve and artery

Superior alveolar plexus

Nerves and arteries of the pterygopalatine fossa

Supra-orbital nerve

Communicating branch

Lacrimal nerve

Zygomaticotemporal nerve

Ophthalmic nerve [V₁]

Trigeminal nerve [V]

Greater petrosal nerve

Mandibular nerve [V₃]

Facial nerve [VII]

Geniculate ganglion

Internal carotid plexus (sympathetic)

Internal carotid nerve

Superior cervical ganglion

Sympathetic trunk

Lacrimal gland

Zygomatic nerve

Maxillary nerve [V₂]

Orbital branches

Nasal nerves

Infra-orbital nerve

Posterior superior alveolar nerve

Nerve of pterygoid canal

Deep petrosal nerve

Cartilage filling foramen lacerum

Internal carotid artery

Pterygopalatine ganglion

Palatine nerves

Pharyngeal nerve in palatovaginal canal

—— Preganglionic parasympathetic
- - - Postganglionic parasympathetic
—— Preganglionic sympathetic
- - - Postganglionic sympathetic

Visceral efferent (motor) pathways through the pterygopalatine fossa

537

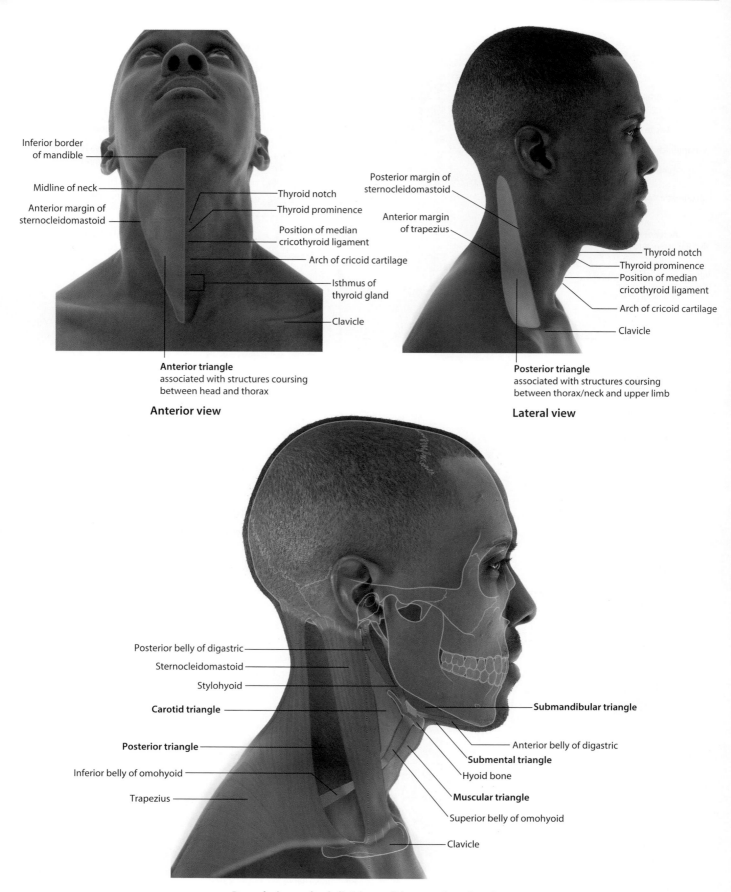

Inferior border of mandible

Midline of neck

Anterior margin of sternocleidomastoid

Thyroid notch

Thyroid prominence

Position of median cricothyroid ligament

Arch of cricoid cartilage

Isthmus of thyroid gland

Clavicle

Anterior triangle
associated with structures coursing between head and thorax

Anterior view

Posterior margin of sternocleidomastoid

Anterior margin of trapezius

Thyroid notch

Thyroid prominence

Position of median cricothyroid ligament

Arch of cricoid cartilage

Clavicle

Posterior triangle
associated with structures coursing between thorax/neck and upper limb

Lateral view

Posterior belly of digastric

Sternocleidomastoid

Stylohyoid

Carotid triangle

Posterior triangle

Inferior belly of omohyoid

Trapezius

Submandibular triangle

Anterior belly of digastric

Submental triangle

Hyoid bone

Muscular triangle

Superior belly of omohyoid

Clavicle

**Boundaries and subdivisions of the anterior triangle
and boundaries of the posterior triangle**

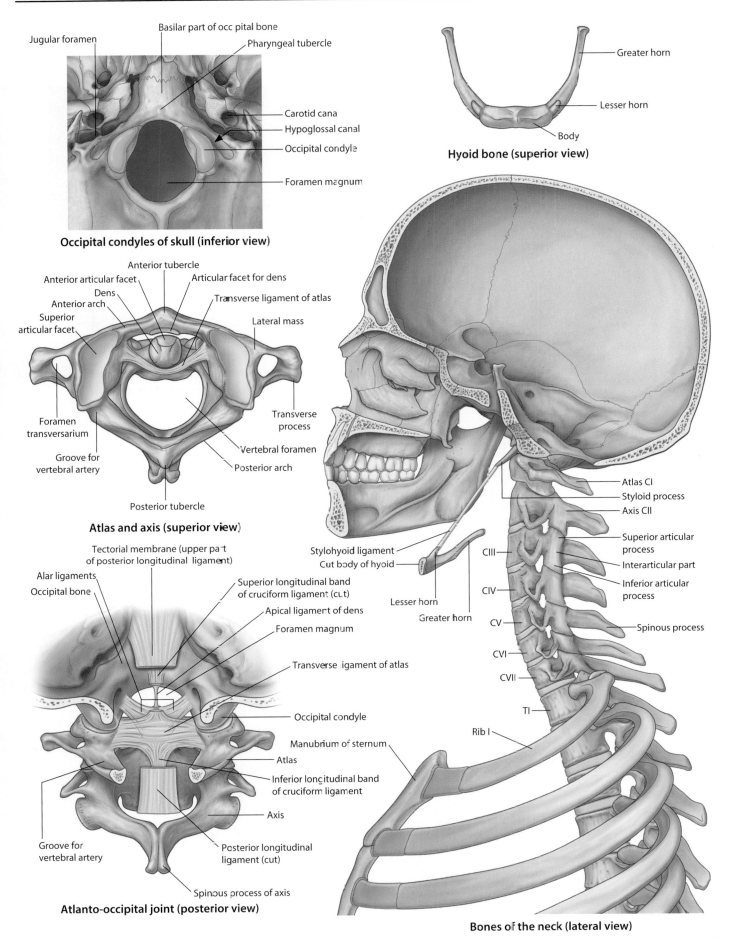

Occipital condyles of skull (inferior view)

Jugular foramen
Basilar part of occipital bone
Pharyngeal tubercle
Carotid canal
Hypoglossal canal
Occipital condyle
Foramen magnum

Hyoid bone (superior view)

Greater horn
Lesser horn
Body

Atlas and axis (superior view)

Anterior tubercle
Anterior articular facet
Dens
Articular facet for dens
Anterior arch
Transverse ligament of atlas
Superior articular facet
Lateral mass
Foramen transversarium
Transverse process
Groove for vertebral artery
Vertebral foramen
Posterior arch
Posterior tubercle

Atlanto-occipital joint (posterior view)

Tectorial membrane (upper part of posterior longitudinal ligament)
Alar ligaments
Occipital bone
Superior longitudinal band of cruciform ligament (cut)
Apical ligament of dens
Foramen magnum
Transverse ligament of atlas
Occipital condyle
Manubrium of sternum
Atlas
Inferior longitudinal band of cruciform ligament
Axis
Groove for vertebral artery
Posterior longitudinal ligament (cut)
Spinous process of axis

Stylohyoid ligament
Cut body of hyoid
Lesser horn
Greater horn
CIII
CIV
CV
CVI
CVII
TI
Rib I

Atlas CI
Styloid process
Axis CII
Superior articular process
Interarticular part
Inferior articular process
Spinous process

Bones of the neck (lateral view)

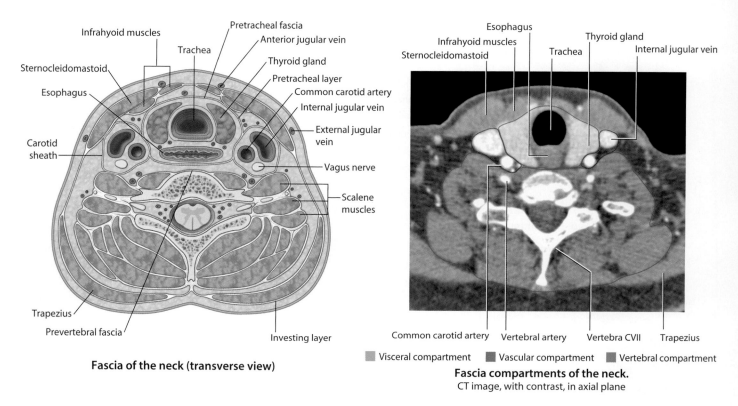

Infrahyoid muscles

Pretracheal fascia

Trachea

Anterior jugular vein

Thyroid gland

Sternocleidomastoid

Pretracheal layer

Esophagus

Common carotid artery

Internal jugular vein

Carotid sheath

External jugular vein

Vagus nerve

Scalene muscles

Trapezius

Prevertebral fascia

Investing layer

Fascia of the neck (transverse view)

Esophagus

Infrahyoid muscles

Thyroid gland

Sternocleidomastoid

Trachea

Internal jugular vein

Common carotid artery

Vertebral artery

Vertebra CVII

Trapezius

☐ Visceral compartment   ☐ Vascular compartment   ☐ Vertebral compartment

Fascia compartments of the neck.
CT image, with contrast, in axial plane

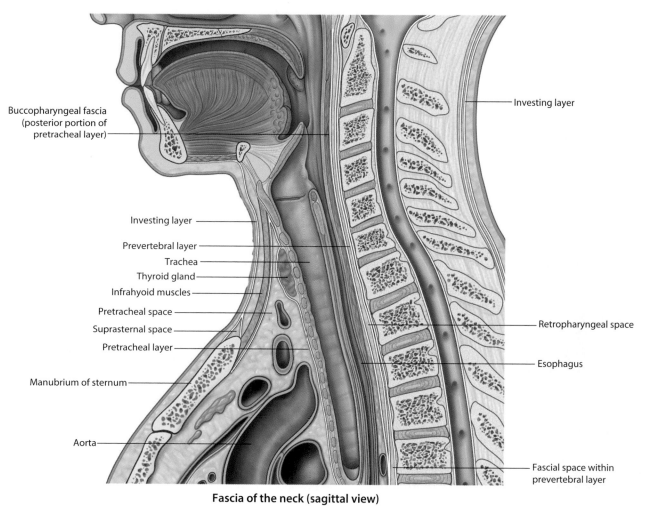

Buccopharyngeal fascia (posterior portion of pretracheal layer)

Investing layer

Investing layer

Prevertebral layer

Trachea

Thyroid gland

Infrahyoid muscles

Pretracheal space

Suprasternal space

Pretracheal layer

Manubrium of sternum

Aorta

Retropharyngeal space

Esophagus

Fascial space within prevertebral layer

Fascia of the neck (sagittal view)

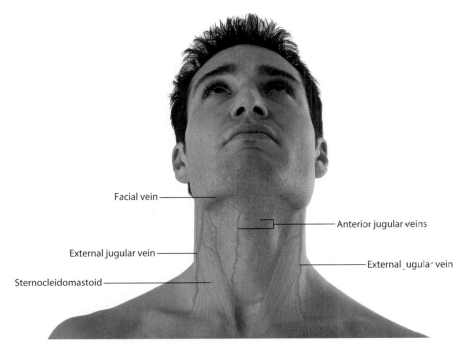

Facial vein

Anterior jugular veins

External jugular vein

External jugular vein

Sternocleidomastoid

**Palpable veins of the neck
(or visible)**

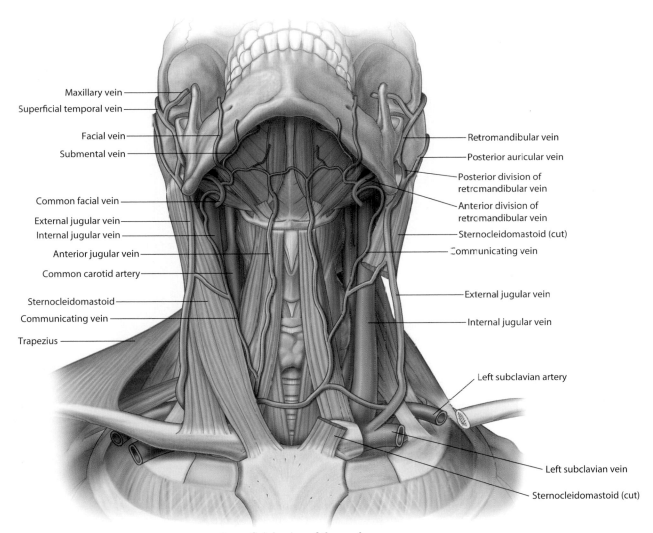

Maxillary vein

Superficial temporal vein

Facial vein

Submental vein

Common facial vein

External jugular vein

Internal jugular vein

Anterior jugular vein

Common carotid artery

Sternocleidomastoid

Communicating vein

Trapezius

Retromandibular vein

Posterior auricular vein

Posterior division of
retromandibular vein

Anterior division of
retromandibular vein

Sternocleidomastoid (cut)

Communicating vein

External jugular vein

Internal jugular vein

Left subclavian artery

Left subclavian vein

Sternocleidomastoid (cut)

Superficial veins of the neck

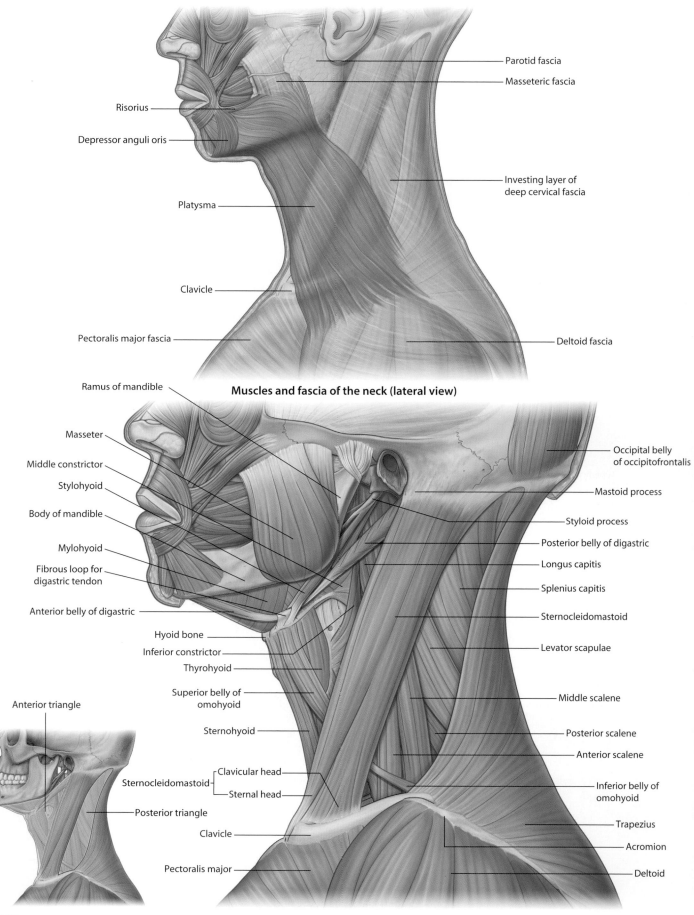

Parotid fascia

Masseteric fascia

Risorius

Depressor anguli oris

Investing layer of
deep cervical fascia

Platysma

Clavicle

Pectoralis major fascia

Deltoid fascia

Muscles and fascia of the neck (lateral view)

Ramus of mandible

Masseter

Middle constrictor

Stylohyoid

Body of mandible

Mylohyoid

Fibrous loop for
digastric tendon

Anterior belly of digastric

Hyoid bone

Inferior constrictor

Thyrohyoid

Superior belly of
omohyoid

Sternohyoid

Anterior triangle

Sternocleidomastoid

Clavicular head

Sternal head

Posterior triangle

Clavicle

Pectoralis major

Occipital belly
of occipitofrontalis

Mastoid process

Styloid process

Posterior belly of digastric

Longus capitis

Splenius capitis

Sternocleidomastoid

Levator scapulae

Middle scalene

Posterior scalene

Anterior scalene

Inferior belly of
omohyoid

Trapezius

Acromion

Deltoid

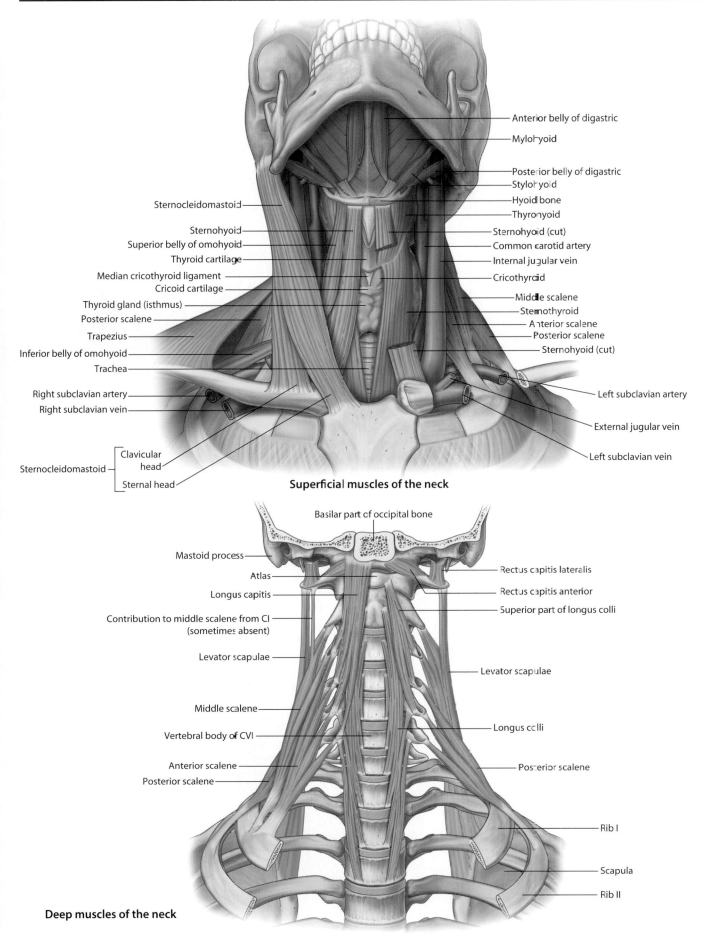

Superficial muscles of the neck

Anterior belly of digastric
Mylohyoid
Posterior belly of digastric
Stylohyoid
Hyoid bone
Thyrohyoid
Sternohyoid (cut)
Common carotid artery
Internal jugular vein
Cricothyroid
Middle scalene
Sternothyroid
Anterior scalene
Posterior scalene
Sternohyoid (cut)
Left subclavian artery
External jugular vein
Left subclavian vein

Sternocleidomastoid
Sternohyoid
Superior belly of omohyoid
Thyroid cartilage
Median cricothyroid ligament
Cricoid cartilage
Thyroid gland (isthmus)
Posterior scalene
Trapezius
Inferior belly of omohyoid
Trachea
Right subclavian artery
Right subclavian vein

Sternocleidomastoid — { Clavicular head / Sternal head }

Deep muscles of the neck

Basilar part of occipital bone
Mastoid process
Atlas
Longus capitis
Contribution to middle scalene from CI (sometimes absent)
Levator scapulae
Middle scalene
Vertebral body of CVI
Anterior scalene
Posterior scalene

Rectus capitis lateralis
Rectus capitis anterior
Superior part of longus colli
Levator scapulae
Longus colli
Posterior scalene
Rib I
Scapula
Rib II

543

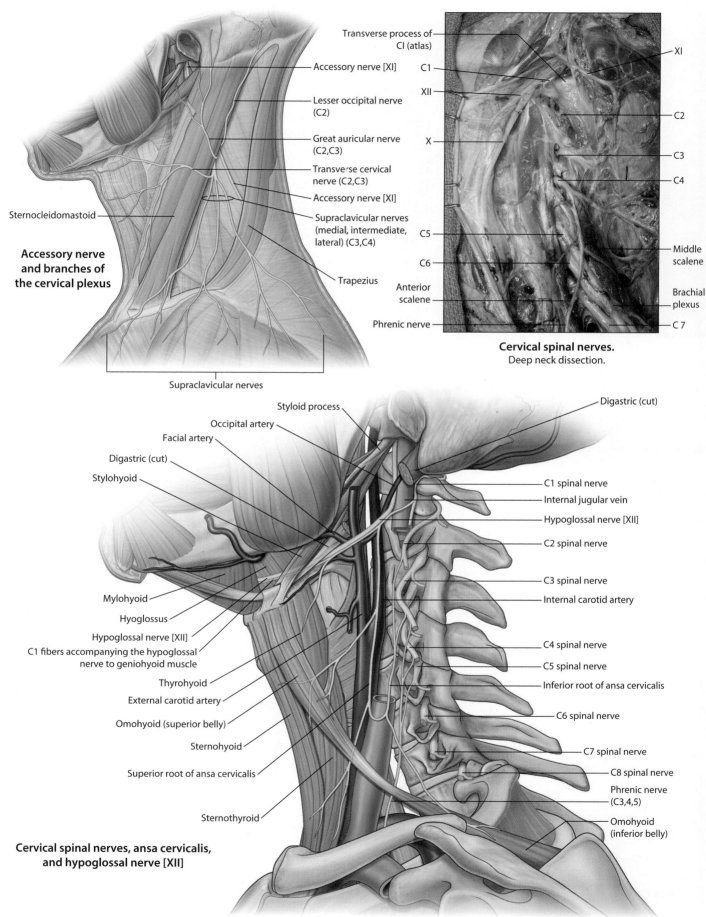

Transverse process of CI (atlas)

XI

C1

XII

X

C2

C3

C4

C5

C6

Accessory nerve [XI]

Lesser occipital nerve (C2)

Great auricular nerve (C2,C3)

Transverse cervical nerve (C2,C3)

Accessory nerve [XI]

Supraclavicular nerves (medial, intermediate, lateral) (C3,C4)

Trapezius

Sternocleidomastoid

Accessory nerve and branches of the cervical plexus

Supraclavicular nerves

Middle scalene

Anterior scalene

Phrenic nerve

Brachial plexus

C 7

Cervical spinal nerves.
Deep neck dissection.

Styloid process

Occipital artery

Facial artery

Digastric (cut)

Stylohyoid

Digastric (cut)

C1 spinal nerve

Internal jugular vein

Hypoglossal nerve [XII]

C2 spinal nerve

C3 spinal nerve

Internal carotid artery

Mylohyoid

Hyoglossus

Hypoglossal nerve [XII]

C1 fibers accompanying the hypoglossal nerve to geniohyoid muscle

Thyrohyoid

External carotid artery

Omohyoid (superior belly)

Sternohyoid

Superior root of ansa cervicalis

Sternothyroid

C4 spinal nerve

C5 spinal nerve

Inferior root of ansa cervicalis

C6 spinal nerve

C7 spinal nerve

C8 spinal nerve

Phrenic nerve (C3,4,5)

Omohyoid (inferior belly)

Cervical spinal nerves, ansa cervicalis, and hypoglossal nerve [XII]

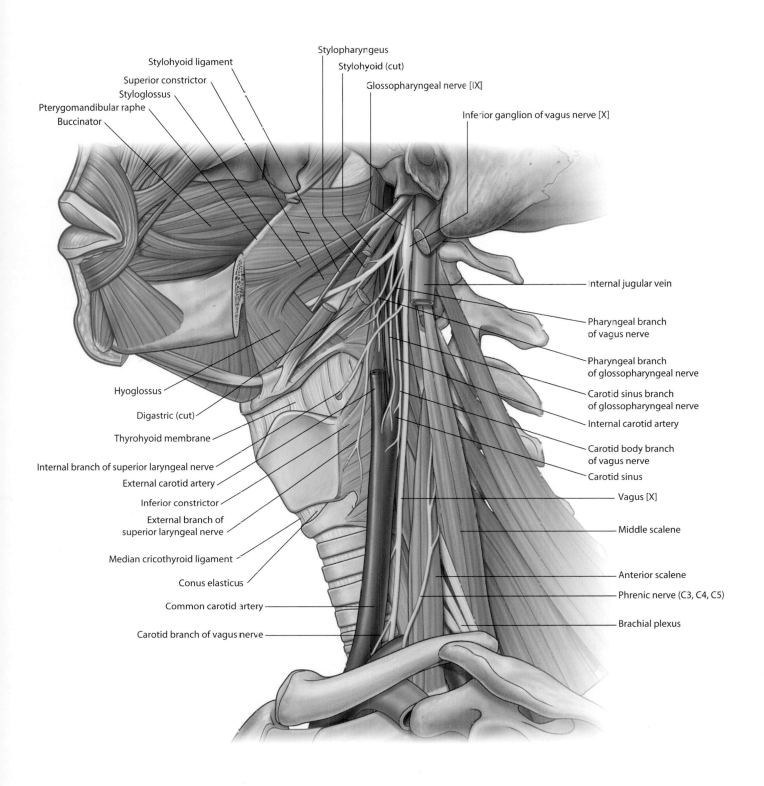

Stylohyoid ligament

Superior constrictor

Styloglossus

Pterygomandibular raphe

Buccinator

Stylopharyngeus

Stylohyoid (cut)

Glossopharyngeal nerve [IX]

Inferior ganglion of vagus nerve [X]

Internal jugular vein

Pharyngeal branch of vagus nerve

Pharyngeal branch of glossopharyngeal nerve

Carotid sinus branch of glossopharyngeal nerve

Internal carotid artery

Carotid body branch of vagus nerve

Carotid sinus

Vagus [X]

Middle scalene

Anterior scalene

Phrenic nerve (C3, C4, C5)

Brachial plexus

Hyoglossus

Digastric (cut)

Thyrohyoid membrane

Internal branch of superior laryngeal nerve

External carotid artery

Inferior constrictor

External branch of superior laryngeal nerve

Median cricothyroid ligament

Conus elasticus

Common carotid artery

Carotid branch of vagus nerve

Branches of glossopharyngeal [IX] and vagus nerves [X] in neck

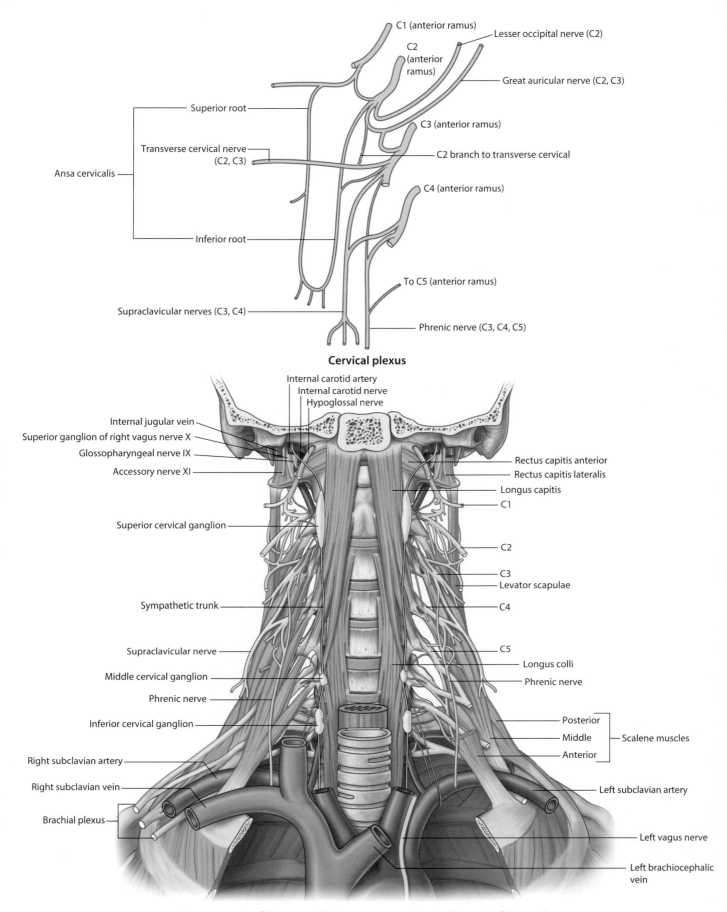

C1 (anterior ramus)

Lesser occipital nerve (C2)

C2 (anterior ramus)

Great auricular nerve (C2, C3)

Superior root

C3 (anterior ramus)

Transverse cervical nerve (C2, C3)

C2 branch to transverse cervical

Ansa cervicalis

C4 (anterior ramus)

Inferior root

To C5 (anterior ramus)

Supraclavicular nerves (C3, C4)

Phrenic nerve (C3, C4, C5)

Cervical plexus

Internal carotid artery
Internal carotid nerve
Hypoglossal nerve

Internal jugular vein

Superior ganglion of right vagus nerve X

Glossopharyngeal nerve IX

Accessory nerve XI

Rectus capitis anterior
Rectus capitis lateralis
Longus capitis
C1

Superior cervical ganglion

C2

C3
Levator scapulae

Sympathetic trunk

C4

Supraclavicular nerve

C5

Middle cervical ganglion

Longus colli
Phrenic nerve

Phrenic nerve

Inferior cervical ganglion

Posterior
Middle — Scalene muscles
Anterior

Right subclavian artery

Right subclavian vein

Left subclavian artery

Brachial plexus

Left vagus nerve

Left brachiocephalic vein

Components of the sympathetic nervous system in the root of the neck

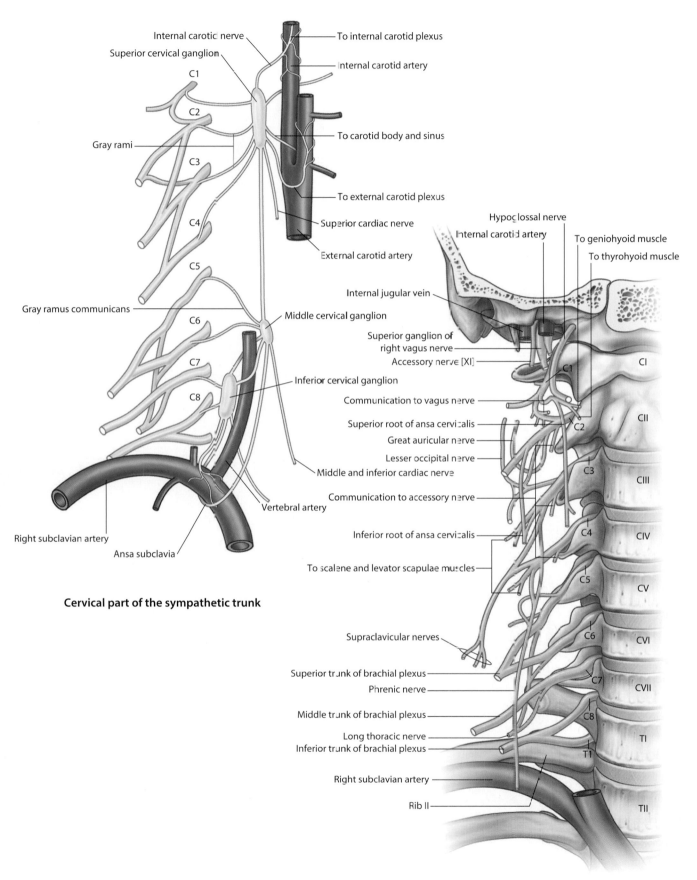

Internal carotic nerve
Superior cervical ganglion
C1
C2
Gray rami
C3
C4
C5
Gray ramus communicans
C6
C7
C8

To internal carotid plexus
Internal carotid artery
To carotid body and sinus
To external carotid plexus
Superior cardiac nerve
External carotid artery
Middle cervical ganglion
Inferior cervical ganglion

Right subclavian artery
Ansa subclavia
Vertebral artery

Cervical part of the sympathetic trunk

Hypoglossal nerve
Internal carotid artery
To geniohyoid muscle
To thyrohyoid muscle
Internal jugular vein
Superior ganglion of right vagus nerve
Accessory nerve [XI]
Communication to vagus nerve
Superior root of ansa cervicalis
Great auricular nerve
Lesser occipital nerve
Middle and inferior cardiac nerve
Communication to accessory nerve
Inferior root of ansa cervicalis
To scalene and levator scapulae muscles
Supraclavicular nerves
Superior trunk of brachial plexus
Phrenic nerve
Middle trunk of brachial plexus
Long thoracic nerve
Inferior trunk of brachial plexus
Right subclavian artery
Rib II

C1
C2
C3
C4
C5
C6
C7
C8
T1

CI
CII
CIII
CIV
CV
CVI
CVII
TI
TII

**Branches of the cervical plexus
(rib I removed)**

547

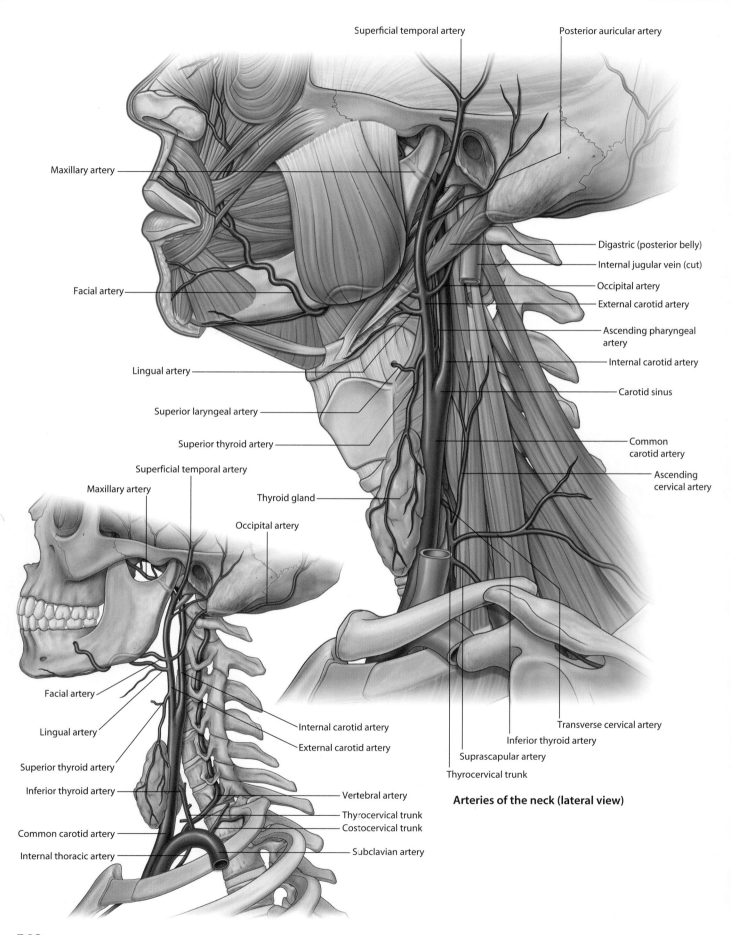

Superficial temporal artery

Posterior auricular artery

Maxillary artery

Digastric (posterior belly)

Internal jugular vein (cut)

Facial artery

Occipital artery

External carotid artery

Ascending pharyngeal artery

Internal carotid artery

Lingual artery

Carotid sinus

Superior laryngeal artery

Superior thyroid artery

Common carotid artery

Superficial temporal artery

Maxillary artery

Thyroid gland

Ascending cervical artery

Occipital artery

Facial artery

Lingual artery

Internal carotid artery

External carotid artery

Superior thyroid artery

Inferior thyroid artery

Transverse cervical artery

Inferior thyroid artery

Common carotid artery

Vertebral artery

Suprascapular artery

Internal thoracic artery

Thyrocervical trunk

Costocervical trunk

Subclavian artery

Thyrocervical trunk

Arteries of the neck (lateral view)

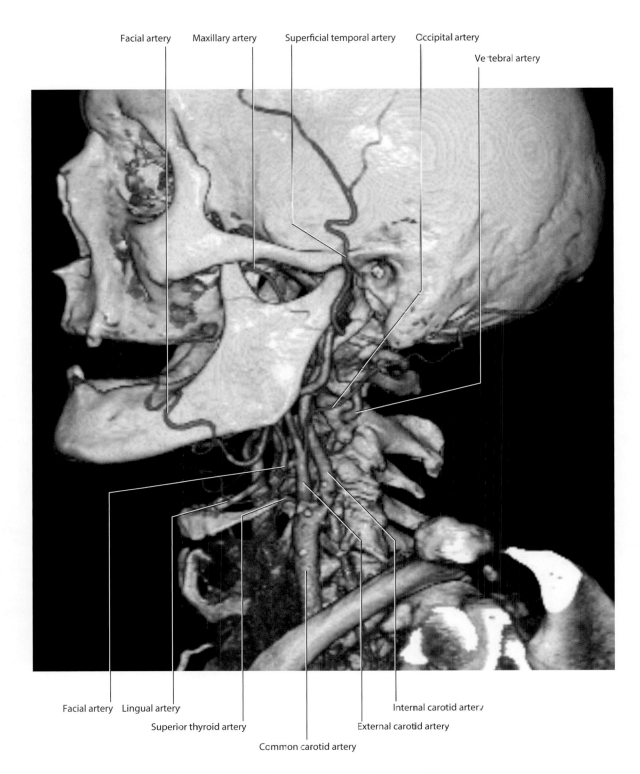

Facial artery Maxillary artery Superficial temporal artery Occipital artery

Vertebral artery

Facial artery Lingual artery

Superior thyroid artery

Common carotid artery

External carotid artery

Internal carotid artery

Lateral view of the branches of the external carotid artery.
Volume-rendered angiographic image with contrast using multidetector CT

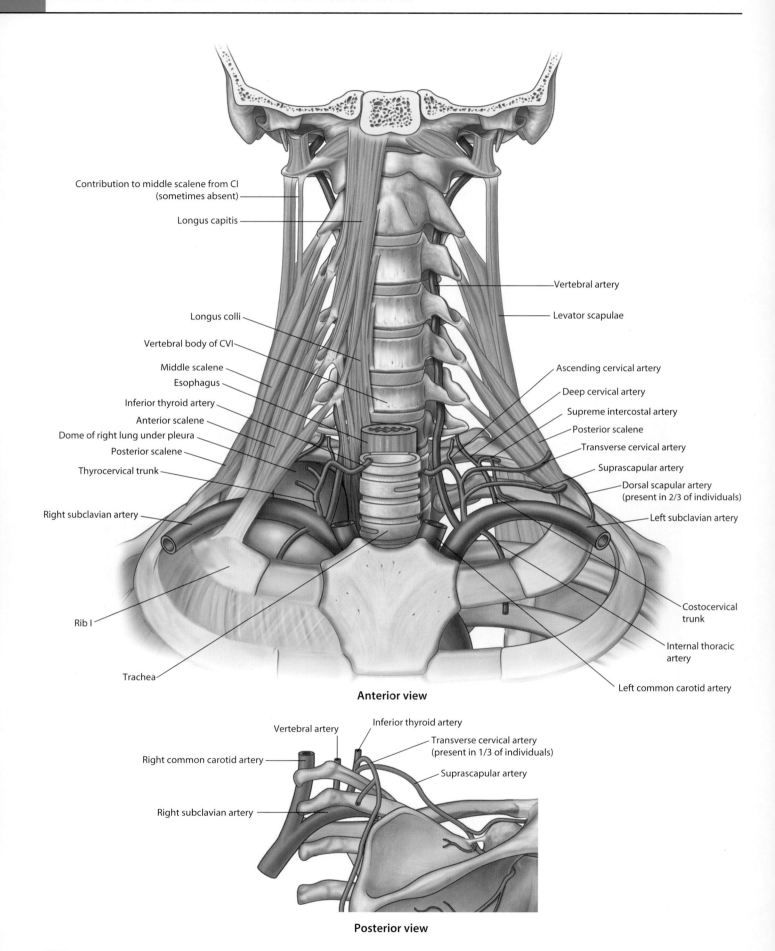

Contribution to middle scalene from CI
(sometimes absent)

Longus capitis

Longus colli

Vertebral body of CVI

Middle scalene

Esophagus

Inferior thyroid artery

Anterior scalene

Dome of right lung under pleura

Posterior scalene

Thyrocervical trunk

Right subclavian artery

Rib I

Trachea

Vertebral artery

Levator scapulae

Ascending cervical artery

Deep cervical artery

Supreme intercostal artery

Posterior scalene

Transverse cervical artery

Suprascapular artery

Dorsal scapular artery
(present in 2/3 of individuals)

Left subclavian artery

Costocervical
trunk

Internal thoracic
artery

Left common carotid artery

Anterior view

Vertebral artery

Inferior thyroid artery

Right common carotid artery

Transverse cervical artery
(present in 1/3 of individuals)

Suprascapular artery

Right subclavian artery

Posterior view

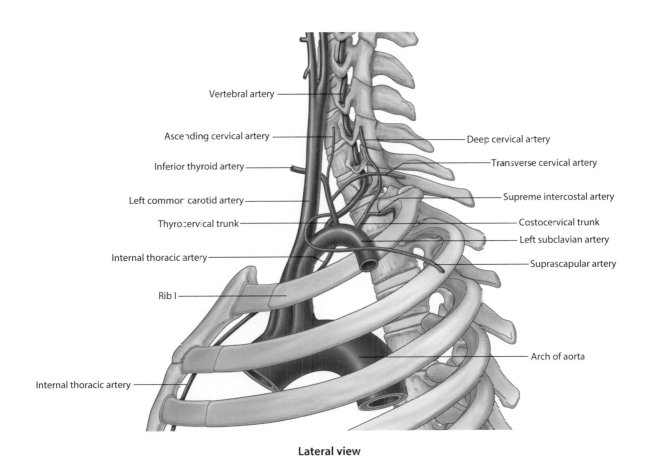

Vertebral artery

Ascending cervical artery

Inferior thyroid artery

Left common carotid artery

Thyrocervical trunk

Internal thoracic artery

Rib I

Internal thoracic artery

Deep cervical artery

Transverse cervical artery

Supreme intercostal artery

Costocervical trunk

Left subclavian artery

Suprascapular artery

Arch of aorta

Lateral view

Vertebral body of CIV

Right vertebral artery

Left vertebral artery

Right common carotid artery

Thyroid gland

Thyrocervical trunk

Costocervical trunk

Right subclavian artery

Right internal thoracic artery

Inferior thyroid artery

Thyrocervical trunk

Left common carotid artery

Left subclavian artery

Anterior view of the root of the neck showing the branches of the subclavian arteries.
Volume-rendered angiographic image with contrast using multidetector CT

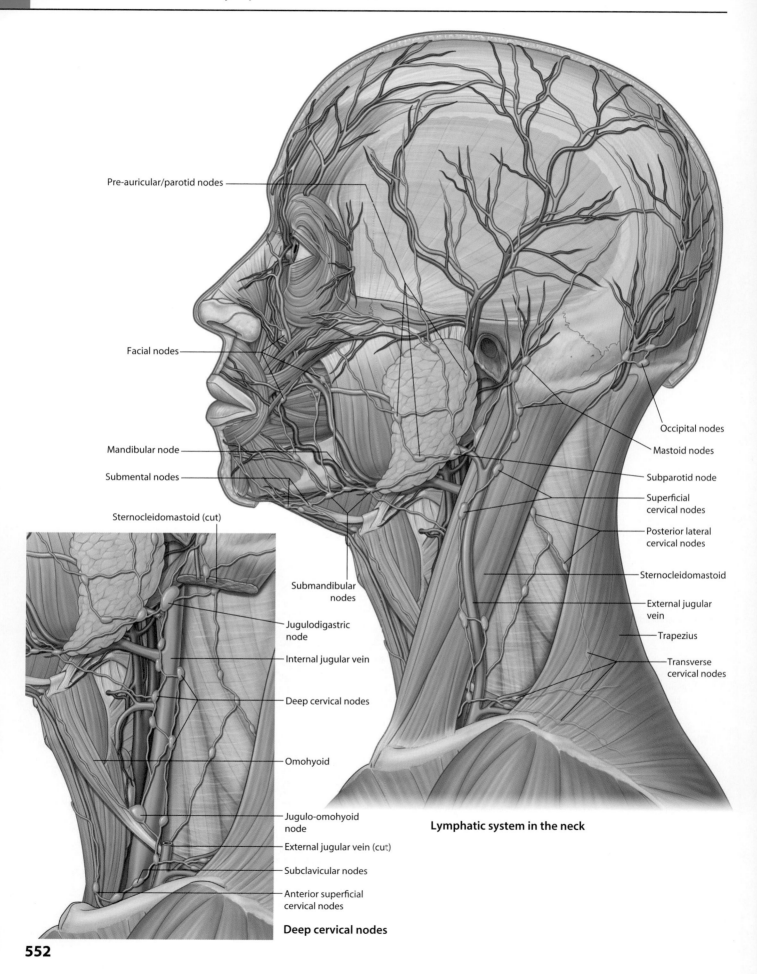

Pre-auricular/parotid nodes

Facial nodes

Mandibular node

Submental nodes

Sternocleidomastoid (cut)

Submandibular nodes

Jugulodigastric node

Internal jugular vein

Deep cervical nodes

Omohyoid

Jugulo-omohyoid node

External jugular vein (cut)

Subclavicular nodes

Anterior superficial cervical nodes

Occipital nodes

Mastoid nodes

Subparotid node

Superficial cervical nodes

Posterior lateral cervical nodes

Sternocleidomastoid

External jugular vein

Trapezius

Transverse cervical nodes

Deep cervical nodes

Lymphatic system in the neck

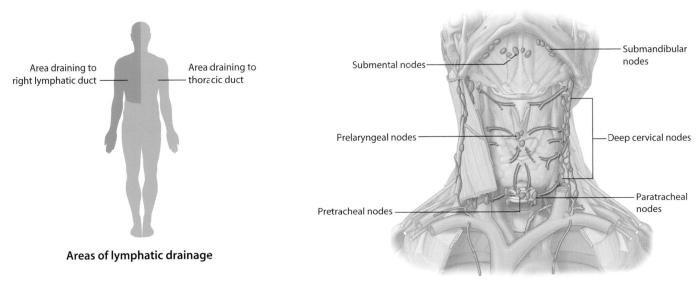

Areas of lymphatic drainage

Area draining to right lymphatic duct

Area draining to thoracic duct

Submental nodes

Submandibular nodes

Prelaryngeal nodes

Deep cervical nodes

Pretracheal nodes

Paratracheal nodes

Lymphatic drainage of the thyroid gland, larynx, and trachea

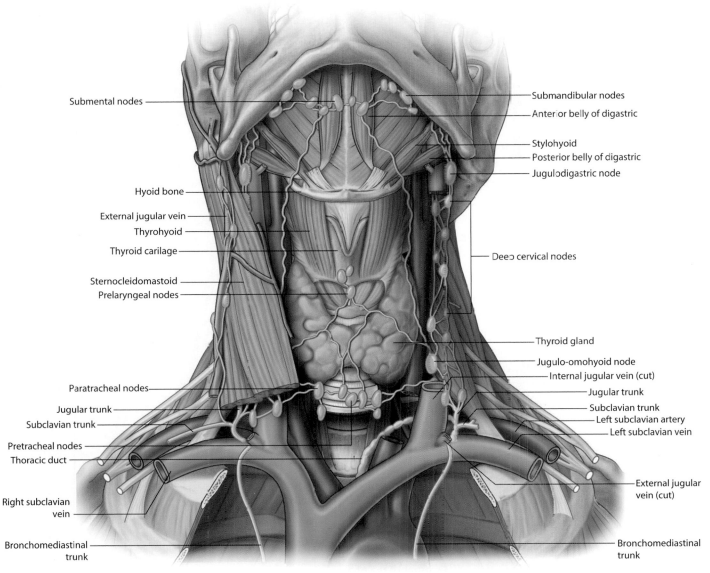

Submental nodes

Submandibular nodes

Anterior belly of digastric

Stylohyoid

Posterior belly of digastric

Jugulodigastric node

Hyoid bone

External jugular vein

Thyrohyoid

Thyroid carilage

Sternocleidomastoid

Prelaryngeal nodes

Deep cervical nodes

Thyroid gland

Jugulo-omohyoid node

Internal jugular vein (cut)

Jugular trunk

Subclavian trunk

Left subclavian artery

Left subclavian vein

Paratracheal nodes

Jugular trunk

Subclavian trunk

Pretracheal nodes

Thoracic duct

Right subclavian vein

External jugular vein (cut)

Bronchomediastinal trunk

Bronchomediastinal trunk

Lymphatic system in the neck

553

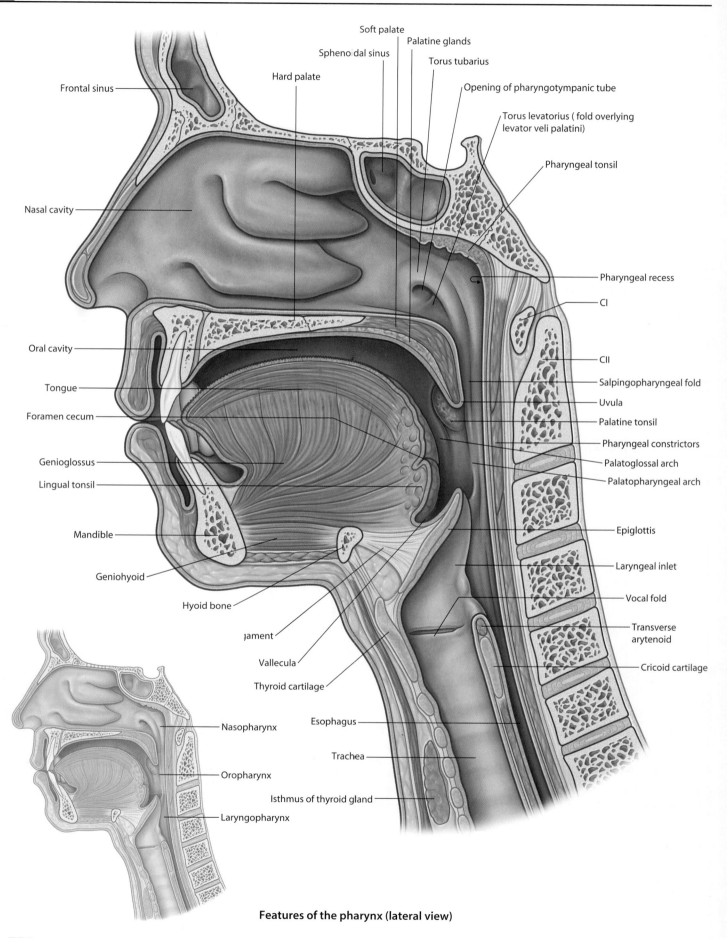

Frontal sinus

Nasal cavity

Oral cavity

Tongue

Foramen cecum

Genioglossus

Lingual tonsil

Mandible

Geniohyoid

Hyoid bone

 just ligament

Vallecula

Thyroid cartilage

Soft palate

Sphenoidal sinus

Hard palate

Palatine glands

Torus tubarius

Opening of pharyngotympanic tube

Torus levatorius (fold overlying levator veli palatini)

Pharyngeal tonsil

Pharyngeal recess

CI

CII

Salpingopharyngeal fold

Uvula

Palatine tonsil

Pharyngeal constrictors

Palatoglossal arch

Palatopharyngeal arch

Epiglottis

Laryngeal inlet

Vocal fold

Transverse arytenoid

Cricoid cartilage

Nasopharynx

Oropharynx

Laryngopharynx

Esophagus

Trachea

Isthmus of thyroid gland

Features of the pharynx (lateral view)

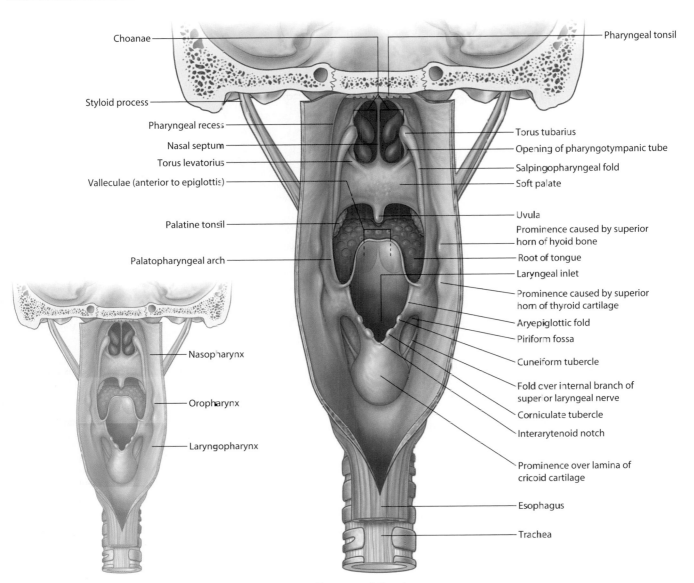

Choanae

Styloid process

Pharyngeal recess

Nasal septum

Torus levatorius

Valleculae (anterior to epiglottis)

Palatine tonsil

Palatopharyngeal arch

Pharyngeal tonsil

Torus tubarius

Opening of pharyngotympanic tube

Salpingopharyngeal fold

Soft palate

Uvula

Prominence caused by superior horn of hyoid bone

Root of tongue

Laryngeal inlet

Prominence caused by superior horn of thyroid cartilage

Aryepiglottic fold

Piriform fossa

Cuneiform tubercle

Fold over internal branch of superior laryngeal nerve

Corniculate tubercle

Interarytenoid notch

Prominence over lamina of cricoid cartilage

Esophagus

Trachea

Nasopharynx

Oropharynx

Laryngopharynx

Features of the pharynx
(posterior view with the pharyngeal wall opened)

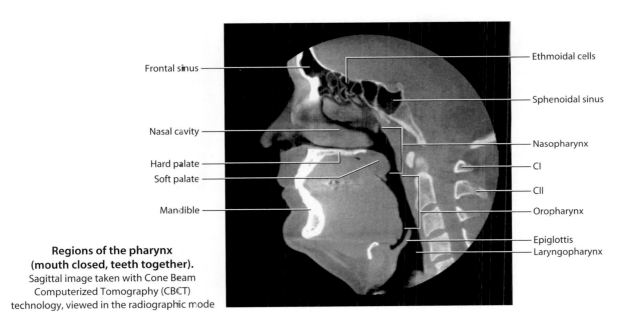

Frontal sinus

Nasal cavity

Hard palate

Soft palate

Mandible

Ethmoidal cells

Sphenoidal sinus

Nasopharynx

CI

CII

Oropharynx

Epiglottis

Laryngopharynx

Regions of the pharynx
(mouth closed, teeth together).
Sagittal image taken with Cone Beam
Computerized Tomography (CBCT)
technology, viewed in the radiographic mode

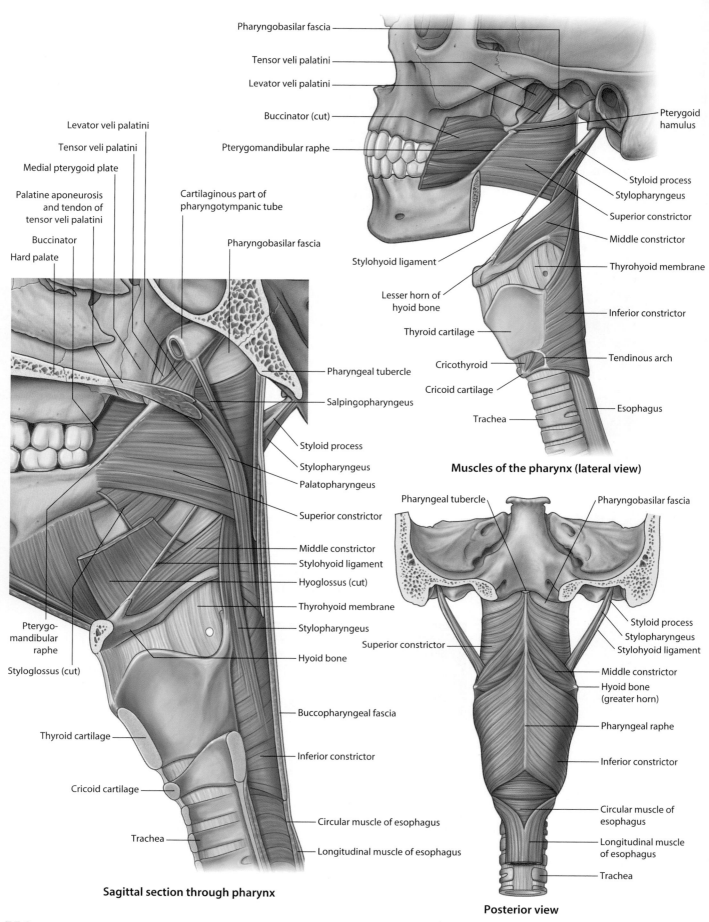

Pharyngobasilar fascia

Tensor veli palatini

Levator veli palatini

Buccinator (cut)

Pterygomandibular raphe

Pterygoid hamulus

Styloid process

Stylopharyngeus

Superior constrictor

Middle constrictor

Stylohyoid ligament

Thyrohyoid membrane

Lesser horn of hyoid bone

Inferior constrictor

Thyroid cartilage

Cricothyroid

Tendinous arch

Cricoid cartilage

Esophagus

Trachea

Muscles of the pharynx (lateral view)

Levator veli palatini

Tensor veli palatini

Medial pterygoid plate

Palatine aponeurosis and tendon of tensor veli palatini

Buccinator

Hard palate

Cartilaginous part of pharyngotympanic tube

Pharyngobasilar fascia

Pharyngeal tubercle

Salpingopharyngeus

Styloid process

Stylopharyngeus

Palatopharyngeus

Superior constrictor

Middle constrictor

Stylohyoid ligament

Hyoglossus (cut)

Thyrohyoid membrane

Stylopharyngeus

Hyoid bone

Pterygo-mandibular raphe

Styloglossus (cut)

Buccopharyngeal fascia

Thyroid cartilage

Inferior constrictor

Cricoid cartilage

Circular muscle of esophagus

Trachea

Longitudinal muscle of esophagus

Sagittal section through pharynx

Pharyngeal tubercle

Pharyngobasilar fascia

Styloid process

Stylopharyngeus

Stylohyoid ligament

Superior constrictor

Middle constrictor

Hyoid bone (greater horn)

Pharyngeal raphe

Inferior constrictor

Circular muscle of esophagus

Longitudinal muscle of esophagus

Trachea

Posterior view

556

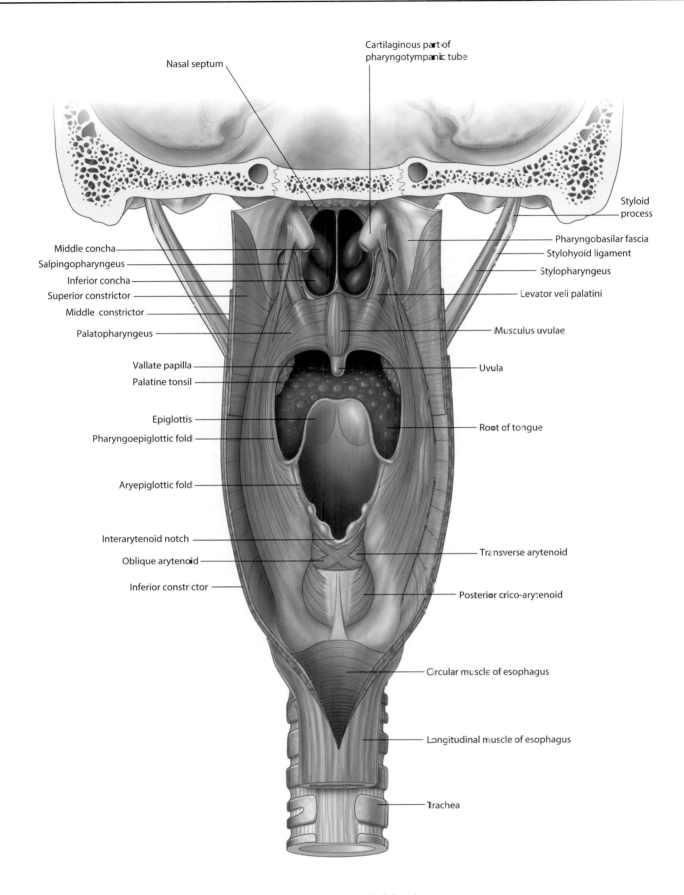

Nasal septum

Cartilaginous part of
pharyngotympanic tube

Styloid
process

Middle concha

Salpingopharyngeus

Inferior concha

Superior constrictor

Middle constrictor

Palatopharyngeus

Vallate papilla

Palatine tonsil

Epiglottis

Pharyngoepiglottic fold

Aryepiglottic fold

Interarytenoid notch

Oblique arytenoid

Inferior constrictor

Pharyngobasilar fascia

Stylohyoid ligament

Stylopharyngeus

Levator veli palatini

Musculus uvulae

Uvula

Root of tongue

Transverse arytenoid

Posterior crico-arytenoid

Circular muscle of esophagus

Longitudinal muscle of esophagus

Trachea

Muscles of the posterior wall of the pharynx

557

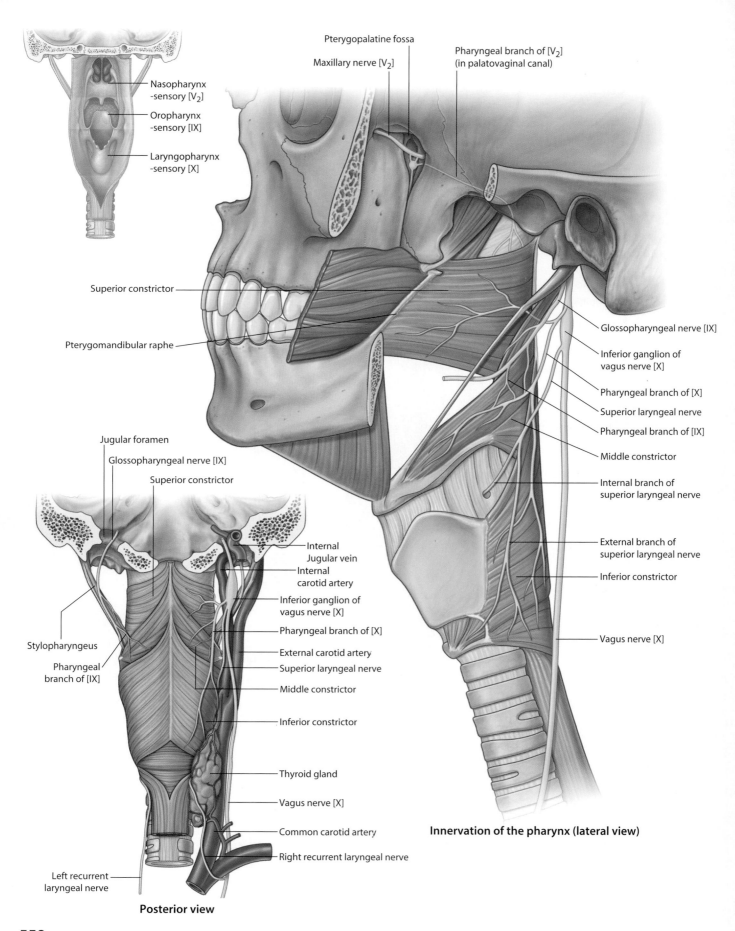

Pterygopalatine fossa

Maxillary nerve [V$_2$]

Pharyngeal branch of [V$_2$]
(in palatovaginal canal)

Nasopharynx
-sensory [V$_2$]

Oropharynx
-sensory [IX]

Laryngopharynx
-sensory [X]

Superior constrictor

Pterygomandibular raphe

Glossopharyngeal nerve [IX]

Inferior ganglion of
vagus nerve [X]

Pharyngeal branch of [X]

Superior laryngeal nerve

Pharyngeal branch of [IX]

Middle constrictor

Internal branch of
superior laryngeal nerve

External branch of
superior laryngeal nerve

Inferior constrictor

Vagus nerve [X]

Jugular foramen

Glossopharyngeal nerve [IX]

Superior constrictor

Internal
Jugular vein

Internal
carotid artery

Inferior ganglion of
vagus nerve [X]

Pharyngeal branch of [X]

External carotid artery

Superior laryngeal nerve

Middle constrictor

Inferior constrictor

Thyroid gland

Vagus nerve [X]

Common carotid artery

Right recurrent laryngeal nerve

Stylopharyngeus

Pharyngeal
branch of [IX]

Left recurrent
laryngeal nerve

Posterior view

Innervation of the pharynx (lateral view)

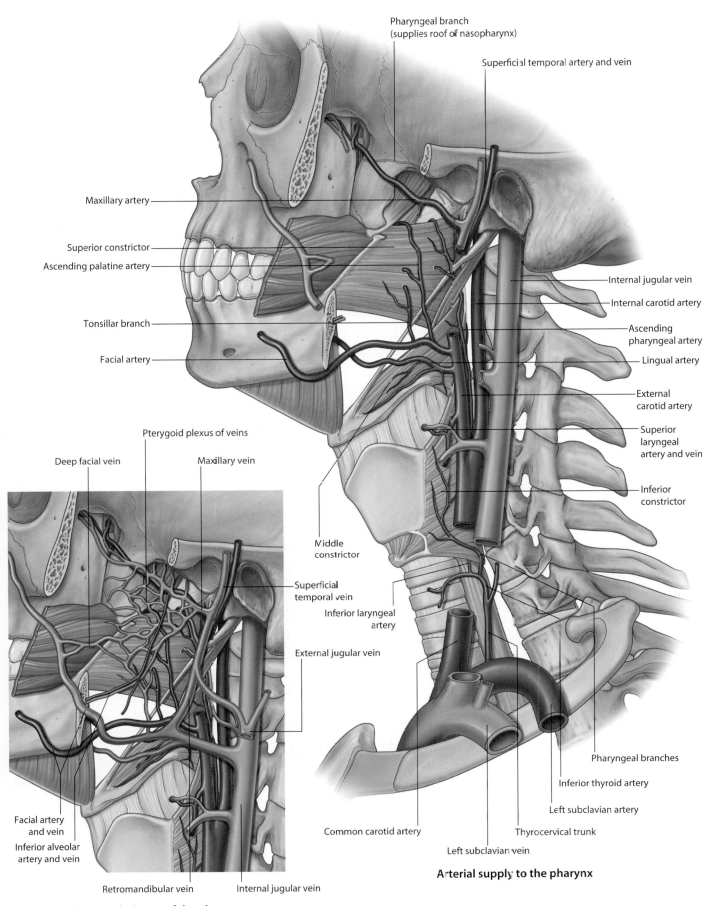

Pharyngeal branch
(supplies roof of nasopharynx)

Superficial temporal artery and vein

Maxillary artery

Superior constrictor

Ascending palatine artery

Tonsillar branch

Facial artery

Internal jugular vein

Internal carotid artery

Ascending
pharyngeal artery

Lingual artery

External
carotid artery

Superior
laryngeal
artery and vein

Inferior
constrictor

Pterygoid plexus of veins

Deep facial vein

Maxillary vein

Middle
constrictor

Superficial
temporal vein

Inferior laryngeal
artery

External jugular vein

Facial artery
and vein

Inferior alveolar
artery and vein

Pharyngeal branches

Inferior thyroid artery

Left subclavian artery

Retromandibular vein

Internal jugular vein

Common carotid artery

Left subclavian vein

Thyrocervical trunk

Arterial supply to the pharynx

Venous drainage of the pharynx

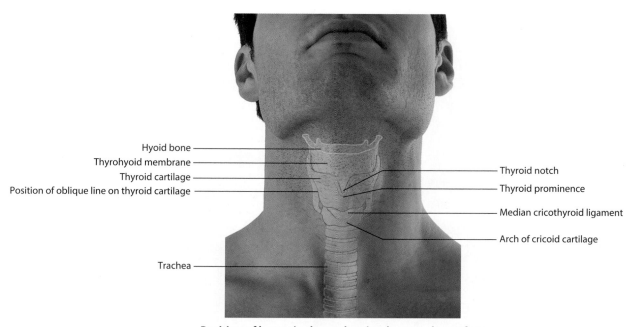

Hyoid bone

Thyrohyoid membrane

Thyroid cartilage

Position of oblique line on thyroid cartilage

Thyroid notch

Thyroid prominence

Median cricothyroid ligament

Arch of cricoid cartilage

Trachea

Position of larynx in the neck as it relates to the surface

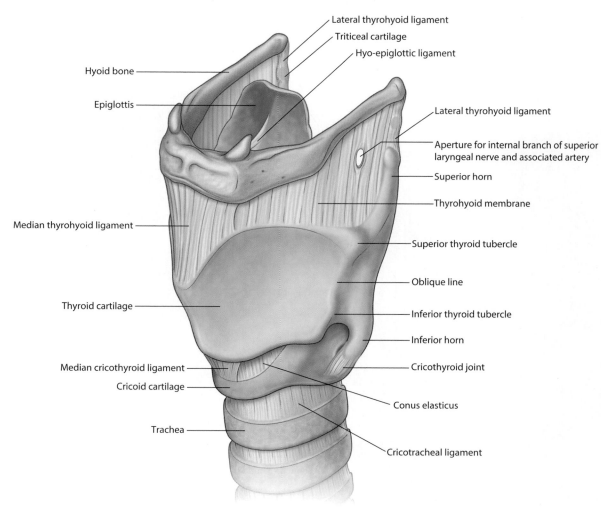

Lateral thyrohyoid ligament

Triticeal cartilage

Hyo-epiglottic ligament

Hyoid bone

Epiglottis

Lateral thyrohyoid ligament

Aperture for internal branch of superior laryngeal nerve and associated artery

Superior horn

Thyrohyoid membrane

Median thyrohyoid ligament

Superior thyroid tubercle

Oblique line

Inferior thyroid tubercle

Thyroid cartilage

Inferior horn

Cricothyroid joint

Median cricothyroid ligament

Cricoid cartilage

Conus elasticus

Trachea

Cricotracheal ligament

External features of the larynx (anterolateral view)

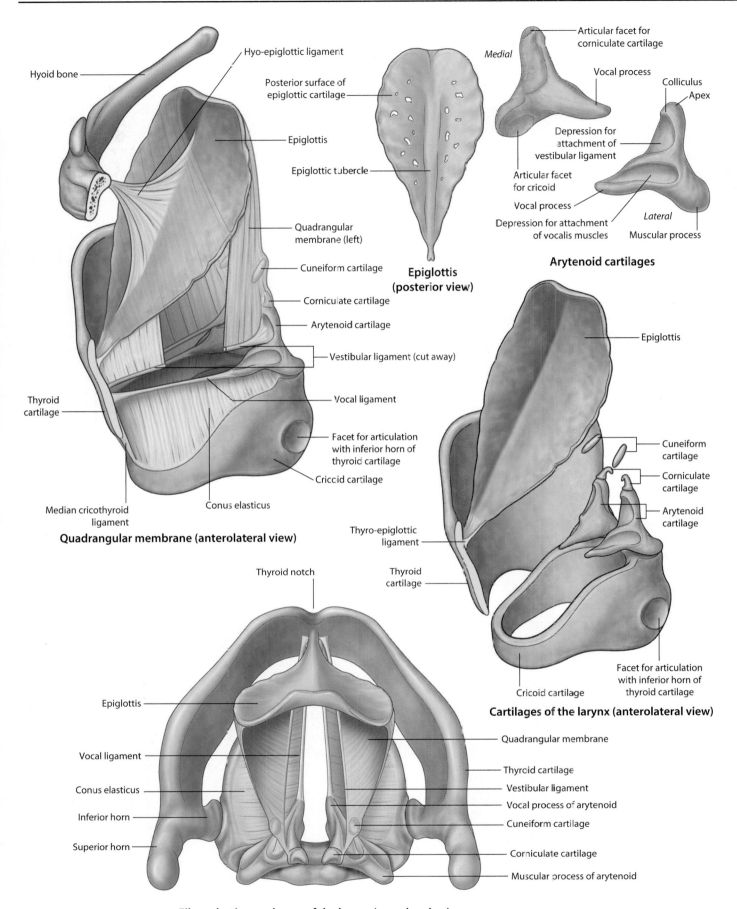

Hyoid bone

Hyo-epiglottic ligament

Posterior surface of epiglottic cartilage

Epiglottis

Epiglottic tubercle

Quadrangular membrane (left)

Cuneiform cartilage

Corniculate cartilage

Arytenoid cartilage

Vestibular ligament (cut away)

Vocal ligament

Facet for articulation with inferior horn of thyroid cartilage

Cricoid cartilage

Thyroid cartilage

Median cricothyroid ligament

Conus elasticus

Quadrangular membrane (anterolateral view)

Epiglottis (posterior view)

Medial

Articular facet for corniculate cartilage

Vocal process

Colliculus

Apex

Depression for attachment of vestibular ligament

Articular facet for cricoid

Vocal process

Depression for attachment of vocalis muscles

Lateral

Muscular process

Arytenoid cartilages

Epiglottis

Cuneiform cartilage

Corniculate cartilage

Arytenoid cartilage

Thyro-epiglottic ligament

Thyroid cartilage

Facet for articulation with inferior horn of thyroid cartilage

Cricoid cartilage

Cartilages of the larynx (anterolateral view)

Thyroid notch

Epiglottis

Vocal ligament

Conus elasticus

Inferior horn

Superior horn

Quadrangular membrane

Thyroid cartilage

Vestibular ligament

Vocal process of arytenoid

Cuneiform cartilage

Corniculate cartilage

Muscular process of arytenoid

Fibro-elastic membrane of the larynx (superior view)

561

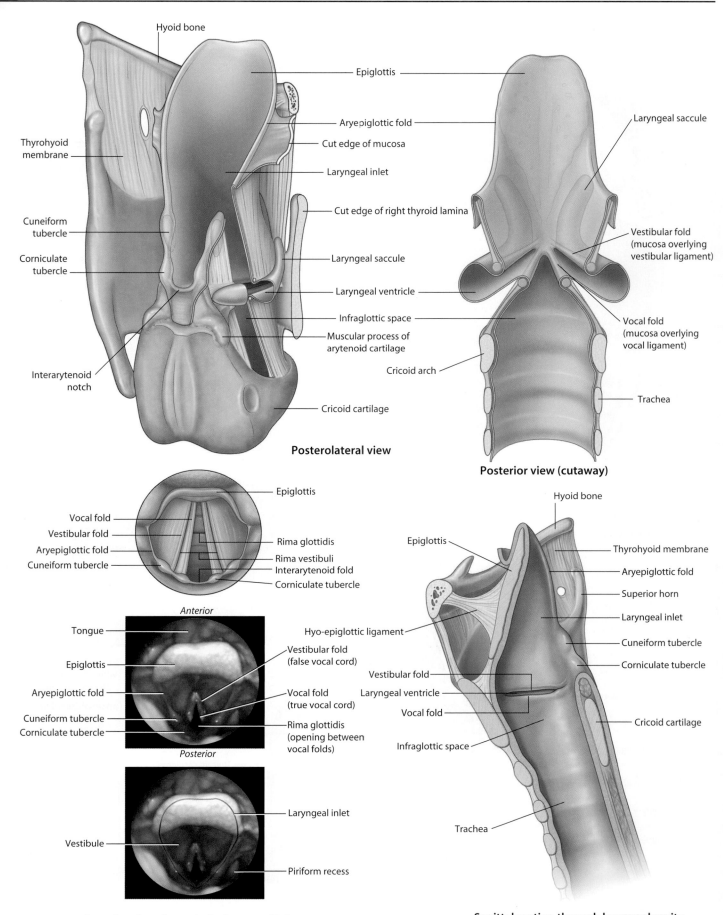

Hyoid bone

Epiglottis

Aryepiglottic fold

Cut edge of mucosa

Laryngeal inlet

Cut edge of right thyroid lamina

Thyrohyoid membrane

Cuneiform tubercle

Corniculate tubercle

Laryngeal saccule

Laryngeal ventricle

Infraglottic space

Muscular process of arytenoid cartilage

Interarytenoid notch

Cricoid cartilage

Posterolateral view

Laryngeal saccule

Vestibular fold (mucosa overlying vestibular ligament)

Vocal fold (mucosa overlying vocal ligament)

Cricoid arch

Trachea

Posterior view (cutaway)

Epiglottis

Vocal fold

Vestibular fold

Aryepiglottic fold

Cuneiform tubercle

Rima glottidis

Rima vestibuli

Interarytenoid fold

Corniculate tubercle

Anterior

Tongue

Epiglottis

Aryepiglottic fold

Cuneiform tubercle

Corniculate tubercle

Vestibular fold (false vocal cord)

Vocal fold (true vocal cord)

Rima glottidis (opening between vocal folds)

Posterior

Vestibule

Laryngeal inlet

Piriform recess

Superior view through the laryngeal inlet

Hyoid bone

Epiglottis

Thyrohyoid membrane

Aryepiglottic fold

Superior horn

Laryngeal inlet

Cuneiform tubercle

Corniculate tubercle

Hyo-epiglottic ligament

Vestibular fold

Laryngeal ventricle

Vocal fold

Infraglottic space

Cricoid cartilage

Trachea

Sagittal section through laryngeal cavity

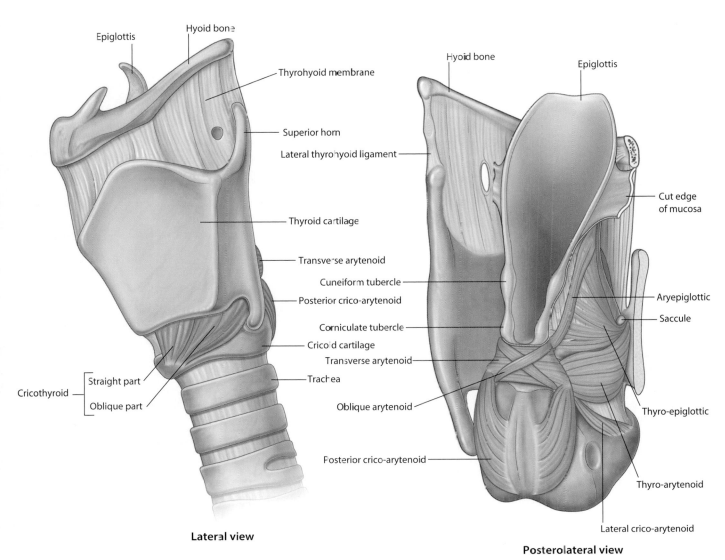

Epiglottis
Hyoid bone
Thyrohyoid membrane
Superior horn
Lateral thyrohyoid ligament
Thyroid cartilage
Transverse arytenoid
Cuneiform tubercle
Posterior crico-arytenoid
Corniculate tubercle
Cricoid cartilage
Transverse arytenoid
Trachea
Cricothyroid
Straight part
Oblique part
Oblique arytenoid
Posterior crico-arytenoid

Lateral view

Hyoid bone
Epiglottis
Cut edge of mucosa
Aryepiglottic
Saccule
Thyro-epiglottic
Thyro-arytenoid
Lateral crico-arytenoid

Posterolateral view

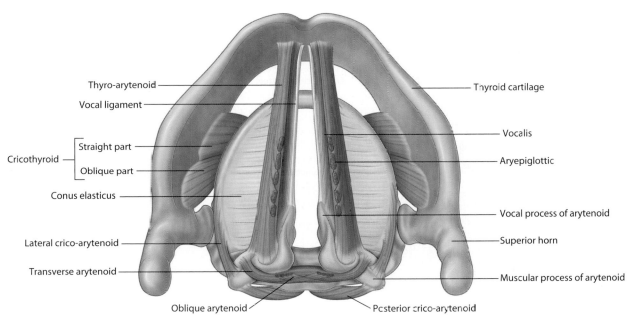

Thyro-arytenoid
Vocal ligament
Cricothyroid
Straight part
Oblique part
Conus elasticus
Lateral crico-arytenoid
Transverse arytenoid
Oblique arytenoid
Posterior crico-arytenoid
Thyroid cartilage
Vocalis
Aryepiglottic
Vocal process of arytenoid
Superior horn
Muscular process of arytenoid

Superior view

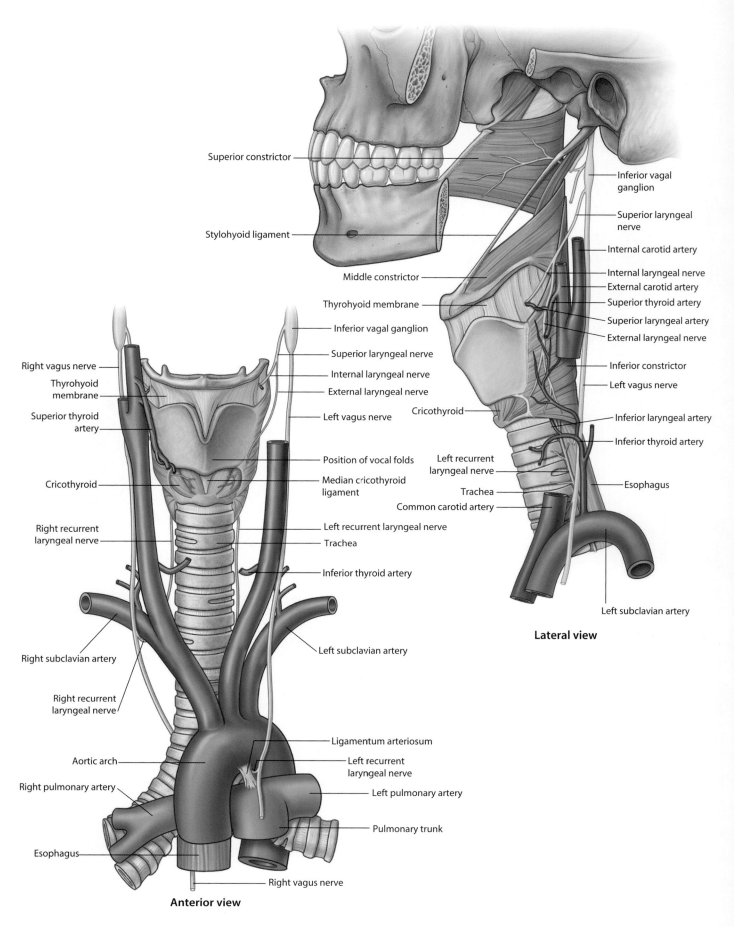

Superior constrictor

Stylohyoid ligament

Middle constrictor

Thyrohyoid membrane

Inferior vagal ganglion

Inferior vagal ganglion

Superior laryngeal nerve

Internal carotid artery

Internal laryngeal nerve

External carotid artery

Superior thyroid artery

Superior laryngeal artery

External laryngeal nerve

Inferior constrictor

Left vagus nerve

Cricothyroid

Inferior laryngeal artery

Inferior thyroid artery

Left recurrent laryngeal nerve

Trachea

Common carotid artery

Esophagus

Left subclavian artery

Lateral view

Right vagus nerve

Thyrohyoid membrane

Superior thyroid artery

Superior laryngeal nerve

Internal laryngeal nerve

External laryngeal nerve

Left vagus nerve

Cricothyroid

Position of vocal folds

Median cricothyroid ligament

Right recurrent laryngeal nerve

Left recurrent laryngeal nerve

Trachea

Inferior thyroid artery

Right subclavian artery

Left subclavian artery

Right recurrent laryngeal nerve

Ligamentum arteriosum

Left recurrent laryngeal nerve

Aortic arch

Right pulmonary artery

Left pulmonary artery

Esophagus

Pulmonary trunk

Right vagus nerve

Anterior view

564

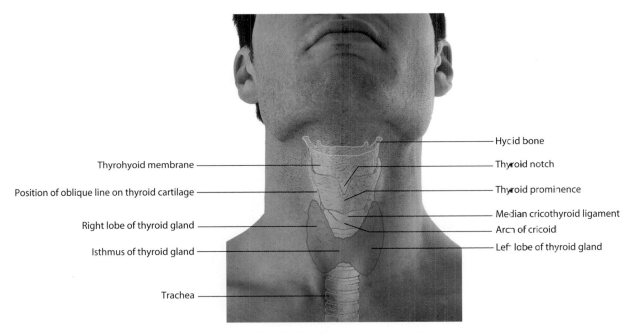

Thyroid gland as it relates to surface

Hyoid bone

Thyrohyoid membrane

Position of oblique line on thyroid cartilage

Right lobe of thyroid gland

Isthmus of thyroid gland

Thyroid notch

Thyroid prominence

Median cricothyroid ligament

Arch of cricoid

Left lobe of thyroid gland

Trachea

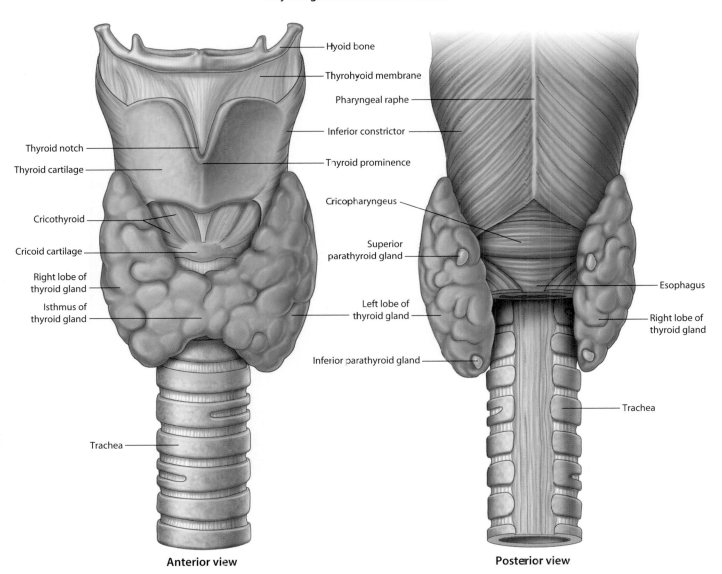

Hyoid bone

Thyrohyoid membrane

Pharyngeal raphe

Inferior constrictor

Thyroid prominence

Thyroid notch

Thyroid cartilage

Cricothyroid

Cricoid cartilage

Right lobe of thyroid gland

Isthmus of thyroid gland

Cricopharyngeus

Superior parathyroid gland

Left lobe of thyroid gland

Inferior parathyroid gland

Esophagus

Right lobe of thyroid gland

Trachea

Trachea

Anterior view

Posterior view

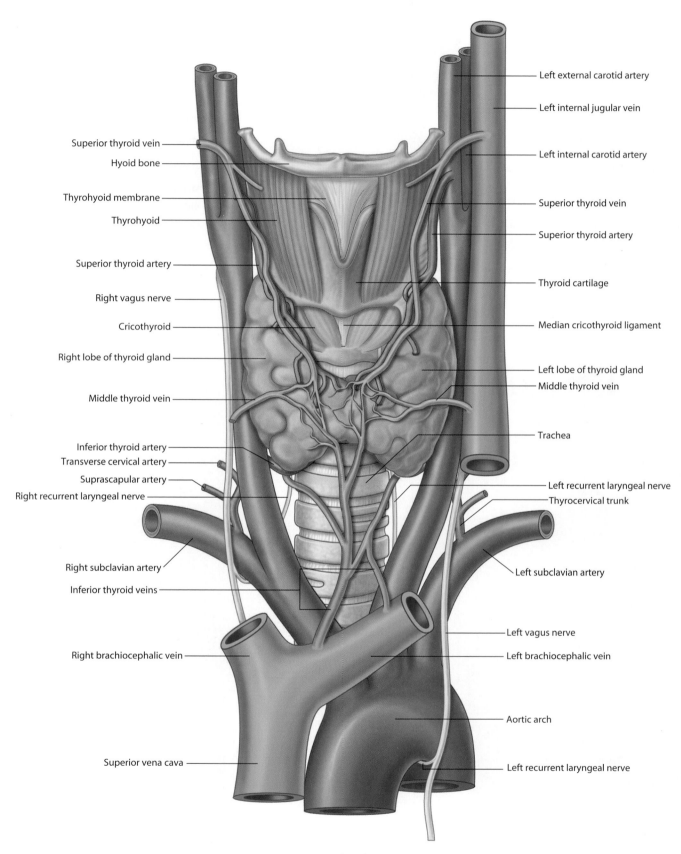

Superior thyroid vein

Hyoid bone

Thyrohyoid membrane

Thyrohyoid

Superior thyroid artery

Right vagus nerve

Cricothyroid

Right lobe of thyroid gland

Middle thyroid vein

Inferior thyroid artery

Transverse cervical artery

Suprascapular artery

Right recurrent laryngeal nerve

Right subclavian artery

Inferior thyroid veins

Right brachiocephalic vein

Superior vena cava

Left external carotid artery

Left internal jugular vein

Left internal carotid artery

Superior thyroid vein

Superior thyroid artery

Thyroid cartilage

Median cricothyroid ligament

Left lobe of thyroid gland

Middle thyroid vein

Trachea

Left recurrent laryngeal nerve

Thyrocervical trunk

Left subclavian artery

Left vagus nerve

Left brachiocephalic vein

Aortic arch

Left recurrent laryngeal nerve

Anterior view

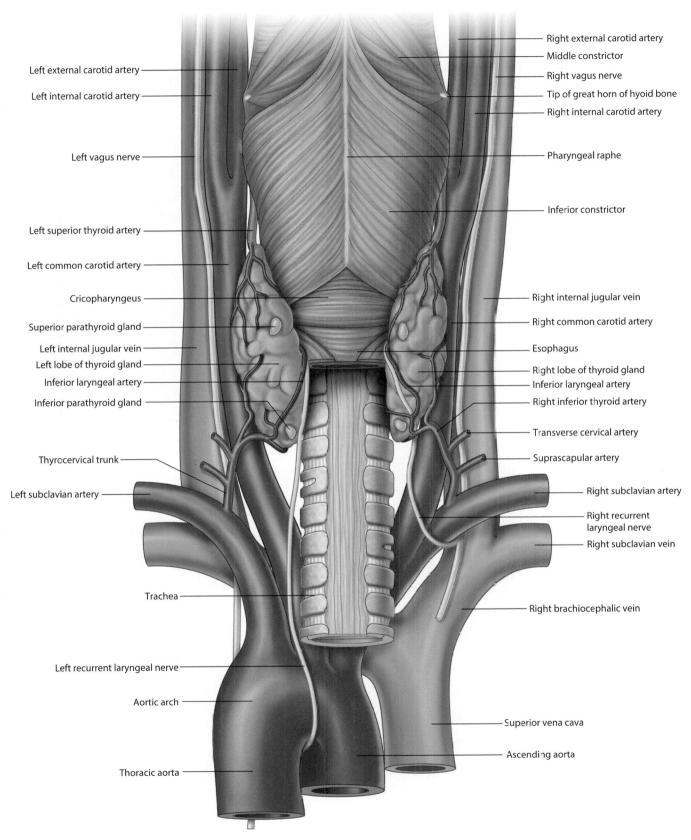

Left external carotid artery

Left internal carotid artery

Left vagus nerve

Left superior thyroid artery

Left common carotid artery

Cricopharyngeus

Superior parathyroid gland

Left internal jugular vein

Left lobe of thyroid gland

Inferior laryngeal artery

Inferior parathyroid gland

Thyrocervical trunk

Left subclavian artery

Trachea

Left recurrent laryngeal nerve

Aortic arch

Thoracic aorta

Right external carotid artery

Middle constrictor

Right vagus nerve

Tip of great horn of hyoid bone

Right internal carotid artery

Pharyngeal raphe

Inferior constrictor

Right internal jugular vein

Right common carotid artery

Esophagus

Right lobe of thyroid gland

Inferior laryngeal artery

Right inferior thyroid artery

Transverse cervical artery

Suprascapular artery

Right subclavian artery

Right recurrent laryngeal nerve

Right subclavian vein

Right brachiocephalic vein

Superior vena cava

Ascending aorta

Posterior view

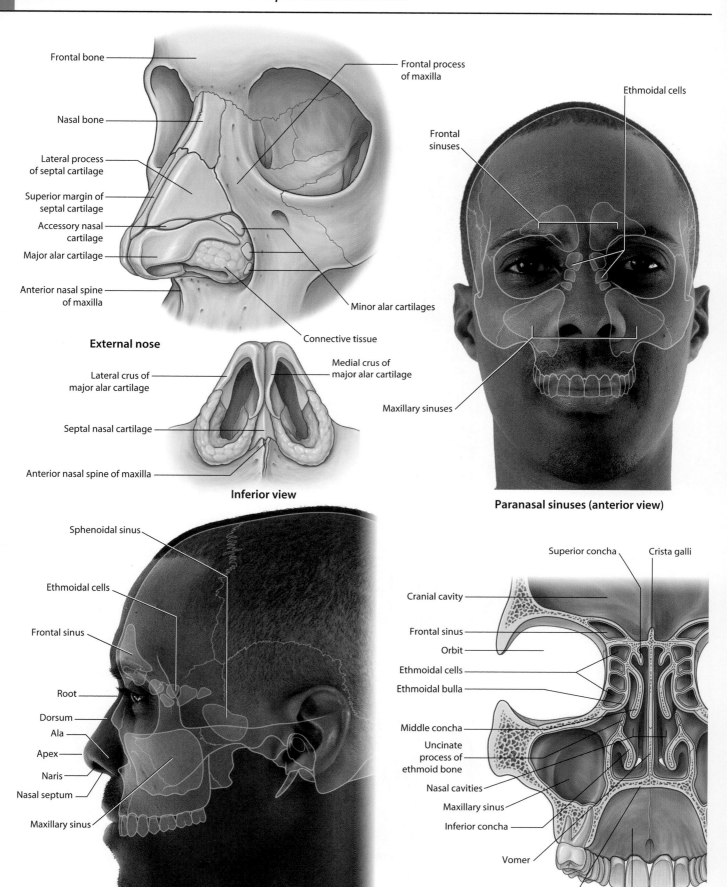

Frontal bone

Frontal process of maxilla

Ethmoidal cells

Nasal bone

Frontal sinuses

Lateral process of septal cartilage

Superior margin of septal cartilage

Accessory nasal cartilage

Major alar cartilage

Anterior nasal spine of maxilla

Minor alar cartilages

Connective tissue

Maxillary sinuses

External nose

Lateral crus of major alar cartilage

Medial crus of major alar cartilage

Septal nasal cartilage

Anterior nasal spine of maxilla

Inferior view

Paranasal sinuses (anterior view)

Sphenoidal sinus

Superior concha

Crista galli

Ethmoidal cells

Cranial cavity

Frontal sinus

Frontal sinus

Orbit

Root

Ethmoidal cells

Dorsum

Ethmoidal bulla

Ala

Middle concha

Apex

Uncinate process of ethmoid bone

Naris

Nasal septum

Nasal cavities

Maxillary sinus

Maxillary sinus

Inferior concha

Vomer

Palatine process of maxillary bone

Oral cavity

Surface anatomy of nose and paranasal sinuses (lateral view)

Coronal section through nasal cavity (posterior view)

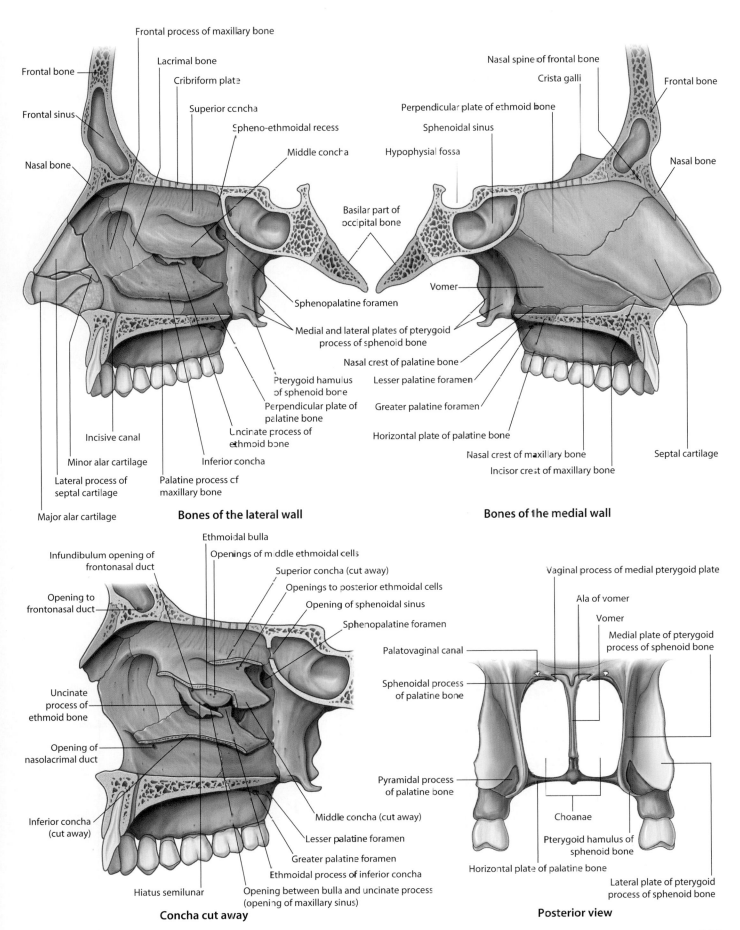

Bones of the lateral wall

Frontal bone
Frontal sinus
Nasal bone
Frontal process of maxillary bone
Lacrimal bone
Cribriform plate
Superior concha
Spheno-ethmoidal recess
Middle concha
Basilar part of occipital bone
Sphenopalatine foramen
Medial and lateral plates of pterygoid process of sphenoid bone
Pterygoid hamulus of sphenoid bone
Perpendicular plate of palatine bone
Uncinate process of ethmoid bone
Inferior concha
Palatine process of maxillary bone
Incisive canal
Minor alar cartilage
Lateral process of septal cartilage
Major alar cartilage

Bones of the medial wall

Nasal spine of frontal bone
Crista galli
Perpendicular plate of ethmoid bone
Sphenoidal sinus
Hypophysial fossa
Frontal bone
Nasal bone
Vomer
Nasal crest of palatine bone
Lesser palatine foramen
Greater palatine foramen
Horizontal plate of palatine bone
Nasal crest of maxillary bone
Incisor crest of maxillary bone
Septal cartilage

Concha cut away

Infundibulum opening of frontonasal duct
Ethmoidal bulla
Openings of middle ethmoidal cells
Superior concha (cut away)
Openings to posterior ethmoidal cells
Opening of sphenoidal sinus
Sphenopalatine foramen
Opening to frontonasal duct
Uncinate process of ethmoid bone
Opening of nasolacrimal duct
Inferior concha (cut away)
Hiatus semilunar
Middle concha (cut away)
Lesser palatine foramen
Greater palatine foramen
Ethmoidal process of inferior concha
Opening between bulla and uncinate process (opening of maxillary sinus)

Posterior view

Vaginal process of medial pterygoid plate
Ala of vomer
Vomer
Medial plate of pterygoid process of sphenoid bone
Palatovaginal canal
Sphenoidal process of palatine bone
Pyramidal process of palatine bone
Choanae
Pterygoid hamulus of sphenoid bone
Horizontal plate of palatine bone
Lateral plate of pterygoid process of sphenoid bone

569

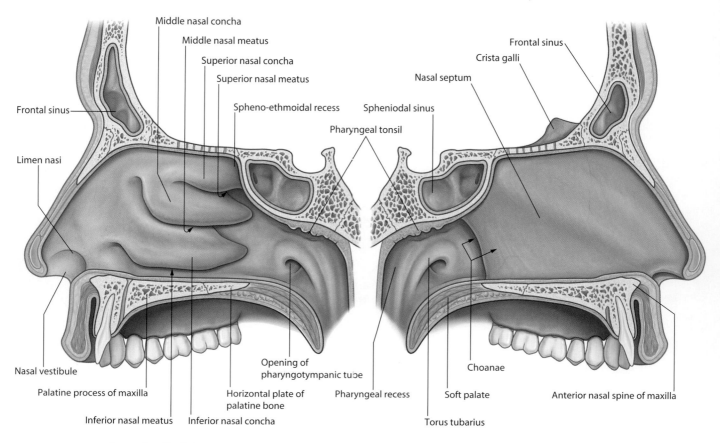

Middle nasal concha
Middle nasal meatus
Superior nasal concha
Superior nasal meatus
Spheno-ethmoidal recess
Pharyngeal tonsil
Frontal sinus
Limen nasi
Spheniodal sinus

Nasal vestibule
Palatine process of maxilla
Inferior nasal meatus
Inferior nasal concha
Horizontal plate of palatine bone
Opening of pharyngotympanic tube

Lateral wall of the nasal cavity

Frontal sinus
Crista galli
Nasal septum

Choanae
Soft palate
Torus tubarius
Pharyngeal recess
Anterior nasal spine of maxilla

Medial wall of the nasal cavity

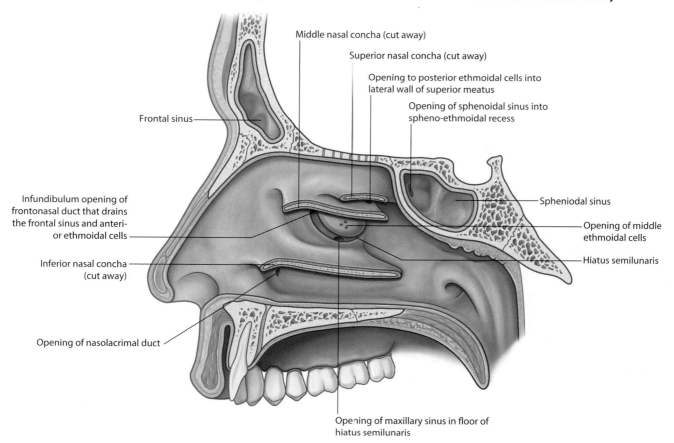

Middle nasal concha (cut away)
Superior nasal concha (cut away)
Opening to posterior ethmoidal cells into lateral wall of superior meatus
Opening of sphenoidal sinus into spheno-ethmoidal recess
Frontal sinus

Infundibulum opening of frontonasal duct that drains the frontal sinus and anterior ethmoidal cells
Inferior nasal concha (cut away)
Opening of nasolacrimal duct
Spheniodal sinus
Opening of middle ethmoidal cells
Hiatus semilunaris

Opening of maxillary sinus in floor of hiatus semilunaris

Lateral wall of the nasal cavity, concha cut away

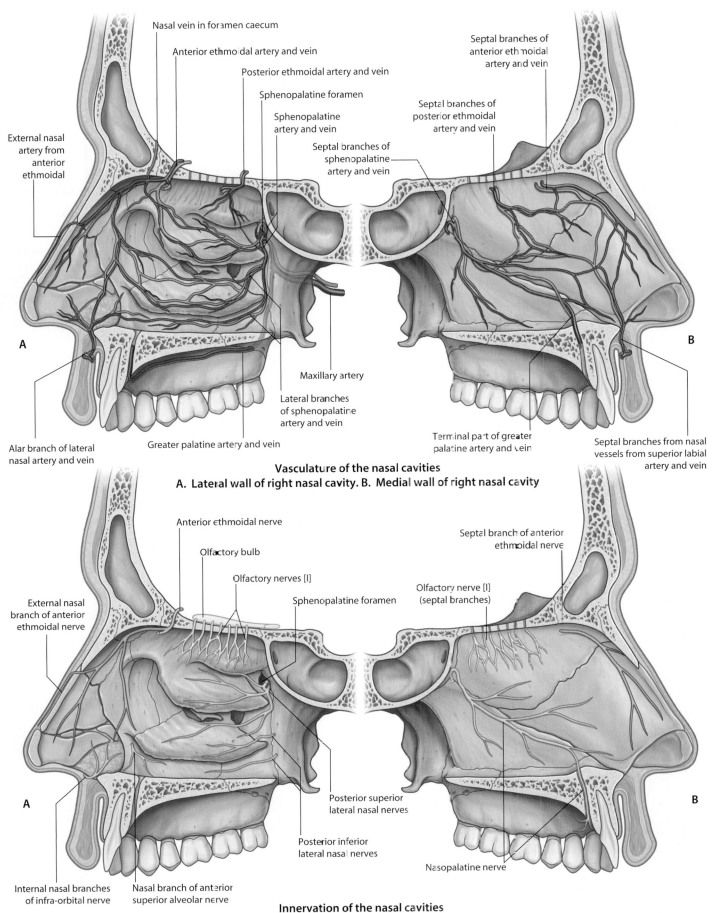

Nasal vein in foramen caecum

Anterior ethmoidal artery and vein

Posterior ethmoidal artery and vein

Sphenopalatine foramen

Sphenopalatine artery and vein

Septal branches of anterior ethmoidal artery and vein

Septal branches of posterior ethmoidal artery and vein

Septal branches of sphenopalatine artery and vein

External nasal artery from anterior ethmoidal

Maxillary artery

Lateral branches of sphenopalatine artery and vein

Alar branch of lateral nasal artery and vein

Greater palatine artery and vein

Terminal part of greater palatine artery and vein

Septal branches from nasal vessels from superior labial artery and vein

A

B

Vasculature of the nasal cavities
A. Lateral wall of right nasal cavity. B. Medial wall of right nasal cavity

Anterior ethmoidal nerve

Olfactory bulb

Olfactory nerves [I]

Sphenopalatine foramen

Septal branch of anterior ethmoidal nerve

Olfactory nerve [I] (septal branches)

External nasal branch of anterior ethmoidal nerve

Posterior superior lateral nasal nerves

Posterior inferior lateral nasal nerves

Nasopalatine nerve

Internal nasal branches of infra-orbital nerve

Nasal branch of anterior superior alveolar nerve

A

B

Innervation of the nasal cavities
A. Lateral wall of right nasal cavity. B. Medial wall of right nasal cavity

571

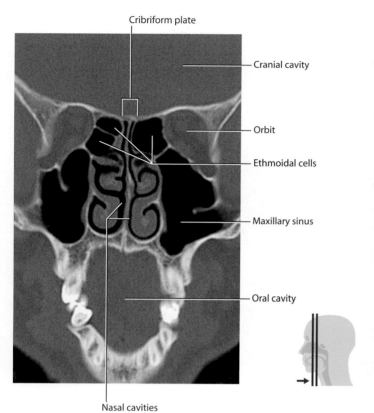

Cribriform plate

Cranial cavity

Orbit

Ethmoidal cells

Maxillary sinus

Oral cavity

Nasal cavities

Anterior view of the maxillary sinus and ethmoidal cells.
CT image in coronal plane

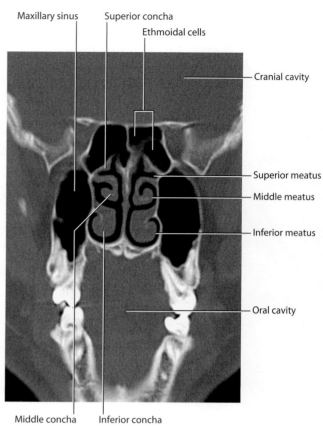

Maxillary sinus

Superior concha

Ethmoidal cells

Cranial cavity

Superior meatus

Middle meatus

Inferior meatus

Oral cavity

Middle concha

Inferior concha

Anterior view looking into the nasal cavity showing the relationship of various structures.
CT image in coronal plane

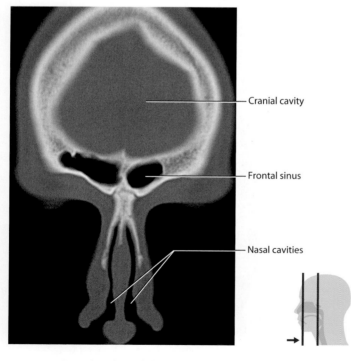

Cranial cavity

Frontal sinus

Nasal cavities

Anterior view of the frontal sinuses.
CT image in coronal plane

Cranial cavity

Sphenoidal sinuses

Nasal cavities

Anterior view of the sphenoidal sinuses showing their relationship to the nasal cavity.
CT image in coronal plane

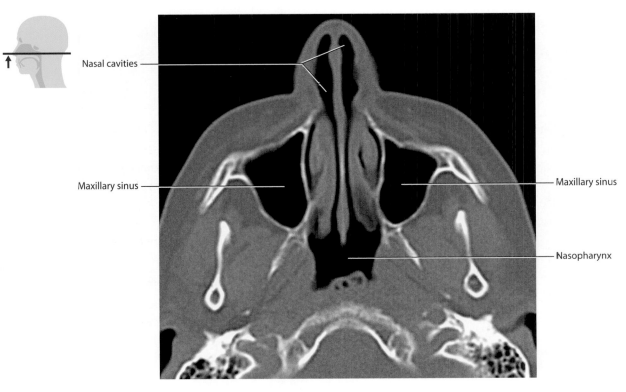

Nasal cavities

Maxillary sinus

Maxillary sinus

Nasopharynx

Axial section showing the relationship between the nasal cavity, nasopharynx, and maxillary sinuses.
CT image in axial plane

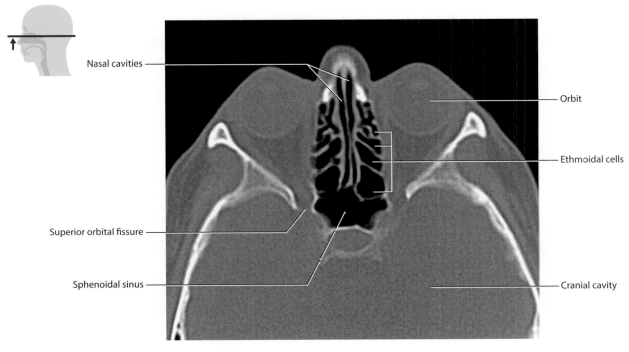

Nasal cavities

Orbit

Ethmoidal cells

Superior orbital fissure

Sphenoidal sinus

Cranial cavity

Axial section showing the ethmoidal cells and the sphenoidal sinuses and the relationship of these structures to the orbit.
CT image in axial plane

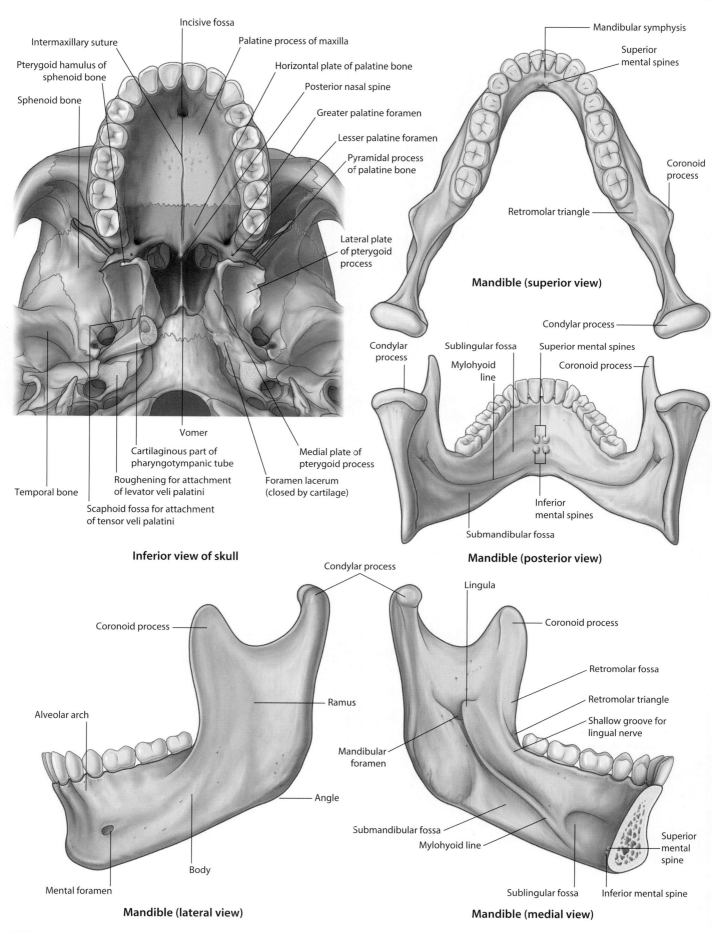

Incisive fossa

Intermaxillary suture

Pterygoid hamulus of sphenoid bone

Sphenoid bone

Palatine process of maxilla

Horizontal plate of palatine bone

Posterior nasal spine

Greater palatine foramen

Lesser palatine foramen

Pyramidal process of palatine bone

Lateral plate of pterygoid process

Vomer

Cartilaginous part of pharyngotympanic tube

Roughening for attachment of levator veli palatini

Temporal bone

Scaphoid fossa for attachment of tensor veli palatini

Medial plate of pterygoid process

Foramen lacerum (closed by cartilage)

Inferior view of skull

Mandibular symphysis

Superior mental spines

Coronoid process

Retromolar triangle

Condylar process

Mandible (superior view)

Condylar process

Sublingular fossa

Mylohyoid line

Superior mental spines

Coronoid process

Inferior mental spines

Submandibular fossa

Mandible (posterior view)

Condylar process

Coronoid process

Alveolar arch

Ramus

Angle

Mental foramen

Body

Mandible (lateral view)

Lingula

Coronoid process

Retromolar fossa

Retromolar triangle

Shallow groove for lingual nerve

Mandibular foramen

Submandibular fossa

Mylohyoid line

Sublingular fossa

Superior mental spine

Inferior mental spine

Mandible (medial view)

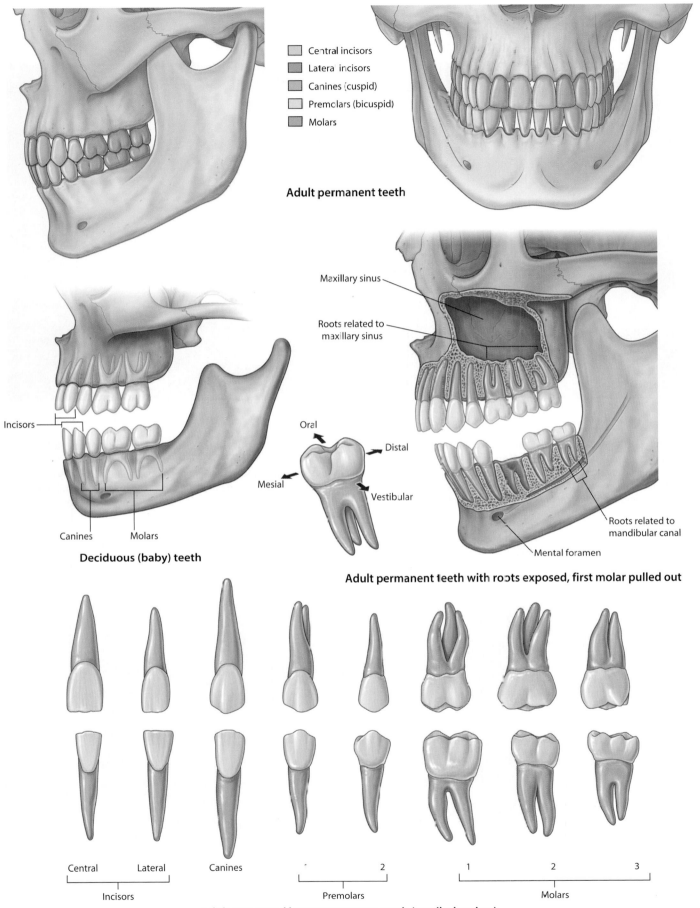

Central incisors
Lateral incisors
Canines (cuspid)
Premolars (bicuspid)
Molars

Adult permanent teeth

Maxillary sinus

Roots related to maxillary sinus

Incisors

Oral

Distal

Mesial

Vestibular

Canines Molars

Deciduous (baby) teeth

Roots related to mandibular canal

Mental foramen

Adult permanent teeth with roots exposed, first molar pulled out

Central Lateral Canines 2 1 2 3

Incisors Premolars Molars

Adult upper and lower permanent teeth (vestibular view)

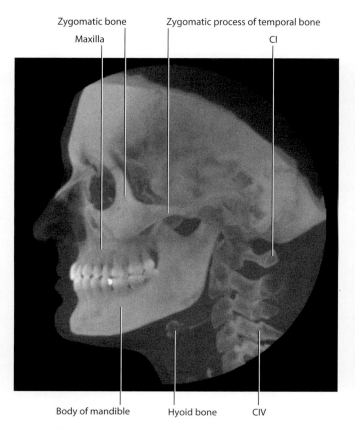

Zygomatic bone
Maxilla
Zygomatic process of temporal bone
CI

Body of mandible
Hyoid bone
CIV

View of the left side of the face showing the craniofacial structures including the teeth.
Image taken with Cone Beam Computerized Tomography (CBCT) technology, viewed in the Maximum Intensity Projection (MIP) mode, which combines a radiographic view with a view of surface structures

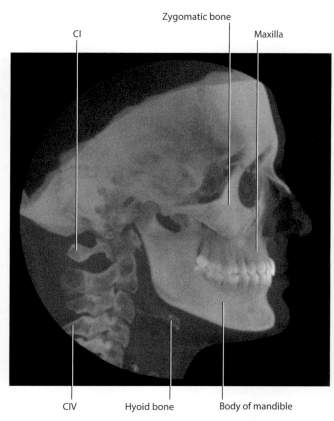

CI
Zygomatic bone
Maxilla

CIV
Hyoid bone
Body of mandible

View of the right side of the face showing the craniofacial structures including the teeth.
Image taken with Cone Beam Computerized Tomography (CBCT) technology, viewed in the Maximum Intensity Projection (MIP) mode, which combines a radiographic view with a view of surface structures

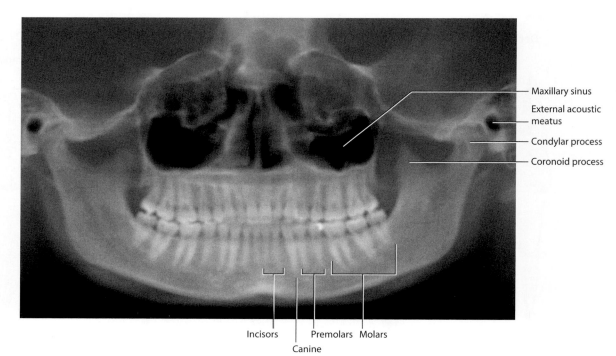

Maxillary sinus
External acoustic meatus
Condylar process
Coronoid process

Incisors
Canine
Premolars Molars

Panoramic view of the teeth (dentition), which also shows the maxillary sinuses and mandibular condylar processes.
Image taken with Cone Beam Computerized Tomography (CBCT) technology

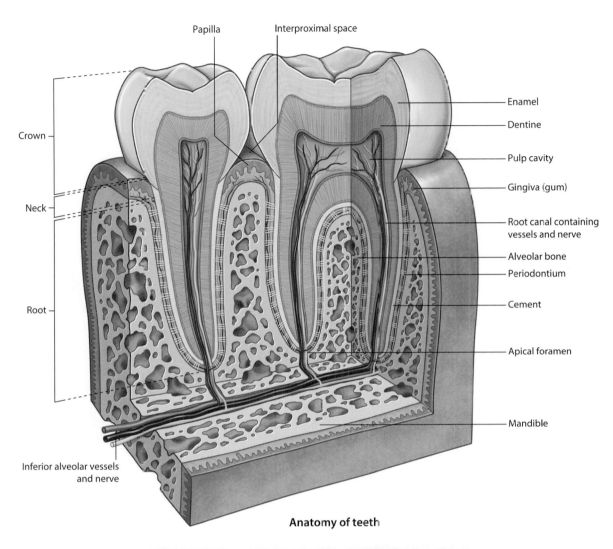

Anatomy of teeth

Papilla

Interproximal space

Crown

Neck

Root

Enamel

Dentine

Pulp cavity

Gingiva (gum)

Root canal containing vessels and nerve

Alveolar bone

Periodontium

Cement

Apical foramen

Mandible

Inferior alveolar vessels and nerve

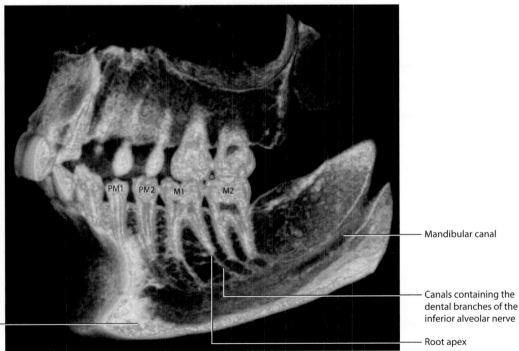

Inside, lingual or sagittal view of the right side of the maxillary and mandibular alveolar processes in occlusion (teeth together).
Image taken with Cone Beam Computerized Tomography (CBCT) technology viewed in the surface mode

PM1   PM 2   M1   M2

Mandibular canal

Canals containing the dental branches of the inferior alveolar nerve

Root apex

Mandible

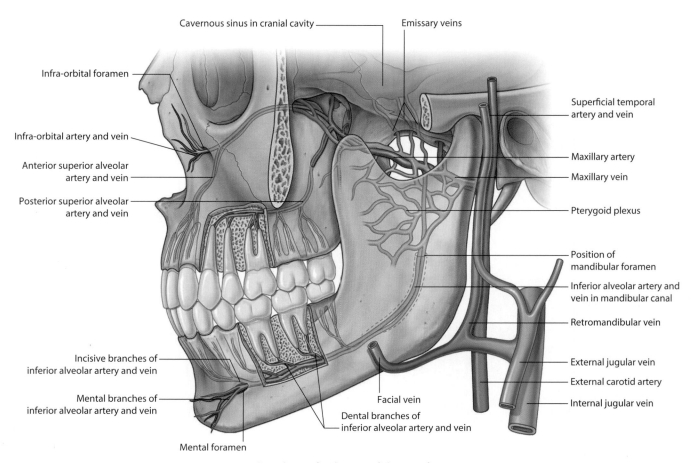

Cavernous sinus in cranial cavity

Emissary veins

Infra-orbital foramen

Infra-orbital artery and vein

Anterior superior alveolar artery and vein

Posterior superior alveolar artery and vein

Superficial temporal artery and vein

Maxillary artery

Maxillary vein

Pterygoid plexus

Position of mandibular foramen

Inferior alveolar artery and vein in mandibular canal

Retromandibular vein

Incisive branches of inferior alveolar artery and vein

Mental branches of inferior alveolar artery and vein

External jugular vein

External carotid artery

Internal jugular vein

Facial vein

Dental branches of inferior alveolar artery and vein

Mental foramen

Arteries and veins supplying teeth

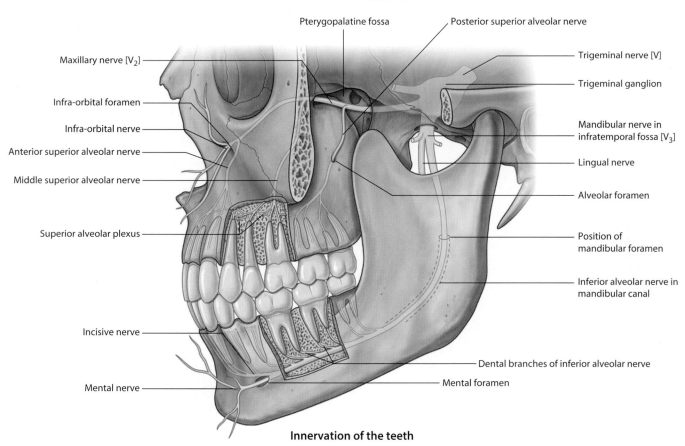

Pterygopalatine fossa

Posterior superior alveolar nerve

Maxillary nerve [V₂]

Infra-orbital foramen

Infra-orbital nerve

Anterior superior alveolar nerve

Middle superior alveolar nerve

Superior alveolar plexus

Trigeminal nerve [V]

Trigeminal ganglion

Mandibular nerve in infratemporal fossa [V₃]

Lingual nerve

Alveolar foramen

Position of mandibular foramen

Inferior alveolar nerve in mandibular canal

Incisive nerve

Mental nerve

Dental branches of inferior alveolar nerve

Mental foramen

Innervation of the teeth

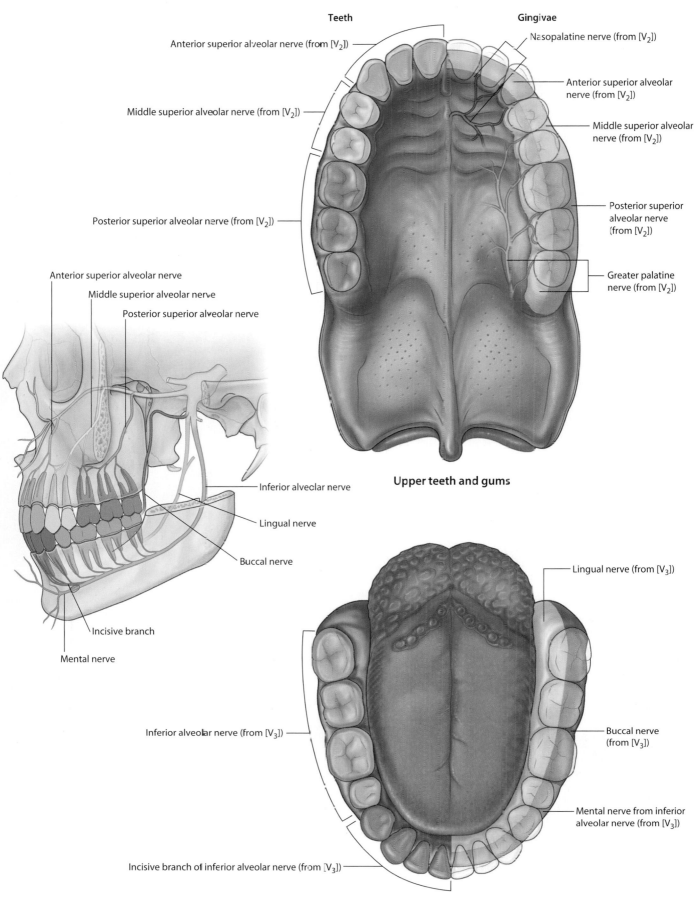

Teeth   **Gingivae**

Anterior superior alveolar nerve (from [V₂])

Nasopalatine nerve (from [V₂])

Middle superior alveolar nerve (from [V₂])

Anterior superior alveolar nerve (from [V₂])

Middle superior alveolar nerve (from [V₂])

Posterior superior alveolar nerve (from [V₂])

Posterior superior alveolar nerve (from [V₂])

Greater palatine nerve (from [V₂])

Anterior superior alveolar nerve

Middle superior alveolar nerve

Posterior superior alveolar nerve

Inferior alveolar nerve

Lingual nerve

Buccal nerve

Incisive branch

Mental nerve

Upper teeth and gums

Lingual nerve (from [V₃])

Inferior alveolar nerve (from [V₃])

Buccal nerve (from [V₃])

Mental nerve from inferior alveolar nerve (from [V₃])

Incisive branch of inferior alveolar nerve (from [V₃])

Lower teeth and gums

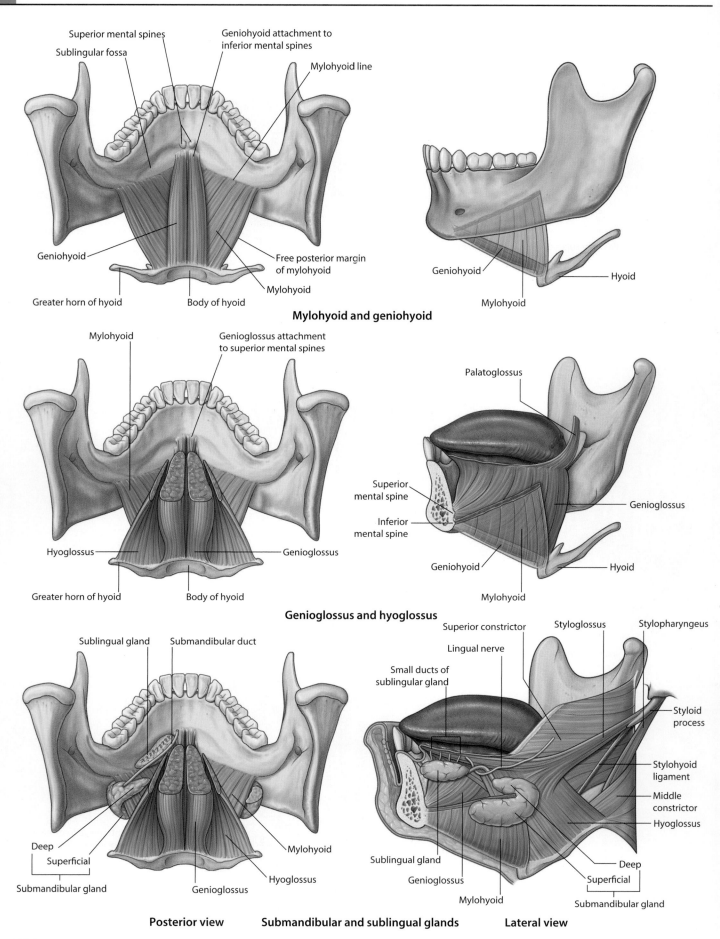

Superior mental spines
Sublingular fossa
Geniohyoid attachment to inferior mental spines
Mylohyoid line
Geniohyoid
Free posterior margin of mylohyoid
Mylohyoid
Greater horn of hyoid
Body of hyoid
Geniohyoid
Mylohyoid
Hyoid

Mylohyoid and geniohyoid

Mylohyoid
Genioglossus attachment to superior mental spines
Palatoglossus
Superior mental spine
Inferior mental spine
Genioglossus
Geniohyoid
Hyoid
Mylohyoid
Hyoglossus
Genioglossus
Greater horn of hyoid
Body of hyoid

Genioglossus and hyoglossus

Sublingual gland
Submandibular duct
Superior constrictor
Styloglossus
Stylopharyngeus
Lingual nerve
Small ducts of sublingual gland
Styloid process
Stylohyoid ligament
Middle constrictor
Hyoglossus
Deep
Superficial
Submandibular gland
Sublingual gland
Mylohyoid
Hyoglossus
Genioglossus
Deep
Superficial
Genioglossus
Mylohyoid
Submandibular gland

Posterior view   **Submandibular and sublingual glands**   **Lateral view**

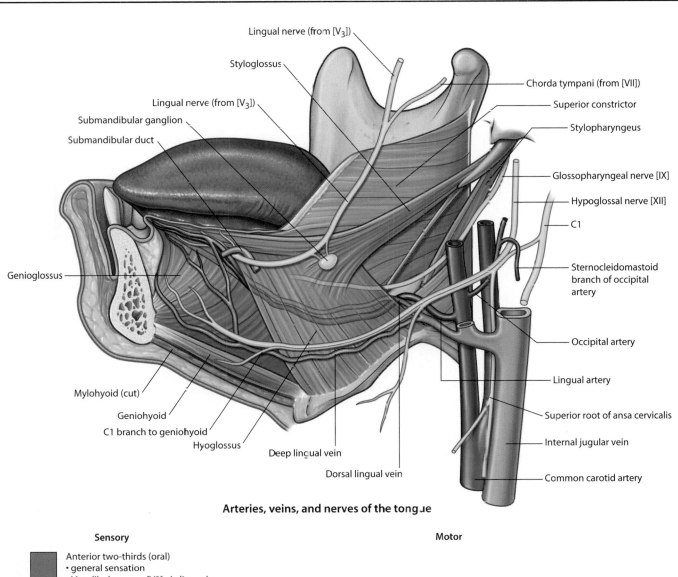

Lingual nerve (from [V₃])

Styloglossus

Lingual nerve (from [V₃])

Submandibular ganglion

Submandibular duct

Genioglossus

Mylohyoid (cut)

Geniohyoid

C1 branch to geniohyoid

Hyoglossus

Deep lingual vein

Dorsal lingual vein

Chorda tympani (from [VII])

Superior constrictor

Stylopharyngeus

Glossopharyngeal nerve [IX]

Hypoglossal nerve [XII]

C1

Sternocleidomastoid branch of occipital artery

Occipital artery

Lingual artery

Superior root of ansa cervicalis

Internal jugular vein

Common carotid artery

Arteries, veins, and nerves of the tongue

Sensory

Anterior two-thirds (oral)
• general sensation
  Mandibular nerve [V3] via lingual nerve
• special sensation (taste)
  Facial nerve [VII] via chorda tympani

Posterior one-third (pharyngeal)
• general and special sensation (taste)
  Glossopharyngeal nerve [IX]

Motor

Palatoglossus – vagus nerve [X]

Styloglossus – hyoglossal nerve [XII]

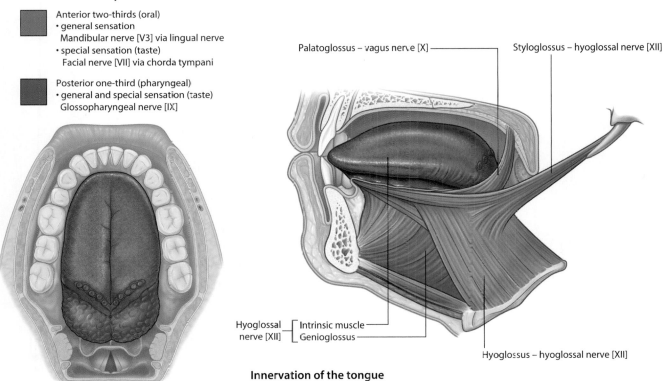

Hyoglossal nerve [XII]

Intrinsic muscle

Genioglossus

Hyoglossus – hyoglossal nerve [XII]

Innervation of the tongue

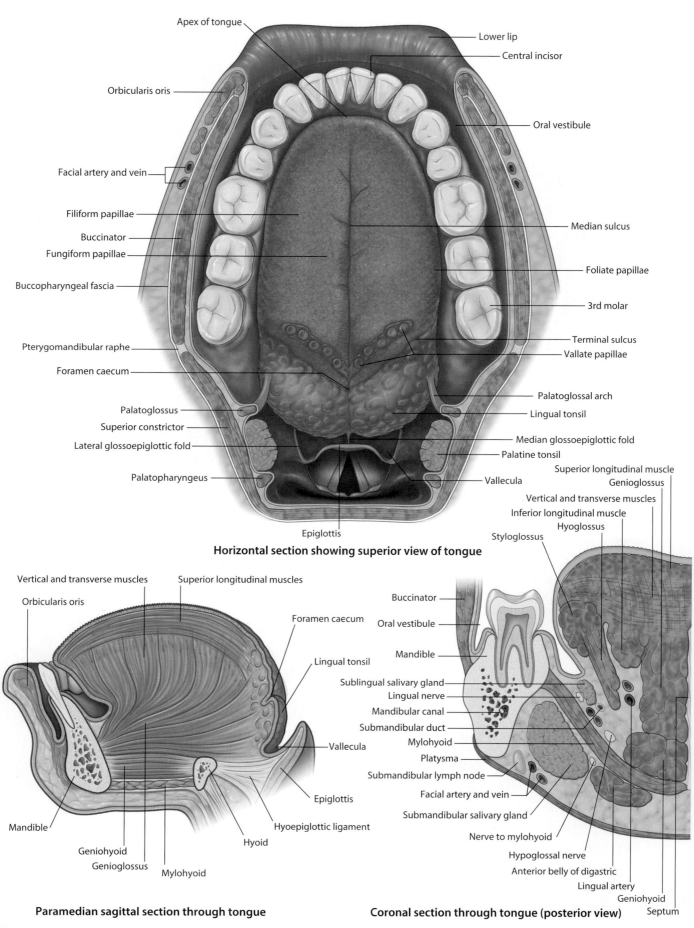

Horizontal section showing superior view of tongue

Apex of tongue

Lower lip

Central incisor

Orbicularis oris

Oral vestibule

Facial artery and vein

Median sulcus

Filiform papillae

Buccinator

Foliate papillae

Fungiform papillae

Buccopharyngeal fascia

3rd molar

Terminal sulcus

Pterygomandibular raphe

Vallate papillae

Foramen caecum

Palatoglossal arch

Palatoglossus

Lingual tonsil

Superior constrictor

Median glossoepiglottic fold

Lateral glossoepiglottic fold

Palatine tonsil

Palatopharyngeus

Vallecula

Superior longitudinal muscle

Genioglossus

Vertical and transverse muscles

Inferior longitudinal muscle

Hyoglossus

Styloglossus

Epiglottis

Paramedian sagittal section through tongue

Vertical and transverse muscles

Superior longitudinal muscles

Orbicularis oris

Foramen caecum

Lingual tonsil

Vallecula

Epiglottis

Mandible

Hyoepiglottic ligament

Geniohyoid

Hyoid

Genioglossus

Mylohyoid

Coronal section through tongue (posterior view)

Buccinator

Oral vestibule

Mandible

Sublingual salivary gland

Lingual nerve

Mandibular canal

Submandibular duct

Mylohyoid

Platysma

Submandibular lymph node

Facial artery and vein

Submandibular salivary gland

Nerve to mylohyoid

Hypoglossal nerve

Anterior belly of digastric

Lingual artery

Geniohyoid

Septum

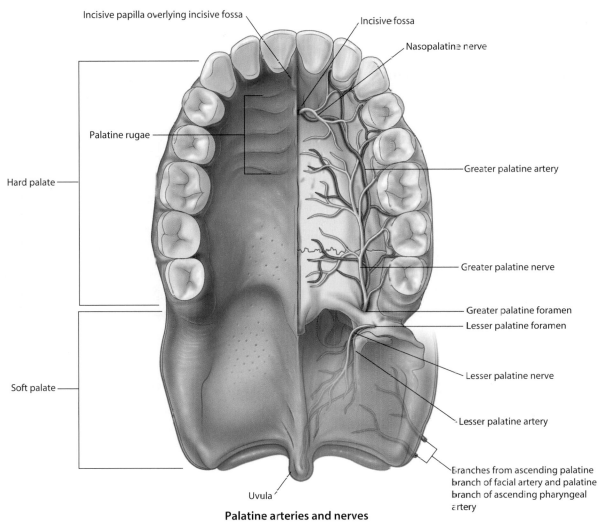

Incisive papilla overlying incisive fossa

Incisive fossa

Nasopalatine nerve

Palatine rugae

Hard palate

Greater palatine artery

Greater palatine nerve

Greater palatine foramen

Lesser palatine foramen

Soft palate

Lesser palatine nerve

Lesser palatine artery

Branches from ascending palatine branch of facial artery and palatine branch of ascending pharyngeal artery

Uvula

Palatine arteries and nerves

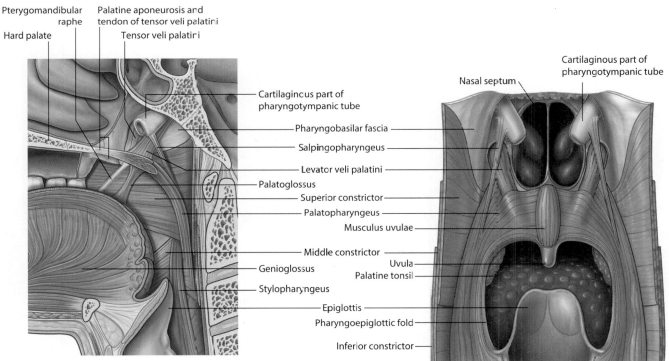

Pterygomandibular raphe

Palatine aponeurosis and tendon of tensor veli palatini

Hard palate

Tensor veli palatini

Cartilaginous part of pharyngotympanic tube

Nasal septum

Cartilaginous part of pharyngotympanic tube

Cartilaginous part of pharyngotympanic tube

Pharyngobasilar fascia

Salpingopharyngeus

Levator veli palatini

Palatoglossus

Superior constrictor

Palatopharyngeus

Musculus uvulae

Middle constrictor

Genioglossus

Uvula

Palatine tonsil

Stylopharyngeus

Epiglottis

Pharyngoepiglottic fold

Inferior constrictor

Muscles of the soft palate (sagittal section)

Muscles of the soft palate (posterior view)

583

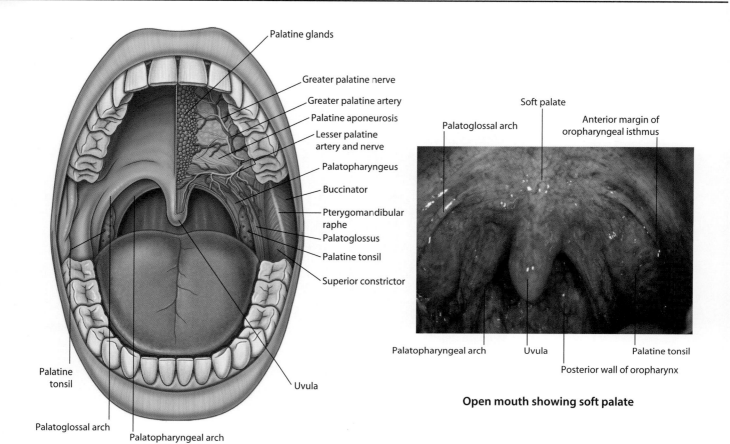

Palatine glands

Greater palatine nerve

Greater palatine artery

Palatine aponeurosis

Lesser palatine artery and nerve

Palatopharyngeus

Buccinator

Pterygomandibular raphe

Palatoglossus

Palatine tonsil

Superior constrictor

Palatine tonsil

Palatoglossal arch

Palatopharyngeal arch

Uvula

Roof of oral cavity

Soft palate

Palatoglossal arch

Anterior margin of oropharyngeal isthmus

Palatopharyngeal arch

Uvula

Palatine tonsil

Posterior wall of oropharynx

Open mouth showing soft palate

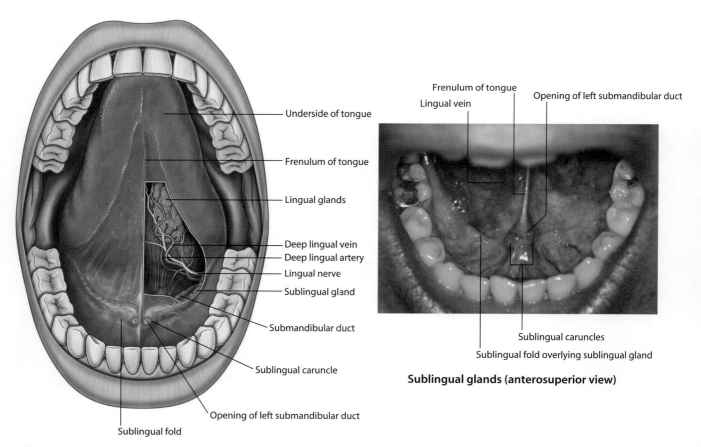

Underside of tongue

Frenulum of tongue

Lingual glands

Deep lingual vein

Deep lingual artery

Lingual nerve

Sublingual gland

Submandibular duct

Sublingual caruncle

Opening of left submandibular duct

Sublingual fold

Inferior surface of tongue and floor of oral cavity

Frenulum of tongue

Lingual vein

Opening of left submandibular duct

Sublingual caruncles

Sublingual fold overlying sublingual gland

Sublingual glands (anterosuperior view)

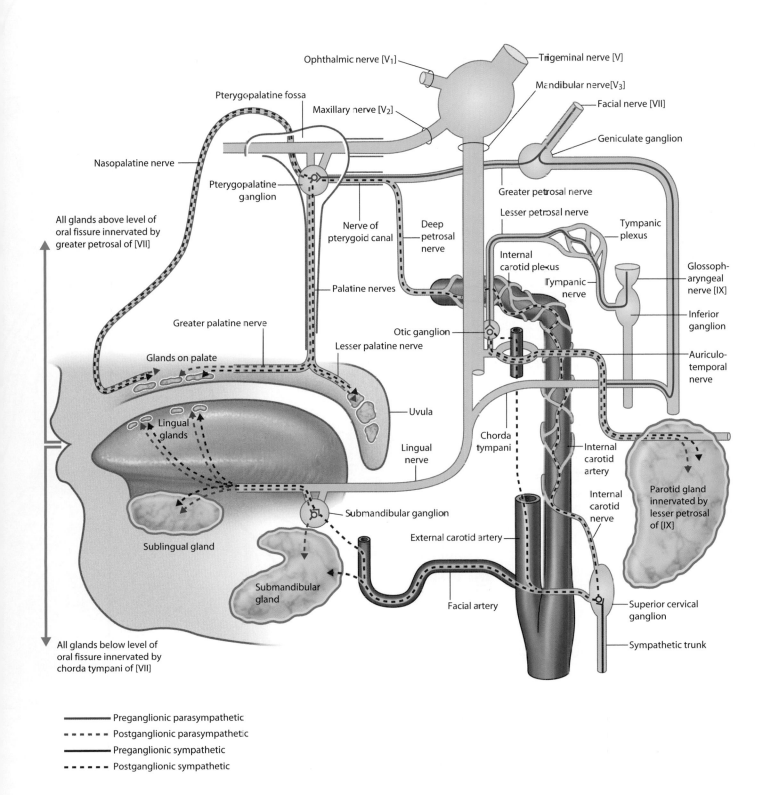

Ophthalmic nerve [V₁]

Trigeminal nerve [V]

Pterygopalatine fossa

Mandibular nerve[V₃]

Maxillary nerve [V₂]

Facial nerve [VII]

Nasopalatine nerve

Geniculate ganglion

Pterygopalatine ganglion

Greater petrosal nerve

Lesser petrosal nerve

All glands above level of oral fissure innervated by greater petrosal of [VII]

Nerve of pterygoid canal

Deep petrosal nerve

Tympanic plexus

Internal carotid plexus

Tympanic nerve

Glossoph-aryngeal nerve [IX]

Palatine nerves

Inferior ganglion

Greater palatine nerve

Otic ganglion

Lesser palatine nerve

Auriculo-temporal nerve

Glands on palate

Lingual glands

Uvula

Lingual nerve

Chorda tympani

Internal carotid artery

Sublingual gland

Submandibular ganglion

Internal carotid nerve

Parotid gland innervated by lesser petrosal of [IX]

External carotid artery

Submandibular gland

Facial artery

Superior cervical ganglion

All glands below level of oral fissure innervated by chorda tympani of [VII]

Sympathetic trunk

———— Preganglionic parasympathetic

- - - - - Postganglionic parasympathetic

———— Preganglionic sympathetic

- - - - - Postganglionic sympathetic

Visceral efferent (motor) innervation of glands related to the oral cavity

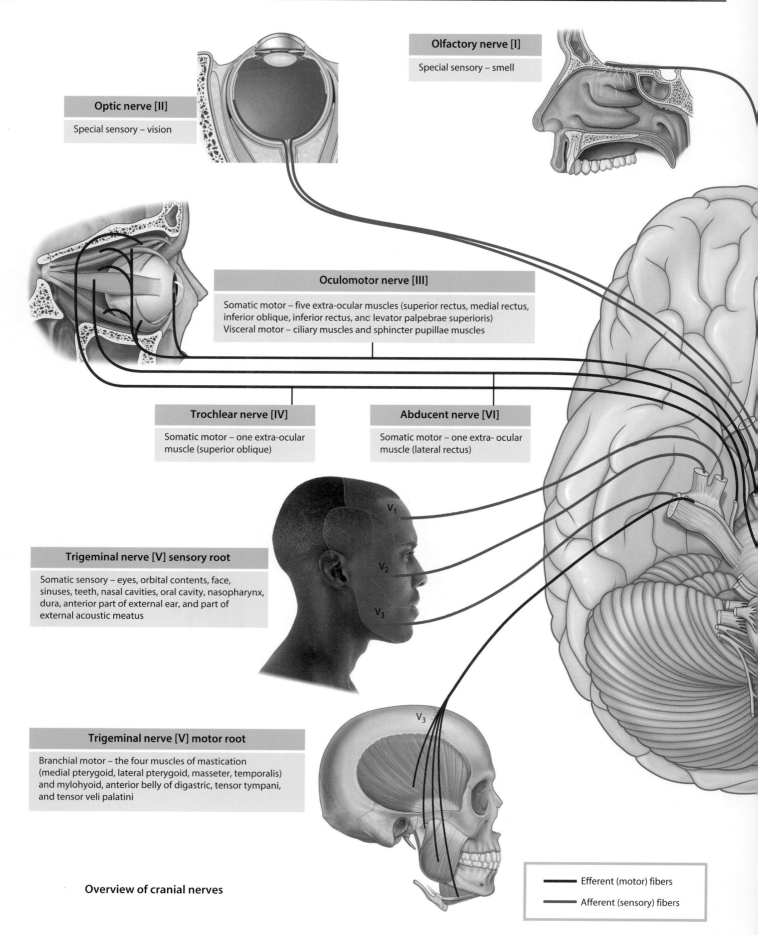

Optic nerve [II]

Special sensory – vision

Olfactory nerve [I]

Special sensory – smell

Oculomotor nerve [III]

Somatic motor – five extra-ocular muscles (superior rectus, medial rectus, inferior oblique, inferior rectus, anc levator palpebrae superioris)
Visceral motor – ciliary muscles and sphincter pupillae muscles

Trochlear nerve [IV]

Somatic motor – one extra-ocular muscle (superior oblique)

Abducent nerve [VI]

Somatic motor – one extra- ocular muscle (lateral rectus)

Trigeminal nerve [V] sensory root

Somatic sensory – eyes, orbital contents, face, sinuses, teeth, nasal cavities, oral cavity, nasopharynx, dura, anterior part of external ear, and part of external acoustic meatus

V_1

V_2

V_3

V_3

Trigeminal nerve [V] motor root

Branchial motor – the four muscles of mastication (medial pterygoid, lateral pterygoid, masseter, temporalis) and mylohyoid, anterior belly of digastric, tensor tympani, and tensor veli palatini

Overview of cranial nerves

—— Efferent (motor) fibers

—— Afferent (sensory) fibers

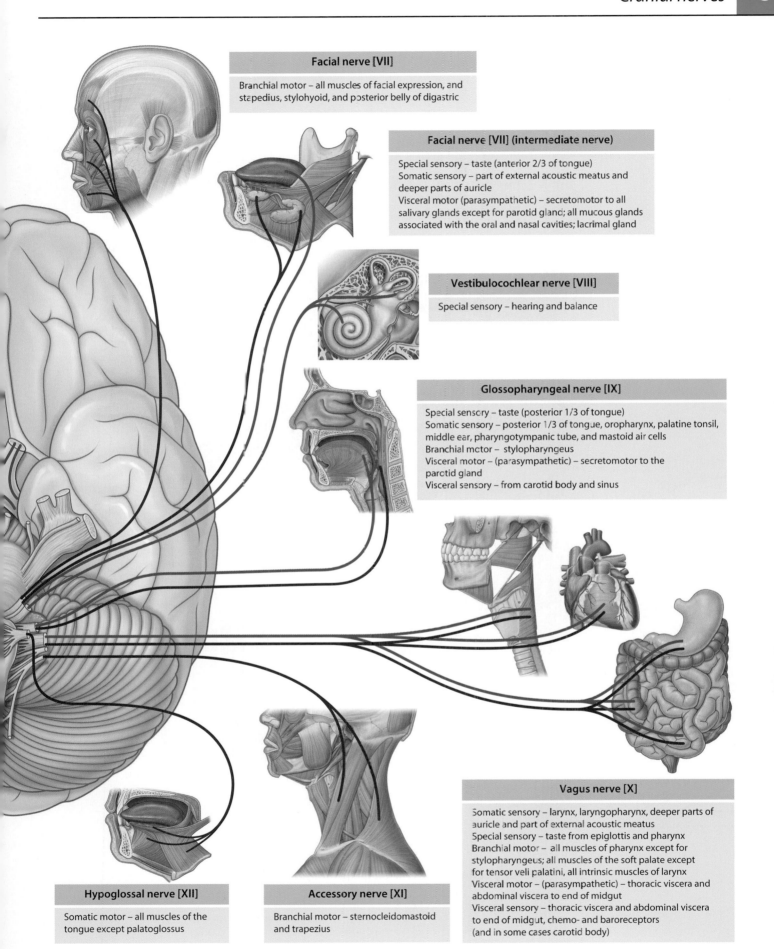

Facial nerve [VII]

Branchial motor – all muscles of facial expression, and stapedius, stylohyoid, and posterior belly of digastric

Facial nerve [VII] (intermediate nerve)

Special sensory – taste (anterior 2/3 of tongue)
Somatic sensory – part of external acoustic meatus and deeper parts of auricle
Visceral motor (parasympathetic) – secretomotor to all salivary glands except for parotid gland; all mucous glands associated with the oral and nasal cavities; lacrimal gland

Vestibulocochlear nerve [VIII]

Special sensory – hearing and balance

Glossopharyngeal nerve [IX]

Special sensory – taste (posterior 1/3 of tongue)
Somatic sensory – posterior 1/3 of tongue, oropharynx, palatine tonsil, middle ear, pharyngotympanic tube, and mastoid air cells
Branchial motor – stylopharyngeus
Visceral motor – (parasympathetic) – secretomotor to the parotid gland
Visceral sensory – from carotid body and sinus

Vagus nerve [X]

Somatic sensory – larynx, laryngopharynx, deeper parts of auricle and part of external acoustic meatus
Special sensory – taste from epiglottis and pharynx
Branchial motor – all muscles of pharynx except for stylopharyngeus; all muscles of the soft palate except for tensor veli palatini, all intrinsic muscles of larynx
Visceral motor – (parasympathetic) – thoracic viscera and abdominal viscera to end of midgut
Visceral sensory – thoracic viscera and abdominal viscera to end of midgut, chemo- and baroreceptors (and in some cases carotid body)

Hypoglossal nerve [XII]

Somatic motor – all muscles of the tongue except palatoglossus

Accessory nerve [XI]

Branchial motor – sternocleidomastoid and trapezius

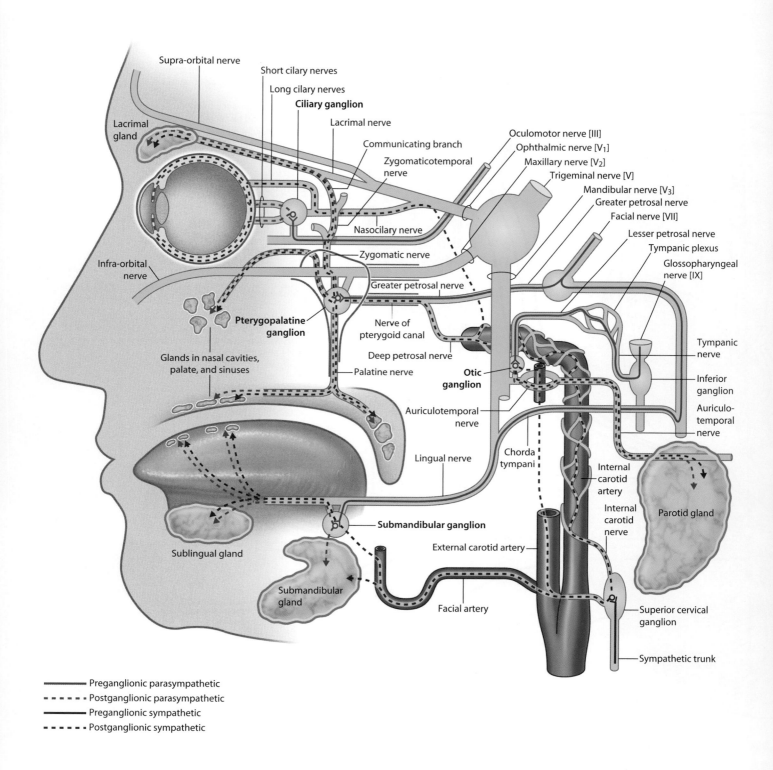

Summary of visceral efferent (motor) pathways in the head

- ——— Preganglionic parasympathetic
- - - - - Postganglionic parasympathetic
- ——— Preganglionic sympathetic
- - - - - Postganglionic sympathetic

External foramina of the skull

Foramen		Structures passing through foramen
Anterior view		
Supra-orbital foramen	1	Supra-orbital nerve and vessels
Infra-orbital foramen	2	Infra-orbital nerve and vessels
Mental foramen	3	Mental nerve and vessels
Lateral view		
Zygomaticofacial foramen	4	Zygomaticofacial nerve
Superior view		
Parietal foramen	5	Emissary veins

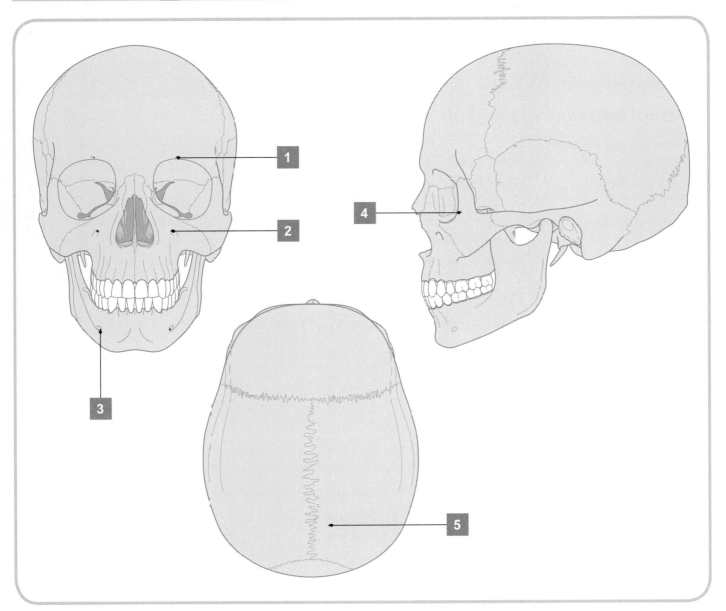

External foramina of the skull

Foramen		Structures passing through foramen
Inferior view		
Incisive foramina	1	Nasopalatine nerve; sphenopalatine vessels
Greater palatine foramen	2	Greater palatine nerve and vessels
Lesser palatine foramina	3	Lesser palatine nerves and vessels
Pterygoid canal	4	Pterygoid nerve and vessels
Foramen ovale	5	Mandibular nerve [V_3]; lesser petrosal nerve
Foramen spinosum	6	Middle meningeal artery
Foramen lacerum	7	Filled with cartilage
Carotid canal	8	Internal carotid artery and nerve plexus
Foramen magnum	9	Continuation of brain and spinal cord; vertebral arteries and nerve plexuses; anterior spinal artery; posterior spinal arteries; roots of accessory nerve [XI]; meninges
Condylar canal	10	Emissary veins
Hypoglossal canal	11	Hypoglossal nerve [XII] and vessels
Jugular foramen	12	Internal jugular vein; inferior petrosal sinus; glossopharyngeal nerve [IX]; vagus nerve [X]; accessory nerve [XI]
Stylomastoid foramen	13	Facial nerve [VII]

Internal foramina of the skull

Foramen		Structures passing through foramen
Anterior cranial fossa		
Foramen cecum	1	Emissary veins to nasal cavity
Olfactory foramina in cribriform plate	2	Olfactory nerves [I]
Middle cranial fossa		
Optic canal	3	Optic nerve [II]; ophthalmic artery
Superior orbital fissure	4	Oculomotor nerve [III]; trochlear nerve [IV]; ophthalmic division of the trigeminal nerve [V_1]; abducent nerve [VI]; ophthalmic veins
Foramen rotundum	5	Maxillary division of the trigeminal nerve [V_2]
Foramen ovale	6	Mandibular division of the trigeminal nerve [V_3]; lesser petrosal nerve
Foramen spinosum	7	Middle meningeal artery
Hiatus for the greater petrosal nerve	8	Greater petrosal nerve
Hiatus for the lesser petrosal nervex	9	Lesser petrosal nerve
Posterior cranial fossa		
Foramen magnum	10	End of brainstem/beginning of spinal cord; vertebral arteries; spinal roots of the accessory nerve; meninges
Internal acoustic meatus	11	Facial nerve [VII]; vestibulocochlear nerve [VIII]; labyrinthine artery
Jugular foramen	12	Glossopharyngeal nerve [IX]; vagus nerve [X]; accessory nerve [XI]; inferior petrosal sinus, sigmoid sinus (forming internal jugular vein)
Hypoglossal canal	13	Hypoglossal nerve [XII]; meningeal branch of the ascending pharyngeal artery
Condylar canal	14	Emissary vein

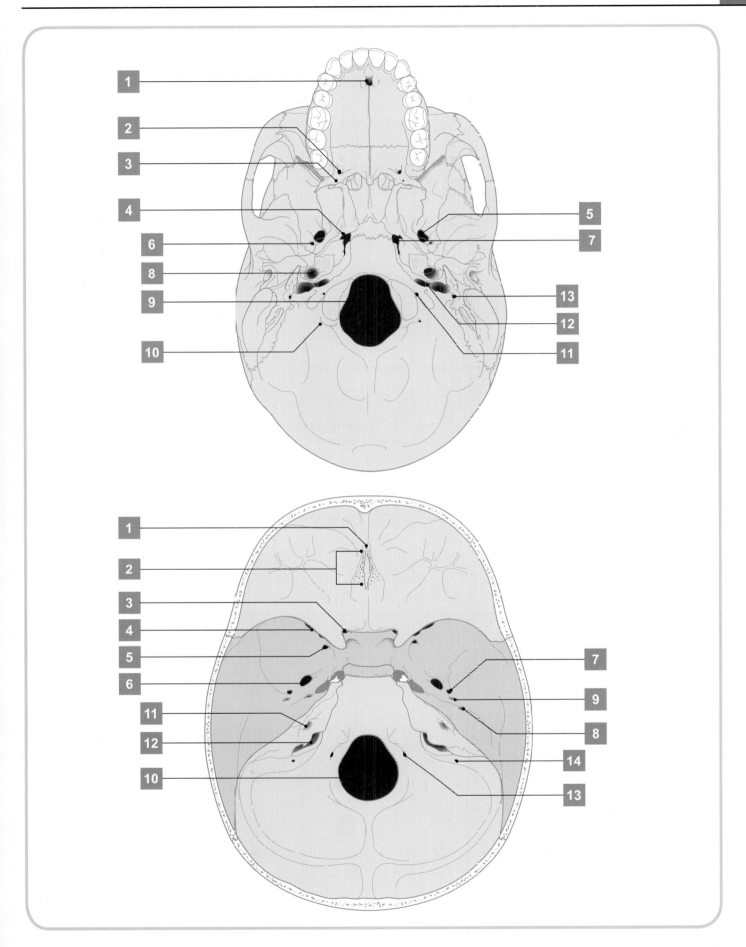

Muscles of the face

Muscle		Origin	Insertion	Innervation	Function
Orbital group					
Orbicularis oculi —Palpebral part	1	Medial palpebral ligament	Lateral palpebral raphe	Facial nerve [VII]	Closes the eyelids gently
—Orbital part	2	Nasal part of frontal bone; frontal process of maxilla; medial palpebral ligament	Fibers form an uninterrupted ellipse around orbit	Facial nerve [VII]	Closes the eyelids forcefully
Corrugator supercilii	3	Medial end of the superciliary arch	Skin of the medial half of eyebrow	Facial nerve [VII]	Draws the eyebrows medially and downward
Nasal group					
Nasalis —Transverse part	4	Maxilla just lateral to nose	Aponeurosis across dorsum of nose with muscle fibers from the other side	Facial nerve [VII]	Compresses nasal aperture
—Alar part	5	Maxilla over lateral incisor	Alar cartilage of nose	Facial nerve [VII]	Draws cartilage downward and laterally opening nostril
Procerus	6	Nasal bone and upper part of lateral nasal cartilage	Skin of lower forehead between eyebrows	Facial nerve [VII]	Draws down medial angle of eyebrows producing transverse wrinkles over bridge of nose
Depressor septi	7	Maxilla above medial incisor	Mobile part of the nasal septum	Facial nerve [VII]	Pulls nose inferiorly

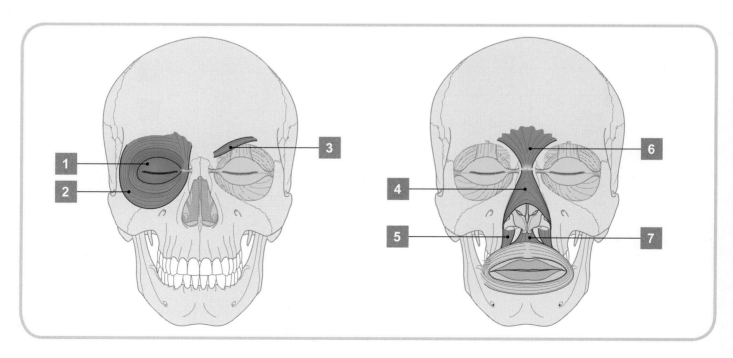

Muscles of the face

Muscle		Origin	Insertion	Innervation	Function
Oral group					
Depressor anguli oris	1	Oblique line of mandible below canine, premolar, and first molar teeth	Skin at the corner of mouth and blending with orbicularis oris	Facial nerve [VII]	Draws corner of mouth down and laterally
Depressor labii inferioris	2	Anterior part of oblique line of mandible	Lower lip at midline; blends with muscle from opposite side	Facial nerve [VII]	Draws lower lip downward and laterally
Mentalis	3	Mandible inferior to incisor teeth	Skin of chin	Facial nerve [VII]	Raises and protrudes lower lip as it wrinkles skin on chin
Risorius	4	Fascia over masseter muscle	Skin at the corner of the mouth	Facial nerve [VII]	Retracts corner of mouth
Zygomaticus major	5	Posterior part of lateral surface of zygomatic bone	Skin at the corner of the mouth	Facial nerve [VII]	Draws the corner of the mouth upward and laterally
Zygomaticus minor	6	Anterior part of lateral surface of zygomatic bone	Upper lip just medial to corner of mouth	Facial nerve [VII]	Draws the upper lip upward
Levator labii superioris	7	Infra-orbital margin of maxilla	Skin of upper lateral half of upper lip	Facial nerve [VII]	Raises upper lip; helps form nasolabial furrow
Levator labii superioris alaeque nasi	8	Frontal process of maxilla	Alar cartilage of nose and upper lip	Facial nerve [VII]	Raises upper lip and opens nostril
Levator anguli oris	9	Maxilla below infra-orbital foramen	Skin at the corner of mouth	Facial nerve [VII]	Raises corner of mouth; helps form nasolabial furrow
Orbicularis oris	10	From muscles in area; maxilla and mandible in midline	Forms ellipse around mouth	Facial nerve [VII]	Closes lips; protrudes lips
Buccinator	11	Posterior parts of maxilla and mandible; pterygomandibular raphe	Blends with orbicularis oris and into lips	Facial nerve [VII]	Presses the cheek against teeth; compresses distended cheeks

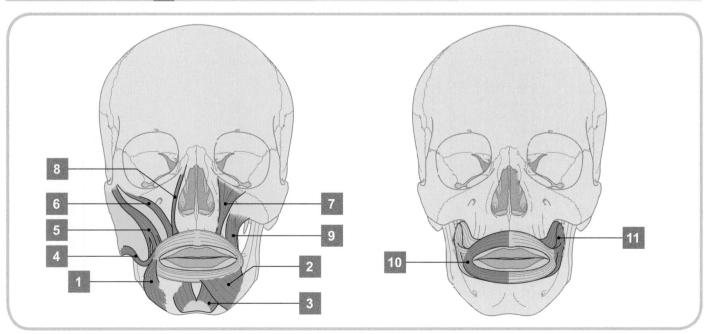

Muscles of the face

Muscle		Origin	Insertion	Innervation	Function
Other muscles or groups					
Anterior auricular	1	Anterior part of temporal fascia	Into helix of ear	Facial nerve [VII]	Draws ear upward and forward
Superior auricular	2	Epicranial aponeurosis on side of head	Upper part of auricle	Facial nerve [VII]	Elevates ear
Posterior auricular	3	Mastoid process of temporal bone	Convexity of concha of ear	Facial nerve [VII]	Draws ear upward and backward
Occipitofrontalis —Frontal belly	4	Skin of eyebrows	Into galea aponeurotica	Facial nerve [VII]	Wrinkles forehead; raises eyebrows
—Occipital belly	5	Lateral part of superior nuchal line of occipital bone and mastoid process of temporal bone	Into galea aponeurotica	Facial nerve [VII]	Draws scalp backward

Extrinsic (extra-ocular) muscles

Muscle		Origin	Insertion	Innervation	Function
Levator palpebrae superioris	1	Lesser wing of sphenoid anterior to optic canal	Anterior surface of tarsal plate; a few fibers to skin and superior conjunctival fornix	Oculomotor nerve [III]—superior branch	Elevation of upper eyelid
Superior rectus	2	Superior part of common tendinous ring	Anterior half of eyeball superiorly	Oculomotor nerve [III]—superior branch	Elevation, adduction, medial rotation of eyeball
Inferior rectus	3	Inferior part of common tendinous ring	Anterior half of eyeball inferiorly	Oculomotor nerve [III]—inferior branch	Depression, adduction, lateral rotation of eyeball
Medial rectus	4	Medial part of common tendinous ring	Anterior half of eyeball medially	Oculomotor nerve [III]—inferior branch	Adduction of eyeball
Lateral rectus	5	Lateral part of common tendinous ring	Anterior half of eyeball laterally	Abducent nerve [VI]	Abduction of eyeball
Superior oblique	6	Body of sphenoid, superior and medial to optic canal	Outer posterior quadrant of eyeball (superior surface)	Trochlear nerve [IV]	Depression, abduction, medial rotation of eyeball
Inferior oblique	7	Medial floor of orbit posterior to rim; maxilla lateral to nasolacrimal groove	Outer posterior quadrant of eyeball (inferior surface)	Oculomotor nerve [III]—inferior branch	Elevation, abduction, lateral rotation of eyeball

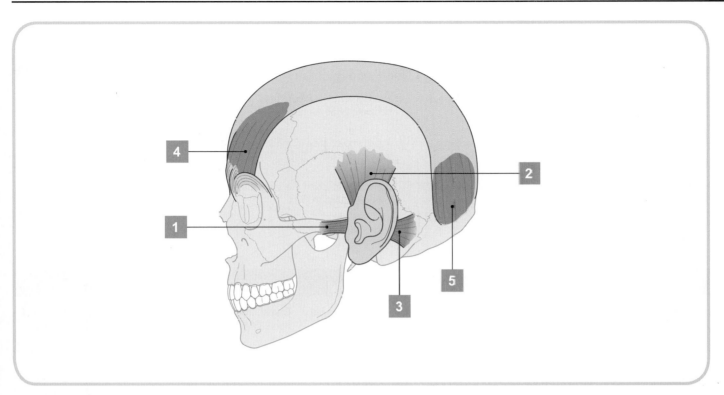

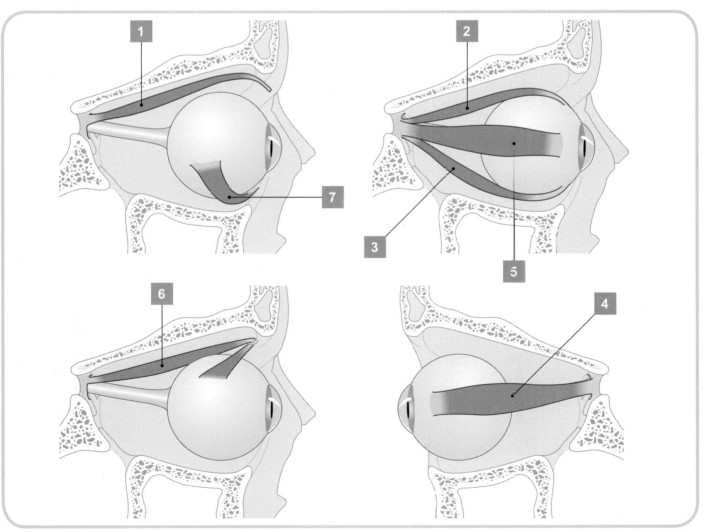

Intrinsic muscles of the eye

Muscle		Location	Innervation	Function
Ciliary	1	Muscle fibers in the ciliary body	Parasympathetics from the oculomotor nerve [III]	Constricts ciliary body, relaxes tension on lens, lens become more rounded
Sphincter pupillae	2	Circularly arranged fibers in the iris	Parasympathetics from the oculomotor nerve [III]	Constricts pupil
Dilator pupillae	3	Radially arranged fibers in the iris	Sympathetics from the superior cervical ganglion (T1)	Dilates pupil

Muscles of the middle ear

Muscle		Origin	Insertion	Innervation	Function
Tensor tympani	1	Cartilaginous part of pharyngotympanic tube, greater wing of sphenoid, its own bony canal	Upper part of handle of malleus	Branch from mandibular nerve [V₃]	Contraction pulls handle of malleus medially, tensing tympanic membrane
Stapedius	2	Attached to inside of pyramidal eminence	Neck of stapes	Branch of facial nerve [VII]	Contraction pulls stapes posteriorly, preventing excessive oscillation

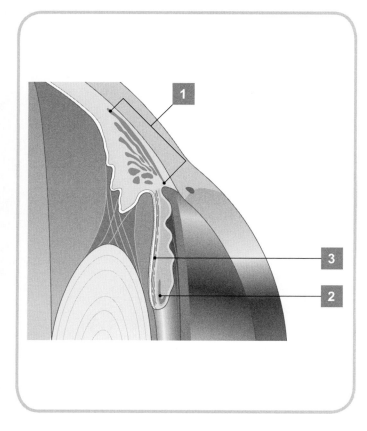

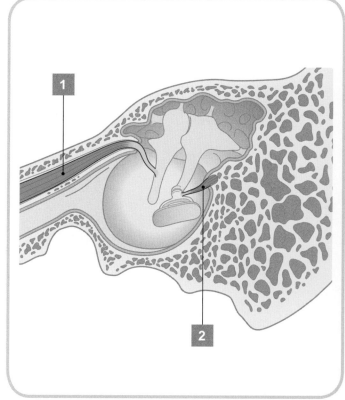

Muscles of mastication

Muscle		Origin	Insertion	Innervation	Function
Masseter	1	Zygomatic arch and maxillary process of the zygomatic bone	Lateral surface of ramus of mandible	Masseteric nerve from the anterior trunk of the mandibular nerve [V$_3$]	Elevation of mandible
Temporalis	2	Bone of temporal fossa and temporal fascia	Coronoid process of mandible and anterior margin of ramus of mandible almost to last molar tooth	Deep temporal nerves from the anterior trunk of the mandibular nerve [V$_3$]	Elevation and retraction of mandible
Medial pterygoid	3	Deep head—medial surface of lateral plate of pterygoid process and pyramidal process of palatine bone; superficial head—tuberosity of the maxilla and pyramidal process of palatine bone	Medial surface of mandible near angle	Nerve to medial pterygoid from the mandibular nerve [V$_3$].	Elevation and side-to-side movements of the mandible
Lateral pterygoid	4	Upper head—roof of infratemporal fossa; lower head—lateral surface of lateral plate of the pterygoid process	Capsule of temporomandibular joint in the region of attachment to the articular disc and to the pterygoid fovea on the neck of mandible	Nerve to lateral pterygoid directly from the anterior trunk of the mandibular nerve [V3] or from the buccal branch	Protrusion and side-to-side movements of the mandible

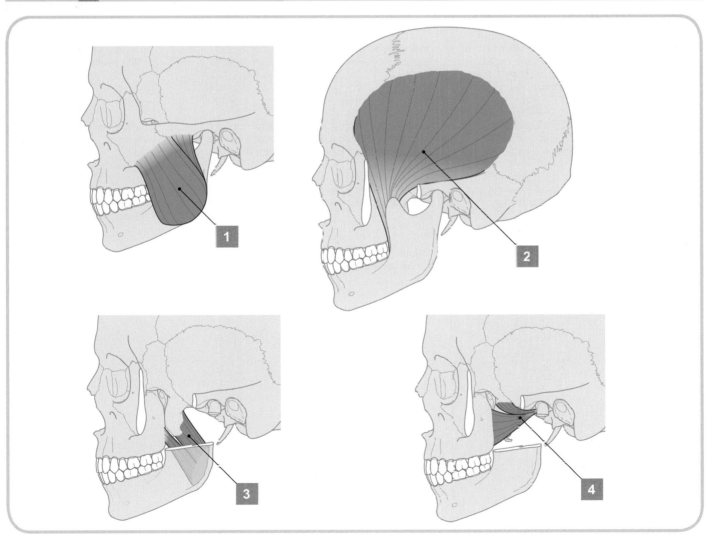

Anterior triangle of neck (suprahyoid and infrahyoid muscles)

Muscle		Origin	Insertion	Innervation	Function
Stylohyoid	1	Base of styloid process	Lateral area of body of hyoid bone	Facial nerve [VII]	Pulls hyoid bone upward in a posterosuperior direction
Digastric —Anterior belly	2	Digastric fossa on lower inside of mandible	Attachment of tendon between two bellies to body of hyoid bone	Mylohyoid nerve from inferior alveolar branch of mandibular nerve [V_3]	Opens mouth by lowering mandible; raises hyoid bone
—Posterior belly	3	Mastoid notch on medial side of mastoid process of temporal bone		Facial nerve [VII]	Pulls hyoid bone upward and back
Mylohyoid	4	Mylohyoid line on mandible	Body of hyoid bone and fibers from muscle on opposite side	Mylohyoid nerve from inferior alveolar branch of mandibular nerve [V_3]	Support and elevation of floor of mouth; elevation of hyoid
Geniohyoid	5	Inferior mental spine on inner surface of mandible	Anterior surface of body of hyoid bone	Branch from anterior ramus of C1 (carried along the hypoglossal nerve [XII])	Fixed mandible elevates and pulls hyoid bone forward; fixed hyoid bone pulls mandible downward and inward
Sternohyoid	6	Posterior aspect of sternoclavicular joint and adjacent manubrium of sternum	Body of hyoid bone medial to attachment of omohyoid muscle	Anterior rami of C1 to C3 through the ansa cervicalis	Depresses hyoid bone after swallowing
Omohyoid	7	Superior border of scapula medial to suprascapular notch	Lower border of body of hyoid bone just lateral to attachment of sternohyoid	Anterior rami of C1 to C3 through the ansa cervicalis	Depresses and fixes hyoid bone
Thyrohyoid	8	Oblique line on lamina of thyroid cartilage	Greater horn and adjacent aspect of body of hyoid bone	Fibers from anterior ramus of C1 carried along hypoglossal nerve [XII]	Depresses hyoid bone, but when hyoid bone is fixed raises larynx
Sternothyroid	9	Posterior surface of manubrium of sternum	Oblique line on lamina of thyroid cartilage	Anterior rami of C1 to C3 through the ansa cervicalis	Draws larynx (thyroid cartilage) downward

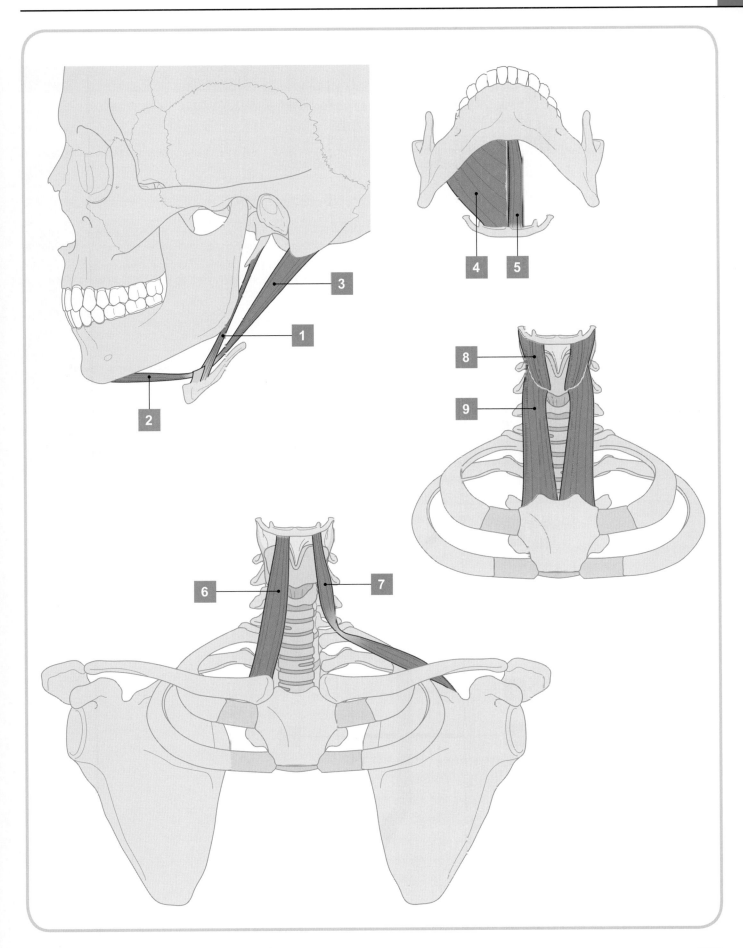

Branches of the external carotid artery

Artery		Parts supplied
Superior thyroid artery	1	Thyrohyoid muscle, internal structures of the larynx, sternocleidomastoid and cricothyroid muscles, thyroid gland
Ascending pharyngeal artery	2	Pharyngeal constrictors and stylopharyngeus muscle, palate, tonsil, pharyngotympanic tube, meninges in posterior cranial fossa
Lingual artery	3	Muscles of the tongue, palatine tonsil, soft palate, epiglottis, floor of mouth, sublingual gland
Facial artery	4	All structures in the face from the inferior border of the mandible anterior to the masseter muscle to the medial corner of the eye, the soft palate, palatine tonsil, pharyngotympanic tube, submandibular gland
Occipital artery	5	Sternocleidomastoid muscle, meninges in posterior cranial fossa, mastoid cells, deep muscles of the back, posterior scalp
Posterior auricular artery	6	Parotid gland and nearby muscles, external ear and scalp posterior to ear, middle and inner ear structures
Superficial temporal artery	7	Parotid gland and duct, masseter muscle, lateral face, anterior part of external ear, temporalis muscle, parietal and temporal fossae
Maxillary artery	8	External acoustic meatus, lateral and medial surface of tympanic membrane, temporomandibular joint, dura mater on lateral wall of skull and inner table of cranial bones, trigeminal ganglion and dura in vicinity, mylohyoid muscle, mandibular teeth, skin on chin, temporalis muscle, outer table of bones of skull in temporal fossa, structures in infratemporal fossa, maxillary sinus, upper teeth and gingivae, infra-orbital skin, palate, roof of pharynx, nasal cavity

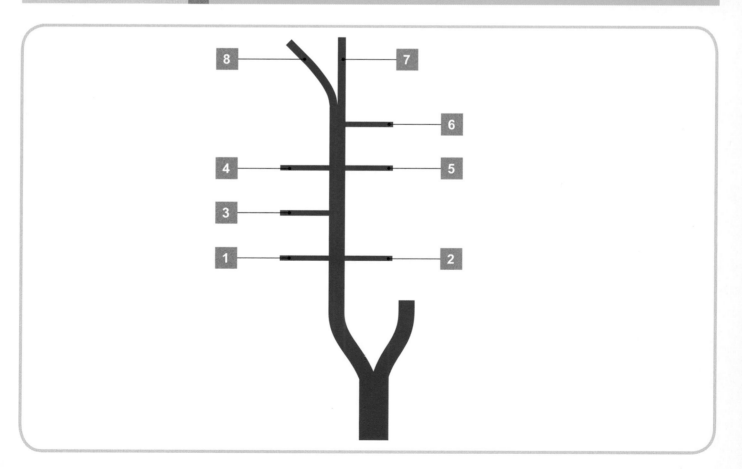

Subdivisions of the anterior triangle of the neck—a regional approach

Subdivision		Boundaries	Contents
Submental triangle (unpaired)	1	Mandibular symphysis; anterior belly of digastric muscles; body of hyoid bone	Submental lymph nodes; tributaries forming the anterior jugular vein
Submandibular triangle (paired)	2	Lower border of mandible; anterior belly of digastric muscle; posterior belly of digastric muscle	Submandibular gland; submandibular lymph nodes; hypoglossal nerve [XII]; mylohyoid nerve; facial artery and vein
Carotid triangle (paired)	3	Posterior belly of digastric muscle; superior belly of omohyoid muscle; anterior border of sternocleidomastoid muscle	Tributaries to common facial vein; cervical branch of facial nerve [VII]; common carotid artery; external and internal carotid arteries; superior thyroid; ascending pharyngeal; lingual, facial, and occipital arteries; internal jugular vein; vagus [X], accessory [XI], and hypoglossal [XII] nerves; superior and inferior roots of ansa cervicalis; transverse cervical nerve
Muscular triangle (paired)	4	Midline of neck; superior belly of omohyoid muscle; anterior border of sternocleidomastoid muscle	Sternohyoid, omohyoid, sternohyoid, and thyrohyoid muscles; thyroid and parathyroid glands; pharynx

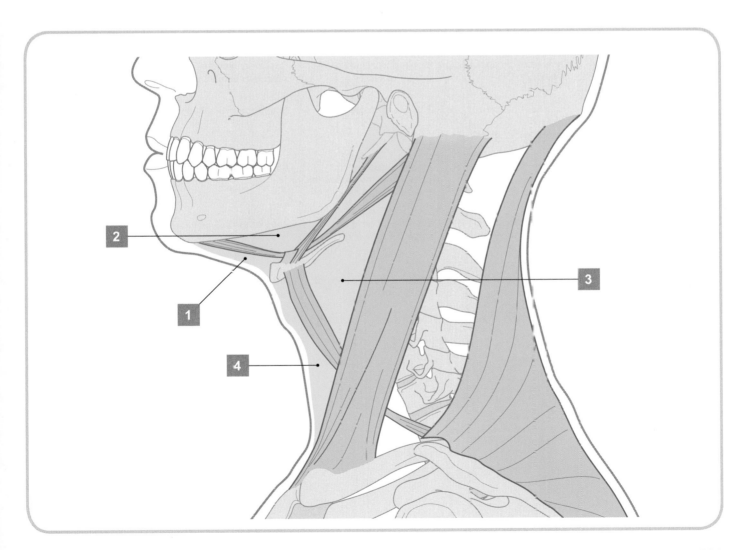

Muscles associated with the posterior triangle of the neck
Parentheses indicate possible involvement

Muscle		Origin	Insertion	Innervation	Function
Sternocleidomastoid—Sternal head	1	Upper part of anterior surface of manubrium of sternum	Lateral one-half of superior nuchal line	Accessory nerve [XI] and branches from anterior rami of C2 to C3 (C4)	Individually—will tilt head toward shoulder on same side rotating head to turn face to opposite side; acting together, draw head forward
—Clavicular head	2	Superior surface of medial one-third of clavicle	Lateral surface of mastoid process		
Trapezius	3	Superior nuchal line; external occipital protuberance; ligamentum nuchae; spinous processes of vertebrae CVII to TXII	Lateral one-third of clavicle; acromion; spine of scapula	Motor—accessory nerve [XI]; proprioception—C3 and C4	Assists in rotating the scapula during abduction of humerus above horizontal; upper fibers—elevate, middle fibers—adduct, lower fibers—depress scapula
Splenius capitis	4	Lower half of ligamentum nuchae; spinous processes of vertebrae CVII to TIV	Mastoid process, skull below lateral one-third of superior nuchal line	Posterior rami of middle cervical nerves	Together, draw head backward; individually, draw and rotate head to one side (turn face to same side)
Levator scapulae	5	Transverse processes of CI to CIV	Upper part of medial border of scapula	C3, C4; and dorsal scapular nerve (C4, C5)	Elevates scapula
Posterior scalene	6	Posterior tubercles of transverse processes of vertebrae CIV to CVI	Upper surface of rib II	Anterior rami of C5 to C7	Elevation of rib II
Middle scalene	7	Transverse processes of vertebrae CII to CVII	Upper surface of rib I posterior to the groove for the subclavian artery	Anterior rami of C3 to C7	Elevation of rib I
Anterior scalene	8	Anterior tubercles of the transverse processes of vertebrae CIII to CVI	Scalene tubercle and upper surface of rib I	Anterior rami of C4 to C7	Elevation of rib I
Omohyoid	9	Superior border of scapula medial to scapular notch	Inferior border of body of hyoid bone	Ansa cervicalis; anterior rami of C1 to C3	Depress the hyoid bone

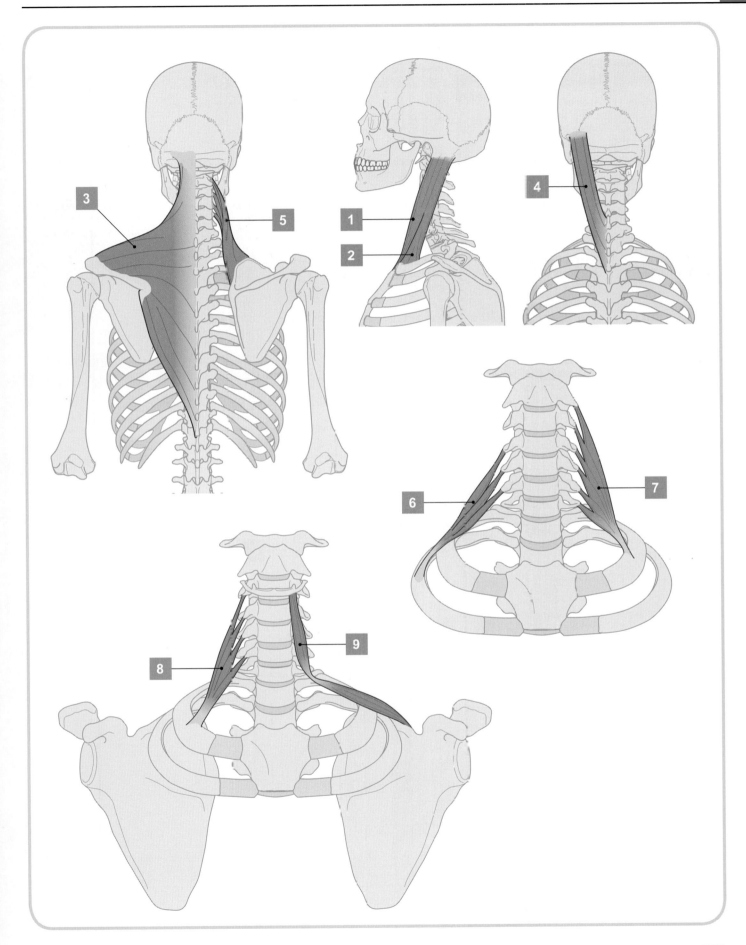

Prevertebral and lateral muscles

Muscle		Origin	Insertion	Innervation	Function
Rectus capitis anterior	1	Anterior surface of lateral part of atlas and its transverse process	Inferior surface of basilar part of occipital bone	Branches from anterior rami of C1, C2	Flexes head at atlanto-occipital joint
Rectus capitis lateralis	2	Superior surface of transverse process of atlas	Inferior surface of jugular process of occipital bone	Branches from anterior rami of C1, C2	Flexes head laterally to same side
Longus colli —Superior oblique part	3	Anterior tubercles of transverse processes of vertebrae CIII to CV	Tubercle of anterior arch of atlas	Branches from anterior rami of C2 to C6	Flexes neck anteriorly and laterally and slight rotation to opposite side
—Inferior oblique part	4	Anterior surface of bodies of vertebrae TI, TII, and maybe TIII	Anterior tubercles of transverse processes of vertebrae CV and CVI		
—Vertical part	5	Anterior surface of bodies of TI to TIII and CV to CVII	Anterior surface of bodies of vertebrae CII to CIV		
Longus capitis	6	Tendinous slips to transverse processes of vertebrae CIII to CVI	Inferior surface of basilar part of occipital bone	Branches from anterior rami of C1 to C3	Flexes the head

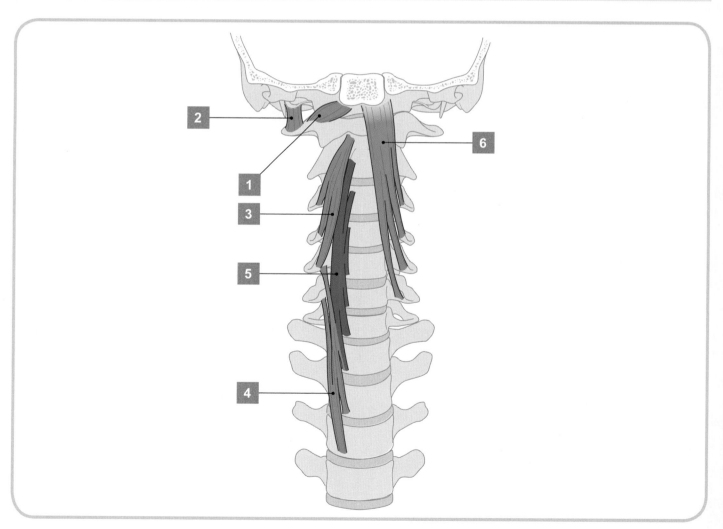

Constrictor muscles of the pharynx

Muscle		Posterior attachment	Anterior attachment	Innervation	Function
Superior constrictor	1	Pharyngeal raphe	Pterygomandibular raphe and adjacent bone on the mandible and pterygoid hamulus	Vagus nerve [X]	Constriction of pharynx
Middle constrictor	2	Pharyngeal raphe	Upper margin of greater horn of hyoid bone and adjacent margins of lesser horn and stylohyoid ligament	Vagus nerve [X]	Constriction of pharynx
Inferior constrictor	3	Pharyngeal raphe	Cricoid cartilage, oblique line of thyroid cartilage, and a ligament that spans between these attachments and crosses the cricothyroid muscle	Vagus nerve [X]	Constriction of pharynx

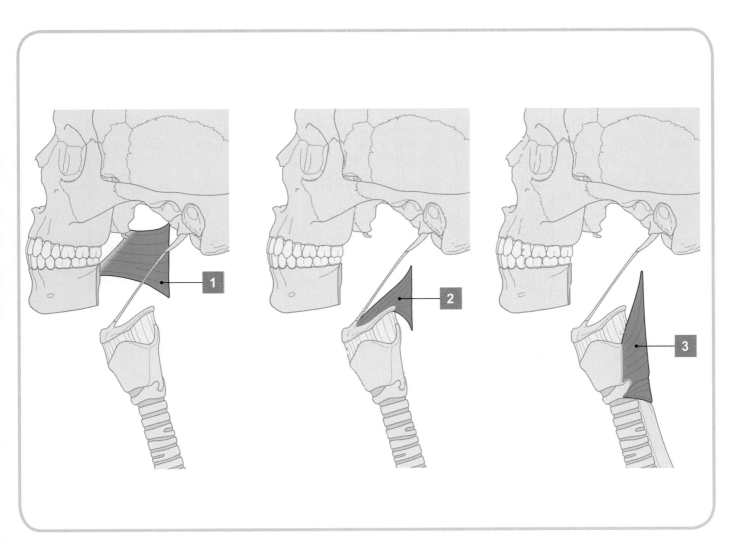

Longitudinal muscles of the pharynx

Muscle		Origin	Insertion	Innervation	Function
Stylopharyngeus	1	Medial side of base of styloid process	Pharyngeal wall	Glossopharyngeal nerve [IX]	Elevation of the pharynx
Salpingopharyngeus	2	Inferior aspect of pharyngeal end of pharyngotympanic tube	Pharyngeal wall	Vagus nerve [X]	Elevation of the pharynx
Palatopharyngeus	3	Upper surface of palatine aponeurosis	Pharyngeal wall	Vagus nerve [X]	Elevation of the pharynx; closure of the oropharyngeal isthmus

Intrinsic muscles of the larynx

Muscle		Origin	Insertion	Innervation	Function
Cricothyroid	1	Anterolateral aspect of arch of cricoid cartilage	Oblique part—inferior horn of the thyroid cartilage; straight part—inferior margin of thyroid cartilage	External branch of superior laryngeal nerve from the vagus nerve [X]	Forward and downward rotation of the thyroid cartilage at the cricothyroid joint
Posterior crico-arytenoid	2	Oval depression on posterior surface of lamina of cricoid cartilage	Posterior surface of muscular process of arytenoid cartilage	Recurrent laryngeal branch of the vagus nerve [X]	Abduction and external rotation of the arytenoid cartilage. The posterior crico-arytenoid muscles are the primary abductors of the vocal folds. In other words, they are the primary openers of the rima glottidis.
Lateral crico-arytenoid	3	Superior surface of arch of cricoid cartilage	Anterior surface of muscular process of arytenoid cartilage	Recurrent laryngeal branch of the vagus nerve [X]	Internal rotation of the arytenoid cartilage and adduction of vocal folds
Transverse arytenoid	4	Lateral border of posterior surface of arytenoid cartilage	Lateral border of posterior surface of opposite arytenoid cartilage	Recurrent laryngeal branch of the vagus nerve [X]	Adduction of arytenoid cartilages
Oblique arytenoid	5	Posterior surface of muscular process of arytenoid cartilage	Posterior surface of apex of adjacent arytenoid cartilage; extends into aryepiglottic fold	Recurrent laryngeal branch of the vagus nerve [X]	Sphincter of the laryngeal inlet
Thyro-arytenoid	6	Thyroid angle and adjacent cricothyroid ligament	Anterolateral surface of arytenoid cartilage; some fibers continue in aryepiglottic folds to the lateral margin of the epiglottis	Recurrent laryngeal branch of the vagus nerve [X]	Sphincter of vestibule and of laryngeal inlet
Vocalis	7	Lateral surface of vocal process of arytenoid cartilage	Vocal ligament and thyroid angle	Recurrent laryngeal branch of the vagus nerve [X]	Adjusts tension in vocal folds

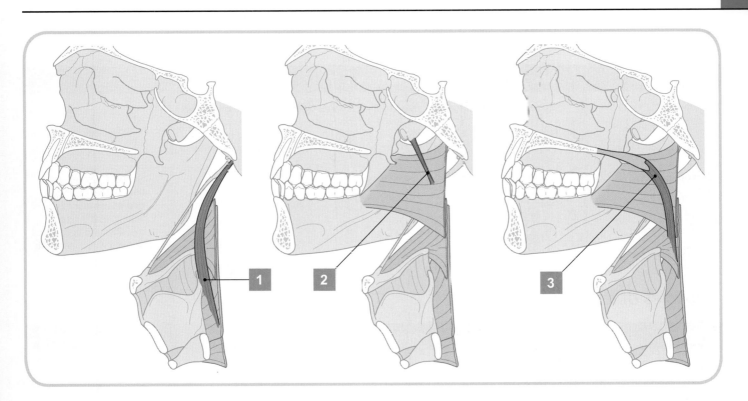

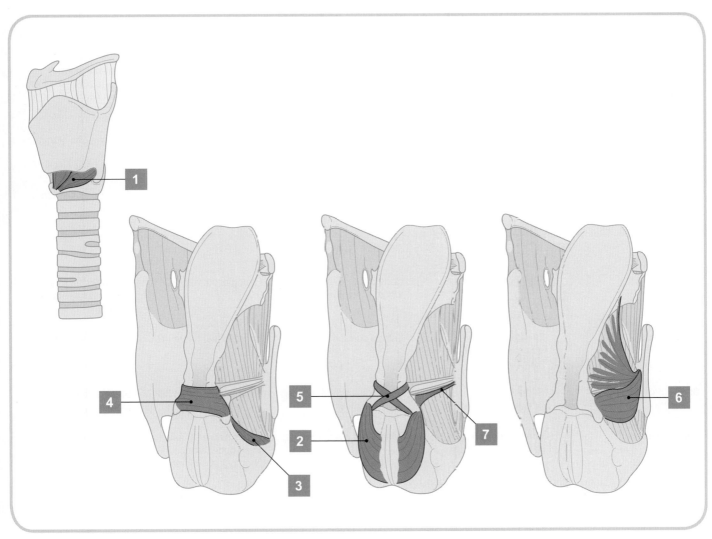

Muscles in the floor of the oral cavity

Muscle		Origin	Insertion	Innervation	Function
Mylohyoid	1	Mylohyoid line of mandible	Median fibrous raphe and adjacent part of hyoid bone	Nerve to mylohyoid from the inferior alveolar branch of mandibular nerve [V$_3$]	
Geniohyoid	2	Inferior mental spines of mandible	Body of hyoid bone	C1	Supports and elevates floor of oral cavity; depresses mandible when hyoid is fixed; elevates and pulls hyoid forward when mandible is fixed

Muscles of the tongue

Muscle		Origin	Insertion	Innervation	Function
Intrinsic					
Superior longitudinal (just deep to surface of tongue)	1	Submucosal connective tissue at the back of the tongue and from the median septum of the tongue	Muscle fibers pass forward and obliquely to submucosal connective tissue and mucosa on margins of tongue	Hypoglossal nerve [XII]	Shortens tongue; curls apex and sides of tongue
Inferior longitudinal (between genioglossus and hyoglossus muscles)	2	Root of tongue (some fibers from hyoid)	Apex of tongue	Hypoglossal nerve [XII]	Shortens tongue; uncurls apex and turns it downward
Transverse	3	Median septum of the tongue	Submucosal connective tissue on lateral margins of tongue	Hypoglossal nerve [XII]	Narrows and elongates tongue
Vertical	4	Submucosal connective tissue on dorsum of tongue	Connective tissue in more ventral regions of tongue	Hypoglossal nerve [XII]	Flattens and widens tongue
Extrinsic					
Genioglossus	5	Superior mental spines	Body of hyoid; entire length of tongue	Hypoglossal nerve [XII]	Protrudes tongue; depresses center of tongue
Hyoglossus	6	Greater horn and adjacent part of body of hyoid bone	Lateral surface of tongue	Hypoglossal nerve [XII]	Depresses tongue
Styloglossus	7	Styloid process (anterolateral surface)	Lateral surface of tongue	Hypoglossal nerve [XII]	Elevates and retracts tongue
Palatoglossus	8	Inferior surface of palatine aponeurosis	Lateral margin of tongue	Vagus nerve [X] (via pharyngeal branch to pharyngeal plexus)	Depresses palate; moves palatoglossal fold toward midline; elevates back of the tongue

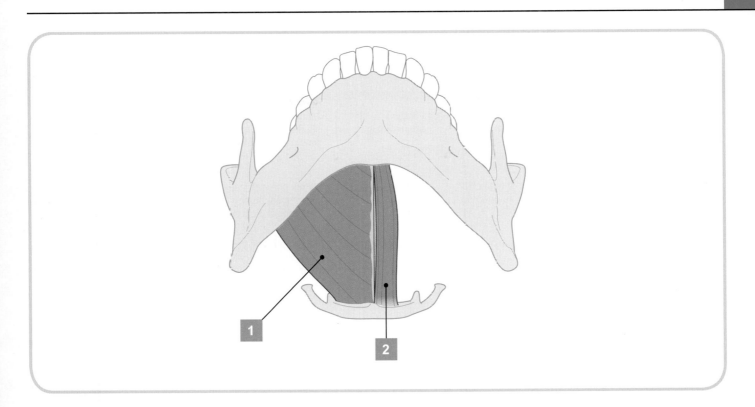

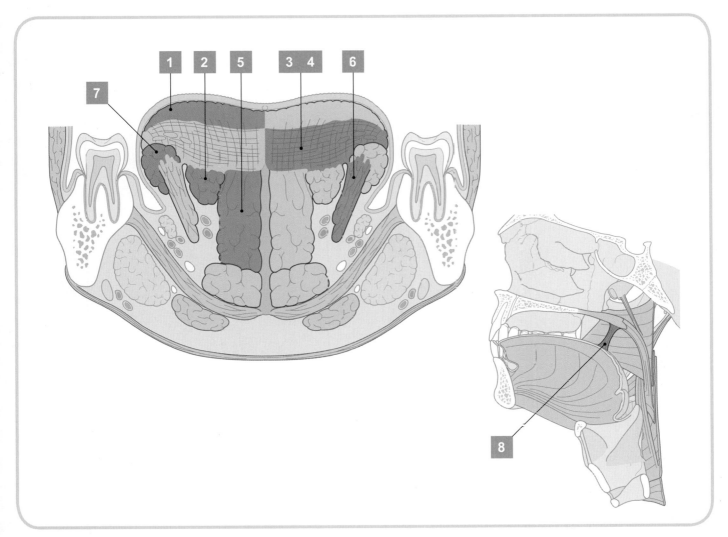

Muscles of the soft palate

Muscle		Origin	Insertion	Innervation	Function
Tensor veli palatini	1	Scaphoid fossa of sphenoid bone; fibrous part of pharyngotympanic tube; spine of sphenoid	Palatine aponeurosis	Mandibular nerve [V₃] via the branch to medial pterygoid muscle	Tenses the soft palate; opens the pharyngotympanic tube
Levator veli palatini	2	Petrous part of temporal bone anterior to opening for carotid canal	Superior surface of palatine aponeurosis	Vagus nerve [X] via pharyngeal branch to pharyngeal plexus	Only muscle to elevate the soft palate above the neutral position
Palatopharyngeus	3	Superior surface of palatine aponeurosis	Pharyngeal wall	Vagus nerve [X] via pharyngeal branch to pharyngeal plexus	Depresses soft palate; moves palatopharyngeal arch toward midline; elevates pharynx
Palatoglossus	4	Inferior surface of palatine aponeurosis	Lateral margin of tongue	Vagus nerve [X] via pharyngeal branch to pharyngeal plexus	Depresses palate; moves palatoglossal arch toward midline; elevates back of the tongue
Musculus uvulae	5	Posterior nasal spine of hard palate	Connective tissue of uvula	Vagus nerve [X] via pharyngeal branch to pharyngeal plexus	Elevates and retracts uvula; thickens central region of soft palate

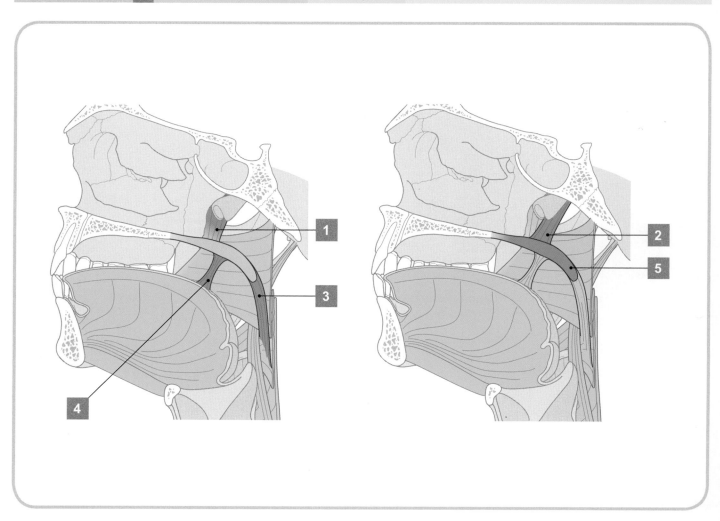